国际经典内科学教科书

第 10 版
Cecil Essentials of Medicine
希氏内科学精要
中英双语版

原　著　**Edward J. Wing, MD, FACP, FIDSA**
Former Dean of Medicine and Biological Sciences
Professor of Medicine
Warren Alpert Medical School of Brown University, Providence, Rhode Island

Fred J. Schiffman, MD, MACP
Sigal Family Professor of Humanistic Medicine
Vice Chair, Department of Medicine
Warren Alpert Medical School of Brown University, Providence, Rhode Island

中英双语版　编辑委员会　主任委员　王　辰

―――――― 第 5 分册 ――――――

血液疾病

主　译　黄晓军　王建祥

北京大学医学出版社

XISHI NEIKEXUE JINGYAO（DI 10 BAN） DI 5 FENCE　XUEYE JIBING（ZHONGYING SHUANGYU BAN）

图书在版编目（CIP）数据

希氏内科学精要：第 10 版 . 第 5 分册，血液疾病：汉、英 ／（美）爱德华·温（Edward J. Wing），（美）弗雷德·谢夫曼（Fred J. Schiffman）原著；黄晓军，王建祥主译 . -- 北京：北京大学医学出版社，2024. 11. -- ISBN 978-7-5659-3254-0

Ⅰ. R5

中国国家版本馆 CIP 数据核字第 20245B23K4 号

北京市版权局著作权合同登记号：图字：01-2024-4518

Elsevier (Singapore) Pte Ltd.
3 Killiney Road, #08-01 Winsland House I, Singapore 239519
Tel: (65) 6349-0200; Fax: (65) 6733-1817

Cecil Essentials of Medicine, Tenth Edition
Copyright © 2022 by Elsevier, Inc. All rights are reserved, including those for text and data mining, AI training, and similar technologies.
Publisher's note: Elsevier takes a neutral position with respect to territorial disputes or jurisdictional claims in its published content, including in maps and institutional affiliations.
Previous editions copyrighted 2016, 2010, 2007, 2004, 2001, 1997, 1993, 1990, and 1986.
ISBN-13: 978-0-323-72271-1

This translation of Cecil Essentials of Medicine, Tenth Edition by Edward J. Wing and Fred J. Schiffman was undertaken by Peking University Medical Press and is published by arrangement with Elsevier (Singapore) Pte Ltd.
Cecil Essentials of Medicine, Tenth Edition by Edward J. Wing and Fred J. Schiffman 由北京大学医学出版社进行翻译，并根据北京大学医学出版社与爱思唯尔（新加坡）私人有限公司的协议约定出版。
《希氏内科学精要（第 10 版） 第 5 分册　血液疾病（中英双语版）》（黄晓军　王建祥　主译）
ISBN: 978-7-5659-3254-0
Copyright © 2024 by Elsevier (Singapore) Pte Ltd. and Peking University Medical Press.
All rights reserved. No part of this publication may be reproduced or transmitted in any form or by any means, electronic or mechanical, including photocopying, recording, or any information storage and retrieval system, without permission in writing from Elsevier (Singapore) Pte Ltd. and Peking University Medical Press.

注　意

本译本由北京大学医学出版社独立完成。相关从业及研究人员必须凭借其自身经验和知识对文中描述的信息数据、方法策略、搭配组合、实验操作进行评估和使用。由于医学科学发展迅速，临床诊断和给药剂量尤其需要经过独立验证。在法律允许的最大范围内，爱思唯尔、译文的原文作者、原文编辑及原文内容提供者均不对译文或因产品责任、疏忽或其他操作造成的人身及（或）财产伤害及（或）损失承担责任，亦不对由于使用文中提到的方法、产品、说明或思想而导致的人身及（或）财产伤害及（或）损失承担责任。

Published in China by Peking University Medical Press under special arrangement with Elsevier (Singapore) Pte Ltd. This edition is authorized for sale in the People's Republic of China only, excluding Hong Kong SAR, Macau SAR and Taiwan. Unauthorized export of this edition is a violation of the contract.

希氏内科学精要（第 10 版）　第 5 分册　血液疾病（中英双语版）

主　　译：黄晓军　王建祥

出版发行：北京大学医学出版社

地　　址：（100191）北京市海淀区学院路 38 号　北京大学医学部院内

电　　话：发行部 010-82802230；图书邮购 010-82802495

网　　址：http://www.pumpress.com.cn

E-mail：booksale@bjmu.edu.cn

印　　刷：北京信彩瑞禾印刷厂

经　　销：新华书店

策划编辑：高　瑾

责任编辑：梁　洁　　　责任校对：靳新强　　　责任印制：李　啸

开　　本：889 mm×1194 mm　1/16　　印张：16　　字数：592 千字

版　　次：2024 年 11 月第 1 版　2024 年 11 月第 1 次印刷

书　　号：ISBN 978-7-5659-3254-0

定　　价：110.00 元

版权所有，违者必究

（凡属质量问题请与本社发行部联系退换）

中英双语版 编辑委员会

主任委员

王 辰

委　　员（按姓氏笔画排序）

王 洁	王伊龙	王建祥	巴 一	代华平	宁 光	宁晓红	朱 兰
任景怡	刘海鹰	李小鹰	李梦涛	李雪梅	杨爱明	张福杰	郑金刚
房静远	赵 晶	赵明辉	郝 伟	姜 辉	栗占国	贾继东	夏维波
黄 慧	黄晓军	曹 彬	彭 斌	潘 慧			

第1分册　内科学概论·呼吸与危重症医学·术前和术后照护
　　　　主译　王 辰　代华平　赵 晶　黄 慧

第2分册　心血管疾病
　　　　主译　郑金刚　任景怡

第3分册　肾脏疾病
　　　　主译　李雪梅　赵明辉

第4分册　胃肠疾病·肝脏与胆道系统疾病
　　　　主译　房静远　杨爱明　贾继东

第5分册　血液疾病
　　　　主译　黄晓军　王建祥

第6分册　肿瘤疾病
　　　　主译　王 洁　巴 一

第7分册　内分泌疾病与代谢疾病·女性健康·男性健康·骨与骨矿物质代谢疾病
　　　　主译　宁 光　朱 兰　姜 辉　夏维波　潘 慧

第8分册　肌肉骨骼与结缔组织疾病
　　　　主译　栗占国　李梦涛

第9分册　感染性疾病
　　　　主译　刘海鹰　张福杰　曹 彬

第10分册　神经疾病·老年医学·缓和医疗·酒精和物质使用
　　　　主译　彭 斌　王伊龙　李小鹰　宁晓红　郝 伟

医学名词审定指导

任慧玲　李晓瑛　冀玉静　张燕舞　李军莲

中英双语版 序言

让我国医学生与国际医学生站在同一起跑线上的首要之事,是为其提供具有世界先进水平的标准教材。我们应争取使每一位医学生都能接触到内容经典、充分代表现代医学水平的国际权威原文教材并力求准确翻译,提供原文与中文双语对照版本,使医学生和医生在学习中形成双语医学词语、概念、概念间逻辑及由此构成的医学知识体系。在这样的思想驱动下,国际经典内科学教科书《希氏内科学精要(第10版)》中英双语版应运而生。

《希氏内科学》原著以其论述严谨准确、系统全面,被誉为"标准的内科学参考书"。自1927年首次出版以来,在内科学领域渐享世界级声誉,成为全球众多优秀医学院校,包括哈佛医学院、斯坦福大学医学院、约翰斯·霍普金斯大学医学院、牛津大学医学部、剑桥大学医学院、墨尔本大学医学院、新加坡国立大学医学院及多伦多大学医学院等普遍采用的内科学参考书。首版《希氏内科学精要》则诞生于1986年,旨在凝炼其全本的精华和要点,以最为简洁明确的方式向以医学生为主体的医学界精辟传达《希氏内科学》的核心信息,包括书中所体现出的人文精神。此后,每版精要本都力求凝炼地反映当时最新医学成果和医疗实践指南,愈来愈成为各国医学生、住院医师、专培医师及教师学习和传授内科学的主要教本,在世界医学教材体系中居引领地位。《希氏内科学》和《希氏内科学精要》两个版本不仅在英语国家被广泛使用,更被翻译为葡萄牙语、西班牙语、希腊语、意大利语、日语、简体中文版,为全球医学界广泛采用。

中国的医学生、住院医师、专培医师需要培养国际专业信息获取能力。将精要本原文引进并准确翻译,以中英文对照的形式呈现,便于读者进行双语对照阅读和学习,使之在学习理解国际标准医学内容的同时,学习好中英文医学词语,为国际医学交流打好基础。相信此举对于提高我国的医学教育水平,培养国际型医学人才至为有益。

《希氏内科学精要》精练地涵盖了内科学的所有主要领域,包括心血管疾病、呼吸疾病与危重症、消化疾病、肾脏疾病、内分泌和代谢疾病、风湿疾病、血液疾病、肿瘤、感染性疾病、神经与老年疾病等,构建了较为系统的知识体系。在翻译引进过程中,我们遵循将相关内容集中的原则,将原书按系统器官拆分为十个分册,使其更具有专科阅读的对应性,以更加灵活轻便的形式为读者提供多样化的阅读选择。

为确保译文质量，我们在译者遴选上采取了严谨的标准。从《希氏内科学（第26版）》翻译团队中择优选取责任心强、译文优质的译者，同时吸纳了临床医学专业"101"计划核心教材的编者团队。每个分册均由主译专家带领各自译者团队完成翻译、审校、交叉互审、通审四级审校工作。这些译者具备扎实的英语与专业能力，他们在翻译过程中，深入理解原文，准确阐述作者思想，并多角度审视译文的准确性、流畅性与风格一致性，确保译文的忠实性、规范性与可读性，在不同的语言和文化间架起坚实的桥梁。尤其值得称赞的是，对原著中疏漏或不够完善之处，译文中以"译者注"的形式加以适当解释和说明，使译文内容在忠实于原著的基础上更为准确。

本书读者定位于具有一定学习能力和基础的高等医学院校医学专业8年制、5年制学生以及相关医学专业人员，可作为医务人员的内科学参考书、住院医师规范化培训和专科医师规范化培训辅导教材、研究生入学考试辅导教材、内科学教师参考书、内科学各专科医师复习回顾其他专科知识的重要读本。

呼吸与危重症医学教授
中国医学科学院院长
北京协和医学院校长
2024年11月

对学习者教科书重要。
对学医者内科学重要。
世界上的内科学教科书，
首推《希氏内科学精要》。

中文是中国医生主要执业用语。
英文是国际医学交流的主要文字。
学习医学，当以双语对应阅读为好。
如此，可获纵横国际之效。

本书力求有助于此。

In Memoriam

Thomas E. Andreoli, MD

Dr. Thomas Andreoli, along with Drs. Lloyd Hollingsworth (Holly) Smith, Jr., Fred Plum, and Charles C.J. Carpenter, was one of the four founding editors of *Cecil Essentials of Medicine*. He served as editor for editions one through eight before he passed away on April 14, 2009. Dr. Andreoli was born in the Bronx, New York, in 1935, attended Catholic primary and high schools, and graduated from St. Vincent College and the Georgetown School of Medicine. He trained as a resident at Duke University under legendary Chair of Medicine Dr. Eugene Stead, who recognized him as a brilliant physician and scientist and encouraged his research career. Dr. Andreoli received his research training at the NIH and then in the laboratory of Dr. Tosteson at Duke. His research focused on the biochemical and biophysical properties of renal tubular cell membranes and their role in water and electrolyte transport. He made fundamental discoveries on the normal renal physiology, illuminating the way to subsequent work by many others on renal health and disease. His research was recognized with numerous awards and election to honorific societies both in the United States and in Europe. Dr. Andreoli also served as editor of *The American Journal of Physiology: Renal Physiology* and Editor in Chief of *Kidney International*.

Tom's national prominence and leadership qualities were recognized early in his career when he became head of Nephrology at the University of Alabama in Birmingham. There he helped faculty and trainees develop outstanding research, organized clinical services, and created a hemodialysis program to build one of the outstanding Divisions of Nephrology in the country. In 1979, Dr. Andreoli was appointed Chair of the Department of Internal Medicine at the University of Texas, Houston, where he assembled an outstanding faculty focused on research, clinical care, and teaching. In 1988, he accepted the position as Chairman of Internal Medicine at the University of Arkansas School of Medicine, a position he held until his death. There he again assembled a distinguished faculty who were outstanding researchers but also dedicated to outstanding clinical care and teaching. Morning report and clinical rounds with Dr. Andreoli were rigorous and riveting, focusing on the individual patient, not only their diagnoses and treatment but also on each patient's personal concerns and well-being. Dr. Andreoli was revered by medical students, his house staff, faculty, and colleagues, and I (EJW) personally can attest to what he regarded as his most cherished role—the mentorship and education of the next generation of physicians.

One of Dr. Andreoli's great interests was *Cecil Essentials of Medicine*, for which he was the editor/chief editor for eight of its ten editions, an interest that reflected his commitment to the education of students, house staff, and other physicians in the "essentials" of Internal Medicine.

Dr. Andreoli was devoted to his family. He was married to Elizabeth Berglund Andreoli from 1987 until his death. He was previously married to Dr. Kathleen Gainor Andreoli, mother of his three children and their ten grandchildren. Being of Italian ancestry and from Bronx, New York, it is not surprising that Dr. Andreoli was a passionate fan of the New York Yankees, Italian opera, which he could sing in Italian, and Frank Sinatra.

Dr. Andreoli's legacy lives on in his numerous previous students, house staff, colleagues, and in this book.

缅 怀

托马斯·安德里奥利博士

托马斯·安德里奥利（Thomas E. Andreoli）博士携手李奥德·霍灵斯沃斯·史密斯［Lloyd Hollingsworth（Holly）Smith］博士、弗雷德·普拉姆（Fred Plum）博士和查尔斯·卡彭特（Charles C.J. Carpenter）博士同为《希氏内科学精要》的创始编者。他在 2009 年 4 月 14 日去世前，曾担任该书第 1 至第 8 版的编者。安德里奥利博士于 1935 年出生于美国纽约布朗克斯区，就读于天主教小学和中学，后毕业于圣文森特学院和乔治城大学医学院。他在杜克大学医学院接受住院医师培训期间师从著名内科主任尤金·斯特德（Eugene Stead）博士，后者将其视为杰出的医生和科学家，并鼓励他投身科研事业。安德里奥利博士在美国国立卫生研究院接受科研训练后，前往杜克大学托斯特森（Tosteson）博士的实验室继续深造。他重点研究肾小管细胞膜的生化和生物物理特性及其在水和电解质转运中所发挥的作用。他在正常肾脏生理学方面的重要发现为后续关于肾脏健康和疾病的研究铺平了道路。安德里奥利博士的研究工作荣获多个学术奖项，并入选美国和欧洲的多个荣誉学会。他还担任《美国生理学杂志：肾脏生理学篇》（*The American Journal of Physiology：Renal Physiology*）的编辑以及《国际肾脏杂志》（*Kidney International*）的主编。

安德里奥利博士担任阿拉巴马大学伯明翰分校肾脏病学系主任后不久，即因其杰出领导力而赢得全美业内声誉。他帮助本校师生们取得科研突破，负责临床业务的组织实施，并因开创血液透析业务而使该科跻身全美顶级肾脏内科之列。1979 年，安德里奥利博士被任命为得克萨斯大学休斯敦分校内科学系主任，他在该系组建了一支科研、临床诊疗和教学并重的优秀教职团队。自 1988 年起，他担任阿肯色大学医学院内科学系主任，直至辞世。在这里他再次组建了一支卓越的教职团队，他们不仅科研工作出色，临床诊疗和教学工作也出类拔萃。安德里奥利博士带领的晨会报告和查房非常严谨而引人入胜，不仅尽心竭力于每位患者的诊断和治疗，还关注到他们每个人的个体情况和福祉。安德里奥利博士深受医学生、住院医师、教职人员和同事的崇敬，我（EJW）可以证明，他最珍视的角色当属培养和教育下一代医生。

安德里奥利博士对《希氏内科学精要》倾注了满腔热忱，先后担任了该书 10 版中 8 版的编者/主编，践行他为医学生、住院医师和其他各科医生们传授内科学"精要"的承诺。

安德里奥利博士高度重视家庭。他与第二任妻子伊丽莎白·伯格兰德·安德里奥利（Elizabeth Berglund Andreoli）的婚姻从 1987 年延续到辞世。他与第一任妻子凯瑟琳·盖娜·安德里奥利（Kathleen Gainor Andreoli）博士育有三个子女和十个孙辈。作为意大利裔和纽约布朗克斯人，安德里奥利博士是纽约洋基队、意大利歌剧（他能用意大利语演唱）和美国著名歌手、演员、主持人弗兰克·辛纳屈（Frank Sinatra）的忠实拥趸。安德里奥利博士将永远被他的众多学生、住院医师和同事怀念，并因本书而流芳百世。

In Memoriam

Charles C.J. Carpenter, MD

Dr. Charles C.J. Carpenter joined Drs. Thomas Andreoli, Lloyd Hollingsworth Smith, Jr., and Fred Plum as a founder of *Cecil Essentials of Medicine.* He served as editor for seven editions and was followed in that role by Dr. Ivor Benjamin and then Dr. Edward Wing. Sadly, Chuck passed away on March 19, 2020, surrounded by his wife and children. He was Professor Emeritus of Medicine at The Warren Alpert Medical School of Brown University and Physician-in-Chief Emeritus at The Miriam Hospital.

Chuck was born in Savannah, Georgia, on January 5, 1931. He attended college at Princeton and medical school at Johns Hopkins where he also did his house staff training, including chief residency, and then joined the Johns Hopkins faculty. With his young family, he travelled to Calcutta, India, where he carried out landmark studies for the treatment of cholera.

Before coming to Brown in 1986, he was Chair of Medicine at Baltimore City Hospital and Case Western Reserve University.

His contributions to medical science and clinical care were many. While in Calcutta, using basic scientific evidence coupled with practical approaches, Dr. Carpenter developed "oral rehydration therapy" to address the cholera epidemic there. This treatment has saved millions of lives. While at Case, one of his innovations was to develop the nation's first Division of Geographic Medicine because of his strong belief that all physicians should be medical citizens of the world. In 1987, as he became deeply involved in the clinical management of persons living with HIV, he initiated a unique program in which Brown University faculty and trainees assumed responsibility for all HIV care in the Rhode Island State prison system.

Dr. Carpenter served as Chairman of the American Board of Internal Medicine and President of the Association of American Physicians. He has been a member of the NIH AIDS Executive Committee, the National Advisory Allergy and Infectious Diseases Council, and the USPHS AIDS Task Force. He was Chair of the Antiretroviral Treatment Panel of the International AIDS Society-USA and authored their recommendations on antiretroviral treatment. He also served as Chair of the Treatment Committee to evaluate the President's Emergency Plan for HIV/AIDS Relief. He became the director of the Brown University International Health Institute and the director of the Lifespan/Brown Center for AIDS Research with several Boston hospitals.

Throughout his career, Dr. Carpenter was the recipient of many international, national, and regional awards, accepting each with characteristic humility. With both small and large groups of learners, Chuck made certain that every member of his team was well educated, and each felt that they contributed to the well-being of their patients. His ability to sit calmly at the bedside, hold the patient's hand, comfort them, and listen in a genuinely focused way, influenced so many physicians. He was truly grateful for the opportunity to care for those less fortunate than he, and the feeling of being privileged to do so was clearly transmitted to all. Dr. Carpenter was a wonderful blend of profound compassion combined with the adherence to scholarship and teaching. Sir William Osler wrote that physicians should "Do the kind thing and do it first." Chuck lived by this precept. Vigor and insight characterized his approach to clinical and ethical challenges, always with younger colleagues at his side. In a recent tribute to him, many emphasized that Dr. Carpenter dedicated his life to his patients, many of whom were the most vulnerable members of society. We hope that we will have some of his strength and use his example as our compass as we are challenged to reduce suffering and improve the health of all for whom we are responsible.

He is survived by his wife of 61 years, Sally; three sons, Charles, Murray, and Andrew; and seven grandchildren.

缅 怀

查尔斯·卡彭特博士

查尔斯·卡彭特（Charles C.J. Carpenter）博士与托马斯·安德里奥利（Thomas E. Andreoli）博士、李奥德·霍灵斯沃斯·史密斯（Lloyd Hollingsworth Smith）博士和弗雷德·普拉姆（Fred Plum）博士共同开创了《希氏内科学精要》。他共担任了7版的编者，嗣后由艾弗·本杰明（Ivor Benjamin）博士和爱德华·温（Edward Wing）博士接任。查尔斯·卡彭特博士于2020年3月19日在妻子和子女们的陪伴下辞世。他曾担任布朗大学沃伦·阿尔珀特医学院的内科学系名誉教授和米里亚姆医院的名誉主任医师。

查尔斯·卡彭特博士于1931年1月5日出生于美国佐治亚州萨凡纳市。他在普林斯顿大学获得学士学位后进入约翰斯·霍普金斯大学医学院，并完成了包括住院总医师在内的住院医师培训，随后加入了约翰斯·霍普金斯大学的教职团队。他曾携妻子和年幼的孩子前往印度加尔各答，在当地对霍乱的治疗进行了具有里程碑意义的研究工作。

在1986年入职布朗大学之前，他曾担任巴尔的摩市医院和凯斯西储大学医学院的内科学主任。

他在医学科学研究和临床诊疗领域建树颇多。在加尔各答期间，基于基础科学证据及临床实践，查尔斯·卡彭特博士开创了"口服补液疗法"以遏制当地的霍乱疫情。这一疗法拯救了数百万人的生命。秉承医生无国界的世界公民理念，他在凯斯西储大学做了一项开创性工作，建立了美国首个地缘医学部（研究地理环境因素对人体健康和疾病影响的学科）。1987年，他深度参与人类免疫缺陷病毒（HIV）携带者的临床管理，并发起了一个独特的项目——由布朗大学教职团队和医学生们承担罗德岛州监狱系统内所有艾滋病相关诊疗工作。

查尔斯·卡彭特博士曾担任美国内科医师委员会主席和美国医师协会主席。他曾是美国国立卫生研究院艾滋病行政委员会、美国国家过敏与传染病咨询委员会以及公共卫生服务部艾滋病工作组的成员。他还曾担任国际艾滋病学会-美国分会抗逆转录病毒治疗组主席，并撰写了抗逆转录病毒治疗建议。他还担任过艾滋病治疗委员会主席，该委员会负责评估美国总统防治艾滋病紧急救援计划；曾担任布朗大学国际健康研究所所长，以及大学与多家波士顿当地医院合办的生命周期/布朗大学艾滋病研究中心主任。

查尔斯·卡彭特博士在职业生涯中获得过诸多国际性、全美和地区性奖项，同时展现其谦逊品格。无论学员人数多寡，查尔斯·卡彭特博士都会确保人人都能受到良好教育，并让他们感到自己也对患者的健康做出了贡献。他能够安静地坐在病床边，握住患者的手，安慰他们，并全神贯注地听取患者倾诉，这一举动深深地感染了许多医生。他十分珍视诊治不幸染病者的机会，并且能够将这种殊荣感传递给所有人。查尔斯·卡彭特博士完美地融汇了对患者的宅心仁厚与对学术和教学的坚守。威廉·奥斯勒（William Osler）爵士曾写道，医生应该"行善事，为人先"，而这正是查尔斯·卡彭特博士一生奉行的信条。他在面对临床和伦理挑战时充满活力和洞察力，始终重视提携年轻同事。许多人的悼词中都重点指出，查尔斯·卡彭特博士将毕生致力于患者福祉，其中许多人属于社会上最弱势群体。我们希望，在我们面临减少患者痛苦及改善其健康状况的挑战时，能够拥有他的力量，并以他为榜样获得指引。

查尔斯·卡彭特博士与妻子萨丽（Sally）共度了61年的婚姻时光，育有查尔斯（Charles）、穆雷（Murray）和安德鲁（Andrew）三子以及七个孙辈。

ABOUT THE EDITORS

Dr. Edward J. Wing was an editor of *Cecil Essentials of Medicine*, editions 8 and 9, and is the lead editor of edition 10. He graduated from Williams College in 1967 and from the Harvard Medical School in 1971. He was a resident in Internal Medicine at the Peter Bent Brigham and completed an Infectious Diseases Fellowship at Stanford University. Joining the faculty at the University of Pittsburgh in 1975, he focused his NIH-funded research on mechanisms of cell-mediated immunity as well as various clinical aspects of Infectious Diseases. From 1990 to 1998, the University and UPMC appointed him as Physician-in-Chief at Montefiore Hospital, then Chief of Infectious Diseases, and finally Interim Chair of Medicine.

In 1998, Dr. Wing became Chair of Medicine at Brown University (1998–2008) where he consolidated the department across hospitals, practice plans, and training programs. As Dean of Medicine and Biological Sciences at Brown University (2008–2013) he strengthened ties with affiliated hospitals (Lifespan and Care New England), increased research, and oversaw the construction of a new medical school building. International exchange programs with medical schools in Kenya, the Dominican Republic, and Haiti were established during his years as chairman and dean. Dr. Wing has cared for patients with HIV since the beginning of the epidemic in outpatient clinics. He continues to be active in research, clinical care, and teaching.

Dr. Fred J. Schiffman, who along with Dr. Edward Wing is editor of *Cecil Essentials of Medicine*, 10th edition, attended Wagner College and then the New York University School of Medicine, from which he graduated in 1973. He performed his early house staff training at Yale-New Haven Hospital and then spent two years at the National Cancer Institute. He returned to Yale as Chief Medical Resident followed by a hematology fellowship. He became Medical Director of Yale's Primary Care Center before coming to Brown University in 1983, where he has been a leader in the medical residency program as well as Associate Physician-in-Chief at The Miriam Hospital.

Dr. Schiffman holds The Sigal Family Professorship in Humanistic Medicine at The Warren Alpert Medical School of Brown University. His scholarly interests include the structure and function of the human spleen and the intersection of the arts and medical care. He has directed or championed many projects and programs, including those that encourage and reinforce wellness and resilience in patients, families, and caregivers. He began a novel program that places medical students and physicians with other nonmedical professionals as they share in the viewing of works of art in the Museum of the Rhode Island School of Design. Dr. Schiffman recently led a Brown University edX course entitled, "Artful Medicine: Art's Power to Enrich Patient Care," with worldwide participation. Dr. Schiffman has also edited texts on hematologic pathophysiology, consultative hematology, and the anemias.

原著主编

爱德华·温（Edward J. Wing）博士是《希氏内科学精要》第 8 版和第 9 版的编者，以及第 10 版的主编。他先后于 1967 年和 1971 年毕业于威廉姆斯学院和哈佛医学院。他曾在彼得·本特·布里格姆医院任内科住院医师，后在斯坦福大学完成了传染病学的专科医师（Fellowship）课程。自 1975 年加入匹兹堡大学医学院以来，他通过美国国立卫生研究院资助的研究项目，探索细胞介导免疫的机制以及传染病学各领域的临床诊疗工作。1990—1998 年期间，他先后被匹兹堡大学及其医学中心任命为蒙特菲奥里医院的主任医师、传染病科主任，后担任内科临聘主任。

1998 年起，温博士担任布朗大学医学院的内科主任（1998—2008 年）。在此期间，他在不同医院、实践计划和培训项目间对内科进行整合。在担任布朗大学医学与生物科学院院长（2008—2013 年）期间，他加强了与各附属医院（Lifespan 医院和 Care New England 医院）间的联系，提升了科研工作的水准，并为医学院建成了一座新楼。在担任主任和院长期间，他还建立了与肯尼亚、多米尼加共和国和海地的医学院的国际交流项目。温博士自艾滋病流行初期便在门诊诊治艾滋病患者，并始终工作在科研、临床和教学一线。

弗雷德·谢夫曼（Fred J. Schiffman）博士与爱德华·温（Edward Wing）博士共同担任《希氏内科学精要》第 10 版的主编。他就读于瓦格纳学院，随后进入纽约大学医学院，并于 1973 年毕业。他在耶鲁大学附属纽黑文医院接受早期住院医师培训，随后在美国国家癌症研究所工作了两年。回到耶鲁大学后，他担任住院总医师，然后完成了血液学专科医师课程，随后成为耶鲁初级保健中心医学主任。他于 1983 年入职布朗大学，领导医学住院医师项目并担任米里亚姆医院的副主任医师。

谢夫曼博士担任布朗大学沃伦·阿尔珀特医学院人文医学系的西格尔家庭医学教授。他的学术兴趣涵盖人体脾脏的结构和功能，以及艺术与医疗的交叉融合。他主持或参与了许多项目和计划，其中包括许多旨在鼓励和加强患者、家人和医护人员的福祉与康复能力的项目。他所创办的一个新项目可以让医学生和医生与其他非医学专业人士一起，共同欣赏罗德岛设计学院博物馆的艺术作品。谢夫曼博士近期还主持了布朗大学名为"艺术与医学：艺术赋能患者照护"的 edX 课程，此课程的参与者来自全球多个国家。谢夫曼博士还出版了有关血液病理生理学、血液科会诊和贫血的著作。

原著者名单

Jinnette Dawn Abbott, MD
Rajiv Agarwal, MD
Marwa Al-Badri, MD
Hyeon-Ju Ryoo Ali, MD
Jason M. Aliotta, MD
Khaldoun Almhanna, MD, MPH
Mohanad T. Al-Qaisi, MD
Zuhal Arzomand, MD
Akwi W. Asombang, MD, MPH
Su N. Aung, MD, MPH
Christopher G. Azzoli, MD
Christina Bandera, MD
Debasree Banerjee, MD
Mashal Batheja, MD
Jeffrey J. Bazarian, MD, MPH
Selim R. Benbadis, MD
Ivor J. Benjamin, MD, FAHA, FACC
Eric Benoit, MD
Marcie G. Berger, MD
Clemens Bergwitz, MD
Nancy Berliner, MD
Jeffrey S. Berns, MD
Pooja Bhadbhade, DO
Ratna Bhavaraju-Sanka, MD
Tanmayee Bichile, MD
Ariel E. Birnbaum, MD
Charles M. Bliss, Jr., MD
Andrew S. Blum, MD, PhD
Bryan J. Bonder, MD
Russell Bratman, MD
Glenn D. Braunstein, MD
Alma M. Guerrero Bready, MD
Richard Bungiro, PhD
Anna Marie Burgner, MD, MEHP
Jonathan Cahill, MD
Andrew Canakis, DO
Benedito A. Carneiro, MD, MS
Brian Casserly, MD
Abdullah Chahin, MD, MA, MSc
Philip A. Chan, MD
Kimberle Chapin, MD
William P. Cheshire, Jr., MD
Waihong Chung, MD, PhD
Emma Ciafaloni, MD

Joaquin E. Cigarroa, MD
Michael P. Cinquegrani, MD
Andreea Coca, MD, MPH
Harvey Jay Cohen, MD
Scott Cohen, MD, MPH
Beatrice P. Concepcion, MD, MS
Nathan T. Connell, MD, MPH
Maria Constantinou, MD
Roberto Cortez, MD
Timothy J. Counihan, MD, FRCPI
Anne Haney Cross, MD
Cheston B. Cunha, MD, FACP
Joanne S. Cunha, MD
Susan Cu-Uvin, MD
Noura M. Dabbouseh, MD
Kwame Dapaah-Afriyie, MD, MBA
Erin M. Denney-Koelsch, MD
Andre De Souza, MD
An S. De Vriese, MD, PhD
Neal D. Dharmadhikari, MD
Leah Dickstein, MD
Don Dizon, MD, FACP, FASCO
Robyn T. Domsic, MD, MPH
Kim A. Eagle, MD
Michael G. Earing, MD
Pamela Egan, MD
Wafik S. El-Deiry, MD, PhD, FACP
Mitchell S. V. Elkind, MD, MS
Tarra B. Evans, MD
Michael B. Fallon, MD
Dimitrios Farmakiotis, MD
Francis A. Farraye, MD
Ronan Farrell, MD
Panayotis Fasseas, MD, FACC
Mary Anne Fenton, MD
Fernando C. Fervenza, MD, PhD
Sean Fine, MD
Arkadiy Finn, MD
Timothy Flanigan, MD
Brisas M. Flores, MD
Andrew E. Foderaro, MD
Theodore C. Friedman, MD, PhD
Joseph Metmowlee Garland, MD, AAHIVM

Eric J. Gartman, MD
Abdallah Geara, MD
Raul Macias Gil, MD
Timothy Gilligan, MD, FASCO
Michael Raymond Goggins, MB BCh BAO, MRCPI
Geetha Gopalakrishnan, MD
Vidya Gopinath, MD
Susan L. Greenspan, MD, FACP
Osama Hamdy, MD, PhD
Johanna Hamel, MD
Sajeev Handa, MD, SFHM
Mitchell T. Heflin, MD, MHS
Robert G. Holloway, MD, MPH
Christopher S. Huang, MD
Zilla Hussain, MD
T. Alp Ikizler, MD
Iris Isufi, MD
Carlayne E. Jackson, MD
Paul G. Jacob, MD, MPH
Matthew D. Jankowich, MD
Niels V. Johnsen, MD, MPH
Jessica E. Johnson, MD
Rayford R. June, MD
Tareq Kheirbek, MD, ScM, FACS
Alok A. Khorana, MD, FACP, FASCO
Sena Kilic, MD
David Kim, MD
James Kleczka, MD
James R. Klinger, MD
Patrick Koo, MD, ScM
Pooja Koolwal, MD
Mary P. Kotlarczyk, PhD
Nicole M. Kuderer, MD
Awewura Kwara, MD
Jennifer M. Kwon, MD, MPH
Richard A. Lange, MD, MBA
Jerome Larkin, MD
Alfred I. Lee, MD, PhD
Daniel J. Levine, MD
David E. Lewandowski, MD
Kelly V. Liang, MD, MS
Kimberly P. Liang, MD, MS
David R. Lichtenstein, MD

扫描二维码了解更多信息

Douglas W. Lienesch, MD
Geoffrey S.F. Ling, MD, PhD
Ester Little, MD, FACP
Yi Liu, MD
Nicole L. Lohr, MD, PhD
John R. Lonks, MD, FACP, FIDSA, FSHEA
Gary H. Lyman, MD, MPH
Jeffrey M. Lyness, MD
Shane Lyons, MD, MRCPI, MRCP(UK)
Diana Maas, MD
Talha A. Malik, MD, MSPH
Sonia Manocha, MD
Susan Manzi, MD, MPH
Frederick J. Marshall, MD
F. Dennis McCool, MD
Russell J. McCulloh, MD
Kelly McGarry, MD, FACP
Eavan Mc Govern, MD, PhD
Robin L. McKinney, MD
Anthony Mega, MD
Shivang Mehta, MD
Douglas F. Milam, MD
Maria D. Mileno, MD
Abhinav Kumar Misra, MBBS, MD
Orson W. Moe, MD
Niveditha Mohan, MBBS
Larry W. Moreland, MD
Alan R. Morrison, MD, PhD
Steven F. Moss, MD
Christopher J. Mullin, MD, MHS
Sinéad M. Murphy, MB, BCh, MD, FRCPI
Sagarika Nallu, MD, FAAP, FAAN, FAASM
Javier A. Neyra, MD, MSCS
Ghaith Noaiseh, MD

Thomas A. Ollila, MD
Steven M. Opal, MD
Biff F. Palmer, MD
Jen Jung Pan, MD, PhD
Anna Papazoglou, MD
Aric Parnes, MD
Nayan M. Patel, DO, MPH
Ari Pelcovits, MD
Mark A. Perazella, MD
Michael F. Picco, MD, PhD
Kate E. Powers, DO
Laura A. Previll, MD, MPH
Nilum Rajora, MD
Adolfo Ramirez-Zamora, MD
John Reagan, MD
Rebecca Reece, MD
Harlan Rich, MD, AGAF, FACP
Jennifer H. Richman, MD
Lisa R. Rogers, DO
Ralph Rogers, MD
Michal G. Rose, MD
James A. Roth, MD
Sharon Rounds, MD
Jason C. Rubenstein, MD
Abbas Rupawala, MD
Jenna Sarvaideo, DO
Ramesh Saxena, MD, PhD
Fred J. Schiffman, MD, MACP
Ruth B. Schneider, MD
Kristin A. Seaborg, MD
Anil Seetharam, MD
Stuart Seropian, MD
Jigme Michael Sethi, MD
Sanjeev Sethi, MD, PhD
Elizabeth Shane, MD
Esseim Sharma, MD

Shani Shastri, MD, MPH
Barry S. Shea, MD
Lauren Shevell, MD, MPH
Joseph A. Smith, Jr., MD
Robert J. Smith, MD
Davendra P.S. Sohal, MD, MPH
Christopher Song, MD, FACC
Thomas Sperry, MD
Jeffrey M. Statland, MD
Emily M. Stein, MD
Jennifer L. Strande, MD, PhD
Rochelle Strenger, MD
Thomas R. Talbot, MD, MPH
Christopher G. Tarolli, MD, MSEd
Yael Tarshish, MD
Pushpak Taunk, MD
Philip Tsoukas, MD
Allan R. Tunkel, MD, PhD
Jeffrey M. Turner, MD
Zoe G.S. Vazquez, MD
Stacie A. F. Vela, MD
Paul M. Vespa, MD, FCCM, FAAN, FANA, FNCS
Wanpen Vongpatanasin, MD
Marcella D. Walker, MD
Eunice S. Wang, MD
Sharmeel K. Wasan, MD
Thomas J. Weber, MD
Brandon J. Wilcoxson, MD
Edward J. Wing, MD, FACP, FIDSA
Ellice Wong, MD
John J. Wysolmerski, MD
Rayan Yousefzai, MD
Thomas R. Ziegler, MD
Rebecca Zon, MD

ACKNOWLEDGMENTS

Dr. Schiffman and I wish to thank first of all, the authors of the 128 chapters that make up the tenth edition of *Cecil Essentials of Medicine*. They have worked diligently to compose the material for each chapter and apply their mastery as they added the newest information, in clear language, to the text. Their efforts are apparent in the excellence of the book, and we are immensely grateful for their work. We wish to also thank Marybeth Thiel, Jennifer Ehlers, and Dan Fitzgerald from Elsevier who guided and supported our work as editors and whose expertise has made this volume possible. Finally, we are always thankful to our wives, Dr. Rena Wing and Ms. Gerri Schiffman, without whose love, support, and especially humor, this book would not have happened.

致　谢

　　谢夫曼博士和我首先要致谢《希氏内科学精要》第 10 版全书 128 章的各位作者。感谢他们精益求精地撰写每一章节，并运用其专业知识，以简明的语言将前沿资讯呈现在书中。正是他们的辛勤努力确保了本书的卓越地位，对他们唯有由衷的感激。我们还要感谢爱思唯尔出版集团的玛丽贝丝·蒂尔（Marybeth Thiel）、詹妮弗·埃勒斯（Jennifer Ehlers）和丹·菲茨杰拉德（Dan Fitzgerald），他们对本书的编辑工作给予了指导和支持，其专业水准保障了本书的完稿。最后，要特别感谢我们的妻子——蕾娜·温（Rena Wing）博士和盖瑞·谢夫曼（Gerri Schiffman）女士，对她们的爱和支持，特别是积极乐观的心态始终心存感激，她们为本书的圆满完成发挥了不可或缺的作用。

总目录

第1分册

第1篇　内科学概论　Introduction to Medicine
第2篇　呼吸与危重症医学　Pulmonary and Critical Care Medicine
第3篇　术前和术后照护　Preoperative and Postoperative Care

第2分册

心血管疾病　Cardiovascular Disease

第3分册

肾脏疾病　Renal Disease

第4分册

第1篇　胃肠疾病　Gastrointestinal Disease
第2篇　肝脏与胆道系统疾病　Diseases of the Liver and Biliary System

第5分册

血液疾病　Hematologic Disease

第6分册

肿瘤疾病　Oncologic Disease

第7分册

第1篇　内分泌疾病与代谢疾病　Endocrine Disease and Metabolic Disease
第2篇　女性健康　Women's Health
第3篇　男性健康　Men's Health
第4篇　骨与骨矿物质代谢疾病　Diseases of Bone and Bone Mineral Metabolism

第 8 分册

肌肉骨骼与结缔组织疾病　Musculoskeletal and Connective Tissue Disease

第 9 分册

感染性疾病　Infectious Disease

第 10 分册

第 1 篇　神经疾病　Neurologic Disease
第 2 篇　老年医学　Geriatrics
第 3 篇　缓和医疗　Palliative Care
第 4 篇　酒精和物质使用　Alcohol and Substance Use

第5分册

血液疾病

第 5 分册译者名单

主　译

黄晓军　王建祥

译　者（按姓氏笔画排序）

马　瑞　北京大学人民医院	邱录贵　中国医学科学院血液病医院
王建祥　中国医学科学院血液病医院	（中国医学科学院血液学研究所）
（中国医学科学院血液学研究所）	张　磊　中国医学科学院血液病医院
代新岳　中国医学科学院血液病医院	（中国医学科学院血液学研究所）
（中国医学科学院血液学研究所）	易树华　中国医学科学院血液病医院
刘　静　北京大学人民医院	（中国医学科学院血液学研究所）
江　浩　北京大学人民医院	高海涛　北京大学人民医院
许兰平　北京大学人民医院	唐菲菲　北京大学人民医院
孙　葳　北京大学人民医院	黄晓军　北京大学人民医院
孙　婷　中国医学科学院血液病医院	阎禹廷　中国医学科学院血液病医院
（中国医学科学院血液学研究所）	（中国医学科学院血液学研究所）
孙于谦　北京大学人民医院	董　焕　中国医学科学院血液病医院
杨仁池　中国医学科学院血液病医院	（中国医学科学院血液学研究所）
（中国医学科学院血液学研究所）	薛　峰　中国医学科学院血液病医院
	（中国医学科学院血液学研究所）

第 5 分册目录

血液疾病　Hematologic Disease

1. Hematopoiesis and Hematopoietic Failure, 4
   造血与造血衰竭，5

2. Clonal Disorders of the Hematopoietic Stem Cell, 30
   造血干细胞克隆性疾病，31

3. Disorders of Red Blood Cells, 68
   红细胞疾病，69

4. Clinical Disorders of Granulocytes and Monocytes, 92
   中性粒细胞和单核细胞相关疾病，93

5. Disorders of Lymphocytes, 102
   淋巴细胞疾病，103

6. Normal Hemostasis, 134
   正常止血，135

7. Disorders of Hemostasis: Bleeding, 150
   止血障碍：出血，151

8. Disorders of Hemostasis: Thrombosis, 190
   止血障碍：血栓形成，191

索引 Index，214

CECIL ESSENTIALS OF MEDICINE

Hematologic Disease

Hematologic Disease

1 Hematopoiesis and Hematopoietic Failure, 4

2 Clonal Disorders of the Hematopoietic Stem Cell, 30

3 Disorders of Red Blood Cells, 68

4 Clinical Disorders of Granulocytes and Monocytes, 92

5 Disorders of Lymphocytes, 102

6 Normal Hemostasis, 134

7 Disorders of Hemostasis: Bleeding, 150

8 Disorders of Hemostasis: Thrombosis, 190

血液疾病

1 造血与造血衰竭，5

2 造血干细胞克隆性疾病，31

3 红细胞疾病，69

4 中性粒细胞和单核细胞相关疾病，93

5 淋巴细胞疾病，103

6 正常止血，135

7 止血障碍：出血，151

8 止血障碍：血栓形成，191

1

Hematopoiesis and Hematopoietic Failure

Eunice S. Wang, Nancy Berliner

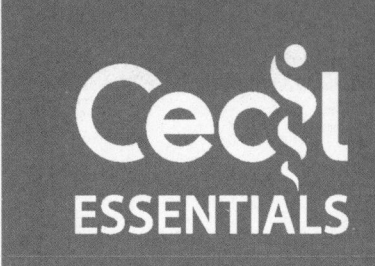

HEMATOPOIESIS

Hematopoiesis is the process of formation and development of blood cells. The constituents of peripheral blood arise by a complex and carefully regulated process of ontogeny. The pluripotent hematopoietic stem cell (HSC) maintains itself by self-renewal and undergoes multilineage differentiation to generate the appropriate numbers and types of cells in the circulating blood compartment (Table 1.1). The hematopoietic system is unique in that it is constantly undergoing this full cycle of maturation by which a primitive cell develops into a variety of highly specialized end-stage cells, all of which have different lifespans and occur in different quantities.

The bone marrow must have the capacity to produce cells to compensate for the normal rapid turnover of hematopoietic cells resulting from senescence, normal use, and migration into tissue spaces. It must have a reserve capacity to produce additional cells in response to unusual demands that arise from bleeding, infection, or other stresses. Understanding the repeated cycle of cellular ontogeny and self-renewal that meets these challenges provides important insights into normal and pathologic mechanisms in hematology.

Hematopoietic Tissues

Hematopoiesis commences in the embryonic yolk sac, in which early erythroblasts in blood islands form the first hemoglobinized cells. After 6 weeks' gestation, the fetal liver begins producing primitive lymphocytoid cells, megakaryocytes, and erythroblasts, and the spleen becomes a secondary site of erythropoiesis. Hematopoiesis then shifts to its definitive long-term site in the bone marrow, the principal site for lifelong hematopoiesis in the normal host.

Early in life, all fetal bones contain regenerative bone marrow, but the marrow becomes progressively replaced by fat with age. In adults, active marrow resides only in the axial skeleton (i.e., sternum, vertebrae, pelvis, and ribs) and in the proximal ends of the femur and humerus. Consequently, bone marrow samples, which are needed for many hematologic diagnoses, are usually obtained from the iliac crest or sternum. Under pathologic conditions that stress the capacity of the marrow space, as seen in diseases associated with marrow fibrosis (e.g., chronic myeloproliferative diseases) or in severe inherited hemolytic anemia (e.g., thalassemia major), extramedullary hematopoiesis may be reestablished in sites of fetal hematopoiesis, especially the spleen.

Stem Cell Theory of Hematopoiesis

All mature hematopoietic cells are hypothesized to originate from a small population of pluripotent stem cells. Comprising less than 1% of all cells in the bone marrow, these cells bear no distinctive morphologic markings and are best defined by their unique functional properties.

Stem cells have two distinctive characteristics. First, they are highly resilient and productive, capable of continuously replenishing huge numbers of granulocytes, lymphocytes, and erythrocytes throughout life. The demand for a continuous, fluctuating supply of blood cells requires a hematopoietic system capable of producing large numbers of selected cells in a short time. For example, overwhelming infection by invading microorganisms triggers the release of neutrophils, whereas hypoxia or acute blood loss leads to increased red blood cell production. Second, HSCs represent a self-renewing cell population that is able to maintain its numbers while providing a continued supply of progenitor cells of many different lineages.

Despite their vast proliferative potential, under normal conditions, most HSCs are quiescent, and few cells undergo expansion or differentiation at any one time. However, their ability to proliferate is striking. Studies with lethally irradiated mice have demonstrated the ability of a few transplanted cells (i.e., spleen colony-forming unit [CFU-S] cells) to regenerate multilineage hematopoiesis.

The signals regulating the differentiation of pluripotent stem cells into committed progenitors are unknown. Data suggest that the first step in lineage commitment is a stochastic (chance) event; subsequent stages of maturation are hypothesized to occur under the influence of growth factors, or cytokines (Table 1.2). Cytokines act on different cells through specific cytokine receptors. Receptor activation induces signal-transduction pathways that lead to changes in gene transcription and eventual cell proliferation and differentiation. These growth factors also act as survival factors for the developing hematopoietic cells by preventing *apoptosis* (i.e., programmed cell death). This process occurs in the cellular milieu of the bone marrow, where hematopoiesis depends in part on the nonhematopoietic cells (i.e., fibroblasts, endothelial cells, osteoblasts, and fat cells) that make up that microenvironment. Research in HSC biology has focused on how these cells are regulated by growth factors, unique cell surface ligands, and key interactions between stem cells and the surrounding microenvironmental cells (i.e., mesenchymal stromal cells, adipocytes, immune cells) within specialized marrow regions termed *stem cell niches*.

Hematopoietic Differentiation Pathway

Hematopoiesis has been hypothesized to proceed along a tightly regulated hierarchy (Fig. 1.1) governed by effects of intrinsic transcription factors and cytokines in the bone marrow microenvironment. As more primitive cells mature under the influence of specific regulatory cytokines, they undergo several cell divisions and become *progenitor cells* committed to one lineage. They also lose their self-renewal capacity. Morphologically, these cells are transformed from nonspecific blast-like cells into cells that can be identified by their color, shape, and granular and nuclear content. Functionally, they acquire distinguishing cell surface receptors and responses to specific signals.

Maturing granulocytes and erythroid cells undergo several more cell divisions in the bone marrow, whereas lymphocytes travel to the thymus and lymph nodes for further development. Megakaryocytes cease cellular

造血与造血衰竭

刘静 译　江浩 审校　黄晓军 通审

造血

造血是血细胞形成和发育的过程。外周血细胞成分在个体发育过程中通过复杂而精细的调节而产生。多能造血干细胞（HSC）通过自我更新来维持自身，并历经多谱系分化，产生适当数量和类型的细胞进入循环血液中（表1.1）。造血系统中一个原始细胞发育成各种高度特异化的终末期细胞，后者各有不同的寿命和数量，这种持续进行的完整的细胞周期，造就了造血系统的独特性。

正常造血细胞因衰老、正常使用和迁移到组织间隙而快速消耗，骨髓必须具备产生细胞以弥补这些消耗的能力。为应对因出血、感染或其他应激情况而产生的异常需求，骨髓必须有生产额外细胞的储备能力。了解血细胞为应对各种挑战不断进行的细胞分化和自我更新，对于理解血液学中的正常和病理学机制非常重要。

造血组织

造血开始于胚胎卵黄囊，在卵黄囊中，血岛中的早期有核红细胞形成了最初的含血红蛋白的细胞。妊娠第6周后，胎儿肝开始产生原始淋巴细胞、巨核细胞和有核红细胞，脾成为产生红细胞的次级器官。随后，造血细胞移行到骨髓，并维持终身，骨髓是正常宿主终身的主要造血器官。

在生命早期，所有胎儿骨骼都含有可再生的骨髓，但随着年龄的增长，骨髓逐渐被脂肪所取代。在成人中，活跃的骨髓仅存在于中轴骨（如胸骨、脊椎、骨盆和肋骨）以及股骨和肱骨近端。因此，许多血液病诊断所需的骨髓样本通常取自髂嵴或胸骨。当出现骨髓纤维化相关疾病（如慢性骨髓增殖性疾病）或严重的遗传性溶血性贫血（如重型地中海贫血）等病理情况时，髓外造血可能会在胎儿时期的造血器官（尤其是脾）中重启。

造血过程的干细胞理论

假设所有的成熟造血细胞均起源于一小部分多能干细胞，这些细胞占骨髓全部细胞的比例不足1%，它们没有特异的形态学特征，只能通过其特有的功能特性进行区分。

干细胞具有两大鲜明特点。第一，它们具有高度的适应力和增殖能力，能够终身持续补充大量粒细胞、淋巴细胞和红细胞。对持续且波动性的血细胞供应需求，要求造血系统具有在短时间内产生大量特定细胞的能力。例如，微生物侵入机体引起的严重感染可促进中性粒细胞释放，而低氧或急性失血可促进红细胞生成。第二，HSC是一组能够自我更新的细胞，在维持自身数量的同时能持续不断地产生多系造血祖细胞。

HSC虽然有很强大的增殖潜能，但在正常情况下，大多数HSC是静止的，每一次仅有极少数细胞扩增或分化。但它们的增殖能力十分惊人。对接受致死辐射量的小鼠进行的研究表明，少数移植细胞［如脾集落形成单位（CFU-S）细胞］具有重建多系造血的能力。

调节多能干细胞分化为定向祖细胞的信号通路尚不明确。数据显示，定向分化的第一步是随机事件，目前假说认为后续的成熟阶段是在生长因子或细胞因子（表1.2）的影响下进行的。细胞因子通过特定的细胞因子受体对不同细胞发挥作用。受体激活可介导信号转导途径，改变基因转录，最终影响细胞增殖和分化。这些生长因子也可通过阻止细胞凋亡（如程序性细胞死亡）而使发育中的造血干细胞得以存活。该过程均在骨髓的细胞环境中进行，造血过程部分依赖于骨髓微环境中的非造血细胞（如成纤维细胞、内皮细胞、成骨细胞和脂肪细胞）。HSC生物学的研究重点集中于干细胞如何被骨髓微环境中的生长因子、特定细胞表面配体及干细胞与其周围微环境中的细胞（如间充质干细胞、脂肪细胞、免疫细胞，这些细胞位于骨髓的特定区域，被称为"干细胞微环境"）之间的相互作用所调控。

造血分化途径

目前认为，造血过程受骨髓微环境中内源性转录因子和细胞因子的严格等级调控（图1.1）。在特定的调节性细胞因子的影响下，随着更多的原始细胞不断成熟，经历数次细胞分裂而成为某系定向祖细胞，祖细胞也失去了自我更新的能力。从形态学上看，祖细胞从非特异性母细胞样细胞转化为能通过染色、形状、颗粒及核内容物识别的特异性细胞。从功能上看，祖细胞获得了特异的细胞表面受体，可对特定信号产生应答。

正在发育中的粒细胞和红系细胞会在骨髓中经历多次细胞分裂，而淋巴细胞则移行至胸腺和淋巴结进一步发育。巨核细胞可停止细胞分裂，但继续进行核

TABLE 1.1 Normal Values for Peripheral Blood Cells

Cell Type and Size	Mean	Range
Hemoglobin	Women: 14 g/dL Men: 15.5 g/dL	Women: 12-16 g/dL Men: 13.5-17.5 g/dL
Hematocrit	Women: 41% Men: 47%	Women: 36-46% Men: 41-53%
Reticulocyte count	60,000/μL (1%)	35,000-85,000/μL (0.5-1.5%)
Mean corpuscular volume		80-100 fL
Platelet count	250,000/μL	150,000-400,000/μL
Total white blood cell count	7400/μL	4500-11,000/μL
Neutrophils	4400/μL (40-60%)	1800-7700/μL
Lymphocytes	2500/μL (20-40%)	1000-4800/μL
Monocytes	300/μL (<5%)	200-950 (4-11%)

TABLE 1.2 Cytokines and Their Activities

Acronym	Name	Effects on Hematopoiesis (and Possible Clinical Applications)
EPO	Erythropoietin	Stimulation of proliferation and maturation of erythroid progenitors; produced by the kidney in response to anemia and hypoxia; important clinically for treatment of anemia associated with low EPO levels (e.g., renal failure, anemia of chronic disease)
G-CSF	Granulocyte colony-stimulating factor	Stimulation of proliferation and maturation of granulocytes; more broad-based effect because also increases release of stem cells in peripheral blood; clinically important for treatment of neutropenia and mobilization of stem cells for transplantation
GM-CSF	Granulocyte-monocyte colony-stimulating factor	Proliferation of granulocyte and monocyte precursors; role unclear in steady-state hematopoiesis (mice deficient in GM-CSF gene still develop normally and no major perturbation of hematopoiesis up to 12 weeks of age)
TPO	Thrombopoietin	Proliferation of megakaryocytes; clinical studies of recombinant TPO were discontinued due to auto-antibody formation in individual patients
M-CSF	Monocyte colony-stimulating factor	Proliferation of monocytes
IL-2	Interleukin-2	Proliferation of T cells
IL-3	Interleukin-3 (multi–colony-stimulating factor)	Proliferation of granulocytes, monocytes; broad-based effects, appearing to increase the proliferation of stem cells; not in use clinically, differentiation of basophils and eosinophils from primitive hematopoietic stem cells
IL-4	Interleukin-4	Proliferation of B cells, differentiation of basophils and eosinophils
IL-5	Interleukin-5	Proliferation of T cells, B cells; proliferation and differentiation of eosinophils, differentiation of basophils and eosinophils
IL-11	Interleukin-11	Proliferation of megakaryocytes; undergoing clinical testing
LIF	Leukemia inhibitory factor	Proliferation of stem cells and megakaryocytes
SCF	Stem cell factor (kit ligand)	Proliferation of progenitor cells; broad-based effects on multiple lineages

division but continue with nuclear replication. Eventually, these cells are released from the marrow as fully functional erythrocytes, mast cells, granulocytes, monocytes, eosinophils, macrophages, and platelets.

Pluripotent Stem Cells

The pluripotent HSC is morphologically indistinguishable and is best identified by its expression of the cell differentiation antigen, CD34, and by its ability to form pluripotent colonies in vitro. Under the influence of interleukin-1 (IL-1), IL-3, IL-6, FMS-like tyrosine kinase 3 (FLT3), and a specific stem cell factor (KIT ligand [KITLG], or steel factor), this cell matures into a myeloid-lineage stem cell (i.e., granulocyte-erythrocyte-macrophage-megakaryocyte colony-forming unit [CFU-GEMM] cell) or a lymphoid-lineage stem cell. In the presence of granulocyte-macrophage colony-stimulating factor (GM-CSF) and

表 1.1　外周血细胞的相关正常值

项目	平均值	范围
血红蛋白	女性：14 g/dl 男性：15.5 g/dl	女性：12～16 g/dl 男性：13.5～17.5 g/dl
血细胞比容	女性：41% 男性：47%	女性：36%～46% 男性：41%～53%
网织红细胞	60 000/μl（1%）	35 000～85 000/μl（0.5%～1.5%）
平均红细胞体积		80～100 fl
血小板	250 000/μl	150 000～400 000/μl
白细胞	7400/μl	4500～11 000/μl
中性粒细胞	4400/μl（40%～60%）	1800～7700/μl
淋巴细胞	2500/μl（20%～40%）	1000～4800/μl
单核细胞	300/μl（<5%）	200～950（4%～11%）

表 1.2　细胞因子及其活性

缩写	全称	对造血的作用（和可能的临床应用）
EPO	红细胞生成素	刺激红系祖细胞增殖和成熟；出现贫血和缺氧时由肾生成；临床上用于治疗低 EPO 水平相关贫血（如肾衰竭、慢性病导致的贫血）
G-CSF	粒细胞集落刺激因子	刺激粒细胞增殖和成熟；还可以增加外周血中干细胞的释放，故作用更广泛；临床上用于治疗中性粒细胞减少症和移植前的干细胞动员
GM-CSF	粒细胞-单核细胞集落刺激因子	促进粒细胞和单核细胞前体细胞增殖；稳态造血时 GM-CSF 的功能尚不明确（GM-CSF 基因缺陷小鼠在 12 周龄之前仍正常发育，且未对造血产生重大干扰）
TPO	血小板生成素	促进巨核细胞增殖；临床研究中由于患者体内产生自身抗体，因此停用重组 TPO
M-CSF	单核细胞集落刺激因子	促进单核细胞增殖
IL-2	白介素-2	促进 T 细胞增殖
IL-3	白介素-3（多集落刺激因子）	促进粒细胞、单核细胞增殖；作用广泛，似乎可促进干细胞增殖；未应用于临床，促进造血干细胞分化为嗜碱性粒细胞和嗜酸性粒细胞
IL-4	白介素-4	促进 B 细胞增殖，促进嗜碱性粒细胞和嗜酸性粒细胞的分化
IL-5	白介素-5	促进 T 细胞和 B 细胞增殖；促进嗜酸性粒细胞的增殖和分化；促进嗜碱性粒细胞和嗜酸性粒细胞的分化
IL-11	白介素-11	促进巨核细胞增殖；正在开展临床试验
LIF	白血病抑制因子	促进干细胞和巨核细胞增殖
SCF	干细胞因子（KIT 配体）	促进祖细胞增殖；对多系具有广泛的作用

复制。最终，这些功能正常的红细胞、肥大细胞、粒细胞、单核细胞、嗜酸性粒细胞、巨噬细胞和血小板从骨髓释放至外周血中。

多能干细胞

多能造血干细胞在形态学上是无法区分的，只能通过表达的细胞分化抗原 CD34 及其在体外形成多能克隆的能力来识别。在白介素-1（IL-1）、IL-3、IL-6、FMS 样酪氨酸激酶（FLT3）和特异性干细胞因子［KIT 配体（KITL），又称 steel 因子］的作用下，多能干细胞分化为髓系干细胞［即粒细胞-红细胞-巨噬细胞-巨核细胞集落形成单位（CFU-GEMM）细胞］或淋巴系干细胞。在粒细胞-巨噬细胞集落刺激因子（GM-CSF）和 IL-3 的作用下，髓系干细胞可进一步分化为不同种系的子细胞

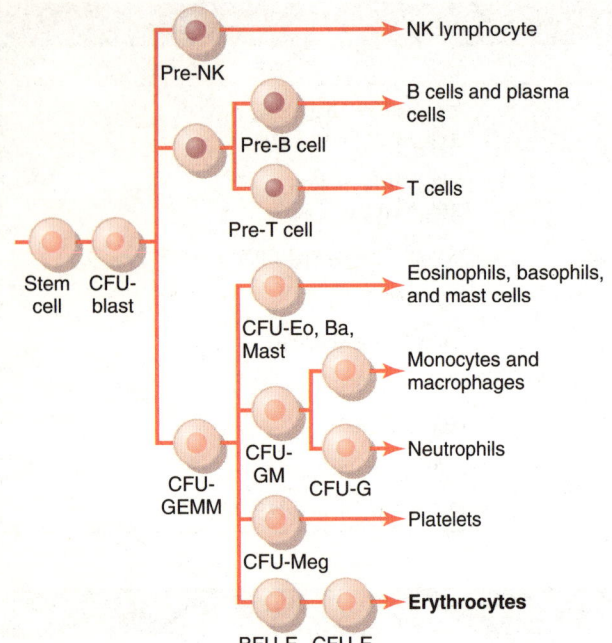

Fig. 1.1 Development of bone marrow cells. *Ba,* Basophil; *BFU,* blast-forming unit; *CFU,* colony-forming unit; *E,* erythroid; *Eo,* eosinophil; *G,* granulocyte; *GEMM,* granulocyte-erythrocyte-macrophage-megakaryocyte; *GM,* granulocyte-macrophage; *Meg,* megakaryocyte; *NK,* natural killer.

TABLE 1.3	Differential Diagnosis Of Pancytopenia

Primary bone marrow disorders
- Aplastic anemia
- Congenital aplastic anemia syndromes
- Fanconi anemia
- Shwachman-Diamond syndrome
- Congenital dyskeratosis
- Acquired aplastic anemia
- Hypocellular myelodysplastic syndrome
- Myelofibrosis
- Paroxysmal nocturnal hemoglobinuria
- Acute leukemias: acute lymphocytic leukemia, acute myeloid leukemia
- Hairy cell leukemia

Systemic diseases with secondary bone marrow effects
- Metastatic solid tumor to marrow
- Autoimmune disorders: systemic lupus erythematosus, Sjögren's syndrome
- Nutritional deficiencies: vitamin B_{12}, folate, alcoholism
- Infections: overwhelming sepsis from any cause, viruses, brucellosis, ehrlichiosis (mycobacteria)
- Storage diseases: Gaucher's disease, Niemann-Pick disease
- Anatomic defects: hypersplenism

IL-3, the myeloid stem cell further differentiates into daughter cells of its named lineages (see Fig. 1.1). The lymphopoietic stem cell becomes a pre-B cell or a prothymocyte (pre-T cell) and leaves the marrow for further maturation.

Erythroid Lineage

Primitive erythroid precursors arising from the myeloid stem cell are called burst-forming unit–erythroid cells. These cells then differentiate into erythroid colony-forming unit (CFU-E) cells, which are the committed progenitor cells of erythrocytes. CFU-E cells express receptors for erythropoietin (EPO), an 18-kD molecule produced by renal interstitial cells in response to low oxygenation states or anemia. EPO upregulates proliferation of CFU-E cells and promotes their maturation into proerythroblasts and reticulocytes, which begin to synthesize hemoglobin (see Table 1.2).

Granulocyte and Monocyte Lineages

Human GM-CSF acts early in the hematopoietic pathway to regulate maturation of the CFU-GEMM stem cell. Differentiation of this myeloid precursor into specific committed progenitors occurs under the direction of granulocyte CSF (G-CSF) and monocyte CSF (see Table 1.2). Granulocyte CFU cells undergo sequential transformation into easily recognizable myeloblasts, myelocytes, and eventually early polymorphonuclear neutrophils with their characteristic polysegmented nuclei. Monocyte CFU cells, in contrast, retain a single nucleus as they mature from monoblasts to promonocytes to monocytes and sometimes to macrophages.

Other Lineages

Eosinophils and basophils develop from CFU-GEMM cells under the influence of IL-5 and IL-3 plus IL-4, respectively. The acquisition of their specific granular contents helps in distinguishing their precursors from those of early monocytes.

The development of platelets is morphologically distinct from the other lineages. CFU-GEMM cells differentiate into megakaryocyte CFU cells, so named because the cells cease cell division early but not nuclear replication. Megakaryocytes are the only cells in the body with the capacity to double their DNA content (i.e., endomitosis). Over the course of several cell cycles, the maturing megakaryocyte eventually acquires several times the nuclear content of other cells in preparation for its eventual dissolution into platelets with a fraction of the cytoplasm of other hematopoietic cells. Two growth factors, thrombopoietin (TPO) and IL-11, increase platelet counts by promoting megakaryocyte development (see Table 1.2).

Stem Cell Plasticity

Provocative data have challenged the conventional paradigm of hierarchical HSC differentiation. Laboratory evidence has demonstrated that HSCs can be induced to dedifferentiate into more immature progenitors that have the ability to cross lineages and transdifferentiate into myriad non-lymphohematopoietic cells such as vascular endothelial precursors, myocytes, hepatocytes, gastrointestinal epithelial cells, and neurons. This plasticity of HSCs constitutes an intrinsic property of adult stem cells and/or fusion of hematopoietic cells with other tissue cells and supports further investigation of adult HSCs as a dynamic, renewable resource for tissue repair and regeneration.

PRIMARY HEMATOPOIETIC FAILURE SYNDROMES

Diseases of the HSC that disrupt the normal regulated pattern of stem cell development can result in underproduction of mature progeny (i.e., aplastic anemia), overproduction of mature progeny (i.e., chronic myeloproliferative disease), or failed differentiation with the production of excess immature forms (i.e., myelodysplasia and acute leukemia). *Hematopoietic failure,* defined as the inability of HSCs to produce normal numbers of mature blood cells, manifests clinically as peripheral pancytopenia (i.e., decreased production of all blood cell lineages).

Although marrow dysfunction producing pancytopenia can result from several hematologic and nonhematologic causes (Table 1.3), primary bone marrow failure disorders are characterized by a profound

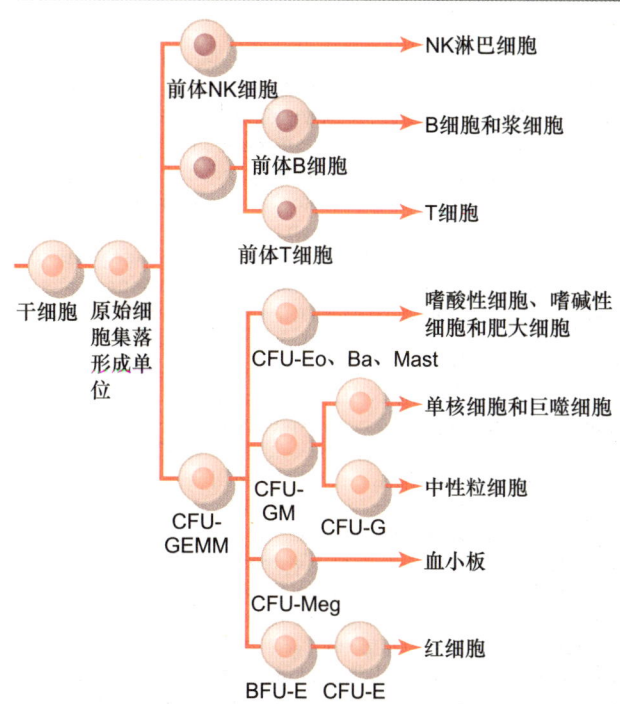

图1.1 骨髓细胞的发育。Ba,嗜碱性粒细胞;BFU,爆式集落形成单位;CFU,集落形成单位;E,红细胞;Eo,嗜酸性粒细胞;G,粒细胞;GEMM,粒细胞-红细胞-巨噬细胞-巨核细胞;GM,粒细胞-巨噬细胞;Mast,肥大细胞;Meg,巨核细胞;NK,自然杀伤

表1.3 全血细胞减少的鉴别诊断
原发性骨髓疾病
• 再生障碍性贫血
• 先天性再生障碍性贫血综合征
• 范科尼贫血
• Shwachman-Diamond 综合征
• 先天性角化不良
• 获得性再生障碍性贫血
• 低增生性骨髓增生异常综合征
• 骨髓纤维化
• 阵发性睡眠性血红蛋白尿症
• 急性白血病:急性淋巴细胞白血病、急性髓系白血病
• 毛细胞白血病
系统性疾病继发的骨髓疾病
• 恶性实体瘤转移至骨髓
• 自身免疫性疾病:系统性红斑狼疮、干燥综合征
• 营养缺乏:维生素 B_{12}、叶酸缺乏、酗酒
• 感染:任何原因引起的严重感染中毒症、病毒感染、布鲁菌病、埃立克体病(分枝杆菌)感染
• 贮积病:戈谢病、尼曼-皮克病
• 解剖异常:脾功能亢进

(图1.1)。淋巴生成干细胞分化为前体 B 细胞或前胸腺细胞(前体 T 细胞),离开骨髓并进一步发育成熟。

红系

源自髓系干细胞的原始红系前体细胞称为红系爆式集落形成单位(BFU-E)细胞。这些细胞进一步分化为红系集落形成单位(CFU-E)细胞,后者为红细胞定向前体细胞。CFU-E 细胞表达红细胞生成素(EPO)受体,EPO 的分子量为 18 kDa,由肾间质细胞在低氧状态或贫血时产生。EPO 可上调 CFU-E 细胞的增殖能力,并促进其成熟为原始红细胞和网织红细胞,后者开始合成血红蛋白(表1.2)。

粒细胞和单核细胞系

人体 GM-CSF 在造血通路早期可调控 CFU-GEMM 干细胞的发育成熟。髓系前体细胞在粒细胞集落刺激因子(G-CSF)和单核细胞集落刺激因子的作用下,可分化为特定的定向前体细胞(表1.2)。G-CFU 细胞经过一系列转化成为易于辨识的原始粒细胞、中幼粒细胞,并最终成为多核中性粒细胞,其具有特征性的多叶核。相比之下,单核 CFU 细胞在由原始单核细胞到幼单核细胞再到单核细胞或巨噬细胞的成熟过程中,始终保持着单个细胞核。

其他细胞系

嗜酸性粒细胞和嗜碱性粒细胞分别在 IL-5 和 IL-3 + IL-4 的作用下由 CFU-GEMM 细胞发育而来。成熟过程中所获得的特异性颗粒内容物可用于区分它们的前体细胞与早期单核细胞。

血小板形态的发育与其他细胞系迥然不同。CFU-GEMM 细胞分化为巨核细胞 CFU 细胞,之所以命名为巨核细胞,是因为这些细胞在早期停止分裂,但核复制仍继续。巨核细胞是机体内唯一具有倍增 DNA 能力的细胞(即核内有丝分裂)。在数个细胞周期中,成熟巨核细胞最终的核内容物是其他细胞的数倍,为其最终分解为血小板做好准备,血小板包含了其他造血细胞的一部分胞质。血小板生成素(TPO)和 IL-11 可通过促进巨核细胞发育来增加血小板数目(表1.2)。

干细胞的可塑性

目前一些研究对传统的 HSC 等级分化模式提出了挑战。HSC 可被诱导去分化为更不成熟的前体细胞,并且可以跨系转变分化为非淋巴造血细胞,如血管内皮前体细胞、肌细胞、肝细胞、胃肠道上皮细胞和神经元。HSC 的这种可塑性是成人干细胞和(或)造血细胞与其他组织细胞融合的内在特性,并支持进一步研究成人 HSC 作为组织修复和再生的动态可再生资源。

原发性造血衰竭综合征

HSC 疾病干扰了干细胞发育的正常模式,导致成熟细胞生成不足(如再生障碍性贫血)、成熟细胞生成过度(如慢性骨髓增殖性疾病)或分化障碍生成过多的幼稚细胞(如骨髓增生异常综合征和急性白血病)。造血衰竭是指 HSC 无法产生正常数量的成熟血细胞,临床表现为外周全血细胞减少(三系生成减低)。

虽然多种血液系统疾病和非血液系统疾病均可引起骨髓功能异常,从而造成全血细胞减少(表1.3),但原发性骨髓衰竭性疾病的主要特点是 HSC 补充干

impairment of the ability of the HSC to replenish the stem cell pool. Marrow failure syndromes can arise from intrinsic HSC defects including germline inherited disposition and age-related clonal hematopoietic mutational events. In other cases, marrow failure disorders are the result of extrinsic damage to normal HSCs. The treatment modalities for primary hematopoietic failure disorders include exogenous growth factor administration, immunosuppressive therapy, and allogeneic stem cell transplantation.

Growth Factors in Clinical Use

Discovery of the factors that influence normal hematopoiesis led to important therapeutic applications for patients with defects in hematopoietic cell production. The finding that committed hematopoietic cells of each lineage can be stimulated to proliferate and differentiate by specific cytokines (see Table 1.2) has been therapeutically useful. Advances in DNA technology led to the synthesis and purification of recombinant human (rh) proteins with similar biologic activity in vivo. Administration of these products to patients enabled successful manipulation of mature cells in the peripheral blood. For example, exogenous EPO has become a mainstay in the management of anemia caused by renal failure, chemotherapy, and marrow failure syndromes. The use of G-CSF or GM-CSF in patients with febrile neutropenia and documented infection or sepsis after chemotherapy or radiation therapy has reduced hospital stays and shortened the period of high infection risk. Administration of GM-CSF is thought to improve host immune responses to fungal infections. High-dose G-CSF also is routinely used to mobilize $CD34^+$ marrow stem cells into the peripheral blood for collection before and after stem cell transplantation in patients with delayed stem cell engraftment (discussed later).

Early trials of TPO growth factors to stimulate platelet production were halted because of development of antihuman TPO antibodies in some patients, leading to severe thrombocytopenia. Second-generation thrombopoietic agents bearing no structural resemblance to TPO but designed to bind and activate the TPO receptor are in clinical use. Romiplostim is a recombinant Fc-peptide fusion protein termed a peptibody that when given as a weekly subcutaneous injection can increase platelet counts, decrease platelet transfusion requirements, and improve quality of life for patients with refractory chronic immune-mediated thrombocytopenia. Eltrombopag is an orally available, small, organic TPO agonist that increases platelet counts and decreases bleeding in similar patients. The clinical utility of eltrombopag when added to immunosuppressive regimens for treatment of aplastic anemia supports its role as an activator of HSC production.

Hematopoietic Stem Cell Transplantation
Types of Transplantations

Improved understanding of HSC biology has fostered the development of techniques to manipulate these cells for therapeutic purposes. The antitumor effects of most chemotherapeutic drugs and radiation therapy are dose dependent, and both cause the major dose-limiting toxicity of myelosuppression. Several modes of stem cell transplantation have been developed.

In *autologous transplantation*, the patient's bone marrow or peripheral blood stem cells (PBSCs) are collected during remission after high-dose chemotherapy or G-CSF administration. These cells are cryopreserved, thawed, and reinfused. This approach incurs a higher risk of relapse as a result of reinfusion of a stem cell product that may remain contaminated with tumor cells and is generally considered therapeutically equivalent to administration of multiple cycles of high-dose chemotherapy with noncurative intent.

In *allogeneic stem cell transplantation (alloSCT)*, abnormally functioning hematopoietic bone marrow is eradicated and replaced with normal bone marrow or stem cells from a compatible source either from a related or unrelated donor. High-dose chemotherapy with or without total body irradiation is used to destroy the patient's marrow, followed by infusion of new stem cells that engraft and restore normal hematopoiesis. Treatment-related mortality and morbidity occurs due to infectious complications during cytopenic periods and development of *graft-versus-host disease (GVHD)*, an autoimmune phenomenon in which intact lymphocytes in the transplanted marrow attack the host tissues. Despite improvements in supportive care and immunomodulatory therapy, mortality rates associated with transplant remain in the range of 10% to 30% even in younger patients. To mitigate the risk of GVHD, all potential donors and patients are tested for compatibility of human leukocyte antigen (HLA) and major and minor histocompatibility complex (MHC) proteins expressed on all cells. Three major HLA class I antigens (i.e., A, B, and C) and three MHC class II antigens (i.e., DP, DQ, and DR) have been identified. The HLA gene loci are tightly linked on chromosome 6 and are almost always inherited on a single cluster of genes, or *haplotype*. All children are a half-match (i.e., haploidentical) to each of their parents, and full siblings have a 25% probability of being HLA identical to one another. HLA-matched, nonrelated transplants have higher rates of GVHD than transplants from HLA-matched, related donors as a result of other minor HLA incompatibilities. Patients who receive an HLA-mismatched stem cell transplantation risk acute GVHD, marrow rejection, and fatal marrow aplasia. Morbidity and mortality rates associated with non–HLA-compatible transplants can be prohibitive. Patients younger than 50 years are considered the best candidates for this intensive therapy, although this is changing in the setting of newer supportive modalities.

It is now believed that the immunologic effects of transplanted allogeneic cells are as important as or more important than cytoreduction in effecting cure of hematologic malignancies. Evidence indicates that the excellent response of patients to alloSCT may largely be related to the active suppression of the patient's original (residual) or relapsing disease by donor immune cells from the newly transplanted donor graft, referred to as the *graft-versus-leukemia (GVL) effect*. Studies have documented that donor lymphocyte infusions (DLI) can restore remission in patients with early evidence of relapse after alloSCT for chronic myelogenous leukemia. Conversely, procedures that minimize the reactivity between donor and host increase disease relapse. For example, there is an increased rate of relapse among patients who undergo syngeneic (identical twin) stem cell transplantation and patients who receive T-cell–depleted marrow in an attempt to reduce GVHD.

Recognition of the immunologic benefits of alloSCT has led to the development of *reduced intensity* (also known as *non-myeloablative*) allogeneic stem cell transplants. These transplants are now standard of care in adult patients otherwise ineligible for traditional myeloablative transplantation regimens due to age (>55 years old) other comorbidities, or without fully HLA-matched donors available. Conditioning and immunosuppressive regimens are administered in doses sufficient to permit donor stem cell engraftment without aggressive cytoreduction. These so-called "mini" transplants result in chimeric marrows (i.e., part patient and part donor) and are not characterized by significant periods of cytopenias or hematopoietic compromise. Most responding patients convert to a fully donor-derived marrow over time. The use of newer immunosuppressive regimens has also allowed patients to receive transplants from related family members who are only 50% HLA matched (so called *haplotype identical* or *haploidentical* transplants). Almost all patients have compatible half-matched parents, siblings, children, or even grandchildren, thereby allowing for multiple family members to serve as donors. Although feasible and well tolerated in many patients, haploidentical transplants are associated with an enhanced risk of relapsed disease due to reduced GVL effects

细胞池的能力严重受损。骨髓衰竭综合征可由内源性 HSC 缺陷引起，包括种系遗传倾向和与年龄相关的克隆性造血突变事件。在其他情况下，骨髓衰竭性疾病可由正常 HSC 遭到外源性破坏导致。原发性造血衰竭疾病的治疗手段包括使用外源性生长因子、免疫抑制治疗和异基因造血干细胞移植。

生长因子的临床应用

对影响正常造血的因素的发现为造血细胞生成减少的患者提供了重要的治疗手段。研究发现不同类型的定向造血细胞可在特定细胞因子的刺激下增殖和分化（表 1.2），这具有重要的临床意义。DNA 技术的进步使人们得以合成和纯化重组人（rh）蛋白，后者与体内蛋白的生物活性相似。在患者中使用这些合成物可以成功调控外周血中的成熟细胞。例如，外源性 EPO 已经成为治疗由肾衰竭、化疗和骨髓衰竭综合征所致的贫血的主要药物。在中性粒细胞减少期发热和放化疗后出现感染中毒症的患者中，使用 G-CSF 或 GM-CSF 可以缩短住院时间和高感染风险的持续时间。使用 GM-CSF 可以改善宿主对真菌感染的免疫应答。大剂量 G-CSF（动员 CD34$^+$ 骨髓干细胞进入外周血）被常规用于延迟移植的患者，以便在干细胞移植前后采集干细胞（见下文）。

在有关 TPO 生长因子刺激血小板生成的早期研究中，由于部分患者产生了抗人 TPO 抗体，引起严重的血小板减少症，因此试验被提前终止。临床正在使用的第二代促血小板生成药物与 TPO 结构不同，但可以结合并激活 TPO 受体。罗米司亭是一种重组 Fc-肽段融合蛋白（即肽体），每周皮下注射 1 次可增加血小板数目、减少血小板输注需求并提高慢性难治性免疫介导的血小板减少症患者的生活质量。艾曲泊帕是一种口服小分子 TPO 激动剂，可在类似患者中增加血小板数目，减少出血事件。作为 HSC 生成的激活剂，艾曲泊帕已被纳入治疗再生障碍性贫血的免疫抑制方案中。

造血干细胞移植

移植类型

对 HSC 生物学的进一步了解促进了通过调控 HSC 用于治疗目的技术的发展。大多数化疗药物和放疗的抗肿瘤效应呈剂量依赖性，两者均会引起骨髓抑制这一主要的剂量限制性毒性。目前已有多种干细胞移植的模式。

自体移植是指在患者接受大剂量化疗后的缓解期或给予 G-CSF 动员后，采集患者的骨髓或外周血造血干细胞（PBSC）。将细胞冷冻保存，后解冻并回输至患者体内。由于这种干细胞采集物中可能混入肿瘤细胞，因此自体移植的复发率高，目前普遍认为自体移植的疗效等同于以非治愈为目标的多疗程大剂量化疗。

异基因干细胞移植（alloSCT）是指根除功能异常的骨髓造血细胞，并予以亲属或非亲缘相合供者来源的正常骨髓或干细胞进行替代。使用大剂量化疗联合或不联合全身放射治疗，以破坏患者的骨髓，然后回输新鲜干细胞，使其植入体内并重建正常造血。治疗相关并发症的死亡率和发病率常由骨髓抑制期合并感染和移植物抗宿主病（GVHD）所致，GVHD 是一种自身免疫现象，指移植物骨髓中的淋巴细胞攻击宿主组织。尽管支持治疗和免疫调节治疗在不断改善 alloSCT 的结局，但即便在年轻患者中，移植相关死亡率仍高达 10%～30%。为了降低 GVHD 的风险，所有可能的供者和患者均应检测人类白细胞抗原（HLA）及所有细胞表面的主要和次要组织相容性复合体（MHC）的相容性。目前已发现 3 种主要的 HLA Ⅰ型抗原（即 A、B、C）和 3 种 MHC Ⅱ型抗原（即 DP、DQ 和 DR）。这些 HLA 基因位点在 6 号染色体上紧密连接，且几乎总是以单组基因遗传，即单倍体基因型。所有的子代和其父母都是半相合的（即单倍体相同），亲兄弟姐妹 HLA 完全相同的概率是 25%。同样是 HLA 相合，非亲缘的移植物较亲缘供者的 GVHD 发生率更高，这是由于前者的其他次要 HLA 不相合。接受 HLA 不相合干细胞移植的患者存在急性 GVHD、移植排斥和致死性造血衰竭的风险。HLA 不相合移植相关的并发症发生率和死亡率非常高。虽然 50 岁以下的患者被认为是这种强化治疗的最佳候选人，但在不断涌现的新支持治疗的模式下这种情况正在发生改变。

目前认为，在治愈血液系统恶性肿瘤方面，同种异体细胞移植的免疫效应与减瘤作用同样重要，甚至更重要。研究发现，患者对 alloSCT 的反应良好，这可能主要是由于移植物中的供者免疫细胞对患者的白血病细胞具有杀伤作用，这种现象被称为移植物抗白血病（GVL）效应。研究发现，alloSCT 后有早期复发迹象的慢性髓系白血病患者进行供者淋巴细胞输注（DLI）后可以再次获得缓解。然而，HLA 差异太小也会使复发率升高。例如，接受同基因（同卵双胞胎）干细胞移植的患者和接受去 T 细胞移植以减少 GVHD 风险的患者，疾病复发率升高。

由于认识到 alloSCT 对免疫方面的益处，减低剂量预处理（即非清髓性）方案的 alloSCT 应运而生。对于因年龄（>55 岁）、其他合并症或没有 HLA 全相合供者而不适合传统清髓性移植的成年患者，这种移植现已成为标准治疗方法。患者接受的预处理和免疫抑制方案的剂量应足以进行供者干细胞植入，同时不引起严重的细胞减灭。这种所谓的"微移植"可产生嵌合骨髓（即部分患者和部分供者），同时不引起严重的全血细胞减少或造血功能障碍。大部分有治疗反应的患者最终会转化为完全供者来源的骨髓。新免疫抑制方案的应用使患者能够接受只有 50% 的 HLA 相合的家庭成员供者的移植（所谓的单倍型相同或单倍体移植）。几乎所有患者都有半相合的父母、兄弟姐妹、子女，甚至孙辈，因此多个亲属均可作为供者。虽然这种方法在多数患者中可

and therefore are best utilized for those with optimal disease control at time of the procedure. Although historically used in the treatment of primary malignant stem cell disorders such as leukemia, the therapeutic potential of alloSCT is now increasingly being employed for patients with nonmalignant hematologic conditions (e.g., aplastic anemia, sickle cell anemia, congenital immunodeficiencies), solid tumors (e.g., renal cell carcinoma, melanoma), and particularly autoimmune diseases (e.g., amyloidosis, systemic lupus, multiple sclerosis).

Hematopoietic Stem Cell Sources

Historically, alloSCT has employed donor bone marrow stem cells aspirated from the posterior iliac crest and intravenously infused after myeloablation and immunosuppressive therapy. The process of engraftment or reconstitution of normal hematopoietic function takes several weeks. Patients often require almost daily platelet and red blood cell transfusions, and they are hospitalized during this period of prolonged neutropenia to minimize life-threatening bacterial, viral, and fungal infections. Other complications include severe mucositis, hemorrhagic cystitis, GVHD, relapsed disease, and graft failure.

The discovery that high-dose G-CSF treatment mobilizes large numbers of $CD34^+$ hematopoietic progenitor and stem cells from bone marrow sites into circulating blood (i.e., 10-fold to 15-fold increase over baseline levels) has led to the routine use of PBSCs collected by apheresis procedures in place of bone marrow stem cells for allogeneic transplantation. Compared with marrow-derived stem cells, PBSCs engraft more rapidly after myeloablation. Patients receiving allogeneic PBSC transplants have decreased neutrophil recovery time, lower transfusion requirements, fewer inpatient hospital days, and similar rates of acute GVHD and long-term survival outcomes as traditional marrow-transplanted patients. Because PBSC collections often contain 3-fold to 4-fold more $CD34^+$ stem cells and 10-fold more lymphoid cells than harvested marrow grafts, higher rates of chronic GVHD may occur.

Umbilical cord blood (UCB) stem cells constitute a rich source of immature $CD34^+$ HSCs. In the past, the less stringent HLA-compatibility requirements for UCB HSC matches has allowed the use of these transplants as a therapy for patients lacking fully compatible HLA-matched donors. Although still considered experimental, some transplantation centers have reported long-term outcomes after UCB HSC transplants similar to those for conventional marrow or peripheral PBSC transplants for primary hematologic diseases. However, the relatively limited numbers of $CD34^+$ stem cells found in harvested UCB units accounts for a much slower hematopoietic recovery after the procedure and a statistically higher risk for nonengraftment compared with other stem cell sources. For this reason, UCB transplantation procedures have been limited to pediatric patients and smaller adults or to adult patients for whom there is more than one HLA-compatible UCB unit.

Aplastic Anemia
Definition and Epidemiology

Aplastic anemia (AA) is a rare disorder characterized by pancytopenia with a markedly hypocellular bone marrow. This disease was first described in 1888 by Paul Ehrlich, who observed that autopsy bone marrow specimens from a young woman who died of severe anemia and neutropenia were extremely hypoplastic. Later studies demonstrated that patients with severe AA possessed only a fraction of normal pluripotent stem cell numbers despite normal functional marrow stromal cells and normal or even elevated levels of stimulatory cytokines. The incidence of AA ranges from 1 to 5 cases per million people in the general population. It occurs predominantly in young adults (20 to 25 years old) and older adults (60 to 65 years old). The incidence is 3-fold higher in developing countries (e.g., Thailand and China) compared with industrialized Western nations (e.g., Europe and Israel), a fact that is not explained by differences in drug or radiation exposure.

Etiology

AA arises as either an inherited disorder or an acquired syndrome or as an idiopathic phenomenon. A small number of cases occur in the context of a congenital bone marrow failure disorder, including Fanconi anemia, Schwachman-Diamond syndrome, and dyskeratosis congenita. The most common of these, Fanconi anemia, is an autosomal recessive disorder arising from mutations in genes encoding DNA repair proteins. The known causes of acquired AA are numerous (Table 1.4) and range from myeloablative radiation exposure to common viruses and medications. Prior bone marrow toxicity from drugs, chemicals (e.g., benzene, cyclic hydrocarbons found in petroleum products, rubber, glue, insecticides, chemical dyes), or radiation predisposes to AA because these agents directly injure proliferating and differentiating HSCs by inducing DNA damage. In contrast, cytotoxic chemotherapy, especially with alkylating agents, and radiation therapy target all rapidly cycling cells and often induce reversible bone marrow aplasia. Despite these many causes, most cases of AA are idiopathic.

The etiology of both acquired and congenital AAs appear to be mechanistically linked through abnormal telomere maintenance. Telomeres are repeated nucleotide sequences that cap and protect chromosome ends from degradation. Cell division leads to normal telomere erosion; when telomeres reach a critically short length, cells cease to proliferate, senesce, and undergo apoptosis, often with accompanying DNA damage and genomic instability. Telomerase enzyme in normal HSCs preserves long telomeres and promotes quiescence and a prolonged cellular lifespan. Patients with autosomal dominant dyskeratosis congenita have mutations in the genes for telomerase complexes, predisposing to premature aging and enhanced marrow failure in the setting of accelerated telomere shortening. One third of patients with acquired AA also have short telomeres, likely due to a combination of genetic, environmental, and epigenetic factors.

Autoreactive host lymphocytes can destroy normal hematopoiesis in AA. Bone marrow stromal cells and cytokine levels in patients with AA are normal. The fact that AA also occurs in diseases of immune dysregulation and after viral infections further suggests an immune-mediated mechanism for the disease. One hypothesis is that drug or viral antigens presented to the immune system trigger cytotoxic T-cell responses that persist and destroy normal stem cells. Only 1 in 100,000 patients develops severe AA as an idiosyncratic drug reaction. Whether these individuals have a genetically predisposed sensitivity to common exposures (e.g., nonsteroidal anti-inflammatory drugs, sulfonamides, Epstein-Barr virus) is unknown.

TABLE 1.4 Causes of Acquired Aplastic Anemia

Drugs (dose related): chemotherapeutic agents, antibiotics (chloramphenicol, trimethoprim-sulfamethoxazole)
Idiosyncratic causes (many unproved): chloramphenicol, quinacrine, nonsteroidal anti-inflammatory drugs, anticonvulsants, gold, sulfonamides, cimetidine, penicillamine
Toxins: benzene and other hydrocarbons, insecticides
Viral infection: hepatitis, Epstein-Barr virus, human immunodeficiency virus (HIV)
Immune disease: graft-versus-host disease in immunodeficiency, hypogammaglobulinemia
Paroxysmal nocturnal hemoglobinuria (PNH)
Radiation exposure
Pregnancy

行且耐受良好，但由于 GVL 效应降低，单倍体移植患者的复发风险增加，因此最适用于手术时疾病得到最佳控制的患者。尽管一直被用于治疗原发性恶性干细胞疾病（如白血病），但 alloSCT 的治疗潜能使其现在越来越多地被用于治疗非恶性血液系统疾病（如再生障碍性贫血、镰状细胞贫血、先天性免疫缺陷），实体瘤（如肾细胞癌、黑色素瘤），尤其是自身免疫性疾病（如淀粉样变性、系统性红斑狼疮、多发性硬化）患者。

造血干细胞的来源

过去，alloSCT 所需的供者骨髓干细胞来源于髂后上棘穿刺，在患者接受清髓性预处理和免疫抑制后输给患者。移植物植入或正常造血功能恢复需要数周。在此期间，患者几乎每天需要输注血小板和红细胞，且在中性粒细胞减少期必须住院以尽量减少危及生命的细菌、病毒和真菌感染。其他并发症包括严重黏膜炎、出血性膀胱炎、GVHD、疾病复发和移植失败。

研究发现，大剂量 G-CSF 治疗可以将骨髓中大量 $CD34^+$ 造血干祖细胞动员释放至外周血中（即较基线水平提高 10～15 倍），这促使人们在异基因移植中常规使用 PBSC（通过白细胞分离术采集）替代骨髓造血干细胞。与骨髓来源的干细胞相比，PBSC 在清髓后植入更快。接受异基因 PBSC 移植的患者中性粒细胞恢复时间缩短、输血需求减小、住院时间缩短，而急性 GVHD 和长期生存预后与传统骨髓来源的移植患者相似。由于 PBSC 采集物中 $CD34^+$ 细胞和淋巴细胞分别比骨髓采集物多 3～4 倍和 10 倍，故慢性 GVHD 发生率可能更高。

脐带血（UCB）干细胞中含有丰富的未成熟 $CD34^+$ HSC。过去，UCB HSC 对 HLA-相容性的要求更为宽松，因此缺乏 HLA 全相合供者的患者可选择采用 UCB HSC。虽然 UCB HSC 移植仍处在试验阶段，一些移植中心已经报道在原发性血液系统疾病患者中 UCB HSC 移植的远期疗效与传统的 PBSC 相似。然而，由于在采集的 UCB 单位中 $CD34^+$ 干细胞数量相对较少，故移植后的造血恢复更慢，且与其他干细胞来源的移植物相比，植入失败率显著升高。因此，UCB 移植仅限于儿童和年轻成人，或有多于 1 个单位 HLA 相合 UCB 的成人。

再生障碍性贫血

定义和流行病学

再生障碍性贫血（AA）是一种以全血细胞减少伴骨髓增生显著降低的少见疾病。该病于 1888 年由 Paul Ehrlich 首次描述，他在一名死于严重贫血和中性粒细胞减少症的年轻女性尸检标本中观察到骨髓显著低增生。后续研究发现，重型 AA 患者尽管骨髓基质细胞功能正常且刺激性细胞因子水平正常甚至升高，但正常多能干细胞数量减少。AA 的发病率为（1～5）/100 万，主要见于年轻人（20～25 岁）和老年人（60～65 岁）。发展中国家（如泰国和中国）的发病率是西方工业国家（如欧洲国家和以色列）的 3 倍以上，这并不能用药物或放射暴露来解释。

病因

AA 可源于遗传性疾病或获得性综合征，或作为特发性现象出现。一小部分 AA 病例发生于先天性骨髓衰竭性疾病，如范科尼贫血、Shwachman-Diamond 综合征和先天性角化不良。其中最常见的范科尼贫血是由编码 DNA 修复蛋白的基因突变导致的常染色体隐性遗传病。获得性 AA 的病因很多（表 1.4），包括放射暴露、常见病毒感染和药物因素等。既往用药、化学物质（如苯、石油中的环烃、橡胶、胶水、杀虫剂和化学染料）或放疗引起的骨髓毒性可增加 AA 的易感性，以上物质可通过诱导 DNA 破坏而直接损伤正在增殖和分化的 HSC。相反，所有针对快速分裂细胞的细胞毒性化疗药物（尤其是烷化剂）和放疗所诱导的骨髓再生障碍通常是可逆的。虽然获得性 AA 有很多病因，但多数是特发的。

获得性和先天性 AA 的病因似乎都与端粒异常相关。端粒是重复的核苷酸序列，在染色体末端形成保护性的帽子结构，以防止其降解。细胞分裂可引起正常的端粒损耗；当端粒非常短时，会出现细胞增殖停止、衰老和细胞凋亡，这一过程通常伴随着 DNA 损伤和基因组不稳定。正常 HSC 中的端粒酶负责保护长端粒，促进休眠并延长细胞寿命。常染色体显性遗传的先天性角化不良患者由于端粒酶复合物基因突变，端粒缩短加速，导致早衰和严重的骨髓衰竭。1/3 的获得性 AA 患者出现端粒缩短，可能由遗传、环境和表观遗传因素的共同作用所致。

AA 患者体内的自身反应性淋巴细胞可破坏正常造血。AA 患者的骨髓基质细胞和细胞因子水平正常。免疫调节异常的疾病和病毒感染后也可发生 AA，这进一步说明了该病的免疫机制。一种假说是药物或病毒抗原提呈给免疫系统后，诱导细胞毒性 T 细胞应答，其持续存在并破坏正常干细胞。只有 1/100 000 的患者由于特异质的药物反应而发生重型 AA。尚不明确这类患者是否对常见病因的暴露（如非甾体抗炎药、磺胺类药、EB 病毒）具有基因易感性。

表 1.4　获得性 AA 的病因

药物（剂量相关）：化疗药物，抗感染药物（氯霉素、甲氧苄啶-磺胺甲噁唑）
特异质原因（很多未经证实）：氯霉素、米帕林、非甾体抗炎药、抗惊厥药、金制剂、磺胺类药、西咪替丁、青霉胺
毒物：苯和其他烃类、杀虫剂
病毒感染：肝炎病毒、EB 病毒、人类免疫缺陷病毒（HIV）感染
免疫病：免疫缺陷患者中的移植物抗宿主病、低丙种球蛋白血症
阵发性睡眠性血红蛋白尿症（PNH）
放射暴露
妊娠

Clinical Presentation

The clinical onset of AA can be insidious or abrupt. Patients often complain of symptoms related to their cytopenias: weakness, fatigue, dyspnea, or palpitations resulting from anemia; gingival bleeding, epistaxis, petechiae, or purpura caused by low platelet counts; or recurrent bacterial infections caused by low or nonfunctioning neutrophils. In some cases, patients will report recent upper respiratory syndrome. Results of the physical examination may be normal or characterized by ecchymoses and bleeding complications. Patients with congenital AA may have various abnormalities.

Diagnosis and Differential Diagnosis

Diagnostic confirmation of AA requires bone marrow biopsy to confirm hypocellularity and to rule out other marrow processes. Normal bone marrow cellularity ranges from 30% to 50% up to age 70 years and is less than 20% after 70 years of age. In contrast, bone marrow cellularity in patients with AA usually ranges from 5% to 15%, with increased fat accumulation and few or no hematopoietic cells and primarily plasma cells and lymphocytes. In AA, hematopoietic progenitor and precursor cells are morphologically normal but number less than 1% of normal levels, and they are markedly dysfunctional, with a decreased ability to form differentiated progenitor cell colonies in vitro. A hypocellular marrow with evidence of increased blasts, dysplastic hematopoietic cells (e.g., pseudo-Pelger-Huët abnormalities, micromegakaryocytes), and clonal cytogenetically abnormal cells in the peripheral blood or marrow are diagnostic of acute leukemia or myelodysplasia, not AA. In young patients, a diagnosis of Fanconi anemia is made by demonstrating enhanced sensitivity of cultured cells to mitomycin or diepoxybutane-induced chromosomal damage on special testing. Although patients with AA typically have a low reticulocyte count from low red blood cell production and a paucity of blood cells and macrocytic red cells on the peripheral blood smear, these features are nondiagnostic because patients with other primary marrow disorders may exhibit similar findings.

Treatment and Prognosis

Treatment of AA is based on the severity of disease and clinical characteristics. Patients with mild cytopenias can be monitored expectantly. However, patients with severe AA based on peripheral blood cell counts (defined as a neutrophil count <500/μL, platelet count <20,000/μL, anemia with corrected reticulocyte count <1%, and marrow cellularity of 5% to 10%) have a poor median survival of 2 to 6 months without treatment. Because most of these patients die of overwhelming infections, supportive care with broad-spectrum antibiotics, antifungal agents, and antiviral agents is warranted for those with advanced neutropenia. Red blood cell and platelet transfusions can help patients who are profoundly symptomatic.

Current therapeutic approaches to AA focus on replacing the defective HSCs by stem cell transplantation and controlling an overactive immune response with HSC activation. All young patients with severe AA and an HLA-compatible bone marrow donor should be considered for alloSCT, which offers the best chance for definitive cure. Conditioning regimens for those AA patients with congenital abnormalities must be carefully considered prior to alloSCT. Although long-term survival is excellent for patients younger than 30 years transplanted from a sibling donor (75% to 90%), morbidity due to the transplant itself and the management of long-term complications are continuing problems. Outcomes for patients older than 40 years or patients without any HLA-matched related donor are poor.

The presumed immune mechanisms for drug-induced aplasia have led to immunosuppressive approaches to the treatment of AA in older patients, those without a compatible donor and/or otherwise ineligible for alloSCT. Treatment of AA with traditional chemotherapy such as high-dose cyclophosphamide usually has proved too toxic. However, immunosuppressive therapy (IST) using a combination of anti-thymocyte globulin (ATG) and cyclosporine (a specific T-cell inhibitor) restores marrow function and independence from red blood cell or platelet transfusions in up to 70% of patients with a 5-year survival of 90%. Side effects of ATG include anaphylaxis and serum sickness as a result of foreign antigens in the antisera and are usually self-limited. Eltrombopag is an oral TPO mimetic drug originally developed for its ability to stimulate platelet production by binding to MPL receptors on megakaryocytes. In vitro data suggested that administration of high doses of exogenous TPO also could stimulate proliferation and maintenance of HSCs expressing TPO receptors in spite of high levels of endogenous TPO in AA patients. Treatment of refractory severe AA patients with eltrombopag led to hematologic responses in 44% of patients. Subsequently, eltrombopag was added to frontline ATG and cyclosporine (CSA) for newly diagnosed AA and resulted in overall response rates of 80% to 94% after 6 months with excellent long-term survival. Complete hematologic responses occurred in numerous patients with markedly improved marrow cellularity and numbers of measured hematopoietic stem and progenitor cells. This three-drug combination (ATG, CSA, and eltrombopag) has now become the standard of care for up-front treatment of severe AA patients.

Because endogenous cytokine production is usually high in patients with AA, the routine use of growth factors such as G-CSF, EPO, or stem cell factor typically is ineffective. Despite high endogenous TPO levels in AA patients with refractory disease, long-term administration of eltrombopag as maintenance therapy with or without other immunosuppression (ATG, CSA) may have some effect in long-term sustained blood cell counts. Patients who survive initial treatment of AA remain at increased risk for the emergence of other primary hematologic disorders, such as myelodysplasia, leukemia, and paroxysmal nocturnal hemoglobinuria (PNH). A proportion of AA patients also may relapse with loss of hematologic responses over time. Recurrence may warrant retreatment with ATG, androgens, and newer immunosuppressive agents.

Paroxysmal Nocturnal Hemoglobinuria
Definition, Epidemiology, and Etiology

PNH is a rare disease characterized by intravascular hemolysis, venous thrombosis, and bone marrow failure. The disease arises from expansion of pluripotent HSCs containing a somatic mutation in the phosphatidylinositol glycan complementation class A *(PIGA)* gene. Loss of *PIGA*, which codes for a membrane lipid moiety (i.e., glycosyl phosphatidylinositol [GPI]), produces abnormal hematopoietic cells deficient in dozens of proteins that are normally attached to the cell surface by the GPI anchor. Disease manifestations of PNH result from lack of the GPI-linked proteins (CD55 and CD59) that usually protect red blood cells and platelets from complement-mediated attack. Loss of CD55 or CD59 leads to increased immune destruction of blood cells. The release of hemoglobin from broken red cells causes disease symptoms, specifically sudden irregular episodes of passing dark colored urine. The name "paroxysmal nocturnal hemoglobinuria" arises from the observation that dark urine occurs more frequently at night or in the early morning because the urine has been concentrated over night during sleep. In reality, hemolysis in this disorder is a continuous process and does not occur solely at night but during the day as well when it may not be as obvious to patients or clinicians.

临床表现

AA起病隐匿或急骤。患者常出现与血细胞减少相关的症状：贫血导致的无力、乏力、气短或心悸；血小板减少引起的牙龈出血、鼻出血、瘀点或紫癜；中性粒细胞过少或无功能引起的反复细菌感染。部分患者可表现为近期的上呼吸道综合征。AA患者体格检查可能无异常或表现为瘀斑和出血并发症。先天性AA患者可能出现多种异常。

诊断和鉴别诊断

确诊AA需要行骨髓活检确定骨髓低增生，并除外其他骨髓疾病。正常的骨髓造血成分为30%～50%，70岁后可能低于20%。AA患者的骨髓造血成分常占5%～15%，同时存在脂肪堆积增多和造血细胞减少或缺如，其余主要为浆细胞和淋巴细胞。在AA患者中，造血祖细胞和前体细胞形态学正常，但数量低于正常水平的1%，并伴有明显的功能异常，在体外形成分化祖细胞克隆的能力明显下降。急性白血病或骨髓增生异常综合征的诊断证据是外周血或骨髓中发现原始细胞、异常增生的造血细胞（如假性Pelger-Huët畸形、小巨核细胞）和克隆性细胞遗传学异常的细胞增多，但AA没有这些异常。年轻患者中范科尼贫血的诊断依据是培养细胞对丝裂霉素或双环氧丁烷介导的染色体损伤的敏感性增高。虽然AA患者由于红细胞生成减少常引起网织红细胞计数下降、全血细胞减少和外周血涂片示血细胞减少及可见大红细胞，但这些特征并非特异性，其他骨髓原发性疾病可能有相似的表现。

治疗和预后

AA的治疗取决于疾病的严重程度和临床特点。血细胞轻度减少的患者可以定期监测。但是，根据外周血细胞计数诊断为重型AA（中性粒细胞计数<500/μl，血小板计数<20 000/μl，校正后网织红细胞计数<1%，骨髓造血成分5%～10%）的患者预后很差，如不治疗则中位生存期为26个月。由于大多数重型AA患者死于严重感染，对于中性粒细胞严重缺乏的患者应使用广谱抗生素、抗真菌和抗病毒药物进行支持治疗。对于症状明显的患者可予红细胞和血小板输注。

目前治疗AA的方法包括通过干细胞移植替代有缺陷的HSC，或控制过度活跃的免疫应答。对于年轻重型AA且有HLA相合骨髓供者的患者，均应考虑alloSCT，这是根治的最佳机会。对于患有先天性异常的AA患者，在进行alloSCT之前，必须仔细考虑预处理方案。年龄<30岁、接受同胞供者移植的患者长期生存率高（75%～90%），但移植合并症和长期并发症的治疗仍是一个问题。年龄>40岁或无HLA相合亲属供者的患者预后较差。

药物引起的AA的免疫机制，促使了在老年患者、没有相合供者的患者和（或）其他不适合进行alloSCT的患者中采用免疫抑制治疗。治疗AA所采用的传统化疗（如大剂量环磷酰胺）已被广泛证实毒性过大。然而，联用抗胸腺细胞球蛋白（ATG）和环孢素（一种特异性T细胞抑制剂）的免疫抑制治疗（IST）使多达70%的患者恢复了骨髓功能，且无需依赖红细胞或血小板输注，5年生存率达到90%。ATG的副作用包括抗血清中外来抗原引起的过敏反应和血清病，但这些副作用一般呈自限性。艾曲泊帕是一种口服的TPO类似物，其可通过结合巨核细胞上的MPL受体来刺激血小板生成。体外数据表明，尽管AA患者体内存在高水平的内源性TPO，给予高剂量外源性TPO仍然可以刺激表达TPO受体的HSC的增殖和维持。艾曲泊帕可使44%的难治性重型AA患者获得血液学反应。随后，艾曲泊帕被列入初诊AA患者的一线治疗方案中，艾曲泊帕、ATG和环孢素（CSA）的联合方案的6个月总体反应率达80%～94%，且具有较高的长期生存率。许多患者出现了完全的血液学反应，骨髓造血容量和可检测的造血干祖细胞数量显著增多。这种联合方案（ATG＋CSA＋艾曲泊帕）现已成为重型AA患者初始治疗的标准治疗。

由于AA患者的内源性细胞因子生成通常较多，常规使用G-CSF、EPO或干细胞因子等生长因子通常是无效的。尽管难治性AA患者的内源性TPO水平较高，但长期使用艾曲泊帕作为维持治疗可能对长期维持血细胞计数有一定疗效，无论是否联用其他免疫抑制剂（如ATG、CSA）。初次治疗后存活的AA患者仍有较高风险出现其他原发性血液疾病，如骨髓增生异常综合征、白血病和阵发性睡眠性血红蛋白尿症（PNH）。部分AA患者也可能随着时间的推移出现血液学反应丢失的复发情况。复发患者可能需要重新使用ATG、雄激素和新的免疫抑制剂进行治疗。

阵发性睡眠性血红蛋白尿症

定义、流行病学和病因学

PNH是以血管内溶血、静脉血栓形成和骨髓衰竭为特点的少见疾病。其发病机制是含有磷脂酰肌醇聚糖A类（PIGA）基因突变的多能HSC扩增。*PIGA*基因编码一种膜脂结构［即糖基磷脂酰肌醇（GPI）］，*PIGA*基因缺失所产生的异常造血细胞上的GPI锚连蛋白减少。PNH的临床表现由GPI锚连蛋白（CD55和CD59）缺乏所致，后者可保护红细胞和血小板免受补体调控的攻击。CD55和CD59的缺失可引起血细胞的免疫破坏增加。破裂的红细胞释放的血红蛋白会引起疾病症状，具体表现为突然出现不规律的深色尿液。PNH的命名源于观察到深色尿液更多在夜间或清晨出现，因为尿液在睡眠期间被浓缩。实际上，这种疾病中的溶血是一个持续的过程，不仅在夜间发生，白天也会发生，只是可能不如夜间明显。

Blood cells arising from abnormal PNH clones can have complete (type III cells) or partial (type II cells) GPI deficiency. The degree of GPI deficiency is associated with the severity of the clinical symptoms. GPI-deficient cells typically coexist in the marrow with various populations of normal GPI-expressing cells (type I cells). Small numbers of abnormal PNH clones in patients with AA or myelodysplastic syndrome (MDS) suggest significant overlap in the causes of these three diseases. This led to reclassification of PNH as classic PNH disease and PNH in the setting of another specified bone marrow disorder. Suppression of normal hematopoiesis by the host immune system directly or indirectly by a preceding or coexistent disorder appears to provide a marrow environment favoring selective expansion of PNH stem cell clones and their deficient blood cell progeny over normal hematopoiesis.

Clinical Presentation

Patients are typically younger individuals with varying chronic complaints of abdominal pain, dysphagia, erectile dysfunction and impotence (in men), and intense lethargy due to smooth muscle dystonia resulting from depletion of circulating nitric oxide levels by free hemoglobin. Not all affected patients exhibit symptoms. Despite the continuous hemolysis, patients may experience acute exacerbations intermittently or frequently during periods of infection, trauma, and stress that may be difficult to manage. In addition to hemolysis, individuals with PNH are susceptible to recurrent potentially life-threatening thromboses and acute as well as chronic renal disease.

Diagnosis and Differential Diagnosis

The diagnosis of PNH is typically made by identification of complete or partial GPI protein deficiency on red cells and granulocytes. Usually this is determined by the loss of CD59, CD55, CD16, or CD24 expression in a clonal population. Laboratory tests reveal ongoing, low-grade intravascular hemolysis with increased lactate dehydrogenase levels correlating with severity of hemolysis and symptoms. Cytopenias, particularly anemia, often render patients transfusion dependent with ongoing hemoglobinuria due to the release of free plasma hemoglobin from intracellular compartments. About 15% of PNH patients have spontaneous resolution of disease without long-term sequelae, suggesting that *PIGA* mutations may appear transiently and disappear spontaneously in normal hematopoietic cell populations for unknown reasons.

Treatment

Eculizumab is a humanized monoclonal antibody that binds with high affinity to the complement protein C5, preventing terminal complement-mediated intravascular hemolysis in patients with PNH. Eculizumab therapy decreases hemolysis and hemoglobinuria, reduces requirements for red blood cell transfusions, improves chronic renal failure, and is associated with significant improvement in quality of life and survival for PNH patients. The incidence of life-threatening thrombotic events is decreased by more than 80%, likely contributing to the significant improvement in overall survival. Although this agent is associated with a theoretical increased risk for meningococcal infections due to complement-mediated blockade, the long-term safety and efficacy of sustained eculizumab therapy administered for more than 5 years appear to outweigh the potential risks of prolonged treatment. A recently developed longer-acting version of eculizumab offers patients who require lifelong therapy with this complement inhibitor increased convenience with less frequent outpatient administration. Newer agents targeting different stages of the complement pathway are currently in clinical investigation for PNH and other complement-activated hemolytic anemias. Other treatment for PNH includes supportive care with transfusions, iron and folic acid supplementation, and alloSCT in selected patients for curative intent. Documented venous thrombosis is treated with lifelong full anticoagulation.

Prognosis

Despite advances in treatment and adequate anticoagulation, PNH remains a life-threatening disease. Venous thrombosis involving the cerebral and intra-abdominal veins occurs in about one half of patients and is the cause of death for up to one third, although the cause of the increased thrombotic risk is not entirely understood. Other causes of morbidity and mortality are side effects of progressive AA and a 5% long-term risk for leukemic transformation. Historically, the median survival from diagnosis is 10 to 15 years, with one third of patients dying within 5 years of the diagnosis. Whether long-term eculizumab therapy can change the natural history of disease is unknown and is the goal of an international registry of PNH patients.

Myelodysplastic Syndrome
Definition and Epidemiology

MDS is a biologically heterogeneous group of marrow disorders characterized by ineffective and disordered hematopoiesis in one or more of the major myeloid cell lines: erythroid cells, neutrophils and their precursors, and megakaryocytes. Patients have one or more cytopenias despite normal or increased numbers of hematopoietic cells in the bone marrow. Disordered maturation is accompanied by increased intramedullary apoptosis, which contributes to the decreased release of mature cells into the periphery. Primary MDS is predominantly a disease of elderly persons and occurs in about 1 of 500 patients between the ages of 60 and 75 years.

Etiology

Prior exposure to radiation therapy, myelotoxic chemotherapy, and organic chemicals such as benzene and formaldehyde has been linked to the development of what is termed "secondary" MDS. This disorder may occur at any age and comprises 10% to 15% of all diagnosed MDS cases. Therapy-related MDS is defined as MDS arising months to years after prior chemotherapy involving any cytotoxic agent but particularly alkylating agents and anthracyclines, ionizing radiation, radiolabeled antibody therapy, or alloSCT for any cancer or noncancer-related condition. Because therapy-related MDS typically evolves swiftly to more aggressive disease, these cases have been reclassified with therapy-related AML and treated accordingly (see Chapter 2).

Although the remaining majority of cases of MDS were previously thought to be idiopathic, emerging data have demonstrated that age-related clonal hematopoiesis underlies the development of MDS in many older individuals. Extensive genomic analyses of peripheral blood samples in otherwise healthy individuals have identified certain clonal molecular abnormalities, such as *DNMT3A, TET2,* and *ASXL1* mutations, present in hematopoietic cells several years prior to the development of overt hematologic disorders or even abnormal blood counts. Individuals who present with a single cytopenia and at least one clonal mutation in an otherwise normal marrow by morphology or who have a clonal marrow karyotype have been designated to have *CCUS (clonal cytopenia of unknown significance)*. Increased number of mutations and specific mutations have been associated with increased risk of evolution to hematologic malignancy with highest risk seen in patients with two or more mutations, *RUNX1, JAK2V617F,* or *p53* mutations. The ideal management of these individuals, a proportion of whom will inevitably develop myeloid malignancies, is not certain but many physicians will choose to monitor these patients closely with intermittent blood cell counts. MDS is also considered a precursor syndrome with an overall risk of transformation to acute myeloid leukemia (AML) of 25% to

源自异常 PNH 克隆的血细胞可存在完全性（Ⅲ型细胞）或部分性（Ⅱ型细胞）GPI 缺乏。GPI 缺乏程度与临床症状的严重程度相关。缺乏 GPI 的细胞通常与骨髓中多种正常表达 GPI 的细胞（Ⅰ型细胞）共存。AA 或骨髓增生异常综合征（MDS）患者存在少量异常 PNH 克隆，说明这 3 种疾病的病因有明显重叠。因此，人们将 PNH 重新分类为经典 PNH 和伴有其他特定骨髓疾病的 PNH。宿主免疫系统对正常造血的抑制（由先前存在的疾病或合并症直接或间接抑制）似乎提供了一种有利于 PNH 干细胞克隆及其缺陷型血细胞后代选择性扩增的骨髓环境，而非正常的造血过程。

临床表现

PNH 常见于年轻人，可伴有多种慢性症状，如腹痛、吞咽困难、勃起功能障碍和阳痿（男性），以及严重嗜睡（由游离血红蛋白消耗循环一氧化氮引起的平滑肌肌张力障碍所致）。并非所有患者都会出现症状。尽管溶血是持续发生的，但在感染、创伤和应激情况下可能出现间歇性或频繁的急性加重，从而使病情难以控制。除溶血外，PNH 患者还容易反复发生可能威胁生命的血栓及急性和慢性肾病。

诊断和鉴别诊断

PNH 的诊断基于确认红细胞和粒细胞表面 GPI 蛋白完全或部分缺失，通常由某一克隆细胞群上 CD59、CD55、CD16 或 CD24 表达缺失而确定。实验室检查可显示持续的轻度血管内溶血，伴有乳酸脱氢酶水平升高，这与溶血的严重程度及症状相关。患者会因血细胞减少（尤其是贫血）而依赖输血，同时由于细胞内结构释放游离血浆血红蛋白而出现血红蛋白尿。约 15% 的 PNH 患者可自发缓解且无远期后遗症，提示 *PIGA* 突变可能是暂时的，可在正常造血细胞中自发消失，原因尚不明确。

治疗

依库珠单抗是一种人源单克隆抗体，与补体蛋白 C5 有高度亲和力，可预防 PNH 患者出现补体终末途径介导的血管内溶血。依库珠单抗治疗可减少溶血和血红蛋白尿，降低红细胞输注需求，改善慢性肾衰竭，并显著改善 PNH 患者的生活质量和生存率。治疗后危及生命的血栓事件发生率下降超过 80%，从而显著提高了总生存率。虽然该药物通过补体调控阻断在理论上会增加脑膜炎双球菌感染的风险，但超过 5 年持续使用依库珠单抗治疗的长期安全性和疗效仍超出长期治疗的潜在风险。近期研发的一种作用时间更长的依库珠单抗制剂为需要终身治疗的患者提供了更大的便利，因为这种补体抑制剂减少了门诊就诊次数。在治疗 PNH 和其他补体激活的溶血性贫血方面，目前正在进行针对补体通路不同阶段的新药临床试验。PNH 的其他治疗方法包括输血、补充铁和叶酸，alloSCT 适用于追求治愈的患者。已确诊的静脉血栓形成患者需进行终身抗凝治疗。

预后

虽然 PNH 的治疗手段已取得进展，并有充分的抗凝治疗，但 PNH 仍是一种危及生命的疾病。血栓风险增加的原因尚未完全明确，约 1/2 的患者会出现累及大脑和腹腔内静脉的静脉血栓事件，占死亡事件的 1/3。其他引起合并症和死亡的病因包括进展性 AA 所带来的负面影响和 5% 的远期白血病转化风险。在过去，诊断 PNH 后的中位生存期为 10 ～ 15 年，1/3 的患者在诊断后 5 年内死亡。长期使用依库珠单抗治疗是否可以改变疾病的自然病程尚不明确，这是 PNH 患者全球登记组的研究目标。

骨髓增生异常综合征

定义和流行病学

MDS 是一组生物学异质性骨髓疾病，以无效及病态造血为特点，累及 1 个或多个主要髓系细胞系：红细胞、中性粒细胞及其前体细胞和巨核细胞。患者骨髓中造血细胞数量正常或增多，但会有单系或多系血细胞减少。成熟障碍伴骨髓内细胞凋亡增多，导致释放至外周的成熟细胞减少。原发性 MDS 主要见于老年人，60 ～ 75 岁人群的发病率约为 1/500。

病因

既往接受过放疗、骨髓毒性化疗及有机化学物质（如苯和甲醛）暴露与"继发性"MDS 有关。该病可发生于任何年龄段，占所有确诊 MDS 病例的 10% ～ 15%。在接受化疗（包括所有细胞毒性药物，尤其是烷化剂和蒽环类药物）、电离辐射、放射标记抗体治疗或 alloSCT（因癌症或非癌症相关疾病）后月至数年均可能发生 MDS，即治疗相关 MDS。由于治疗相关 MDS 通常会在起病后快速转化为更具侵袭性的疾病，因此这些疾病被重新分类为治疗相关 AML 并给予相应治疗（见第 2 章）。

尽管其余绝大多数 MDS 既往被认为是特发性的，但越来越多的数据表明，许多老年 MDS 的发生与年龄相关的克隆造血相关。在其他健康个体中，对外周血样本进行的广泛基因组分析已经鉴定出一些克隆分子异常，如 *DNMT3A*、*TET2* 和 *ASXL1* 突变，这些突变在明显的血液学疾病发生前或血常规异常前就已存在数年。单系血细胞减少且至少有 1 个克隆性突变（通过形态或骨髓核型分析检测）但未诊断其他血液学疾病的患者被定义为 CCUS（意义未明的克隆性血细胞减少）。突变的数量增加和特异性突变与进展为恶性血液系统肿瘤的风险增加有关，其中存在 *RUNX1*、*JAK2V617F* 或 *p53* 突变中至少 2 个突变的患者风险最高。这类患者中一部分将不可避免地进展为髓系恶性肿瘤，对这些患者的理想管理并不确定，但是许多医生会选择密切监测血细胞计数。MDS 也被认为是前驱综合征，其转化为急性髓系白血病

30%. It is now clear that progression from clonal myeloid HSC injury to multilineage hematopoietic failure and enhanced myeloblast growth reflects a continuum of disease ranging from clonal hematopoiesis to MDS and subsequent AML (see Chapter 2).

Clinical Presentation

Most patients with MDS are referred for evaluation of an incidental finding of peripheral cytopenia. Symptomatic patients usually exhibit findings related to the secondary effects of cytopenias: bleeding and bruising caused by thrombocytopenia, infection caused by leukopenia, or fatigue and dyspnea related to anemia. Physical examination is usually unremarkable, although 25% or more of patients may have splenomegaly. In some patients with MDS, development of skin lesions with fever (i.e., acute febrile neutrophilic dermatosis [Sweet syndrome]) may herald the transformation of MDS into acute leukemia. The disease course of MDS varies widely based on specific prognostic information (see later) including number and severity of cytopenias and karyotypic abnormalities. Although lower-risk MDS patients may live normal lifespans, most patients will eventually die prematurely of cytopenia-related complications, marrow failure, or evolution to AML with a median survival ranging from months to less than 2 years in the highest risk disease.

Diagnosis and Differential Diagnosis

Diagnosis of MDS requires evidence of dysplasia of at least 10% of marrow myeloid hematopoietic cells or 5% to 19% marrow blasts, the presence of peripheral cytopenia in one or more myeloid lineages, and absence of other known causes for the cytopenia. The World Health Organization (WHO) also defines MDS in any marrow regardless of morphology, which contains pathognomonic karyotypic abnormalities, for example, aberrations in chromosome 5 and 7, or 3 or greater aberrations (complex karyotype).

Morphologic evidence of dysplastic changes diagnostic of MDS often require specialized hematopathology review. Review of the peripheral blood smear may show characteristic morphologic abnormalities in addition to cytopenias. Erythroid cells are usually macrocytic, often with basophilic stippling. Neutrophils are often hypogranular and hypolobulated with a characteristic bilobed nuclear morphology called *pseudo-Pelger-Huët abnormality*. This anomaly should be anticipated when automated differential cell counts report unusually large numbers of bands. The bone marrow in MDS is usually normocellular or hypercellular, although 10% of patients may have a hypocellular marrow. Dysplastic changes usually occur in all three cell lines. Erythroid cells appear megaloblastic, with multinucleated cells or asynchronous nuclear-cytoplasmic development. Extremely small micromegakaryocytes and agranular megakaryocytes also may be seen. The myeloid series shows poor maturation with a left shift to earlier hypogranulated myeloid forms. Although elevated numbers of myeloid blasts are common, increasing blast numbers indicate progression to acute leukemia. Electron microscopy of the marrow shows cellular changes (i.e., prominent nuclear chromatin, cytoplasmic vacuoles, and blebs) characteristic of increased apoptosis.

In the past, MDS was classified based on dysplastic marrow morphology and percentage of blasts as one of five subtypes: refractory anemia (RA), refractory anemia with ringed sideroblasts (RARS), refractory anemia with excess blasts (RAEB), refractory anemia with excess blasts in transformation (RAEBT), and chronic myelomonocytic leukemia (CMML). Later, these five subtypes were expanded to eight subtypes, with recognition of multilineage dysplasia as an important feature (e.g., refractory cytopenia with multilineage dysplasia, refractory cytopenia with multilineage dysplasia and ringed sideroblasts) and the reclassification of CMML as myeloproliferative-myelodysplastic syndrome (MPN/MDS) (Table 1.5). MDS with an isolated 5q− cytogenetic abnormality was established as a distinct clinical syndrome. Therapy-related MDS/AML is defined as evidence of marrow dysplasia after prior chemotherapy, radiation therapy, or other myeloablative therapy. Although MDS patients with refractory anemia and excess blasts or refractory cytopenia with multilineage dysplasia usually fare poorly, morphologic classification of MDS correlates only approximately with overall survival.

The natural history and treatment of some MDS subtypes is more closely associated with specific cytogenetic and molecular abnormalities, demanding that careful molecular studies be performed during initial evaluation. For example, MDS characterized by deletion of the short arm of chromosome 7 (7p−) or complex cytogenetic abnormalities such as monosomy 7 or trisomy 8 often have mutations in the p53 tumor suppressor genes and universally poor clinical outcomes. In contrast, patients with MDS featuring an isolated deletion in the long arm of chromosome 5 (i.e., 5q− syndrome) are predominantly older women with a refractory macrocytic anemia, normal or elevated platelet counts, and an overall better clinical prognosis. These patients often live for several years with intermittent red blood cell transfusions, have a low risk of leukemic transformation, and often respond to therapy with lenalidomide (see later).

For the one third to one half of patients with cytopenia and myeloid dysplasia with normal marrow karyotype, the diagnosis of MDS should be one of exclusion after other potential causes of marrow failure and pancytopenia have been evaluated (see Table 1.3). MDS should never be diagnosed in acute disease states, during chronic hospitalization, or within 6 months of known myelotoxic therapy including irradiation or chemotherapy for any cancer or noncancer-related indication(s). Other causes such as vitamin B_{12} or folate deficiency, chronic alcohol use, over-the-counter medications or supplements, and infections including human immunodeficiency virus (HIV) infection should be considered. Patients with possible MDS and a hypocellular bone marrow should also be evaluated for AA and/or PNH.

Prognosis

Although several risk classification systems have been developed to predict outcomes of MDS patients, accurate prediction of MDS prognosis remains a work in progress. The original classification (WHO) was developed by an international working group to be employed at initial disease detection and partitions patients based on age, cytopenias, karyotype, and marrow blasts into different risk categories (see Table 1.5). Based on criticism that the original classification relies only on characteristics of patients at disease onset and includes cases now considered to be acute myeloid leukemia, another WHO classification–based prognostic scoring system (WPSS) was devised emphasizing morphology, karyotype, and transfusion dependence at any time during the MDS disease course (Table 1.6). The International Prognostic Scale (IPSS) divides MDS patients into five new risk categories and was validated to predict for overall survival and leukemic evolution for MDS at any follow-up time (Table 1.7). To further complicate things, data derived from multiple international databases and encompassing 7012 patients was analyzed to generate yet another new classification system, the Revised International Prognostic Scoring System (R-IPSS) including more comprehensive karyotypic abnormalities (Table 1.8). In general, using any of these systems, MDS patients can be divided into three general risk categories: low, intermediate (low to high), or high to very high-risk disease and treated accordingly.

Whole-genome sequencing of untreated MDS samples has revealed that at least 78% of patients carry one or more oncogenic

（AML）的总体风险为 25%～30%。目前已明确从克隆性髓系 HSC 损伤进展到多系造血衰竭和髓系原始细胞增殖加剧，反映了从克隆性造血进展到 MDS 以及随后的 AML 的连续性疾病过程（见第 2 章）。

临床表现

大多数 MDS 患者是因偶然发现外周血细胞减少而被转诊进行评估。患者症状通常与外周血细胞减少的继发效应相关：血小板减少引起出血和瘀斑，白细胞减少引起感染，贫血引起乏力和呼吸困难。体格检查通常无异常，虽然超过 25% 的患者可能有脾大。在部分 MDS 患者中，出现皮肤病变和发热［即急性发热性嗜中性细胞皮肤病（Sweet 综合征）］可能是 MDS 转化为急性白血病的前驱表现。MDS 的病程多样化，取决于特定预后信息（见下文），包括血细胞减少的数量和严重程度及核型异常。虽然低危 MDS 患者寿命正常，但多数患者因血细胞减少相关的并发症、骨髓衰竭或进展至 AML 而过早死亡，其中最高危患者中位生存期 < 2 年。

诊断和鉴别诊断

MDS 的诊断需要至少 10% 的骨髓髓系造血细胞增生异常或 5%～19% 的骨髓原始细胞，同时外周血中单系或多系血细胞减少，且排除其他可能导致血细胞减少的原因。世界卫生组织（WHO）对 MDS 的定义是，无论形态学如何，骨髓包含病理学特异的核型异常，如 5 号和 7 号染色体异常，或 3 个及以上染色体异常（复杂核型）。

诊断 MDS 骨髓增生异常的形态学证据需要专门的血液病理学检查。MDS 患者的外周血涂片检查可见血细胞减少和特征性的形态学异常。红系细胞通常为大细胞性，伴有嗜碱性点彩。中性粒细胞通常颗粒减少，核分叶少，有特征性的双叶核形态，被称为假性 Pelger-Huët 畸形。当血细胞分类计数回报异常的大量杆状核粒细胞时，需警惕假性 Pelger-Huët 畸形。MDS 时骨髓通常是增生正常或活跃，虽然 10% 的患者骨髓可能为增生低下。三系均可出现增生异常。红系细胞可出现巨幼红细胞，伴有多核细胞或核-质发育不同步。同时可观察到小巨核细胞和无颗粒型巨核细胞。髓系核左移至较早期的少颗粒髓系形态，提示成熟不良。虽然髓系原始细胞数目增多较常见，但原始细胞数目不断增加则提示疾病进展至急性白血病。骨髓电镜检查可见细胞成分改变（即核染色质明显、胞质空泡和水泡）是细胞凋亡增加的特征表现。

既往根据病态造血的骨髓形态和原始细胞比例将 MDS 分为 5 个亚型：难治性贫血（RA）、难治性贫血伴环形铁粒幼细胞（RARS）、难治性贫血伴原始细胞增多（RA with excess blasts, RAEB）、难治性贫血伴原始细胞增多转化型（RAEBT）、慢性粒-单核细胞白血病（CMML）。随着对多系增生异常重要性的认识（如难治性血细胞减少伴多系病态造血、难治性贫血伴多系病态造血及环形铁粒幼细胞），以及重新将 CMML 分类为骨髓增殖性肿瘤/骨髓增生异常综合征（MPN/MDS）后，以上 5 个亚型扩展为 8 个亚型（表 1.5）。MDS 伴单纯 5q 缺失（5q−）的细胞遗传学异常是另一种临床综合征。既往接受放化疗或其他清髓治疗后出现骨髓病态造血者应考虑为治疗相关性 MDS/AML。虽然难治性贫血伴原始细胞增多或难治性血细胞减少伴多系病态造血的患者往往预后不佳，但 MDS 的形态学分类仅大致和总生存率相关。

部分 MDS 亚型的自然病程和治疗与特定的细胞遗传学和分子学异常密切相关，因此在初始评估时需要进行详细的骨髓分子生物学检查。例如，存在 7 号染色体短臂缺失（7p−）或复杂细胞遗传学异常（如 7 号染色体单体或 8 号染色体三体）的 MDS 患者通常存在 p53 肿瘤抑制基因突变，临床结局均不佳。仅有 5 号染色体长臂缺失（即 5q 综合征）的 MDS 患者总体临床预后较好，该病主要见于老年女性，存在难治性大细胞贫血、血小板计数正常或升高。这些患者往往需要在数年内间断接受红细胞输注，白血病转化风险较低，来那度胺治疗通常有效（见下文）。

对于存在血细胞减少和髓系病态造血但染色体核型正常的患者（占 1/3～1/2），MDS 诊断为排除性诊断，鉴别诊断时需要评估其他骨髓衰竭和全血细胞减少的可能原因（表 1.3）。在急性疾病状态、长期住院期间或已知 6 个月内接受骨髓毒性治疗（包括用于治疗任何癌症或非癌症相关适应证的放疗或化疗）时，不应诊断 MDS。其他应考虑的病因包括维生素 B_{12} 或叶酸缺乏、慢性酒精使用、非处方药或补充剂使用、感染［包括人类免疫缺陷病毒（HIV）感染］。对于可能患 MDS 且骨髓低增生的患者，应评估 AA 和（或）PNH 的可能性。

预后

尽管已经开发了多个风险分层系统用于预测 MDS 患者的预后，但精准预测 MDS 预后的工作仍在进行中。国际工作组制定的早期分类（WHO）可用于初始疾病检测，并根据年龄、血细胞减少、染色体核型和骨髓原始细胞将患者分为不同的风险类别（表 1.5）。由于最初的分类仅依赖于患者发病时的特点，并且包含了目前已被列为 AML 的疾病，因此人们对该评分标准提出质疑，另一种基于 WHO 分类的预后评分系统（WPSS）强调了形态学、染色体核型和 MDS 病程中任意时间的输血依赖情况（表 1.6）。国际预后评分系统（IPSS）将 MDS 患者分为 5 个新的风险类别，并已经过验证可在任意随访时间预测 MDS 患者的总生存率和白血病进展情况（表 1.7）。在对纳入 7012 例患者的多个国际数据库数据进行分析后，制定了另一个包含染色体核型异常的新评分系统——修订的国际预后评分系统（R-IPSS）（表 1.8）。一般来说，使用其中任意一个评分系统均可将 MDS 患者分为 3 种风险类别：低危、中危、高危至极高危，并据此制订治疗方案。

未经治疗患者的 MDS 样本全基因组测序显示，至少有 78% 的患者携带 1 个或多个致癌基因突变。虽然

TABLE 1.5 World Health Organization Classification of Myelodysplastic Syndromes

Class	Definition
Refractory anemia	Blood: anemia, no or rare blasts BM: erythroid dysplasia only, <5% blasts, and <15% ringed sideroblasts
Refractory anemia with ringed sideroblasts (RARS)	Blood: anemia, no blasts BM: ≥15% ringed sideroblasts, erythroid dysplasia only, <5% blasts
Refractory cytopenia with multilineage dysplasia (RCMD)	Blood: cytopenias (bicytopenia or pancytopenia), no or rare blasts, <1 × 10^9/L monocytes BM: dysplasia in ≥10% of the cells of two or more myeloid cell lines, <5% blasts, no Auer rods, <15% ringed sideroblasts
Refractory cytopenia with multilineage dysplasia and ringed sideroblasts (RCMD-RS)	Blood: cytopenias (two or more), no or rare blasts, no Auer rods, and <1 × 10^9/L monocytes BM: dysplasia in ≥10% of the cells of two or more myeloid cell lines, <5% blasts, ≥15% ringed sideroblasts, no Auer rods
Refractory anemia with excess blasts type 1 (RAEB-1)	Blood: cytopenias, <5% blasts, no Auer rods, <1 × 10^9/L monocytes BM: unilineage or multilineage dysplasia, 5-9% blasts, no Auer rods
Refractory anemia with excess blasts type 2 (RAEB-2)	Blood: cytopenias, 5-19% blasts, Auer rods ± <1 × 10^9/L monocytes BM: unilineage or multilineage dysplasia, 10-19% blasts, ± Auer rods
Myelodysplastic syndrome–unclassified (MDS-U)	Blood: cytopenias, no or rare blasts, no Auer rods BM: unilineage dysplasia in one myeloid line, <5% blasts, no Auer rods
MDS associated with isolated del(5q)	Blood: anemia, usually normal or increased platelet count, <5% blasts BM: normal to increased megakaryocytes with hypolobulated nuclei, <5% blasts, isolated cytogenetic abnormality of deletion 5q, no Auer rods

BM, Bone marrow.

TABLE 1.6 World Health Organization Classification-Based Prognostic Scoring System (WPSS) for Myelodysplastic Disorders

	SCORING[a]			
Factor	0	1	2	3
WHO category	RA, RARS, 5q–	RCMD, RCMD-RS	RAEB-1	RAEB-2
Karyotype[b]	Good	Intermediate	Poor	—
Transfusion requirement[c]	No	Regular	—	—

5q–, Myelodysplastic syndrome with isolated del(5q) and marrow blasts less than 5%; *MDS*, myelodysplastic syndrome; *RA*, refractory anemia; *RARS*, refractory anemia with ringed sideroblasts; *RCMD*, refractory cytopenia with multilineage dysplasia; *RCMD-RS*, refractory cytopenia with multilineage dysplasia and ringed sideroblasts; *RAEB-1*, refractory anemia with excess of blasts type 1; *RAEB-2*, refractory anemia with excess of blasts type 2; *WHO*, World Health Organization.

[a]Risk groups were determined as follows: very low (total score = 0), low (1), intermediate (2), high (3 to 4), and very high (5 to 6).
[b]Karyotype was as follows: good: normal, –Y, del(5q), del(20q); poor: complex (≥3 abnormalities), chromosome 7 anomalies; and intermediate: other abnormalities.
[c]Red blood cell (RBC) transfusion dependency was defined as having at least one RBC transfusion every 8 weeks over a period of 4 months.

TABLE 1.7 International Prognostic Scoring System for Myelodysplastic Disorders (IPSS)

Score	Blasts	Karyotype	Cytopenias[a]	Overall Score	Median Survival (Yr)
0	<5%	Normal, –Y, 5q–, 20q–	0-1 cytopenias	0	5.7
0.5	5-10%	All other abnormalities	2-3 cytopenias	0.5-1.0	3.5
1.0		Abnormal 7, >3 abnormalities		1.5-2.0	1.2
1.5	11-20%			2.5 or higher	0.4
2.0	21-30%				

[a]Cytopenias are defined as hemoglobin <10 g/dL, neutrophils <1500/μL, platelets <100,000/μL.

mutations. Although more than 40 genes are recurrently mutated in MDS, most are altered in less than 5% of MDS patients, reflecting the enormous biologic heterogeneity of this disorder. Genes implicated in MDS are involved in cell signaling, DNA methylation, chromatin regulation, and most importantly, RNA splicing. Several studies have shown that several individual gene mutations, including *EZH2, DNMT3A, SF3B1, TET2, NRAS, TP53, RUNX1,* and *ASXL1*, predict MDS outcomes independent of IPSS classification and can improve on prognostication based on clinical features alone. However, none of the current prognostic models for MDS, such as the revised IPSS,

表 1.5 MDS 的 WHO 分类

分类	定义
难治性贫血（RA）	外周血：贫血，无或罕见原始细胞 骨髓：仅有红系病态造血，原始细胞 < 5%，环形铁粒幼细胞 < 15%
难治性贫血伴环形铁粒幼细胞（RARS）	外周血：贫血，无原始细胞 骨髓：环形铁粒幼细胞 ≥ 15%，仅有红系病态造血，原始细胞 < 5%
难治性血细胞减少伴多系病态造血（RCMD）	外周血：血细胞减少（两系或三系），无或罕见原始细胞，单核细胞 < 1×10⁹/L 骨髓：至少两系髓系细胞病态造血 ≥ 10%，原始细胞 < 5%，无 Auer 小体，环形铁粒幼细胞 < 15%
难治性血细胞减少伴多系病态造血和环形铁粒幼细胞（RCMD-RS）	外周血：血细胞减少（两系或三系），无或罕见原始细胞，无 Auer 小体，单核细胞 < 1×10⁹/L 骨髓：至少两系髓系细胞病态造血 ≥ 10%，原始细胞 < 5%，环形铁粒幼细胞 ≥ 15%，无 Auer 小体
难治性贫血伴原始细胞增多 1 型（RAEB-1）	外周血：血细胞减少，原始细胞 < 5%，无 Auer 小体，单核细胞 < 1×10⁹/L 骨髓：单系或多系病态造血，原始细胞 5%～9%，无 Auer 小体
难治性贫血伴原始细胞增多 2 型（RAEB-2）	外周血：血细胞减少，原始细胞 5%～19%，Auer 小体 ± 单核细胞 < 1×10⁹/L 骨髓：单系或多系病态造血，原始细胞 10%～19% ± Auer 小体
骨髓增生异常综合征-不能分类（MDS-U）	外周血：血细胞减少，无或罕见原始细胞，无 Auer 小体 骨髓：髓系细胞单系病态造血，原始细胞 < 5%，无 Auer 小体
MDS 伴单纯 5q 缺失	外周血：贫血，血小板计数通常正常或增多，原始细胞 < 5% 骨髓：巨核细胞计数正常或增多，伴核分叶减少，原始细胞 < 5%，细胞遗传学异常为单纯 5q 缺失，无 Auer 小体

表 1.6 基于 WHO 分类的预后评分系统（WPSS）

参数	积分[a]			
	0 分	1 分	2 分	3 分
WHO 分类	RA、RARS、5q−	RCMD、RCMD-RS	RAEB-1	RAEB-2
染色体核型[b]	良好	中等	差	—
输血需求[c]	无	依赖	—	—

5q−，MDS 伴单纯 5q 缺失且骨髓原始细胞 < 5%；MDS，骨髓增生异常综合征；RA，难治性贫血；RARS，难治性贫血伴环形铁粒幼细胞；RCMD，难治性血细胞减少伴多系病态造血；RCMD-RS，难治性血细胞减少伴多系病态造血和环形铁粒幼细胞；RAEB-1，难治性贫血伴原始细胞增多 1 型；RAEB-2，难治性贫血伴原始细胞增多 2 型；WHO，世界卫生组织。
[a] 风险类别包括：极低危（总分 = 0 分）、低危（1 分）、中危（2 分）、高危（3～4 分）和极高危（5～6 分）。
[b] 染色体核型如下：良好［正常核型，−Y，del(q)，del(20q)］；差［复杂核型（≥ 3 种异常），7 号染色体异常］；中等（其他核型异常）。
[c] 红细胞输注依赖是指在 4 个月内至少需要每 8 周输注 1 次红细胞。

表 1.7 MDS 的国际预后评分系统（IPSS）

积分	骨髓原始细胞	染色体核型	血细胞减少[a]	总积分	中位生存期（年）
0	< 5%	正常，−Y，5q−，20q−	0～1 系细胞减少	0	5.7
0.5	5%～10%	其他异常	2～3 系细胞减少	0.5～1.0	3.5
1.0		7 号染色体异常，> 3 种异常		1.5～2.0	1.2
1.5	11%～20%			≥ 2.5	0.4
2.0	21%～30%				

[a] 血细胞减少的定义是血红蛋白 < 10 g/dl，中性粒细胞 < 1500/μl，血小板 < 100 000/μl。

有 40 多个基因在 MDS 中反复出现突变，但大多数突变见于不足 5% 的 MDS 患者，这反映了 MDS 极大的生物学异质性。MDS 涉及的基因参与细胞信号、DNA 甲基化、染色质调控，以及最重要的 RNA 剪切。多项研究显示，多种单基因突变（包括 *EZH2*、*DNMT3A*、*SF3B1*、*TET2*、*NRAS*、*TP53*、*RUNX1* 和 *ASXL1*）可以独立于 IPSS 分类而预测 MDS 结局，并可仅根据临床特征改善预后评估。然而，目前针对 MDS 的预后模型

TABLE 1.8 Revised International Prognostic Scoring System for Myelodysplastic Syndromes (R-IPSS)

Prognostic Subgroups (% of Patients)	Cytogenetic Abnormalities	Median Survival (Yr)[a]	Median Evolution to AML, 25%[b] (Yr)[a]	Hazard Ratios OS/AML[a]	Hazard Ratios OS/AML[c]
Very good (3-4%[c])	–Y, del(11q)	5.4	NR	0.7/0.4	0.5/0.5
Good (66-72%)	Normal, del(5q), del(12p), del(20q), double including del(5q)	4.8	9.4	1/1	1/1
Intermediate (13-19%[c])	del(7q), +8, +19, i(17q), any other single or double independent clones	2.7	2.5	1.5/1.8	1.6/2.2
Poor (4-5%[c])	–7, inv(3)/t(3q)/del(3q), double including –7/del(7q), complex: 3 abnormalities	1.5	1.7	2.3/2.3	2.6/3.4
Very poor (7%[c])	Complex: >3 abnormalities	0.7	0.7	3.8/3.6	4.2/4.9

Data from Schanz J, Tüchler H, Solé F, et al: New comprehensive cytogenetic scoring system for primary myelodysplastic syndromes and oligoblastic AML following MDS derived from an international database merge, J Clin Oncol 30:820-829, 2012.

AML, Acute myeloid leukemia; *NR*, not reached; *OS*, overall survival.
[a]Multivariate analysis, N = 7012; data from patients in the International Working Group for Prognosis in MDS (IWG-PM) database.
[b]AML, 25% indicates time for 25% of patients to develop AML.
[c]N = 2754.

currently consider somatic mutations. The development of novel prognostic models incorporating mutational signatures is eagerly awaited in order to further refine prognosis and treatment of MDS patients in the near future.

Treatment

Insights into the pathophysiology of ineffective hematopoiesis characterizing MDS has led to several therapeutic options that ideally should be individualized based on patient preference, performance status, disease biology, and importantly, prognostic risk category.

Low to intermediate-low risk patients

Transfusions, iron chelation, and growth factors. Because most patients with MDS are elderly individuals who may not tolerate or desire aggressive intervention without hope of cure, those patients with asymptomatic low-risk disease who remain transfusion independent are typically observed expectantly. Those with symptomatic anemia and thrombocytopenia can receive supportive red blood cell and platelet transfusions to maintain quality of life. Special care should be taken to initiate iron chelators (deferoxamine or oral deferiprone) to prevent complications of iron overload caused by the delivery of between 200 and 250 mg of iron with each unit of transfused red blood cells. Accumulation of excess iron initially in macrophages and eventually in the hepatic parenchyma, myocardium, skin, and pancreas can lead to secondary hemochromatosis or transfusional iron overload with clinical symptoms of liver and heart failure, hyperpigmentation, and diabetes mellitus. To mitigate this, transfusion-dependent patients with low endogenous serum EPO levels often receive recombinant EPO growth factor to reduce transfusion needs. Similarly, chronic neutropenic individuals with recurrent or refractory infections may benefit from G-CSF or GM-CSF treatment given alone or in addition to EPO and antibiotic regimens to prevent life-threatening infections.

Luspatercept is a first-in-class recombinant fusion protein derived from human activin receptor linked to a protein derived from immunoglobulin G. This agent works by binding to select TGF-β superfamily ligands to reduce aberrant signaling and enhance late-stage erythropoiesis. By interfering with the signals that suppress RBC production, this drug improves patients' ability to manufacture their own RBCs, therefore reducing the need for transfusions. In a randomized clinical trial, luspatercept safely and effectively reduced transfusion burden in over half of patients with lower risk MDS (defined as very low, low, and intermediate risk) with ring sideroblasts who had not previously responded to or were ineligible for erythropoiesis-stimulating agents.

Immunosuppressive therapy. Certain MDS disease subgroups exhibit significant overlap with AA and PNH because hematopoietic failure in all of these conditions is mediated in part by autoimmune cells selectively targeting the destruction of normal HSCs. Young patients with low-risk MDS disease and exhibiting an HLA-DR15 haplotype have demonstrated a 30% to 50% improvement in counts after T-cell immunosuppressive therapy with ATG or cyclosporine. MDS patients with isolated trisomy 8 with and without demonstrated PNH clones have also been reported to respond to treatment with immunosuppression with or without eculizumab therapy.

5q minus syndrome. Patients with lower-risk MDS characterized by deletions in the long arm of chromosome 5 (5q– aberration) typically have anemia with preserved platelet counts. Many have a disease subtype that is extraordinarily sensitive to therapy with lenalidomide, an immunomodulatory agent that exerts antigrowth effects on MDS cells and their surrounding marrow microenvironment. Complete and durable responses after lenalidomide therapy occur in up to 66% of 5q– syndrome MDS patients and are accompanied by disappearance of the abnormal cytogenetic clone in the marrow in some patients. Defects in ribosomal protein function, specifically the ribosomal subunit protein RPS14, have been identified as the cause of 5q– syndrome MDS, paralleling findings implicating a different ribosomal subunit (RPS19) in the congenital bone marrow syndrome Diamond-Blackfan anemia. Studies have demonstrated that lenalidomide targets aberrant signaling pathways caused by haploinsufficiency of specific genes in a commonly deleted region on chromosome 5 (i.e., *SPARC*,

表 1.8　MDS 的修订的国际预后评分系统（IPSS-R）

预后亚组（患者百分比）	细胞遗传学异常	中位生存期（年）[a]	进展至 AML，25%[b] 的中位时间（年）[a]	风险比 OS/AML[a]	风险比 OS/AML[c]
极好（3%～4%[c]）	－Y、del（11q）	5.4	NR	0.7/0.4	0.5/0.5
好（66%～72%）	正常、del（5q）、del（12p）、del（20q）+另一种异常	4.8	9.4	1/1	1/1
中等（13%～19%[c]）	Del（7q）、+8、+19、i（17q）、其他 1 个或 2 个独立克隆的染色体异常	2.7	2.5	1.5/1.8	1.6/2.2
差（4%～5%[c]）	－7、inv（3）/t（3q）/del（3q）、－7/del（7q）+另一种异常、复杂异常（3 个）	1.5	1.7	2.3/2.3	2.6/3.4
极差（7%[c]）	复杂异常：> 3 个	0.7	0.7	3.8/3.6	4.2/4.9

引自 Schanz J, Tüchler H, Solé F, et al: New comprehensive cytogenetic scoring system for primary myelodysplastic syndromes and oligoblastic AML following MDS derived from an international database merge, J Clin Oncol 30：820-829，2012.
AML，急性髓系白血病；NR，未达到；OS，总生存期。
[a] 多因素分析，N = 7012；患者数据来源于 MDS 预后国际工作组（IWG-PM）数据库。
[b] AML，25% 是指有 25% 的患者进展为 AML 的时间。
[c] N = 2754。

（如 R-IPSS）均未考虑体细胞突变。为了在不久的将来进一步改善 MDS 患者的预后和治疗，迫切需要开发包含突变特征的新型预后模型。

治疗

对以无效造血为特征的 MDS 病理生理学的深入研究已产生了多种治疗方案，理想的治疗是基于患者的意愿、体能状况、疾病生物学和预后风险分层的个体化治疗。

低危和中低危患者

输血、铁螯合剂和生长因子　由于大多数 MDS 患者是老年患者，无法耐受或接受积极的干预，且无治愈意愿，因此对于低危无症状且不需要输血的患者，通常予以定期观察。对于存在症状性贫血和血小板减少症的患者，可以采用输注红细胞和血小板支持治疗，以维持生活质量。应特别注意使用铁螯合剂（去铁胺或口服去铁酮），以防止铁过载（因为每输注 1 个单位红细胞会输入 200～250 mg 铁）。过量的铁最初储存在巨噬细胞，最终在肝实质、心肌、皮肤和胰腺累积，引起继发性血色病或输注后铁过载，临床症状包括肝衰竭、心力衰竭、色素沉着和糖尿病。为了缓解这种情况，血清内源性 EPO 水平低的输血依赖患者通常会接受重组 EPO 生长因子治疗，以减少输血需求。同样，伴有反复或难治性感染的慢性中性粒细胞减少症患者可能会受益于 G-CSF 或 GM-CSF 治疗，这些治疗可以单独使用或与 EPO 和抗感染药物方案结合使用，以防止危及生命的感染。

罗特西普是一种首创的重组融合蛋白，由人激活素受体与免疫球蛋白 G 来源的蛋白质连接而成。该药物通过结合选择性 TGF-β 超家族配体，减少异常信号传导，并增加晚期红细胞生成。通过干扰抑制红细胞生成的信号，该药物可改善患者自身红细胞的生成能力，从而减少输血需求。在一项随机临床试验中，罗特西普在超过 1/2 的具有环形铁粒幼细胞的低危 MDS（定义为极低危、低危和中危）患者中安全且有效地减少了输血负担，这些患者既往对红细胞生成刺激剂无应答或不耐受。

免疫抑制治疗　特定 MDS 亚型与 AA 和 PNH 表现出显著的重叠，因为在这些情况下，造血衰竭部分是由自身免疫细胞选择性靶向破坏正常 HSC 所介导的。低危和表现为 HLA-DR15 单倍体基因型的年轻 MDS 患者，在使用 ATG 或环孢素进行 T 细胞免疫抑制治疗后，30%～50% 患者的血细胞计数得到改善。研究显示，单纯 8 号染色体三体伴或不伴 PNH 克隆的 MDS 患者对免疫抑制药物治疗（联用或不联用依库珠单抗）存在应答。

5q 缺失综合征　以 5 号染色体长臂缺失（5q－）为特征表现的低危 MDS 患者常出现贫血，但血小板计数正常。很多 MDS 亚型对来那度胺治疗特别敏感，来那度胺是一种免疫调节剂，对 MDS 细胞及其周围骨髓微环境具有抗生长作用。接受来那度胺治疗后，约 66% 的 5q 缺失综合征 MDS 患者可以获得完全且持续的缓解，部分患者骨髓中的异常细胞遗传学克隆消失。核糖体蛋白功能缺陷（特别是核糖体亚基蛋白 RPS14）是 5q 缺失综合征 MDS 的病因，这与另一种核糖体亚基（RPS19）在先天性骨髓综合征 Diamond-Blackfan 贫血中的作用相似。研究表明，来那度胺可靶向作用于 5 号染色体常见缺失区域中特定基因（如 *SPARC*、*RPS14*、*CDC25C* 和 *PPP2CA*）单倍剂量不足性引起的异常信号通路。该药物特异性靶向作用于 del（5q）克

TABLE 1.9 Suggested Therapies for Bone Marrow Failure Syndromes

Patient Population	Recommended Treatment
Low-risk MDS (LR-MDS)	Transfusions (first line), growth factors, iron chelation, clinical trials (hypomethylating agents)
Low-risk MDS with ringed sideroblasts	Luspatercept (with ringed sideroblasts) (not yet commercially available), transfusions, iron chelation
Del(5q) MDS	Lenalidomide
Hypoplastic MDS	Immunosuppressive therapy (ATG)
Intermediate- to high-risk MDS (HR-MDS)	Hypomethylating agents (azacitidine, decitabine) or intensive AML-based induction chemotherapy (see Chapter 2) ± allogeneic stem cell transplantation, transfusion support, iron chelation, clinical trials
TP53 mutant MDS	Decitabine (10-day regimen)
Therapy-related MDS	Treatment for therapy-related AML (see Chapter 2), hypomethylating agents, allogeneic stem cell transplantation
IDH1/IDH2 mutant MDS	Clinical trials (ivosidenib, enasidenib, venetoclax-based therapy)
Paroxysmal nocturnal hemoglobinuria (PNH)	Eculizimab, anticoagulation (prior thromboses)
Severe aplastic anemia	Immunosuppressive therapy (ATG, CSA, eltrombopag), Danazol (telomere abnormalities), allogeneic stem cell transplant
Clonal hematopoiesis of indeterminate potential (CHIP)/clonal cytopenia of unknown significance (CCUS)	Close monitoring of complete blood cell counts with consideration of marrow biopsy and repeat mutational profiling if progressive cytopenia develop, modification of cardiovascular risk factors

RPS14, *CDC25C*, and *PPP2CA*). The agent specifically targets del(5q) clones while also promoting erythropoiesis and repopulation of the bone marrow in normal cells. Lenalidomide induces responses in up to one third of non-5q– MDS patients who demonstrate a specific defect in erythroid differentiation on gene expression profiling.

Intermediate to high risk MDS patients
Epigenetic therapy. The recognition that epigenetic modifications of the abnormal HSC clones in MDS affect cell growth and apoptosis and are central to disease pathogenesis has led to the successful therapeutic application of two DNA methyltransferase inhibitors (i.e., azacitidine and decitabine) for this disease. These two agents, termed *hypomethylating agents (HMA)*, are hypothesized to reverse the abnormal hypermethylation and gene silencing in abnormal HSCs. Although not curative, HMA are a cornerstone of therapy for higher-risk MDS patients ineligible for and/or unwilling to pursue alloSCT. In a phase III clinical trial of intermediate-2 to high-risk MDS patients, azacitidine significantly prolonged overall survival as compared with cytotoxic chemotherapy or supportive care only. Azacitidine delayed the time to leukemic transformation in two thirds of patients with transfusion-dependent MDS, reduced transfusion requirements, and improved quality of life compared with transfusion support alone. These results were the first to demonstrate that any therapy could alter the natural history of MDS and established azacitidine as the gold standard for treatment. Decitabine, a related compound to azacytidine, is an alternative hypomethylating agent approved for high-risk MDS patients based on the results of multiple studies showing that this agent induced higher remission rates and reduced transfusion needs as compared with supportive care and historical controls. Although decitabine has not yet resulted in an overall survival benefit in MDS patients, the shorter duration of administration (5 days for decitabine vs. 7 days for azacytidine) and the more myelosuppressive nature of this agent has led it to be preferred for some patients with higher-risk MDS with increased white blood cell count and/or blasts.

Hypomethylating therapy resulting in chronic (epigenetic) modification of MDS cells differs from cytotoxic chemotherapy in several ways. Prolonged administration of HMA is needed to induce and maintain efficacy. Therapeutic responses are often not seen until at least 4 to 6 months after treatment initiation and, once achieved, require ongoing monthly administration to maintain response and transfusion-independence. Moreover, marrow responses are not required as MDS patients receiving azacitidine who did not achieve a defined complete remission still survived significantly longer than patients treated with supportive care alone. Whether outcomes of hypomethylating therapy differ based on mutational status of MDS patients is not clear. One study reported more favorable outcomes in poor prognosis MDS patients characterized by TP53 mutations who received a 10-day decitabine regimen. Despite the positive results of HMA therapy in many individuals with MDS, no patients are ultimately cured of their disease, and durable remissions are infrequent. Patients whose disease has progressed on HMA therapy have short overall survival and therefore ideally should be referred for investigational agents and/or allogeneic stem cell transplantation.

Stem cell transplantation. As in other hematologic stem cell disorders, the only curative therapy for MDS patients remains alloSCT, ideally performed at complete remission. All MDS patients younger than 40 years with an available HLA-matched sibling donor are typically offered transplantation at diagnosis. Long-term disease-free survival rates for patients with low-risk disease are greater than 50%; however, the high transplantation-related mortality, morbidity, and relapse rates associated with mismatched or unrelated donor transplants or with transplantation in older MDS patients have usually limited the use of these transplants to patients with high-risk disease. In the past, patients with intermediate-2 or high-risk MDS (i.e., MDS with cytogenetic abnormalities predisposing to leukemic transformation or high levels of blasts or intermediate-2 or higher scores on IPSS classification systems) (see Tables 1.5, 1.6, 1.7, 1.8, and 1.9) have been offered acute leukemia-based chemotherapy regimens (see Chapter 2) designed to eradicate rapidly proliferating blast cells, not dysfunctional MDS cells. Because such therapy for MDS patients is associated with a high relapse rate within 12 to 18 months and no significant prolongation of overall survival, even for patients who achieve remission, such patients are now increasingly being offered hypomethylating agents. Regardless, subsequent

表 1.9 骨髓衰竭综合征的推荐治疗	
患者类型	推荐治疗
低危 MDS（LR-MDS）	输血（一线治疗）、生长因子、铁螯合剂、临床试验（去甲基化药物）
低危 MDS 伴环形铁粒幼细胞	罗特西普（伴环形铁粒幼细胞患者；尚未上市）、输血、铁螯合剂
5q 缺失综合征 MDS	来那度胺
低增生性 MDS	免疫抑制治疗（ATG）
中高危 MDS（HR-MDS）	去甲基化药物（阿扎胞苷、地西他滨）或用于 AML 的强化诱导治疗（见第 2 章）± 异基因造血干细胞移植、输血、铁螯合剂、临床试验
伴 TP53 突变的 MDS	地西他滨（10 天方案）
治疗相关性 MDS	治疗相关性 AML 的治疗（见第 2 章）、去甲基化药物、异基因造血干细胞移植
伴 IDH1/IDH2 突变的 MDS	临床试验（基于艾伏尼布、恩西地平、维奈克拉的治疗）
阵发性睡眠性血红蛋白尿症（PNH）	依库珠单抗、抗凝治疗（既往血栓形成）
重型再生障碍性贫血	免疫抑制治疗（ATG、CSA、艾曲泊帕）、达那唑（端粒异常）、异基因造血干细胞移植
潜能未定克隆性造血（CHIP）/意义未明的克隆性血细胞减少（CCUS）	密切监测全血细胞计数，如果出现进行性血细胞减少，应考虑进行骨髓活检和重复突变分析、改善心血管危险因素

隆，同时可促进红细胞生成和骨髓中正常细胞的再增殖。来那度胺可诱导约 1/3 的非 5q-MDS 患者获得治疗应答，这些患者在基因表达谱中显示红系分化存在特定缺陷。

中高危患者

表观遗传学治疗 随着人们认识到异常 HSC 克隆的表观遗传学修饰影响细胞生长和凋亡是 MDS 发病机制的核心，两种 DNA 甲基转移酶抑制剂（即阿扎胞苷和地西他滨）被成功应用于该病的治疗。这两种药物被称为去甲基化药物（HMA），并被认为可以逆转异常 HSC 的过度甲基化和基因沉默。尽管不能治愈，但 HMA 是不适合或不愿意接受 alloSCT 的较高危 MDS 患者的治疗基石。在一项针对中危-2 至高危 MDS 患者的Ⅲ期临床试验中，与细胞毒性化疗或单纯支持治疗相比，阿扎胞苷显著延长了总体生存期。阿扎胞苷可延长 2/3 的输血依赖性 MDS 患者的白血病转化时间，减少输血需求，并改善生活质量。上述结果首次证明了该治疗可以改变 MDS 的自然病程，并确立了阿扎胞苷作为治疗的金标准。地西他滨（阿扎胞苷的相关化合物）是高危 MDS 患者的另一种治疗选择，多项研究结果显示，与支持治疗和历史对照相比，地西他滨在较高危 MDS 患者中的缓解率更高，并能减少输血需求。尽管地西他滨尚未在 MDS 患者中表现出总体生存获益，但其较短的给药时间（地西他滨为 5 天，阿扎胞苷为 7 天）和更强的骨髓抑制特性，使其成为白细胞增多和（或）原始细胞增多的较高危 MDS 患者的首选药物。

导致 MDS 细胞慢性（表观遗传学）修饰的 HMA 治疗与细胞毒性化疗有以下几个方面的不同。HMA 需要长期使用才能诱导和维持疗效。治疗应答通常在治疗开始后至少 4~6 个月才会出现，一旦出现治疗应答，需要持续每月给药以维持疗效和脱离输血。此外，骨髓缓解不是必需的，因为接受阿扎胞苷治疗的 MDS 患者即使没有达到定义的完全缓解，生存时间仍显著长于仅接受支持治疗的患者。目前尚不清楚 HMA 治疗的疗效是否因 MDS 患者的突变状态而有所不同。一项研究报告，接受 10 天地西他滨方案的 TP53 突变、预后不良的 MDS 患者具有更好的治疗结果。尽管去甲基化治疗在许多 MDS 患者中取得了积极的结果，但最终不能治愈疾病，持久缓解也很少见。在 HMA 治疗过程中疾病进展的患者总体生存期较短，因此理想情况下应转诊至接受研究性药物和（或）alloSCT。

干细胞移植 与其他血液干细胞疾病相同，对于 MDS 患者，唯一能够治愈 MDS 的手段仍然是 alloSCT，且最好在完全缓解时进行。对于所有年龄＜40 岁且有 HLA 相合的同胞供者的 MDS 患者，通常在确诊时推荐进行移植。较低危患者的长期无病生存率＞50%；然而，不相合或非亲缘供者移植或老年患者与较高的移植相关死亡率、并发症发生率和复发率相关，因此对于上述情况，仅推荐对高危患者进行移植治疗。在过去，中危-2 或高危 MDS（即伴有白血病转化高风险细胞遗传学异常或原始细胞水平高的 MDS 或 IPSS 评分为中危-2 或更高）的患者（表 1.5 至表 1.9）通常被推荐使用急性白血病的化疗方案（见第 2 章），旨在消除快速增殖的原始细胞，而非功能失调的 MDS 细胞。由于这种治疗与 12~18 个月内的高复发率相关，且未能显著延长总体生存期（即使在达到缓解的患者中），这类患者现在越来越多地被推荐使用 HMA。无论如何，随后的 alloSCT 仍然是绝大多数 MDS 患者获得长期最

alloSCT offers the best long-term outcome in the majority of MDS patients.

Outcomes following alloSCT can be predicted based on molecular biology of the MDS disease. Over 90% of MDS patients proceeding to alloSCT will have at least one somatic mutation with certain mutations such as *TP53*, *RAS*, and *JAK2V617F* associated with shorter survival and increased risk of disease recurrence following transplant. Persistence or clearance of any pretransplant MDS-associated gene mutation is also important. Detection of a mutation with a variant allele frequency of at least 0.5% at 30 days after transplant correlated with disease progression. These findings point to the importance of enhancing treatment options for MDS prior to alloSCT for optimal outcomes.

PROSPECTUS FOR THE FUTURE

Modern genomic sequencing technologies have revolutionized research in stem cell biology and marrow failure syndromes by allowing parallel assessment of hundreds of genes, pathways, and biologic processes. The study of HSC function in marrow failure syndromes provides hints of specific molecular pathways disturbed in many diseases of hematopoietic and nonhematopoietic stem cells. These observations are furthering our knowledge about the complex interplay among AA, PNH, and MDS. Understanding stem cells' plasticity and regulatory roles promises new therapeutic avenues for a wide array of diseases.

Characterization of the complex genomic landscape of MDS has revealed that almost 80% of cases are characterized by at least one oncogenic mutation, and more than 40 unique genes are recurrently mutated. Much research remains to be done to determine how best to incorporate this vast amount of information into the prognosis of MDS patients. In addition, it is estimated that up to 10% to 15% of patients with MDS, particularly younger individuals, have disease arising from inherited familial genetic predisposition syndromes with germline mutations in genes such as *DDX1* and *RUNX1* that promote aberrant myeloid cell development. Careful acquisition of personal and family history is therefore key for any individual with marrow failure disorders. Routine referral of MDS patients younger than 50 years of age and/or with appropriate family history or specific gene mutations detected on molecular testing is strongly recommended.

Multiple agents targeting the unique biologic features of ineffective hematopoiesis in marrow failure syndromes have moved into the forefront of treatment for these diseases over the last few years. These include eculizumab in PNH, immunosuppressive drugs and eltrombopag in AA and MDS subsets, azacitidine and decitabine in higher-risk MDS, and lenalidomide in 5q– MDS. Advances in allogeneic stem cell transplantation, specifically the now widespread use of reduced intensity and haploidentical transplantation protocols, has made this option a reality for many individuals who would not have been eligible for this life-extending procedure in the past.

Current clinical trials are actively investigating a new wave of tailored therapies for specific MDS biologic signatures. Examples of this include a p53 reactivating agent (APR-246) for p53 mutant MDS, a telomerase inhibitor (imetelstat) for lower-intermediate-risk MDS, a CD123-directed antibody-toxin conjugate (tagraxofusp) for MPN/MDS, and multiple immune checkpoint inhibitors added to hypomethylating therapy for higher-risk MDS. Ongoing clinical trials are also exploring the potential translation of multiple agents recently approved for acute myeloid leukemia to high-risk MDS patients, given the significant clinical and biological overlap of these two disease states. These included enasidenib for *IDH2* mutant MDS, ivosidenib for *IDH1* mutant MDS, and most importantly, venetoclax plus azacytidine or decitabine or low-dose cytarabine for MDS independent of mutation status (see Chapter 2).

Finally, the contribution of hematopoietic stem cells to global health issues is increasingly being recognized and explored. Genomic sequencing has allowed us to discern that many healthy individuals without overt hematologic abnormalities in fact have clonal somatic gene mutations in hematopoietic stem and progenitor cells (termed *clonal hematopoiesis of indeterminate potential* or *CHIP*). The incidence of CHIP appears to increase with age of the individual, likely due to mutational events over time and other yet to be determined genetic and environmental predisposing factors. Over time, individuals with CHIP have an increased risk of developing overt hematologic cancers, particularly therapy-related MDS/AML following exposure to myelosuppressive agents (chemotherapy or radiation) and depending on the specific mutation identified. In many individuals, identification of new cytopenias in these patients (termed *clonal cytopenias of unknown significance* or *CCUS*) may represent the next step in the continuum to development of MDS. CHIP has been associated with other health problems. In one study, presence of CHIP was linked to almost twice the risk of developing coronary heart disease in individuals without other risk factors. Preclinical models of CHIP in mice have demonstrated that CHIP is linked to accelerated atherosclerosis potentially due to higher baseline underlying inflammatory processes. Studies exploring how best to utilize this information for preventive and/or therapeutic purposes are ongoing.

For a deeper discussion of these topics, please see Chapter 147, "Hematopoiesis and Hematopoietic Growth Factors," in *Goldman-Cecil Medicine*, 26th Edition.

SUGGESTED READINGS

Bejar R, Stevenson KE, Caughey BA, et al: Validation of a prognostic model and the impact of mutations in patients with lower-risk myelodysplastic syndromes, J Clin Oncol 30:3376–3382, 2012.

Duncavage EJ, Jacoby MA, Chang GS, et al: Mutation clearance after transplantation for myelodysplastic syndrome, N Engl J Med 379(11):1028–1041, 2018.

Fenaux P, Mufti GJ, Hellstrom-Lindberg E, et al: Efficacy of azacitidine compared with that of conventional care regimens in the treatment of higher-risk myelodysplastic syndromes: a randomised, open-label, phase III study, Lancet Oncol 10(3):223–232, 2009.

Fenaux P, Platzbecker U, Mufti GJ, et al. The MEDALIST trial: results of a phase 3, randomized, double-blind, placebo-controlled study of Luspatercept to treat anemia in patients with very low-, low-, or intermediate-risk myelodysplastic syndromes (MDS) with ring sideroblasts (RS) who require red blood cell (RBC) transfusions. Abstract #1. Presented at the 2018 ASH Annual Meeting, December 2, 2018, San Diego, CA.

Germing U, Schroeder T, Kaivers J, et al: Novel therapies in low- and high-risk myelodysplastic syndromes, Expert Rev Hematol 12(10):893–908, 2019.

Hillmen P, Muus P, Roth A, et al.: Long-term safety and efficacy of sustained eculizumab treatment in patients with paroxysmal nocturnal haemoglobinuria, Br J Haematol 162:2–73, 2013.

Jaiswal S, Natarajan P, Silver AJ, et al: N Engl J Med 377(2):111–121, 2017.

Krönke J, Fink EC, Hollenbach PW, et al.: Lenalidomide induces ubiquination and degradation of CK1alpha in del(5q) MDS, Nature 523(7559):183–188, 2015.

Lindsley RC, Saber W, Mar BG, et al: Prognostic mutations in myelodysplastic syndrome after stem cell transplantation, N Engl J Med 376(6):536–547, 2017.

Olnes MJ, Scheinberg P, Calvo KR, et al: Eltrombopag and improved hematopoiesis in refractory aplastic anemia, N Engl J Med 367:11–19, 2012.

Papaemmanuil E, Gerstung M, Malcovati L, et al: Clinical and biological implications of driver mutations in myelodysplastic syndromes, Blood 122:3616–3627, 2013.

Platzbecker U: Treatment of MDS, Blood 133(10):1096–1107, 2019.

佳结局的治疗手段。

MDS 患者接受 alloSCT 后的结局可以通过分子生物学检查来预测。超过 90% 接受 alloSCT 的 MDS 患者会有至少 1 种体细胞突变，其中一些突变（如 TP53、RAS 和 JAK2V617F）与移植后较短的生存期和较高的疾病复发风险相关。移植前 MDS 相关基因突变是持续存在还是清除也很重要。在移植后 30 天检测到突变的变异等位基因频率 ≥ 0.5% 与疾病进展相关。这些发现表明，MDS 患者在 alloSCT 前的治疗选择对获得最佳结局非常重要。

未来展望

现代基因组测序技术可同时对数百个基因、通路和生物过程进行评估，从而彻底改变了干细胞生物学和骨髓衰竭综合征的研究。对骨髓衰竭综合征中 HSC 功能的研究揭示了许多造血和非造血干细胞疾病中涉及的特定分子通路。这些发现加深了人们对 AA、PNH 和 MDS 之间复杂相互作用的认识。理解干细胞的可塑性和调控作用有望为更多的疾病提供新的治疗途径。

MDS 复杂的基因组图谱特征揭示，近 80% 的患者至少存在 1 种致癌基因突变，且超过 40 个基因反复发生突变。目前关于如何将这些海量信息融入 MDS 患者的预后评估中，仍需进行大量研究工作。此外，据估计，在多达 10%～15% 的 MDS 患者（尤其是年轻患者）中，该病源于家族遗传易感综合征中的生殖系基因突变，如 DDX1 和 RUNX1 突变促进髓系细胞异常发育。因此，仔细收集个人史和家族史对于骨髓衰竭综合征疾病患者十分重要。强烈建议对 50 岁以下的 MDS 患者和（或）具有相关家族史或在分子检测中发现特定基因突变的患者进行常规转诊。

近年来，针对骨髓衰竭综合征中无效造血的多种药物已成为治疗此类疾病的前沿药物。这些药物包括用于治疗 PNH 的依库珠单抗、用于治疗 AA 和 MDS 部分亚型的免疫抑制药和艾曲泊帕、用于治疗较高危 MDS 的阿扎胞苷和地西他滨，以及用于治疗 5q－MDS 的来那度胺。alloSCT 的进展，特别是目前广泛使用的减低剂量预处理和半相合移植方案，使得许多过去无法移植的患者有机会接受移植。

目前临床试验正在积极研究针对 MDS 特异性生物标志物的新一代个体化治疗。例如，用于治疗 p53 突变型 MDS 的 p53 反应激活剂（APR-246）、用于治疗低中危 MDS 的端粒酶抑制剂（伊美司他）、用于治疗 MPN/MDS 的 CD123 靶向抗体－毒素结合物（tagraxofusp），以及多种用于治疗较高危 MDS 的加入 HMA 治疗中的免疫检查点抑制剂。正在进行的临床试验还在探索近期获批用于 AML 的多种药物在较高危 MDS 患者中转化应用的潜能，因为这两种疾病状态在临床和生物学上有显著的重叠。这些药物包括用于治疗 IDH2 突变型 MDS 的恩西地平、用于治疗 IDH1 突变型 MDS 的艾伏尼布，以及用于治疗 MDS（无论突变状态如何）的维奈克拉＋阿扎胞苷或地西他滨或低剂量阿糖胞苷（见第 2 章）。

造血干细胞对全球健康问题的贡献正逐渐被认识和探索。基因组测序使我们能够发现许多没有明显血液学异常的健康个体的造血干祖细胞中具有克隆性体细胞基因突变［即潜能未定克隆性造血（CHIP）］。CHIP 的发生率似乎随年龄的增长而升高，这可能是由于突变事件增多和其他尚未确定的遗传及环境易感因素。随着时间的推移，具有 CHIP 的个体进展为明显的血液学肿瘤的风险增加，特别是在接受化疗或放疗后可能发生治疗相关性 MDS/AML，具体风险取决于特定突变。在许多患者中，出现新发血细胞减少［即意义未明的克隆性血细胞减少（CCUS）］可能提示进展到 MDS 进程的下一个阶段。CHIP 与其他健康问题有关。一项研究发现，具有 CHIP 的患者在没有其他危险因素的情况下，冠心病的发病风险几乎增加了两倍。CHIP 小鼠的临床前模型显示，由于潜在炎症的基线水平更高，CHIP 与加速动脉粥样硬化有关。探讨如何优化利用这些信息以便预防和（或）治疗的研究正在进行中。

有关此专题的深入讨论，请参阅 *Goldman-Cecil Medicine* 第 26 版第 147 章"造血和造血生长因子"。

推荐阅读

Bejar R, Stevenson KE, Caughey BA, et al: Validation of a prognostic model and the impact of mutations in patients with lower-risk myelodysplastic syndromes, J Clin Oncol 30:3376–3382, 2012.

Duncavage EJ, Jacoby MA, Chang GS, et al: Mutation clearance after transplantation for myelodysplastic syndrome, N Engl J Med 379(11):1028–1041, 2018.

Fenaux P, Mufti GJ, Hellstrom-Lindberg E, et al: Efficacy of azacitidine compared with that of conventional care regimens in the treatment of higher-risk myelodysplastic syndromes: a randomised, open-label, phase III study, Lancet Oncol 10(3):223–232, 2009.

Fenaux P, Platzbecker U, Mufti GJ, et al. THE MEDALIST trial: results of a phase 3, randomized, double-blind, placebo-controlled study of Luspatercept to treat anemia in patients with very low-, low-, or intermediate-risk myelodysplastic syndromes (MDS) with ring sideroblasts (RS) who require red blood cell (RBC) transfusions. Abstract #1. Presented at the 2018 ASH Annual Meeting, December 2, 2018, San Diego, CA.

Germing U, Schroeder T, Kaivers J, et al: Novel therapies in low- and high-risk myelodysplastic syndromes, Expert Rev Hematol12(10):893–908, 2019.

Hillmen P, Muus P, Roth A, et al..: Long-term safety and efficacy of sustained eculizumab treatment in patients with paroxysmal nocturnal haemoglobinuria, Br J Haematol 162:2–73, 2013.

Jaiswal S, Natarajan P, Silver AJ, et al: N Engl J Med 377(2):111–121, 2017.

Krönke J, Fink EC, Hollenbach PW, et al..: Lenalidomide induces ubiquination and degradation of CK1alpha in del(5q) MDS, Nature 523(7559):183–188, 2015.

Lindsley RC, Saber W, Mar BG, et al: Prognostic mutations in myelodysplastic syndrome after stem cell transplantation, N Engl J Med 376(6):536–547, 2017.

Olnes MJ, Scheinberg P, Calvo KR, et al: Eltrombopag and improved hematopoiesis in refractory aplastic anemia, N Engl J Med 367:11–19, 2012.

Papaemmanuil E, Gerstung M, Malcovati L, et al: Clinical and biological implications of driver mutations in myelodysplastic syndromes, Blood 122:3616–3627, 2013.

Platzbecker U: Treatment of MDS, Blood 133(10):1096–1107, 2019.

Risitano AM: Paroxysmal nocturnal hemoglobinuria and the complement system: recent insights and novel anticomplement strategies, Adv Exp Med Biol 735:155–172, 2013.

Steensma DP, Bejar R, Jaiswal S, et al: Clonal hematopoiesis of indeterminate potential and its distinction from myelodysplastic syndrome, Blood 126(1):9–16, 2015.

Townsley DM, Scheinberg P, Winkler T, et al: Eltrombopag for treatment of thrombocytopenia-associated disorders, N Engl J Med 376(16):1540–1550, 2017.

Welch JS, Petti AA, Miller CA, et al: TP53 and decitabine in acute myeloid leukemia and myelodysplastic syndrome, N Engl J Med 375(21):2023–2036, 2016.

Risitano AM: Paroxysmal nocturnal hemoglobinuria and the complement system: recent insights and novel anticomplement strategies, Adv Exp Med Biol 735:155–172, 2013.

Steensma DP, Bejar R, Jaiswal S, et al: Clonal hematopoiesis of indeterminate potential and its distinction from myelodysplastic syndrome, Blood 126(1):9–16, 2015.

Townsley DM, Scheinberg P, Winkler T, et al: Eltrombopag for treatment of thrombocytopenia-associated disorders, N Engl J Med 376(16):1540–1550, 2017.

Welch JS, Petti AA, Miller CA, et al: TP53 and decitabine in acute myeloid leukemia and myelodysplastic syndrome, N Engl J Med 375(21):2023–2036, 2016.

Clonal Disorders of the Hematopoietic Stem Cell

Eunice S. Wang, Nancy Berliner

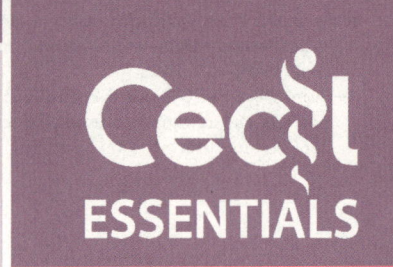

INTRODUCTION

Malignant transformation involves combined defects in cellular maturation and differentiation. The multistep theory of oncogenesis suggests that these defects are often separable and contribute to a stepwise progression from a normal to a fully transformed cell. The continuous cycling of hematopoietic cells provides a milieu for the development of clonal genetic abnormalities that supports the multistep model. Clonal defects of the hematopoietic stem cell give rise to an array of premalignant and malignant disorders. Primary defects of maturation give rise to the myelodysplastic disorders (see Chapter 1), whereas loss of normal control of proliferation results in myeloproliferative disease encompassing chronic and acute leukemias.

MYELOPROLIFERATIVE NEOPLASMS

Definition and Etiology

Myeloproliferative neoplasms (MPN), previously known as chronic myeloproliferative diseases, are clonal stem cell disorders characterized by leukocytosis, thrombocytosis, erythrocytosis, splenomegaly, and bone marrow hypercellularity. The hallmark of MPN is the failure of a transformed multipotent stem cell to respond to normal feedback mechanisms regulating hematopoietic cell mass. Stem cells from patients with MPN demonstrate clonal colony growth in vitro when they are grown in serum without the addition of exogenous cytokines, and this technique historically was used as a diagnostic test for MPN. MPN have traditionally been divided into four classic disorders based on the predominant hyperproliferative cell type: polycythemia vera (PV), essential thrombocytosis (ET), primary myelofibrosis (PMF; i.e., idiopathic myelofibrosis or agnogenic myeloid metaplasia), and chronic myelogenous leukemia (CML). Hypereosinophilic syndrome, mast cell disease, and other less common diseases characterized by profuse myeloid cell proliferation are also considered MPN but are not traditionally included among these "classic" disease subsets (Table 2.1).

The pathogenesis of MPN arises from mutational and biologic processes resulting in dysfunctional kinases that promote unabated myeloid growth and expansion. This is often accompanied by aberrant cytokine production affecting the marrow microenvironment, a gradual shift in hematopoietic cell production from the bone marrow to extramedullary sites in the liver and spleen, and altered coagulation. In CML, a well-described reciprocal translocation between chromosomes 9 and 22 termed the "Philadelphia chromosome" results in an Abelson (ABL) leukemia virus–breakpoint cluster region (BCR) fusion protein (BCR/ABL) with constitutive kinase activity. In PV, PMF, and ET, a mutation involving the substitution of a valine for phenylalanine at position 617 (V617F) in the *Janus kinase 2 (JAK2)* has been identified in most patients and accounts for the abnormal growth properties that characterize these stem cell disorders. In those patients with MPN lacking an actual *JAK2V617F* mutation, upregulation of JAK-STAT signaling pathways has been demonstrated due to other etiologies, supporting common mechanisms of action in all MPN. Other mutations commonly identified in MPN cells include *CALR*, *ASXL1*, and *RUNX1*.

Clinical complications of MPN arise from the overproduction of one or more lineages in the blood. Over time, all MPN can undergo clonal evolution with acquisition of additional cytogenetic and molecular events leading to blastic transformation and eventually acute leukemia. With the exception of CML, this is an infrequent and late complication. Although all MPN are mechanistically related, significant differences still exist in each clinical disease presentation warranting specific therapeutic considerations for each type as will be discussed.

POLYCYTHEMIA VERA

Definition and Epidemiology

PV, literally meaning "increased numbers of red blood cells in the blood," is a syndrome characterized by significantly increased red blood cell mass in the peripheral blood resulting from a clonal multipotent hematopoietic stem cell (HSC) defect. PV is relatively uncommon with an incidence of 1 to 3 of 100,000 people and a median age at diagnosis of 65 years.

Clinical Presentation

PV is a primary clonal stem cell disorder of unknown origin that is characterized by predominant erythrocytosis associated with other hematopoietic abnormalities. Although one half of patients have concurrent leukocytosis or thrombocytosis, erythrocytosis is the hallmark and the cause of the most serious clinical complications of this disease. Typically, patients complain of headache, visual problems, mental clouding, and pruritus after bathing. Occlusive vascular events such as stroke, transient ischemic attacks, myocardial ischemia, and digital pain, paresthesias, or gangrene are common. Pulmonary, deep vein, hepatic, and portal vein thromboses may occur. Paradoxically, patients are also predisposed to hemorrhagic events such as gastrointestinal and mucosal bleeding caused by abnormal platelet function and also ischemic necrosis downstream from vascular occlusion. Physical examination may show retinal vein occlusion, ruddy cyanosis, digital ischemia, and splenomegaly.

Diagnosis and Differential Diagnosis

When patients are first diagnosed with an elevated hemoglobin concentration per unit volume (i.e., erythrocytosis), the initial evaluation

造血干细胞克隆性疾病

孙葳 译 孙于谦 审校 黄晓军 通审

引言

造血细胞发生分化和成熟异常可导致恶性转化。肿瘤发生的多步骤理论认为，分化和成熟异常通常先后发生，逐步积累，导致肿瘤发生。造血细胞的持续分裂为克隆性遗传变异提供了基础，从而支持肿瘤发生的多步骤理论。造血干细胞的克隆异常可导致一系列白血病前期和白血病的发生。原发性造血细胞成熟异常可导致骨髓增生异常性疾病（见第1章），而细胞增殖调控异常可导致骨髓增生性疾病，包括急性和慢性白血病。

骨髓增殖性肿瘤

定义和病因学

骨髓增殖性肿瘤（MPN）又称慢性骨髓增生性疾病（MPD），是以白细胞增多、血小板增多、红细胞增多、脾大和骨髓增生活跃为特征的克隆性干细胞疾病。MPN的标志是转化的多能干细胞不受正常的造血调控。MPN患者的造血干细胞在不添加外源性细胞因子的血清中进行体外培养时可以呈现克隆性集落生长，该技术曾被作为MPN的诊断性检查。传统上，根据主要的过度增殖细胞类型，MPN可分为4种典型疾病：真性红细胞增多症（PV）、原发性血小板增多症（ET）、原发性骨髓纤维化（PMF；即特发性骨髓纤维化）和慢性髓细胞性白血病（CML）。此外还包括高嗜酸性粒细胞增多综合征（HES）、肥大细胞病和其他罕见疾病，这些罕见疾病以大量髓系细胞增殖为特征，虽也被认为是MPN，但传统上不包括在这些"典型"疾病亚群中（表2.1）。

MPN的发病机制源于导致激酶功能失调的突变和生物过程，从而促进髓系持续生长和扩张。这通常伴随着影响骨髓微环境的异常细胞因子生成，造血细胞生成从骨髓产生逐渐转移到髓外部位（如肝和脾），并改变凝血功能。在CML中，9号和22号染色体（即费城染色体）之间的相互易位导致具有组成型激酶活性的Abelson（ABL）白血病病毒-断裂点丛集区（BCR）融合蛋白（BCR/ABL）的形成。大多数PV、PMF和ET患者可检测出Janus激酶2基因（JAK2）V617F突变，导致该位点缬氨酸被苯丙氨酸所取代，该突变可以解释这些干细胞疾病的异常生长特性。在缺乏JAK2V617F突变的MPN患者中，由其他病因导致的JAK-STAT信号通路上调已得到证实，这支持了所有MPN的共同作用机制。MPN细胞中常见的其他突变基因包括CALR、ASXL1和RUNX1。

MPN的临床并发症由血液中单系或多系细胞过度生成所致。随着时间的推移，所有MPN都会经历克隆进化，并获得额外的细胞遗传学和分子事件，引起原始细胞转化，最终导致急性白血病。除CML外，转化为急性白血病是少见的晚期并发症。尽管所有MPN在机制上都是相关的，但每种临床疾病的表现仍然存在显著差异，需要针对每种类型选择特定的治疗（见下文）。

真性红细胞增多症

定义和流行病学

真性红细胞增多症（PV）是指血液中红细胞数量增多，是由克隆性多能造血干细胞异常引起的外周血中红细胞增多的综合征。PV的发病率为（1~3）/10 000，诊断时的中位年龄为65岁。

临床表现

PV是一种原发性克隆性干细胞疾病，病因不明，其特征主要为与造血异常相关的红细胞增多。虽然1/2的患者合并白细胞增多或血小板增多，但红细胞增多是该病的特征和严重并发症的原因。患者可出现头痛、视觉问题、精神错乱和沐浴后瘙痒。闭塞性血管事件较为多见，如卒中、短暂性脑缺血发作、心肌缺血和指端疼痛、感觉异常或坏疽。也可能出现肺静脉、深静脉、肝静脉和门静脉血栓。矛盾的是，患者也易发生出血事件（如胃肠道出血和黏膜出血），这可能是由于血小板功能异常和血管阻塞导致的缺血性坏死。体格检查通常提示视网膜静脉阻塞、皮肤呈绛紫色和脾大。

诊断和鉴别诊断

当患者首次被发现血红蛋白水平升高（即红细

TABLE 2.1 World Health Organization 2016 Classification of Myeloid Neoplasms

1. Acute myeloid leukemia
2. MDS
3. MPNs
   a. Chronic myelogenous leukemia
   b. Polycythemia vera
   c. Essential thrombocythemia
   d. Primary myelofibrosis
   e. Chronic neutrophilic leukemia
   f. Chronic eosinophilic leukemia, not otherwise categorized
   g. Hypereosinophilic syndrome
   h. Mast cell disease
   i. MPNs, unclassifiable
4. MDS, MPN
5. Myeloid neoplasms associated with eosinophilia and abnormalities of PDGF-RA, PDGF-RB, or FGF-R1

From Swerdlow SH, Campo E, Harris NL, Jaffe ES, Pileri SA, Stein H, Thiele J. WHO Classification of Tumours of Haematopoietic and Lymphoid Tissues (Revised Fourth Edition), IARC, 2016.
FGF-R1, Fibroblast growth factor receptor 1; MDS, myelodysplastic syndrome; MPN, myeloproliferative neoplasm; PDGF-RA, platelet-derived growth factor receptor-α polypeptide; PDGF-RB, platelet-derived growth factor receptor-β polypeptide.

TABLE 2.2 Causes of Erythrocytosis

I. Relative or spurious erythrocytosis (normal red cell mass)
   A. Hemoconcentration due to dehydration (e.g., diarrhea, diaphoresis, diuretics, water deprivation, emesis, ethanol, hypertension, preeclampsia, pheochromocytoma, carbon monoxide intoxication)
II. True or absolute erythrocytosis
   A. Polycythemia vera
   B. Primary congenital polycythemia
   C. Secondary erythrocytosis due to
      1. Congenital causes (e.g., activating mutation of erythropoietin receptor)
      2. Hypoxia caused by carbon monoxide poisoning, high oxygen affinity hemoglobin, high-altitude residence, chronic pulmonary disease, hypoventilation syndromes such as sleep apnea, right-to-left cardiac shunt, neurologic defects involving the respiratory center
      3. Nonhypoxic causes with pathologic erythropoietin production
         a. Renal disease (e.g., cysts, hydronephrosis, renal artery stenosis, focal glomerulonephritis, renal transplantation)
         b. Tumors (e.g., renal cell cancer, hepatocellular carcinoma, cerebellar hemangioblastoma, uterine fibromyoma, adrenal tumors, meningioma, pheochromocytoma)
      4. Drug-associated causes
         a. Androgen therapy
         b. Exogenous erythropoietin growth factor therapy

Modified from Hoffman R, Benz EJ, Shattil SJ, et al, editors: Hematology: basic principles and practice, ed 2, New York, 1995, Churchill Livingstone.

TABLE 2.3 World Health Organization 2016 Diagnostic Criteria for Polycythemia Vera

Major criteria[a,b]
1. Hemoglobin (Hgb) >16.5 g/dL (men), >16.0 (women); or hematocrit (Hct) >49% (men), >48% (women) or increased red cell mass (RCM) (more than 25% above mean normal predicted value)
2. Bone marrow biopsy showing hypercellularity for age with trilineage growth (panmyelosis) including prominent erythroid, granulocytic, and megakaryocytic proliferation with pleomorphic, mature megakaryocytes (differences in size)
3. Presence of JAK2 or JAK2 exon 12 mutation

Minor criteria
1. Subnormal serum erythropoietin level

From Swerdlow SH, Campo E, Harris NL, Jaffe ES, Pileri SA, Stein H, Thiele J. WHO Classification of Tumours of Haematopoietic and Lymphoid Tissues (Revised Fourth Edition), IARC, 2016.
[a]PV diagnosis requires meeting either all three major criteria or the first two major criteria and one minor criterion.
[b]Criterion number 2 (bone marrow biopsy) may not be required in cases with sustained absolute erythrocytosis: hemoglobin levels 18.5 g/dL in men (hematocrit 55.5%) or 16.5 g/dL in women (hematocrit 49.5%) if major criterion 3 and the minor criterion are present. However, initial myelofibrosis (present in up to 20% of patients) can only be detected by performing a bone marrow biopsy; this finding may predict a more rapid progression to overt myelofibrosis (post-PV MF).

should focus on whether this increase reflects an enhanced red cell mass (i.e., absolute erythrocytosis or polycythemia) or a normal red cell mass in the setting of a decreased plasma volume (i.e., relative erythrocytosis caused by reduced intravascular volume or other causes). The latter condition is not true polycythemia (Table 2.2). Polycythemia or absolute erythrocytosis is an absolute increase in red cell mass caused by increased red blood cell production. Under normal conditions, the body's ability to increase red blood cell production in states of hypoxemia, anemia, hemolysis, and acute blood loss ensures continuous oxygen delivery to tissues. In response to physiologic stimuli, pluripotent stem cell precursors are activated by erythropoietin (EPO) to differentiate into erythroid progenitor cells and eventually into hemoglobin-carrying erythrocytes. When numbers of mature red blood cells are adequate, a negative feedback mechanism suppresses further EPO production, and the serum hemoglobin level remains normal.

Diagnosis of PV was formerly one of exclusion based on an elevated red cell mass, splenomegaly, thrombocytosis, leukocytosis, lack of hypoxemia and other secondary causes of polycythemia, and elevated levels of leukocyte alkaline phosphatase and serum vitamin B_{12}–binding protein levels. Red blood cells in the peripheral blood often appear microcytic, with or without iron deficiency. Bone marrow examination shows a hypercellular marrow with pronounced hyperplasia of erythroid lineage cells. Cytogenetic features at the time of diagnosis are usually normal. The development of clonal cytogenetic abnormalities heralds transformation in the later stages of disease. The discovery of JAK2 gene mutations in 97% of patients with PV as well as other mutations (such as CALR and ASXL1) and findings elucidating the underlying disease pathophysiology led to new diagnostic criteria (Table 2.3). A suspected diagnosis of PV can now be confirmed in individuals with elevated hemoglobin and/or hematocrit levels by testing for a JAK2 mutation, bone marrow demonstrating trilineage proliferation, and documentation of subnormal serum EPO levels.

Treatment and Prognosis

Early recognition and treatment of PV are important because untreated patients with PV suffer significant morbidity and mortality from thromboembolic complications involving the cerebral, coronary, and mesenteric circulations. Twenty percent of patients show symptoms of arterial and venous thrombosis, and thrombosis remains the most common cause of death. Without treatment, up to one half of patients

表 2.1　髓系肿瘤的 WHO 2016 分类

1. 急性髓系白血病
2. MDS
3. MPN
   a. 慢性髓细胞性白血病
   b. 真性红细胞增多症
   c. 原发性血小板增多症
   d. 原发性骨髓纤维化
   e. 慢性中性粒细胞白血病
   f. 慢性嗜酸性粒细胞白血病，非特指型
   g. 嗜酸性粒细胞增多综合征
   h. 肥大细胞病
   i. MPN，非特指型
4. MDS/MPN
5. 与嗜酸性粒细胞增多和 PDGF-RA、PDGF-RB 或 FGF-R1 异常相关的髓系肿瘤

引自 Swerdlow SH, Campo E, Harris NL, Jaffe ES, Pileri SA, Stein H, Thiele J. WHO Classification of Tumours of Haematopoietic and Lymphoid Tissues (Revised Fourth Edition), IARC, 2016.
FGF-R1，成纤维细胞生长因子受体 1；MDS，骨髓增生异常综合征；MPN，骨髓增殖性肿瘤；PDGF-RA，血小板衍生生长因子受体 α；PDGF-RB，血小板衍生生长因子受体 β。

表 2.2　红细胞增多症的原因

I. 相对或假性红细胞增多症（红细胞数量正常）
   A. 脱水引起的血液浓缩（如腹泻、出汗、利尿剂、缺水、呕吐、乙醇、高血压、先兆子痫、嗜铬细胞瘤、一氧化碳中毒）
II. 真性或绝对红细胞增多症
   A. 真性红细胞增多症
   B. 原发性先天性红细胞增多症
   C. 继发性红细胞增多症
      1. 先天性病因（如促红细胞生成素受体突变）
      2. 缺氧，由一氧化碳中毒、高氧亲和性血红蛋白、高原居住、慢性肺部疾病、低通气综合征（如睡眠呼吸暂停）、心脏右向左分流、累及呼吸中枢的神经性损伤引起的
      3. 非缺氧病因导致病理性生成红细胞生成素
         a. 肾病（如囊肿、肾盂积水、肾动脉狭窄、局灶性肾小球肾炎、肾移植）
         b. 肿瘤（如肾细胞癌、肝细胞癌、小脑血管母细胞瘤、子宫纤维肌瘤、肾上腺肿瘤、脑膜瘤、嗜铬细胞瘤）
      4. 药物相关病因
         a. 雄激素治疗
         b. 外源性促红细胞生成素生长因子治疗

改编自 Hoffman R, Benz EJ, Shattil SJ, et al, editors: Hematology: basic principles and practice, ed 2, New York, 1995, Churchill Livingstone.

表 2.3　PV 的 WHO 2016 诊断标准

主要标准 [a, b]
1. 血红蛋白（Hb）> 165 g/L（男性）、> 160 g/L（女性）；或血细胞比容（HCT）> 49%（男性）、> 48%（女性）或红细胞计数（RCM）增多（高于平均正常预测值的 25% 以上）
2. 骨髓活检显示与年龄相关的三系增生活跃（全髓细胞增殖），包括显著的红系、粒系和巨核细胞增殖伴多形性、成熟巨核细胞（细胞大小存在差异）
3. 存在 JAK2 或 JAK2 12 号外显子突变

次要标准
1. 血清促红细胞生成素水平低于正常

引自 Swerdlow SH, Campo E, Harris NL, Jaffe ES, Pileri SA, Stein H, Thiele J. WHO Classification of Tumours of Haematopoietic and Lymphoid Tissues (Revised Fourth Edition), IARC, 2016.
[a] PV 诊断要求符合 3 项主要标准，或前 2 项主要标准和 1 项次要标准。
[b] 如果存在主要标准 3 和次要标准，则在持续绝对红细胞增多症［男性血红蛋白 185 g/L（血细胞比容 55.5%）或女性血红蛋白 165 g/L（血细胞比容 49.5%）］的情况下可能不需要主要标准 2（骨髓活检）。然而，首发表现为骨髓纤维化的患者（约占 20%）只能通过骨髓活检来诊断；这可能预示着更快进展为显著的骨髓纤维化（PV 后骨髓纤维化）。

增多症）时，初始评估应着重鉴别绝对红细胞增多症（红细胞总量增多）和相对红细胞增多症（即由脱水或其他原因引起的血浆容量减少导致血液浓缩，而红细胞总量不变）。后者并非真正的红细胞增多症（表 2.2）。PV 或绝对红细胞增多症是因红细胞生成增多引起的红细胞总量绝对增加。正常情况下，机体在低氧血症、贫血、溶血和急性失血的状态下生成红细胞的能力增强，从而确保能持续输送氧气至各组织。在生理性刺激下，多能干祖细胞被红细胞生成素（EPO）活化，进而分化为红系祖细胞，并最终分化为携带血红蛋白的红细胞。当成熟红细胞的数量足够多时，机体的负反馈机制将会抑制 EPO 的生成，从而维持血清血红蛋白的正常水平。

在过去，PV 的诊断基于红细胞总量增多、脾大、血小板增多、白细胞增多，以及碱性磷酸酶和血清维生素 B_{12} 结合蛋白水平升高，并除外低氧血症和其他引起继发性红细胞增多症的原因。外周血通常出现红细胞体积小，伴或不伴铁缺乏。骨髓穿刺可见红系显著增生。诊断时细胞遗传学多为正常核型。克隆细胞遗传学异常的出现预示着疾病进展。近年来发现 97% 的 PV 患者存在 JAK2 基因突变或其他基因突变（如 CALR 和 ASXL1），并在此基础上完善了新的诊断标准（表 2.3）。目前，对于血红蛋白和（或）血细胞比容水平升高的患者，可以通过检测 JAK2 基因突变、低血清 EPO 水平、骨髓三系增生来确诊 PV 的疑似病例。

治疗和预后

PV 的早期识别和治疗非常重要，因为未经治疗的 PV 患者罹患颅内、冠状动脉和肠系膜循环血栓栓塞的发病率和死亡率明显高于接受治疗者。20% 的患者表现出动脉和静脉血栓形成的症状，血栓是最常见的死亡原因。若未经治疗，50% 的患者在诊断 PV 后的 18 个月内死于血栓并发症。个体患者发生危及生命的血

with PV may die of thrombotic complications within 18 months of diagnosis. Realization of an individual patient's risk for life-limiting thrombotic complications dictates whether therapy is required to render PV into a chronic, progressive disease.

Low-dose aspirin and treatment of asymptomatic thrombocytosis decrease thromboembolic events in low- and high-risk PV patients and are especially important in older patients with significant cardiovascular risk factors. In younger patients, nonsteroidal anti-inflammatory drugs and antiplatelet agents should be used judiciously because of the risk of gastrointestinal hemorrhage. Patients with advanced age (>60 years), prior history of thrombosis, leukocytosis, high hematocrit values, and clinical cardiovascular factors are at high risk for subsequent vascular events. Although possible, the risk of transformation of PV to acute myeloid leukemia remains relatively low with rates of 2.3% at 10 years and 5.5% at 15 years.

Therapy varies based on risk criteria. For younger patients with lower cardiovascular risk factors, intermittent phlebotomy and aspirin prophylaxis remain the mainstays of treatment and usually result in iron deficiency anemia, which further reduces the rate of red blood cell production.

Cytoreductive therapy is indicated for patients who cannot tolerate and/or fail phlebotomy, older patients with a prior history of and/or coexisting risk factors for cardiovascular events, and those with symptomatic splenomegaly. Commonly used therapies include hydroxyurea (i.e., a low-dose oral cytotoxic agent that does not appear to increase leukemic risk), pegylated interferon-α (i.e., for young patients and women during pregnancy), and anagrelide (i.e., an oral megakaryotoxic agent for treating refractory thrombocytosis). Choice of therapy is often individualized to the patient to best meet their lifestyle requirements given the chronicity of this disease. The main goal of therapy in higher-risk individuals with PV is long-term reduction of red blood cell mass as reflected in maintenance of hematocrit values less than 45% in men (and commonly less than 42% in women). In a multicenter, prospective clinical trial, adult PV patients (largely men) randomized to maintaining a therapeutic hematocrit target of less than 45% using hydroxyurea, phlebotomy, or both had a significantly lower rate of cardiovascular death (2.7% vs. 9.8%) and major thrombosis than those with a hematocrit target maintained at a higher level between 45% and 50%. As with all myeloproliferative disorders, initiation of cytoreductive therapy may precipitate hyperuricemia that results in secondary gout and uric acid stones, warranting treatment with allopurinol.

Although low-dose chemotherapeutic agents (e.g., chlorambucil, busulfan) have historically been used to treat leukocytosis and thrombocytosis not responding to hydroxyurea, these agents have fallen out of favor due to increased toxicity and risk of secondary acute myeloid or myelogenous leukemia (AML). A randomized clinical trial of ruxolitinib, a receptor tyrosine kinase inhibitor targeting constitutively active JAK1/2 signaling pathways, in patients with PV failing prior hydroxyurea therapy, confirmed that this agent is effective in reducing phlebotomy frequency and splenomegaly in refractory patients. Reductions in white blood cell and platelet counts following ruxolitinib therapy were also reported. With effective therapy, the long-term survival of PV patients remains excellent.

ESSENTIAL THROMBOCYTHEMIA

Definition and Epidemiology

ET (also known as primary thrombocythemia) is a pluripotent stem cell disorder predominantly resulting in elevated levels of platelets and white blood cells. Platelet function and length of survival remain normal. ET is an uncommon disorder, with an increasing number of cases found on routine laboratory testing of asymptomatic patients. Although the median age at diagnosis is 60 to 65 years, 10% to 25% of patients are younger than 40 years.

TABLE 2.4 World Health Organization 2016 Diagnostic Criteria for Essential Thrombocythemia

Major criteria[a]
1. Platelet count ≥450 × 10^9/L
2. Bone marrow biopsy showing proliferation mainly of the megakaryocyte lineage with increased numbers of enlarged mature megakaryocytes with hyperlobulated nuclei. No significant left-shift of neutrophil granulopoiesis or erythropoiesis and very rarely minor (grade 1) increase in reticulin fibers
3. Not meeting WHO criteria for *BCR-ABL1+* CML, PV, PMF, MDS, or other myeloid neoplasms
4. Presence of JAK2, CALR, or MPL mutation

Minor criteria
1. Presence of a clonal marker (e.g., abnormal karyotype) or absence of evidence for reactive thrombocytosis

From Swerdlow SH, Campo E, Harris NL, Jaffe ES, Pileri SA, Stein H, Thiele J. WHO Classification of Tumours of Haematopoietic and Lymphoid Tissues (Revised Fourth Edition), IARC, 2016.
CML, Chronic myelogenous leukemia; *MDS,* myelodysplastic syndrome; *PMF,* primary myelofibrosis; *PV,* polycythemia vera; *WHO,* World Health Organization.
[a]ET diagnosis requires meeting all four major criteria or first three major criteria and one minor criterion.

Clinical Presentation

Up to two thirds of patients are symptomatic. Vasomotor symptoms include headache, dizziness, visual changes, and erythromelalgia (i.e., burning pain and erythema of feet and hands). Serious arterial thrombotic complications such as transient ischemic attacks, strokes, seizures, angina, and myocardial infarctions may occur. Patients may rarely have purpuric skin lesions or hematomas. The risk for gastrointestinal bleeding is less than 5%.

Diagnosis and Differential Diagnosis

Elevated platelet counts (thrombocytosis) can result as a reactive process arising from other causes (e.g., bacterial infections, sepsis, iron deficiency, autoimmune diseases, malignant diseases), which must be excluded before a diagnosis of ET is considered. The diagnosis requires a platelet count exceeding 450,000 × 10^9/L with mutations in *JAK2, CALR,* or *MPL* genes and no evidence of reactive thrombocytosis. Bone marrow histology typically displays predominant proliferation involving the megakaryocytic lineage and little or no granulocytic or erythroid proliferation or reticulin fibrosis. Marrow immunohistochemical and cytogenetic studies are essential to exclude myelodysplasia, myelofibrosis, or the Philadelphia chromosome, which are diagnostic of CML (Table 2.4). Unlike PV, the *JAK2 V617F* mutation is only found in one half of samples from patients with ET but the presence of other clonal markers such as an abnormal karyotype can aid in making the diagnosis.

Treatment and Prognosis

Patients with ET have the most favorable outcomes of all patients with MPN with typical long-term survival rates similar to those of age-matched healthy control patients. Similar to PV, shortened overall survival is associated with high-risk features including advanced age (>60 years), prior history of thrombosis, and leukocytosis. The risk of leukemic transformation is extremely low (3% to 4%) compared with other MPNs. However, morbidity from recurrent hemorrhagic and thrombotic complications is high and cannot be reliably predicted from the platelet count or platelet function abnormalities. Because treatment requires

栓并发症的风险决定了其是否需要治疗，从而避免 PV 转变为慢性进展性疾病。

小剂量阿司匹林的应用和对无症状血小板增多症的治疗降低了 PV 患者血栓栓塞事件的发生率，尤其是对于有心血管危险因素的老年患者。对年轻患者而言，应慎用非甾体抗炎药和抗血小板药物，谨防胃肠道出血的风险。高龄（＞60岁）、既往有血栓史、白细胞增多症和高血细胞比容、有临床心血管危险因素的患者后续发生血管事件的风险更高。尽管存在可能性，但 PV 在 10 年内和 15 年内转化为急性髓系白血病（AML）的风险分别仅为 2.3% 和 5.5%。

治疗方法根据风险分层情况而有所不同。对于心血管危险因素较少的年轻患者，间歇性静脉切开术（静脉放血）和阿司匹林预防仍然是主要治疗方法，但通常会导致缺铁性贫血，进而降低红细胞生成速度。

降细胞治疗适用于不能耐受和（或）未能进行静脉放血、具有心血管事件病史和（或）危险因素的老年患者、症状性脾大患者。常用治疗包括羟基脲（即低剂量口服细胞毒性药物，不会增加白血病风险）、聚乙二醇干扰素 α（适用于年轻患者和妊娠期妇女）和阿那格雷（治疗难治性血小板增多症的口服巨核细胞毒性药物）。鉴于该病的慢性特点，首选治疗是针对患者的生活方式需求进行个体化治疗。较高风险的 PV 患者的治疗目标是长期保持男性血细胞比容＜45%，女性＜42%。在一项多中心前瞻性临床试验中，成年 PV 患者（主要为男性）被随机分配到使用羟基脲、静脉放血或兼用两种方式三组中，结果显示，与血细胞比容为 45%～50% 的患者相比，血细胞比容＜45% 的患者心血管事件死亡率（2.7% vs. 19.8%）和主要血栓形成发生率显著降低。与所有骨髓增殖性疾病一样，降细胞治疗可导致高尿酸血症，从而引起继发性痛风和尿酸结石，需要采用别嘌醇治疗。

虽然小剂量化疗药（如苯丁酸氮芥、白消安）既往被用于羟基脲治疗无效的白细胞增多症和血小板增多症，但这些药物可增加毒性和继发性 AML 的风险，故已不再使用。一项随机临床试验显示，芦可替尼（一种靶向持续活跃的 JAK1/2 信号通路的受体酪氨酸激酶抑制剂）在羟基脲治疗失败的难治性 PV 患者中可有效降低静脉放血频率，并有效缩小脾体积。此外，芦可替尼治疗后白细胞和血小板计数也相应减少。经过有效治疗，PV 患者的长期生存率仍然很高。

原发性血小板增多症

定义和流行病学

原发性血小板增多症（ET）是一种主要引起血小板和白细胞水平升高的多能干细胞疾病。ET 患者的血小板功能和寿命仍保持正常。ET 是一种少见疾病，许多患者在体格检查中被发现。虽然诊断时的中位年龄为 60～65 岁，但 10%～25% 的患者年龄＜40 岁。

表 2.4 原发性血小板增多症的 WHO 2016 诊断标准

主要标准 [a]
1. 血小板计数 ≥ 450×10^9/L
2. 骨髓活检显示以巨核细胞系增殖为主，伴成熟巨核细胞增多，核分叶过多。粒系、红系无显著增生或左移，极少见网状纤维轻微增生（1 级）
3. 不符合 *BCR-ABL1*＋CML、PV、PMF、MDS 或其他髓系肿瘤的 WHO 诊断标准
4. 携带 *JAK2*、*CALR* 或 *MPL* 突变

次要标准
1. 存在克隆标记（如异常核型）或没有反应性血小板增多症的证据

引自 Swerdlow SH, Campo E, Harris NL, Jaffe ES, Pileri SA, Stein H, Thiele J. WHO Classification of Tumours of Haematopoietic and Lymphoid Tissues (Revised Fourth Edition), IARC, 2016.
CML，慢性髓细胞性白血病；MDS，骨髓增生异常综合征；PMF，原发性骨髓纤维化；PV，真性红细胞增多症；WHO，世界卫生组织。
[a] ET 诊断要求符合所有 4 项主要标准，或前 3 项主要标准和 1 项次要标准。

临床表现

2/3 的 ET 患者有临床症状，血管舒缩症状包括头痛、头晕、视力变化和红斑性肢痛症（即足和手的灼痛和红斑）。PV 患者可发生严重动脉血栓，如短暂性脑缺血发作、卒中、癫痫发作、心绞痛和心肌梗死，极少数情况下可发生紫癜或血肿。胃肠道出血的风险低于 5%。

诊断和鉴别诊断

ET 的诊断需除外其他原因（如细菌感染、感染中毒症、铁缺乏、自身免疫病、恶性疾病）引起的血小板增多。ET 的诊断需满足血小板计数 ≥ 450×10^9/L 伴有 *JAK2*、*CALR* 或 *MPL* 突变，且除外反应性血小板增多症。骨髓组织学以巨核细胞系增殖为主，成熟巨核细胞增多，很少或没有粒系或红系增殖及网状纤维化。骨髓免疫组织化学和细胞遗传学检查对于排除骨髓增生异常、骨髓纤维化或费城染色体（用于诊断 CML）必不可少（表 2.4）。与 PV 不同，仅有 1/2 的 ET 患者呈 *JAK2 V617F* 突变阳性，但如果存在其他克隆标志物（如异常核型），可协助诊断。

治疗和预后

在所有 MPN 患者中，ET 患者的预后最佳，其寿命与同年龄段健康对照人群相似。与 PV 类似，其总体生存期缩短与高龄（＞60岁）、血栓形成史和白细胞增多有关。与其他 MPN 相比，ET 转化为白血病的风险极低（3%～4%）。然而，反复出血和血栓并发症的发病率高，且无法根据血小板计数或血小板功能异常准确预测。由于该病的治疗需要终身管理，因此危险因素评估、临床体征和症状病史决定着治疗选择。所

lifelong administration for disease control, assessment of risk factors and a history of clinical signs and symptoms dictate therapeutic choices. All patients benefit from aggressive management of cardiovascular risk factors including smoking, hypertension, obesity, and hypercholesterolemia.

Although low-dose enteric coated aspirin may be used in all patients to relieve neurologic symptoms and carries a minimal risk for bleeding, excessive thrombocytosis (platelet count >1000 × 10^9/L) can be associated with excessive bleeding due to an acquired von Willebrand syndrome.

Although young and pregnant patients are often not treated until they become symptomatic, older patients (>60 years) and those with a history of thrombosis, long disease duration, or significant cardiovascular risk factors are most likely to benefit from the addition of platelet-lowering agents. Hydroxyurea, an oral cytotoxic and myelosuppressive agent, is the most common first-line agent and is usually well tolerated with low long-term leukemogenic risks. Anagrelide, an oral antiplatelet agent that inhibits platelet aggregation and megakaryocyte maturation, is also used, primarily as a second-line agent after hydroxyurea failure. This agent is associated with acute side effects such as fluid retention, palpitations, hemorrhage with concomitant aspirin use, and an increased risk of transformation to myelofibrosis. Both agents are known teratogens and therefore cannot be used in the significant fraction of patients with ET who are young women of childbearing age. Because patients with ET have a high incidence of fetal wastage, interferon-α (a cytokine that alters the biologic mechanisms of the malignant clone but does not cross the placenta) with low-dose heparin or aspirin prophylaxis is recommended to improve pregnancy outcomes in these patients.

PRIMARY (IDIOPATHIC) MYELOFIBROSIS

Definition and Epidemiology

PMF, also known as idiopathic myelofibrosis or previously as agnogenic myeloid metaplasia, is a clonal stem cell disorder characterized by abnormal excessive marrow fibrosis leading to marrow failure and organomegaly. PMF is a rare chronic disease that usually is seen in elderly persons. The annual incidence of PMF is 0.5 cases per 100,000 people.

Etiology

An abnormal myeloid precursor is thought to give rise to dysplastic megakaryocytes that produce increased levels of angiogenic and fibroblast growth factors. These cytokines act on normal fibroblasts and other stromal cells, a process that stimulates excessive proliferation and collagen deposition. Over time, increasing fibrosis of the bone marrow leads to premature release of multipotent hematopoietic precursors into the periphery. These cells then migrate and reestablish themselves in other sites, thereby shifting hematopoiesis out of the bone marrow and into other tissues, specifically the spleen and liver. This process is called extramedullary hematopoiesis. Approximately 5% to 10% of cases of MF arise in individuals with prior diagnoses of PV or ET whose disease evolves over time to MF. These cases are referred to as secondary or post-PV/ET MF and are characterized by the same disease biology and clinical symptoms.

Diagnosis and Differential Diagnosis

Early in the disease, patients may be asymptomatic, with incidental findings of abnormal blood counts on routine laboratory tests. Although low blood counts may occur, overall platelet and red blood cell numbers at diagnosis may be increased or normal depending on the degree of compensatory extramedullary hematopoiesis. Review of the peripheral blood profile commonly reveals leukoerythroblastic changes characterized by teardrop-shaped erythrocytes, giant platelets, and nonleukemic immature myeloid, erythroid, and leukocyte cells.

TABLE 2.5 Causes of Bone Marrow Fibrosis

I. Neoplastic causes
  a. Chronic myeloproliferative disorders: chronic idiopathic myelofibrosis, chronic myelogenous leukemia, polycythemia vera
  b. Acute megakaryoblastic leukemia
  c. Myelodysplasia with myelofibrosis
  d. Hairy cell leukemia
  e. Acute lymphoblastic leukemia
  f. Multiple myeloma
  g. Metastatic carcinoma
  h. Systemic mastocytosis
II. Non-neoplastic causes
  a. Granulomatous diseases: mycobacterial infections, fungal infections, sarcoidosis
  b. Paget's disease of bone
  c. Hypoparathyroidism or hyperparathyroidism
  d. Renal osteodystrophy
  e. Osteoporosis
  f. Vitamin D deficiency
  g. Autoimmune diseases: systemic lupus erythematosus, systemic sclerosis

Diagnosis of PMF is made by demonstration of bone marrow fibrosis with markedly increased reticulin or collagen fibers or increased marrow cellularity. Other underlying causes of neoplastic and non-neoplastic bone marrow fibrosis (Table 2.5) should be ruled out. Testing for *JAK2*, *BCR/ABL*, or other diagnostic mutations and cytogenetic markers should be performed before a diagnosis of PMF is made (Table 2.6). In some cases, early prefibrotic changes in the marrow have been noted that signify an early phase of MF development.

Clinical Presentation

Although many patients are asymptomatic at diagnosis, most complain over time of progressive fatigue and dyspnea related to anemia or early satiety and left upper quadrant pain associated with splenomegaly and splenic infarction. More than one half of these patients develop massive hepatosplenomegaly due to extramedullary hematopoiesis. Patients with more advanced disease typically have constitutional symptoms such as fever, weight loss, night sweats, cachexia, pruritus, and bone pain, which may be debilitating. As the bone marrow failure evolves, complications of neutropenia, thrombocytopenia, and anemia develop as a result of ineffective hematopoiesis due to fibrotic changes and loss of marrow cellularity. Bleeding from occult disseminated intravascular coagulation is a risk as are infections arising from neutropenia. Extramedullary hematopoiesis in the peritoneal and pleural cavities and in the central nervous system (CNS) may also cause symptoms.

Treatment and Prognosis

Median survival of patients with PMF is poor, ranging from 2 to 5 years after diagnosis. The most commonly accepted adverse prognostic factors at onset include age greater than 65 years, hemoglobin concentration of less than 10 g/dL, leukocyte count of more than 25 × 10^9/L, a high percentage of circulating blasts (≥1%), and constitutional symptoms. Other important clinical factors are leukopenia, thrombocytopenia (platelets <100 × 10^9/L), massive hepatosplenomegaly, red cell transfusion needs, and unfavorable cytogenetic abnormalities. Over time, the disease may progress from a chronic phase to an accelerated phase, with acute leukemic transformation in 8% to 20% of patients. Treatment of PMF-related AML

有患者均可受益于对心血管危险因素（如吸烟、高血压、肥胖症、高胆固醇症）的积极管理。

虽然低剂量肠溶性阿司匹林可用于所有患者，可减轻神经系统症状且出血风险较低，但血小板过度增多（$>1000\times10^9/L$）者的出血风险增大，与获得性 von Willebrand 综合征有关。

年轻患者和妊娠患者在出现症状前通常无须治疗，而对于老年（>60 岁）、有血栓史、疾病持续时间长、有严重心血管危险因素的患者，降血小板治疗可能有益。羟基脲（一种口服细胞毒性药，可导致骨髓抑制）是最常用的一线药物，通常耐受性良好，长期白血病转化风险低。阿那格雷（一种抑制血小板聚集和巨核细胞成熟的口服抗血小板药物）是羟基脲治疗无效者的二线药物。该药具有急性副作用，如液体潴留、心悸、出血（联用阿司匹林），且发生骨髓纤维化的风险增加。这两种药物都具有致畸作用，因此不能用于育龄期 ET 女性患者。由于 ET 患者的胎儿流产率高，因此推荐妊娠期患者使用干扰素 α（一种细胞因子，可以改变恶性克隆的生物学机制，但不能穿过胎盘）联合低剂量肝素或阿司匹林。

原发性（特发性）骨髓纤维化

定义和流行病学

原发性骨髓纤维化（PMF）又称特发性骨髓纤维化或原因不明的髓样化生，是以异常过度的骨髓纤维化导致骨髓衰竭和器官肿大为特征的干细胞克隆性疾病。PMF 是一种罕见的慢性疾病，多见于老年人。PMF 的年发病率为 0.5/100 000。

病因

髓系前体细胞异常可导致巨核细胞发育异常，使血管源性生长因子和成纤维细胞生长因子生成增加，这些细胞因子作用于正常的成纤维细胞和其他基质细胞，刺激其过度增殖和胶原沉积。随着骨髓纤维化的增加，多能造血祖细胞过早释放至外周。这些细胞随后在其他部位重建，使得这些组织也具有造血功能，特别是脾和肝。该过程被称为髓外造血。5%～10% 的骨髓纤维化发生在既往被诊断为 PV 或 ET 的个体中，随着时间的推移，疾病会演变为骨髓纤维化。这些病例被称为继发性骨髓纤维化或 PV/ET 后骨髓纤维化，其具有相同的疾病生物学特征和临床症状。

诊断和鉴别诊断

在疾病早期，患者可能无症状，仅在常规实验室检查时偶然发现血细胞计数异常。尽管可能发生血细胞计数降低，但根据代偿性髓外造血的程度，诊断时的总体血小板和红细胞数量可能增加或正常。外周血涂片通常可见幼粒幼红细胞改变，其特征包括泪滴状红细胞、巨血小板、非白血病性幼红细胞和幼粒细胞增多、白细胞增多。

PMF 的诊断需满足以下条件：骨髓纤维化伴网硬蛋白或胶原纤维显著增多或骨髓细胞增多。应排除肿瘤性和非肿瘤性原因所致的骨髓纤维化（表 2.5）。此外，诊断 PMF 之前还需检测 *JAK2*、*BCR/ABL* 或其他诊断性突变和细胞遗传学标志物（表 2.6）。某些情况下，在骨髓纤维化发展的早期阶段可观察到骨髓中有纤维化早期改变。

表 2.5 骨髓纤维化的病因

I. 肿瘤原因
  a. 慢性骨髓增殖性疾病：慢性特发性骨髓纤维化、慢性粒细胞白血病、真性红细胞增多症
  b. 急性巨核细胞白血病
  c. 骨髓增生异常伴骨髓纤维化
  d. 毛细胞白血病
  e. 急性淋巴细胞白血病
  f. 多发性骨髓瘤
  g. 转移癌
  h. 系统性肥大细胞增多症

II. 非肿瘤原因
  a. 肉芽肿性疾病：分枝杆菌感染、真菌感染、结节病
  b. 骨佩吉特病
  c. 甲状旁腺功能减退症或甲状旁腺功能亢进症
  d. 肾性骨营养不良
  e. 骨质疏松症
  f. 维生素 D 缺乏
  g. 自身免疫病：系统性红斑狼疮、系统性硬化症

临床表现

虽然许多患者在诊断时无症状，但随着时间的推移，大多数患者会出现与贫血相关的进行性疲劳和呼吸困难，或因脾大和脾梗死导致的早饱和左上腹疼痛。超过 50% 的患者因髓外造血而出现肝脾大。晚期 PMF 患者可有全身症状，如发热、体重减轻、盗汗、恶病质、瘙痒和骨痛等。随着骨髓衰竭的进展，患者会出现无效造血的并发症，包括中性粒细胞减少、血小板减少和贫血。患者也存在隐匿性弥散性血管内凝血导致出血的风险和中性粒细胞减少症导致的感染风险。腹膜腔、胸膜腔和中枢神经系统（CNS）中的髓外造血也可能引起相应症状。

治疗和预后

PMF 患者的中位生存期较短，通常为诊断后 2～5 年。最常见的不良预后因素包括年龄＞65 岁、血红蛋白＜10 g/dl、白细胞计数＞$25\times10^9/L$、外周血原始细胞百分比高（≥1%）和有全身症状。其他临床因素包括白细胞减少、血小板减少（血小板计数＜$100\times10^9/L$）、肝脾大、需要输血和不利的细胞遗传学异常。该病可从慢性期进展到加速期，8%～20% 的患者会转化为急性白血病。PMF 相关性 AML 对常规治疗无效，其他非

TABLE 2.6 World Health Organization 2016 Diagnostic Criteria for Primary Myelofibrosis

Primary Myelofibrosis (PMF): Prefibrotic/Early PMF (pre-PMF)
Major criteria[a]
1. Megakaryocyte proliferation and atypia **without reticulin fibrosis > grade 1**, accompanied by increased age-adjusted bone marrow cellularity, granulocytic proliferation, and often decreased erythropoiesis
2. Not meeting WHO criteria for *BCR-ABL1+* CML, PV, MDS, or other myeloid neoplasm
3. Presence of *JAK2, CALR, or MPL* mutation or in the absence of minor reactive bone marrow reticulin fibrosis

Minor criteria
1. Presence of one or more of the following, confirmed in two consecutive determinations
   a. Anemia not attributed to a comorbid condition
   b. Leukocytosis ≥11 × 10^9/L
   c. Palpable splenomegaly
   d. LDH level above the upper limit of the institutional reference range

Primary Myelofibrosis (PMF)
Major criteria[a]
1. Megakaryocyte proliferation and atypia accompanied by either reticulin and/or collagen fibrosis (grade 2 to 3)
2. Not meeting WHO criteria for *BCR-ABL1+* CML, PV, MDS, or other myeloid neoplasm
3. Presence of *JAK2, CALR, or MPL* mutation or in the absence, the presence of another clonal marker[b] or absence of evidence for reactive bone marrow fibrosis

Minor criteria
1. Presence of one or more of the following, confirmed in two consecutive determinations
   a. Anemia not attributed to a comorbid condition
   b. Leukocytosis ≥11 × 10^9/L
   c. Palpable splenomegaly
   d. LDH level above the upper limit of the institutional reference range
   e. Leukoerythroblastosis

From Swerdlow SH, Campo E, Harris NL, Jaffe ES, Pileri SA, Stein H, Thiele J. WHO Classification of Tumours of Haematopoietic and Lymphoid Tissues (Revised Fourth Edition), IARC, 2016.
[a]Diagnosis of prefibrotic/early PMF requires all three major criteria and at least one minor criterion. Diagnosis of overt PMF requires meeting all three major criteria and at least one minor criterion.
[b]In the absence of any of the three major clonal mutations, the search for the most frequent accompanying mutations *(ASXL1, EZH2, TET2, IDH1/IDH2, SRFS2, SF3B1)* are of help in determining the clonal nature of the disease.

---

is usually ineffective. Other causes of nonleukemic death include heart failure, infection, intracranial hemorrhage, and pulmonary embolism.

Medical therapy for PMF is predicated on the risk category of patients. Low-risk, asymptomatic patients may be treated expectantly. All patients with symptomatic anemia benefit from palliative transfusions and administration of recombinant EPO, androgens (e.g., danazol), or low-dose thalidomide or thalidomide derivatives (i.e., lenalidomide) with or without steroids to maintain adequate red blood cell levels. Symptoms caused by excess thrombocytosis and leukocytosis or progressive extramedullary hematopoiesis may be managed with hydroxyurea as a first-line agent or pegylated interferon-α in younger or pregnant patients. Enlarging splenomegaly is best managed with medical therapy because open splenectomy is associated with significant operative morbidity and mortality, and splenic irradiation is poorly tolerated except as a palliative approach. Young patients with intermediate- to high-risk PMF and possible HLA-matched donors should be considered for potentially curative allogeneic stem cell transplantation (SCT) at academic medical centers.

Although not all patients with PMF have the *JAK2 V617F* mutation, almost all have constitutive activation of the JAK1 and JAK2 signaling pathways, rendering them potentially responsive to treatment with novel JAK1/2 inhibitors. Ruxolitinib is the first oral JAK inhibitor approved for the treatment of patients with intermediate- or high-risk myelofibrosis independent of *JAK2* mutational status, including PMF and myelofibrosis arising from prior PV or ET. In two prospective, randomized, phase III clinical trials, ruxolitinib therapy for myelofibrosis patients was compared with placebo (COMFORT-I trial) and with best available therapy (COMFORT-II trial), respectively. Patients receiving ruxolitinib had significantly greater spleen volume reduction and overall symptom improvement in abdominal pain, early satiety, night sweats, and muscle pain, all of which correlated with overall improvement in quality of life. Updates from both trials have demonstrated significantly prolonged overall survival in the ruxolitinib-treated patients compared with control arms although neither study was designed with this as an end point. Side effects of ruxolitinib include cytopenias, specifically anemia, occurring in the first 6 to 8 weeks of therapy as well as headache, dizziness, and increased risk of herpes simplex virus (HSV) reactivation. Recently a second JAK2 inhibitor, fedratinib, was approved for the treatment of intermediate and high-risk MF as an alternative to and/or failing prior ruxolitinib therapy. Other JAK2 inhibitors are in active clinical development as single agents. Combination therapies evaluating the safety and efficacy of novel mechanistic agents alone and in addition to JAK2 inhibitors are also underway with preliminary results suggesting that even more effective therapies for PMF may be on the horizon.

CHRONIC MYELOGENOUS LEUKEMIA

Definition, Epidemiology, and Pathology

CML is the most common MPN, accounting for 15% to 20% of all leukemias and occurring in 1 of 100,000 people. The median age at diagnosis is 53 years, but patients of any age may be affected. CML is characterized by a predominant increase in the granulocytic cell line associated with concurrent erythroid and platelet hyperplasia. It is

表 2.6　原发性骨髓纤维化的 WHO 2016 诊断标准

原发性骨髓纤维化（PMF）：前纤维化/早期 PMF（前 PMF）
主要标准[a]
1. 有巨核细胞增殖和异型巨核细胞，无显著的网硬蛋白纤维化（MF-1），伴有年龄调整的骨髓增生程度增高、粒细胞增殖，常有红细胞生成减少
2. 不符合 *BCR-ABL1*⁺ CML、PV、MDS 或其他髓系肿瘤的 WHO 诊断标准
3. 存在 *JAK2*、*CALR* 或 *MPL* 突变，或不存在轻微反应性骨髓网硬蛋白纤维化

次要标准
1. 在 2 次连续检测中确认存在以下 1 种或多种情况
    a. 贫血（并非由合并症导致）
    b. 白细胞 ≥ 11×10⁹/L
    c. 可触及的脾大
    d. LDH 水平高于正常值上限

原发性骨髓纤维化（PMF）
主要标准[a]
1. 巨核细胞增殖和异型巨核细胞，伴网硬蛋白和（或）胶原蛋白纤维化（2～3 级）
2. 不符合 *BCR-ABL1*⁺ CML、PV、MDS 或其他髓系肿瘤 WHO 诊断标准
3. 存在 *JAK2 V617F*、*CALR*、*MPL* 基因突变，或如果没有这些突变，需有其他克隆性标志[b]，或缺乏反应性骨髓纤维化的证据

次要标准
1. 在 2 次连续检测中确认存在以下 1 种或多种情况
    a. 贫血（并非由合并症导致）
    b. 白细胞 ≥ 11×10⁹/L
    c. 可触及的脾大
    d. LDH 水平高于正常值上限
    e. 幼粒幼红现象

引自 Swerdlow SH, Campo E, Harris NL, Jaffe ES, Pileri SA, Stein H, Thiele J. WHO Classification of Tumours of Haematopoietic and Lymphoid Tissues (Revised Fourth Edition), IARC, 2016.
[a] 前纤维化/早期 PMF 的诊断需要满足 3 项主要标准和至少 1 项次要标准。明显 PMF 的诊断需要符合所有 3 项主要标准和至少 1 项次要标准。
[b] 如果不存在 3 种主要克隆突变中的任何一种，寻找最常见的伴随突变（*ASXL1*、*EZH2*、*TET2*、*IDH1/IDH2*、*SRFS2*、*SF3B1*）有助于确定疾病的克隆性质。

白血病性死亡原因包括心力衰竭、感染、颅内出血和肺栓塞。

PMF 的治疗取决于患者的风险分层。低危且无症状的患者可观察等待。有症状性贫血的患者可受益于输血、重组 EPO、雄激素（如达那唑）、低剂量沙利度胺或沙利度胺衍生物（如来那度胺），联合或不联合糖皮质激素治疗，以维持红细胞水平。因血小板增多和白细胞增多或髓外造血引起的症状可通过羟基脲（一线药物）来缓解，年轻或妊娠期女性可使用聚乙二醇干扰素 α 治疗。脾大的最佳治疗是羟基脲，因为开放性脾切除术会显著增加手术并发症发病率和死亡率，且脾放疗很难耐受，除非作为姑息性治疗。中高危的年轻 PMF 患者可考虑进行 HLA 相合的异基因造血干细胞移植（alloSCT）。

虽然不是所有 PMF 患者都存在 *JAK2 V617F* 突变，但几乎都具有 JAK1 和 JAK2 信号通路的激活，这使得 JAK1/2 抑制剂可能有效。芦可替尼是第一种被批准用于治疗中高危骨髓纤维化（包括 PMF 和 PV 或 ET 引起的骨髓纤维化，无论 *JAK2* 突变状态如何）的口服 JAK 抑制剂。在两项随机前瞻性Ⅲ期临床试验中，分别比较了使用芦可替尼和安慰剂（COMFORT-Ⅰ试验）及最佳治疗（COMFORT-Ⅱ试验）对骨髓纤维化患者的疗效。结果发现，接受芦可替尼治疗的患者脾缩小和症状改善（如腹痛、早饱、盗汗、肌痛）更显著，从而改善了患者的生活质量。两项试验的更新数据显示，与对照组相比，芦可替尼治疗后骨髓纤维化明显改善、总体生存期显著延长，尽管这两项研究均未将此作为研究终点。芦可替尼的副作用包括血细胞减少（特别是贫血；发生在治疗的前 6～8 周）、头痛、头晕和单纯疱疹病毒（HSV）再激活风险增加。目前第二种 JAK2 抑制剂菲卓替尼已被批准用于治疗芦可替尼无效的中高危 MF 和（或）替代芦可替尼治疗。其他 JAK2 抑制剂作为单药正处于积极的临床研发阶段。对新机制药物单药治疗或联用 JAK2 抑制剂的联合治疗的安全性和有效性评估正在进行中，初步结果表明，更有效的 PMF 治疗方法值得期待。

慢性髓细胞性白血病

定义、流行病学和病理学

慢性髓细胞性白血病（CML）是最常见的 MPN，占所有白血病的 15%～20%，发生率约为 1/100 000。诊断时的中位年龄为 53 岁，但任何年龄段人群均可患 CML。CML 的特征为粒系细胞显著增加，伴红细胞和

TABLE 2.7   Definition of Phases of Chronic Myeloid Leukemia

Phase	Definition	Goal of Therapy
Chronic phase (CP)	<10% blasts <20% peripheral blood basophils	Prevent progression to AP/BP, eradicate molecular *BCR-ABL*
Accelerated phase (AP)	Peripheral blood myeloblasts ≥10% and <20% Peripheral blood myeloblasts and promyelocytes combined ≥30% Peripheral blood basophils ≥20% Platelet count ≤100 × 10^9/L unrelated to therapy	Control CBC, bring back to CP and avoid progression to BP
Blast phase (BP)	Additional clonal cytogenetic abnormalities in Ph+ cells ≥20% blasts (myeloid or lymphoid) in peripheral blood, marrow, or both Extramedullary infiltrates of leukemic cells	Acute leukemia therapy, bridge to allogeneic stem cell transplant

unique among the MPNs in its etiology and natural history, including an inevitable transformation to acute leukemia if untreated. CML was the first malignant hematologic disease shown to be associated with a specific chromosomal abnormality. More than 95% of patients with CML have a clonal expansion of a stem cell that has acquired the Philadelphia chromosome, a balanced translocation between chromosomes 9 and 22 designated as t(9;22) (q34;q11). This translocation juxtaposes the *ABL* gene from chromosome 9 (region q34) to the *BCR* gene on chromosome 22 (region q11) and generates an oncogenic *BCR/ABL* fusion gene. The gene product, the BCR/ABL protein, is a deregulated, constitutively active cytoplasmic receptor tyrosine kinase that induces a leukemic phenotype in hematopoietic stem cells. Expression of the BCR/ABL fusion protein activates multiple downstream signal transduction pathways which permits proliferation independent of cytokine and stromal regulation and renders cells resistant to chemotherapy and normal programmed cell death.

Diagnosis and Differential Diagnosis

Laboratory tests for CML patients typically demonstrate a markedly elevated white blood cell count (median, 170 × 10^9/L), with low leukocyte alkaline phosphatase levels, high uric acid and lactate dehydrogenase levels, and thrombocytosis. Review of the peripheral blood smear in chronic phase CML demonstrates a full complement of myeloid cells in all stages of granulocytic development, including immature myeloblasts (usually <5%), myelocytes, metamyelocytes, basophils, eosinophils, bands, and neutrophils. In contrast, the peripheral blood smear in reactive granulocytic hyperplastic states (i.e., leukemoid reaction) caused by acute infection or sepsis consists predominantly of mature neutrophils and bands with few myelocytes, basophils, or eosinophils. The bone marrow in CML is densely hypercellular, with an overwhelming predominance of myeloid cells at all developmental stages. The differential diagnosis of CML includes reactive leukocytosis (e.g., in active infection or sepsis with a profound neutrophilic response) and other MPNs (e.g., myelofibrosis).

Detection of the Philadelphia chromosome on standard cytogenetic studies and/or abnormal BCR/ABL transcripts using reverse transcription–polymerase chain reaction (RT-PCR) or fluorescent in situ hybridization (FISH) analysis is required for the diagnosis of CML. Assessment of the *BCR/ABL* fusion gene by the same methods is used to monitor disease and response to therapy. Exquisitely sensitive and quantitative RT-PCR procedures allow detection of up to a single BCR/ABL-positive cell in 10^5 to 10^6 peripheral cells and permit measurement of disease status in peripheral blood and marrow samples. A subset of patients with CML lacking a detectable Philadelphia chromosome was found to possess detectable BCR/ABL fusion products by RT-PCR, indicating a subchromosomal translocation resulting in the same pathologic gene product.

Clinical Presentation

Up to 40% of newly diagnosed CML patients are initially asymptomatic with diagnoses made on incidental laboratory results. Other patients exhibit fatigue, lethargy, shortness of breath, weight loss, easy bruising, and early satiety. Physical examination usually detects splenomegaly.

The natural history of CML is divided into three phases: chronic, accelerated, and blast phases (Table 2.7). The majority of patients are typically diagnosed during the *chronic phase of CML*, an indolent stage lasting 3 to 7 years. Peripheral white blood cell counts are elevated, with eosinophilia and basophilia (>20%) but few peripheral or marrow blasts (<5%). With control of peripheral blood cell counts, patients are essentially asymptomatic during this period.

Eventually, the disease enters the *accelerated phase*, which is characterized by fever, weight loss, worsening splenomegaly, and bone pain related to rapid marrow cell turnover. The white blood cell count rises with increased numbers of circulating or marrow blasts ranging from 10% to 19%. The increased percentage of peripheral blood basophils (>20%) results in histamine production, with symptoms of pruritus, diarrhea, and flushing. During this phase, patients may develop increasing splenomegaly, persistent thrombocytopenia, or thrombocytosis and leukocytosis, with new clonal cytogenetic abnormalities found in marrow cells.

CML blast crisis phase marks the evolution to acute leukemia, in which marrow is replaced by 20% or more immature myeloid or lymphoid blasts, with accompanying loss of normal mature cellular elements in the marrow and periphery and extramedullary blast proliferation. Untreated patients typically die in a few weeks to months. Of note, two thirds of patients develop acute myeloid leukemia, whereas the others develop acute lymphoblastic leukemia, a finding confirming that the initial neoplastic cell is an early stem cell capable of multilineage differentiation.

Treatment

Chronic Phase CML

Historically, oral cytotoxic agents such as hydroxyurea and busulfan effectively reduced myeloid cell numbers in patients with chronic phase CML but did not alter the long-term prognosis or prevent progression to blast crises.

Oral receptor tyrosine inhibitors of BCR-ABL are the mainstay of current therapy for CML. The first identified inhibitor, imatinib mesylate (formerly known as STI-571), was heralded as the first successful targeted therapy for cancer and ushered in a new era of cancer therapy. Imatinib is a rationally designed competitive oral inhibitor of multiple tyrosine kinases, including ABL, BCR/ABL, platelet-derived growth-factor receptor (PDGFR), and KIT. Inhibition of phosphorylation of BCR/ABL results in blockade of downstream signaling and growth pathways and induces apoptosis of *BCR-ABL*-positive cells. Preclinical studies demonstrated that imatinib potently inhibited the

表 2.7 CML 分期的定义		
分期	定义	治疗目标
慢性期（CP）	原始细胞＜10% 外周血嗜碱性粒细胞＜20%	预防进展至加速期/急变期，分子学 BCR-ABL 清零
加速期（AP）	外周血原始细胞≥10%且＜20% 外周血原始细胞和早幼粒细胞比例之和≥30% 外周血嗜碱性粒细胞≥20% 血小板计数≤100×10^9/L，与治疗无关 Ph$^+$细胞的其他克隆性细胞遗传学异常	控制血常规，恢复至慢性期并避免进展至急变期
急变期（BP）	外周血和（或）骨髓中原始细胞（髓系或淋巴系）≥20% 白血病细胞髓外浸润	急性白血病治疗，桥接同种异体干细胞移植

血小板增多。这在 MPN 的病因和自然病程中是独一无二的，包括未经治疗将不可避免地转化为急性白血病。CML 是第一个被发现具有特定染色体异常的恶性血液病。超过 95% 的 CML 患者具有获得性费城染色体的干细胞克隆扩增，费城染色体为 9 号和 22 号染色体之间的平衡易位被称为 t（9;22）(q34;911)。这种易位将 9 号染色体（q34 区域）上的 *ABL* 基因与 22 号染色体（q11 区域）上的 *BCR* 基因连接，形成致癌的 *BCR/ABL* 融合基因。该融合基因产物 BCR/ABL 蛋白定位于胞质，是一种失调的具有活性的酪氨酸激酶，可诱导造血干细胞的白血病表型。BCR/ABL 融合蛋白的表达可激活下游多个信号转导通路，使得细胞不再受细胞因子和基质的调控而大量增殖，从而抵抗化疗药物和正常的细胞程序性死亡，导致 CML 的发生。

诊断和鉴别诊断

CML 患者的实验室检查通常可见白细胞计数显著增多（中位数为 170×10^9/L）、碱性磷酸酶水平降低、尿酸和乳酸脱氢酶水平升高，以及血小板增多。CML 慢性期患者的外周血涂片可见粒系发育的所有阶段，包括原始粒细胞（通常＜5%）、中幼粒细胞、晚幼粒细胞、嗜碱性粒细胞、嗜酸性粒细胞、杆状核粒细胞和中性粒细胞。相反，由急性感染或感染中毒症引起的反应性粒细胞增殖状态（即类白血病反应）患者的外周血涂片中主要为成熟的中性粒细胞和少量中幼粒细胞、嗜碱性粒细胞或嗜酸性粒细胞。CML 患者的骨髓检查显示骨髓增生极度活跃，其中处于各个发育阶段的髓系细胞占主导地位。CML 的鉴别诊断包括反应性白细胞增多症（如具有显著中性粒细胞反应的活动性感染或感染中毒症）和其他 MPN（如骨髓纤维化）。

CML 的诊断需要通过标准细胞遗传学检查来检测费城染色体和（或）通过逆转录聚合酶链反应（RT-PCR）或荧光原位杂交（FISH）技术来检测异常 BCR/ABL 转录。通过评估 *BCR/ABL* 融合基因定量水平，可以监测疾病进展和治疗反应。敏感性极高的定量 RT-PCR 可在 10^5～10^6 个细胞中检测出 1 个 BCR/ABL 阳性细胞，从而评估外周血和骨髓中的白血病负荷。部分 CML 患者体内虽无法检测到费城染色体，但利用 RT-PCR 可检测到 BCR/ABL 融合产物，提示亚染色体易位产生同样的病理性基因产物。

临床表现

新诊断的 CML 患者中 40% 最初是无症状的。常见临床表现为疲劳、嗜睡、气短、体重减轻、皮肤易淤血和早饱。体格检查通常可发现脾大。

CML 的自然病程包括慢性期、加速期和急变期（表 2.7）。绝大多数患者在 CML 慢性期被诊断，持续 3～7 年。患者外周血白细胞增多伴嗜酸性粒细胞和嗜碱性粒细胞增多（＞20%），但原始细胞较少（＜5%）。通过控制外周血细胞计数，患者在此期间基本无症状。

最终，疾病进入加速期，表现为发热、体重减轻、进行性脾大和骨髓细胞快速增殖相关的骨痛。白细胞计数随着外周原始细胞数量的增加（10%～19%）而增多。外周血嗜碱性粒细胞比例增大（＞20%）可导致组胺生成，患者表现为瘙痒、腹泻和潮红。在 CML 加速期，患者可能出现进行性脾大、持续性血小板减少或血小板增多和白细胞增多，骨髓细胞中可发现新的细胞遗传学异常克隆。

CML 急变期危象标志着病情进展为急性白血病，患者骨髓的 20% 或更多被髓系或淋巴系原始细胞替代，同时伴随骨髓、外周血中正常成熟细胞丢失和髓外原始细胞增殖。未经治疗的患者可在急变期后数周至数月死亡。应注意，2/3 的 CML 患者会进展为 AML，而其他则发展为急性淋巴细胞白血病（ALL），表明初始肿瘤细胞是能够向多系分化的早期干细胞。

治疗

慢性期 CML

历史上，口服细胞毒性药物（如羟基脲和白消安）可有效减少慢性期 CML 患者的髓系细胞数目。尽管这些药物降低了急性疾病并发症的发生率，但并未改变预后或减缓向急变期的进展。

BCR-ABL 的口服酪氨酸激酶抑制剂是当前 CML 的主要治疗方式。BCR-ABL 抑制剂甲磺酸伊马替尼（既往被称为 STI-571）是第一个成功治疗癌症的口服靶向药物，开创了癌症治疗的新纪元。伊马替尼是多种酪氨酸激酶的竞争性抑制剂，包括 ABL、BCR/ABL、血小板源性生长因子受体（PDGFR）和 KIT。伊马替尼可通过抑制 BCR/ABL 的磷酸化来阻断下游信号转导通路，从而诱导 *BCR/ABL* 阳性细胞的调亡。临床前研

TABLE 2.8 Criteria for Hematologic, Cytogenetic, and Molecular Response and Relapse in Chronic Myeloid Leukemia

Complete hematologic response
- Complete normalization of peripheral blood counts with leukocyte count $<10 \times 10^9$/L
- Platelet count $<450 \times 10^9$/L
- No immature cells, such as myelocytes, promyelocytes, or blasts in peripheral blood
- No signs and symptoms of disease with resolution of palpable splenomegaly

Cytogenetic response
- Complete cytogenetic response (CCyR): No Ph-positive metaphases
- Major cytogenetic response (MCyR): 0-35% Ph-positive metaphases
- Partial cytogenetic response (PCyR): 1-35% Ph-positive metaphases
- Minor cytogenetic response: >35-65% Ph-positive metaphases

Molecular response
- Early molecular response (EMR): *BCR-ABL1* (IS) ≤10% at 3 and 6 months
- Major molecular response (MMR): *BCR-ABL1* (IS) ≤0.1% or ≥3-log reduction in *BCR-ABL1* mRNA from the standardized baseline, if qPCR (IS) is not available
- Complete molecular response (CMR) is variably described and is best defined by the assay's level of sensitivity (e.g., MR4.5)

Relapse
- Any sign of loss of response (defined as hematologic or cytogenetic relapse)
- 1-log increase in *BCR-ABL1* transcript levels with loss of MMR should prompt bone marrow evaluation for loss of CCyR but is not itself defined as relapse (e.g., hematologic or cytogenetic relapse)

TABLE 2.9 Oral BCR-ABL1 Inhibitors for CML Therapy

Drug Name	Drug Dose	Toxicity Profile
Imatinib mesylate	400 mg po daily	Nausea, vomiting, diarrhea, peripheral and periorbital edema, myalgias, myelosuppression, increased liver function tests, rash, pleural and pericardial effusion
Dasatinib	100 mg po daily	Pulmonary arterial hypertension, pleural and pericardial effusions, headache, myelosuppression, cerebral hemorrhage (rare), ascites, peripheral or pulmonary edema
Nilotinib	400 mg po twice a day (avoid food 2 hrs before and 1 hr after drug)	Peripheral arterial occlusive disease, QTC prolongation, pancreatitis, hepatotoxicity, myelosuppression, hyperglycemia, sudden death, rash
Bosutinib	500 mg po daily	Diarrhea, myelosuppression, liver function abnormalities, fluid retention (pulmonary or peripheral edema, pleural and pericardial effusion), GI upset, rash
Ponatinib	15-45 mg po daily (45 mg daily until remission, then 15-30 mg)	Arterial and venous thrombosis and occlusions including fatal myocardial infarction and stroke (up to 35% of patients), heart failure, hepatotoxicity, cardiovascular risk, severe skin rash, pancreatitis, hepatotoxicity, hemorrhage (cerebral, gastrointestinal), cardiac arrhythmias, fluid retention, hypertension, rash, myelosuppression
Ascimimab (phase 1 trial)	Not yet determined	Pancreatitis, increased lipase levels, fatigue, headache, arthralgias, hypertension, thrombocytopenia

growth of BCR/ABL-expressing CML cell lines and progenitor cells in vitro and prolonged survival in animal tumor models.

Responses to BCR-ABL1 inhibitor treatment for CML are defined as hematologic (i.e., restoration of normal peripheral blood cell counts), cytogenetic (i.e., loss of the Philadelphia chromosome determined by normal karyotypic or FISH analysis), and molecular (i.e., a three log or greater reduction of detectable *BCR/ABL* transcripts below a standard baseline by RT-PCR) remissions (Table 2.8). After diagnosis, patients are typically started on tyrosine kinase inhibitor (TKI) therapy with careful interim monitoring for toxicities and clinical response. Standardized RT-PCR assays for *BCR/ABL* are used to measure disease response on a molecular level at 3, 6, and 12 months after therapy initiation. Initial clinical trials of imatinib in 1998 were notable for a hematologic remission rate of 96% in patients receiving a dose greater than 300 mg per day for 4 weeks. One third of individuals obtained cytogenetic remission after 8 weeks. Imatinib was shown to be superior to these prior therapies in individuals with newly diagnosed chronic phase CML with complete cytogenetic responses in almost 90% of patients and an overall survival of 89%. The fact that patients achieving remission could have stable disease for years, even decades, demonstrated conclusively that this agent could effectively alter the natural history of this disease.

Despite these results, most patients achieving cytogenetic responses on imatinib demonstrate persistence of *BCR/ABL*-positive leukemic CML stem cells by sensitive molecular testing. Lifelong imatinib therapy may be required to control disease, and even patients with excellent control of chronic phase CML on imatinib therapy remain at risk for eventual disease progression and therapy failure due to development of imatinib-resistant CML cells and/or non-compliance. It is estimated that up to one third of chronic phase CML patients initiated on imatinib therapy will eventually discontinue the drug due to long-term intolerance of drug-induced side effects (e.g., nausea, vomiting, gastrointestinal issues, peripheral and periorbital edema) or development of imatinib resistance.

To address these issues, four new generation TKIs of BCR/ABL have been developed for the treatment of CML: dasatinib, nilotinib, bosutinib, and ponatinib (Table 2.9). All display increased in vitro potency against the BCR/ABL kinase compared with imatinib. At present, four (imatinib, dasatinib, nilotinib, bosutinib) are indicated for initial therapy of chronic phase CML. Multiple randomized clinical

表 2.8　CML 的血液学缓解、细胞遗传学缓解、分子学缓解及复发标准

完全血液学缓解
- 外周血细胞计数完全恢复正常，白细胞计数 $< 10 \times 10^9$/L
- 血小板计数 $< 450 \times 10^9$/L
- 外周血中无未成熟细胞，如中幼粒细胞、早幼粒细胞或原始细胞
- 无疾病体征和症状，可触及的脾大消退

细胞遗传学缓解
- 完全细胞遗传学缓解（CCyR）：无 Ph^+ 中期分裂相
- 主要细胞遗传学缓解（MCyR）：0%～35% Ph^+ 中期分裂相
- 部分细胞遗传学缓解（PCyR）：1%～35% Ph^+ 中期分裂相
- 次要细胞遗传学缓解：> 35%～65% Ph^+ 中期分裂相

分子学缓解
- 早期分子学缓解（EMR）：第 3 个月和第 6 个月时 BCR-ABL1（IS）≤ 10%
- 主要分子学缓解（MMR）：如果 qPCR（IS）不可行，则 BCR-ABL1（IS）≤ 0.1% 或 BCR-ABL1 mRNA 较标准基线水平下降 ≥ 3 个对数级
- 完全分子学缓解（CMR）的定义各不相同，最好通过各个检测的灵敏度水平（如 MR4.5）来定义

复发
- 任何缓解消失的体征（定义为血液学或细胞遗传学复发）
- MMR 丧失的情况下，BCR-ABL1 转录水平增加 1 个对数级时应立即进行骨髓评估，以确定是否丧失 CCyR，但其本身并不能定义复发（如血液学或细胞遗传学复发）

表 2.9　用于治疗 CML 的口服 BCR-ABL1 抑制剂

药物名称	药物剂量	毒性特征
甲磺酸伊马替尼	400 mg，口服，1 次/日	恶心、呕吐、腹泻、外周和眶周水肿、肌痛、骨髓抑制、肝功能异常、皮疹、胸腔积液和心包积液
达沙替尼	100 mg，口服，1 次/日	肺动脉高压、胸腔积液和心包积液、头痛、骨髓抑制、脑出血（罕见）、腹腔积液、外周或肺水肿
尼洛替尼	400 mg，口服，2 次/日（服药前 2 h 和服药后 1 h 避免进食）	外周动脉闭塞性疾病、QTc 间期延长、胰腺炎、肝毒性、骨髓抑制、高血糖、猝死、皮疹
博舒替尼	500 mg，口服，1 次/日	腹泻、骨髓抑制、肝功能异常、液体潴留（肺或外周水肿、胸腔和心包积液）、胃肠道不适、皮疹
普纳替尼	每日 15～45 mg，口服（45 mg/d 直至缓解，随后剂量为 15～30 mg/d）	动脉和静脉血栓形成和闭塞［包括致死性心肌梗死和卒中（高达 35% 的患者）］、心力衰竭、肝毒性、心血管风险、严重皮疹、胰腺炎、肝毒性、出血（脑和胃肠道）、心律失常、液体潴留、高血压、皮疹、骨髓抑制
Ascimimab（I 期试验）	尚未确定	胰腺炎、脂肪酶水平升高、疲劳、头痛、关节痛、高血压、血小板减少症

究表明，伊马替尼在体外可有效抑制 BCR/ABL 阳性的 CML 细胞系和祖细胞的生长，并延长了动物肿瘤模型的生存期。

CML 患者对 BCR-ABL1 抑制剂有治疗反应被定义为血液学缓解（即外周血细胞计数恢复正常）、细胞遗传学缓解（即通过正常核型或 FISH 技术检测到费城染色体的丢失）和分子学缓解（即通过 RT-PCR 检测到的 BCR/ABL 基因转录物比标准基线降低 ≥ 3 个对数级）（表 2.8）。确诊后，患者通常开始接受酪氨酸激酶抑制剂（TKI）进行治疗，并密切监测药物毒性和临床反应。应在治疗开始后第 3 个月、第 6 个月和第 12 个月时采用标准化 RT-PCR 检测 BCR/ABL，以评估分子学疗效。伊马替尼最初的临床试验（1998 年）显示，96% 的患者（口服剂量 > 300 mg/d，使用 4 周）达到血液学缓解，1/3 的患者在 8 周后获得细胞遗传学缓解。后续数据显示，伊马替尼治疗初诊的慢性期 CML 患者的疗效优于非 TKI 治疗组，近 90% 的慢性期 CML 患者获得完全细胞遗传学缓解，总体存活率约 89%。获得缓解的患者可以在数年甚至数十年内保持疾病稳定，这一事实最终证明该药物可有效改变 CML 的自然病程。

尽管如此，大多数使用伊马替尼获得细胞遗传学缓解的患者仍可持续检测到 BCR/ABL 阳性的白血病干细胞。患者可能需要终身服用伊马替尼来控制病情，即使是病情控制良好的慢性期 CML 患者，由于出现对伊马替尼耐药的 CML 细胞和（或）依从性问题，仍然存在最终疾病进展和治疗失败的风险。据估计，高达 1/3 的慢性期 CML 患者由于不耐受药物诱导的副作用（如恶心、呕吐、胃肠道问题、外周水肿和眶周水肿）或对伊马替尼产生耐药而停药。

为了解决这些问题，目前已研发了 4 种新一代 TKI 用于治疗慢性期 CML：达沙替尼、尼洛替尼、博舒替尼和普纳替尼（表 2.9）。与伊马替尼相比，这 4 种药物的体外试验均显示对 BCR/ABL 激酶的抑制作用明显增强。伊马替尼、达沙替尼、尼洛替尼和博舒

TABLE 2.10 Scoring Systems for Risk Calculation in Newly Diagnosed Chronic Myeloid Leukemia

Risk Score	Calculation	Risk Category
Sokal score[1]	Exp 0.0116 × (age − 43.4) + 0.0345 × (spleen − 7.51) + 0.188 × [(platelet count ÷ 700)2 − 0.563] + 0.0887 × (blasts − 2.10)	Low <0.8 Intermediate 0.8 – 1.2 High >1.2
Hasford (EURO) score[2]	(0.6666 × age [0 when age <50 years; 1, otherwise] + 0.042 × spleen size [cm below costal margin] + 0.0584 × percent blasts + 0.0413 × percent eosinophils + 0.2039 × basophils [0 when basophils <3%; 1, otherwise] + 1.0956 × platelet count [0 when platelets <1500 × 109/L; 1, otherwise]) × 1000	Low ≤780 Intermediate >780-≤1480 High >1480
EUTOS long-term 3 survival (ELTS) score	0.0025 × (age/10)3 + 0.0615 × spleen size cm below costal margin + 0.1052 × blasts in peripheral blood + 0.4104 × (platelet count/1000) − 0.5	Low ≤1.5680 Intermediate >1.5680 but ≤2.2185 High >2.2185

Online calculator for the ELTS score can be found at: https://www.leukemia-net.org/content/leukemias/cml/elts_score/index_eng.html. Calculation of relative risk based on Sokal or Hasford (EURO) score can be found at: https://www.leukemia-net.org/content/leukemias/cml/euro__and_sokal_score/index_eng.html.

trials comparing imatinib versus dasatinib or nilotinib or bosutinib in patients with newly diagnosed chronic phase CML confirmed that these newer generation TKIs outperformed imatinib as reflected by significantly higher numbers of patients achieving complete cytogenetic and molecular responses at specific time points as compared with imatinib-treated individuals. To date, however, none of these newer TKIs have significantly improved long-term overall or transformation-free survival over imatinib. Moreover, while each of these new generation TKIs have been compared in a randomized fashion with imatinib, none have been compared with any TKI other than imatinib. For this reason, recently available generic imatinib formulations continue to be recommended as the mainstay of upfront therapy for chronic phase CML.

Different scoring systems (Table 2.10) have been developed to predict the outcomes of newly diagnosed chronic phase CML patients. These scores use patient age, spleen size, platelet number, and percentage of myeloblasts as well as peripheral basophilia and eosinophilia to divide patients into low-, intermediate-, and high-risk disease. In the current era of TKI therapy, achievement of cytogenetic and molecular milestones within the first year of therapy has proven to be much more predictive of clinical outcome than these scoring systems. However, calculation of these scores has proven useful to guide selection of upfront therapy at initial presentation. Patients with low and intermediate risk scores may be assigned to standard dose imatinib while higher-risk, particularly younger patients, presenting with very high white blood cell counts and/or massive splenomegaly, may be considered for second-generation TKIs (dasatinib, nilotinib, bosutinib). Alternatively, if imatinib is used in higher-risk patients, closer monitoring for need to switch to another TKI may be warranted. Lastly, given the myriad of TKI agents available for upfront therapy, the excellent overall response (>90% for all TKIs), and the possibility that patients may need to remain on therapy for years if not the rest of their lives, consideration of other factors impacting long-term tolerability and compliance are now given increased importance in drug selection. These include patient preference (i.e., for once a day vs. twice a day administration, with food vs. empty stomach), other medical comorbidities (i.e., cardiovascular vs. pulmonary vs. gastrointestinal) that may be exacerbated by specific TKI associated toxicities, and drug-drug interactions (i.e., proton pump inhibitors and dasatinib) (see Table 2.9).

Perhaps the best indicator of the clinical success of BCR-ABL inhibitor therapy for CML is the fact that it is now possible (with careful monitoring) to permanently discontinue TKI therapy in a proportion of patients with chronic phase disease who have achieved optimal durable molecular responses on therapy. Candidates for "TKI discontinuation therapy" are individuals with chronic phase CML treated with an approved TKI agent for at least 3 years and who have obtained major molecular responses lasting for at least 2 years. Importantly, patients should have no history of accelerated or blast phase CML or demonstrated clinical or mutational resistance to prior TKI therapy. They must also be willing to undergo monthly to bimonthly visits for at least 2 years after drug discontinuation for frequent molecular testing. Although nilotinib is the only TKI with a regulatory indication for drug discontinuation, results of multiple clinical trials suggest that stopping any TKI in patients meeting these criteria results in 40% to 50% success rate (i.e., patients able to eventually permanently stop therapy). The remaining 50% to 60% will experience recurrence of disease as reflected by reemergence of molecular detectable disease by qPCR. If detected early, almost all (detected by reemergent *BCR-ABL* transcripts off therapy) can resume TKI therapy with re-achievement of major molecular remission. Some patients develop mild to severe musculoskeletal symptoms after discontinuing TKI (termed "TKI withdrawal syndrome"), which is managed with symptomatic medications.

The most common therapeutic strategy for chronic phase CML patients intolerant of or resistant to first-line TKI therapy based on lack of achievement of molecular and cytogenetic milestones is to switch to another TKI. Mutational analysis at the time of relapse (see Table 2.9) is essential because up to one half of CML patients who develop resistance to imatinib have cancer cells carrying single-nucleotide mutations in the *BCR/ABL* gene. These mutations result in conformational changes of the BCR/ABL kinase, altering drug binding and inhibitory effects. For this reason, it is recommended that patients requiring second-line therapy or beyond undergo testing for identification of mutations as a potential guide to therapy. CML patients with disease associated with a mutation at *T315I* are known to be resistant to imatinib, nilotinib, dasatinib, and bosutinib, but not to ponatinib, a third-generation BCR/ABL inhibitor. Use of ponatinib, a highly potent third-generation BCR-ABL inhibitor, is restricted to individuals with chronic, accelerated or blast phase CML who have failed and/or been intolerant to at least two prior TKI therapies or whose mutational testing demonstrates a *BCR-ABL T315I* tyrosine kinase domain mutation conferring resistance to all other TKIs. Ponatinib is not recommended for the treatment of patients with newly diagnosed chronic phase CML due to adverse events of arterial occlusion (including fatal myocardial infarction, stroke, and severe peripheral vascular disease occurring in up to 35% of patients), venous thromboembolism, heart

表 2.10　初诊 CML 风险计算的评分系统

风险评分	计算方法	风险类别
Sokal 评分 1	0.0116×（年龄－43.4）+0.0345×（脾大小－7.51）+0.188×[（血小板计数÷700）×2－0.563]+0.0887×（原始细胞－2.10）	低危＜0.8 中危 0.8～1.2 高危＞1.2
Hasford（EURO）评分 2	[0.6666×年龄（年龄＜50 岁时为 0；否则为 1）+0.042×脾大小（肋缘下厘米数）+0.0584×原始细胞百分比+0.0413×嗜酸性粒细胞百分比+0.2039×嗜碱性粒细胞（嗜碱性粒细胞＜3% 时为 0；否则为 1）+1.0956×血小板计数（血小板＜1500×10^9/L 时为 0；否则为 1）]×1000	低危≤780 中危＞780 且≤1480 高危＞1480
EUTOS 长期生存（ELTS）评分 3	0.0025×（年龄/10）3+0.0615×脾大小（肋缘下厘米数）+0.1052×外周血原始细胞+0.4104×（血小板计数/1000）－0.5	低危≤1.5680 中危＞1.5680 且≤2.2185 高危＞2.2185

ELTS 评分的在线计算器参见：https://www.leukemia-net.org/content/leukemias/cml/elts_score/index_eng.html。
基于 Sokal 或 Hasford（EURO）评分的相对风险参见：https://www.leukemia-net.org/content/leukemias/cml/euro__and_sokal_score/index_eng.html。

替尼已被批准用于慢性期 CML 的初始治疗。多项随机临床试验比较了达沙替尼与伊马替尼或尼洛替尼与伊马替尼治疗初诊 CML 患者的疗效，结果显示，第二代 TKI 在特定时间点的完全细胞遗传学缓解率和分子学缓解率更高。然而，迄今为止，与伊马替尼相比，这些第二代 TKI 均未显著改善长期总体生存率或无转化生存期。此外，虽然这些新一代 TKI 均已在随机试验中与伊马替尼进行了比较，但尚未与伊马替尼以外的其他 TKI 进行比较。因此，近期上市的伊马替尼仿制药仍被推荐作为慢性期 CML 前期治疗的主要药物。

目前已开发出不同的评分系统（表 2.10）来预测初诊慢性期 CML 患者的临床结局。这些评分利用患者年龄、脾大小、血小板计数、髓系原始细胞百分比及外周血嗜碱性粒细胞增多和嗜酸性粒细胞增多将患者分为低危、中危和高危组。在当前的 TKI 治疗时代，治疗第 1 年内实现细胞遗传学和分子学缓解被证明比这些评分系统更能预测临床结局。然而，这些评分有助于指导初次就诊时前期治疗的选择。低危和中危患者可使用标准剂量伊马替尼，而高危患者[白细胞计数极高和（或）巨脾]，特别是年轻患者，可考虑使用第二代 TKI（达沙替尼、尼洛替尼和博舒替尼）。此外，高危患者使用伊马替尼时可能需要密切监测是否需要改用另一种 TKI。考虑到目前多种 TKI 药物可用于前期治疗、总体反应率非常高（所有 TKI 均＞90%），以及患者可能需要持续治疗数年，因此其他影响长期耐受性和依从性的因素在药物选择中变得越来越重要。这些因素包括患者偏好（如 1 次 / 日 vs. 2 次 / 日给药、随餐服用 vs. 空腹服用）、可能因特定 TKI 相关毒性而加重的合并症（如心血管疾病 vs. 肺部疾病 vs. 胃肠道疾病）和药物间相互作用（如质子泵抑制剂和达沙替尼）（表 2.9）。

BCR-ABL 抑制剂成功治疗 CML 的最佳指标可能是部分已持续达到最佳分子学缓解的慢性期 CML 患者可以永久停止 TKI 治疗（在密切监测下）。"TKI 停药治疗"的候选患者是指接受已获批准的 TKI 药物治疗至少 3 年且已持续获得主要分子反应至少 2 年的慢性期 CML 患者。重要的是，患者不应有加速期或急变期 CML 病史，或表现出对既往 TKI 治疗的临床耐药或突变耐药。此外，还必须在停药后至少 2 年内每 1～2 个月进行 1 次 BCR-ABL 水平检测。虽然尼洛替尼是唯一具有停药监管指征的 TKI，但多项临床试验结果表明，符合上述标准的住院患者停 TKI 的成功率（即患者最终能够永久停止治疗）为 40%～50%。其余 50%～60% 的患者会出现疾病复发（可通过 qPCR 检测到 BCR-ABL 基因复阳）。如果及早发现，几乎所有患者再次使用 TKI 治疗后可重新实现主要分子学缓解。一些患者在停用 TKI 后出现轻度至重度肌肉骨骼症状（被称为"TKI 戒断综合征"），可通过对症药物进行治疗。

对一线 TKI 治疗耐药或不耐受副作用的慢性期 CML 患者通常可改用另一种药物。出现复发时需行突变分析（表 2.9），因为约 1/2 的伊马替尼耐药者存在 BCR/ABL 基因单核苷酸突变，引起 BCR/ABL 激酶的构象变化，改变药物结合和抑制作用。因此，对于需要接受二线治疗或更高剂量治疗的患者，检测突变是必需的。目前发现具有 T315I 突变的 CML 患者对伊马替尼、尼罗替尼、达沙替尼和博舒替尼均耐药，但对第三代 BCR-ABL 抑制剂普纳替尼不耐药。普纳替尼为第三代强效 BCR-ABL 抑制剂，限用于既往至少 2 种 TKI 治疗失败和（或）不耐受或其突变分析表明 BCR-ABL T315I 酪氨酸激酶结构域突变导致对所有其他 TKI 耐药的慢性期、加速期或急变期 CML 患者。由于其可能造成动脉闭塞不良事件（高达 35% 的患者可能发生致命的心肌梗死、卒中和严重周围血管疾病）、静脉血栓栓塞、心力衰竭和肝毒性，不推荐普纳替尼用于治疗初诊慢性期 CML 患者。在≥3 种 TKI 治疗失败的 CML 患者中，阿西米尼（一种新型 BCR-ABL 变构

failure, and hepatotoxicity. In patients with CML that has failed three or more TKIs, treatment with asciminib, a novel allosteric inhibitor of BCR-ABL, has shown promising activity. This agent binds a myristoyl site of BCR-ABL1 protein and thereby locks BCR-ABL1 into an inactive conformation through a mechanism distinct from all other ABL kinase inhibitors. Because asciminib targets both native and mutated BCR-ABL1, it is also effective against CML cells harboring the gatekeeper *T315I* mutation. In a phase 1 trial, almost half (48%) of patients achieved a major molecular response in 12 months, including 8 of 14 patients with prior intolerance or resistance to ponatinib.

Patients whose disease does not respond and/or who are intolerant of multiple TKIs also may receive treatment with omacetaxine mepesuccinate, a natural alkaloid product with proven antitumor activity and efficacy in CML. Its mechanisms of action are distinct from the TKIs and involve inhibition of protein synthesis and induction of apoptosis in tumor cells. Several clinical trials have confirmed the activity of this agent in patients with CML failing multiple TKIs and/or carrying the T315I mutation. A major drawback is the need for subcutaneous injections administered twice daily for 7 to 14 days of every 28 days per month and treatment-associated myelosuppression that may warrant dose reduction or interruption.

Accelerated and Blast Phase CML

Unfortunately, the majority of patients with accelerated or blast phase CML treated with new-generation TKI therapies experience only transient hematologic and cytogenetic responses. For these patients, the optimal treatment modality remains TKI therapy with newer-generation agents with or without additional chemotherapy or clinical trials followed by allogeneic stem cell transplantation (alloSCT). The novel allosteric BCR-ABL inhibitor, asciminib, reportedly induced hematologic responses in seven of eight patients with accelerated phase CML with a median duration of response of greater than 11 months. Blast phase CML patients often undergo induction chemotherapy with acute leukemia regimens with concomitant BCR/ABL inhibition. Transplantation, however, remains the only known curative therapy for these patients. Prior to the advent of targeted BCR/ABL kinase inhibitor therapy, young patients with an HLA-matched donor were routinely offered potentially curative alloSCT at the time of diagnosis of chronic phase CML. Evidence indicated that the excellent response (50% to 75%) of CML patients to SCT was partly related to the active suppression of the disease by the newly transplanted graft, called the *graft-versus-leukemia effect*. At present, in the face of the excellent control and low overall toxicity of long-term BCR/ABL inhibitors for chronic phase CML, together with the known 20% to 30% mortality and morbidity rates after alloSCT, transplantation is now viewed as an option only for patients with accelerated or blast phase disease or chronic phase CML failing multiple lines of prior therapy. Following alloSCT, it is now considered standard of care to resume TKI maintenance therapy for at least 12 months in the post-transplant setting to prevent disease relapse.

Prognosis

Overall, the transformation of CML from a progressively fatal cancer to one in which almost 90% of patients are alive with stable disease on oral kinase therapy and 10% can permanently discontinue therapy after 5 years remains one of the crowning achievements in cancer therapy in the past decade. The median overall survival for chronic phase CML patients has risen dramatically from a few months to a few years in the first half of the 20th century to 6 years for interferon-treated patients. In the era of BCR/ABL inhibition therapy, overall lifespan is expected to be almost normal for most patients on long-term TKI therapy with multiple studies demonstrating that the risk of death in these individuals occurs not due to CML-related complications but rather to increased cardiac and vascular causes. For this reason, a focus of current CML practice is determining how best to balance the long-term toxicities of TKI therapy with its benefits. Although standard of care for CML patients who are responding optimally to treatment remains indefinite continuation of TKI therapy, selected individuals with sustained excellent molecular responses to TKI therapy for at least 3 years are now eligible to discontinue therapy with a 40% to 50% long-term success rate. Despite this therapeutic advance, a true cure for CML disease remains elusive for the majority of patients. Ongoing clinical studies are focused on strategies to further enhance this percentage by targeting CML stem cells and via combinatorial TKI approaches.

ACUTE LEUKEMIAS

Definition and Epidemiology

The acute leukemias are clinically aggressive clonal hematopoietic diseases arising from the malignant transformation of an early hematopoietic stem cell. In adults, acute leukemias are relatively uncommon and occur in 8 to 10 of 100,000 people (compared with 42 of 100,000 for prostate cancer and 62 of 100,000 for breast cancer). Acute leukemias are classified by cell lineage as AML or acute lymphocytic or lymphoblastic leukemia (ALL) based on morphology, cytogenetics, cell surface and cytoplasmic markers, and molecular studies. Between 80% and 90% of leukemia diagnoses in adults are AML. In contrast, 80% to 90% of leukemias in infants and children are ALL, and they constitute the most common cancer diagnosed in this age group.

Pathology

The pathogenesis of acute leukemia is complex and characterized by a high degree of biologic heterogeneity. Many patients with acute leukemia have detectable characteristic clonal chromosomal abnormalities and mutations that drive malignant transformation of normal hematopoietic stem cells bearing myeloid or lymphoid lineage markers. The resultant unchecked proliferation of these immature cells incapable of further differentiation (i.e., blasts) results in marrow replacement by malignant cells, peripheral leukocytosis, with and without severe cytopenias, and rapid hematopoietic failure. Known risk factors for leukemia include high-dose radiation exposure and occupational exposure to chemicals including benzene. Up to 10% of patients with prior malignancies treated with myelosuppressive chemotherapy and/or radiation develop "therapy-related" AML (t-AML). Individuals with t-AML with previous chemotherapy have usually received alkylating agents (e.g., chlorambucil, melphalan, nitrogen mustard) or topoisomerase II inhibitors (e.g., epipodophyllotoxins). Patients with chromosomal instability disorders such as Down syndrome, Bloom syndrome, Fanconi anemia, and ataxia telangiectasia also have an increased incidence of leukemia.

Diagnosis and Differential Diagnosis

To make the distinction between AML and ALL is crucial diagnostically, therapeutically, and prognostically. AML can be distinguished from ALL by cell morphology and the finding of Auer rods (sometimes multiple ones in acute promyelocytic leukemia cells), which are formed by the aggregation of myeloid granules. Further immunophenotyping of blast cells using cell surface antigens, cytochemistry, and immunohistochemistry confirms cells as having a myeloid or lymphoid origin. Morphologic subgroups of ALL and AML were originally defined by the French-American-British (FAB) classification and most recently by the 2016 World Health Organization (WHO) classification, which incorporates newer biologic information, specifically mutations and recurrent cytogenetic aberrations (Table 2.11).

抑制剂）显示出良好的治疗活性。该药物结合 BCR-ABL1 蛋白的肉豆蔻酰位点，从而通过与其他 ABL 激酶抑制剂不同的机制将 BCR-ABL1 锁定为非活性构象。由于阿西米尼同时靶向天然和突变的 BCR-ABL1，因此它也能有效对抗携带 T315I 突变的 CML 细胞。在一项 I 期临床试验中，近 1/2（48%）的患者在 12 个月内实现了主要分子学缓解，其中包括 14 名既往对普纳替尼不耐受或耐药患者中的 8 名。

无治疗反应和（或）对多种 TKI 不耐受的患者也可使用高三尖杉酯碱，这是一种天然生物碱产物，在 CML 中具有抗肿瘤活性和疗效。其作用机制与 TKI 不同，涉及抑制肿瘤细胞的蛋白质合成和诱导细胞凋亡。多项临床试验已证实，该药物对多种 TKI 治疗失败和（或）携带 T315I 突变的 CML 患者具有治疗活性。该药的主要缺点是需要每天皮下注射 2 次，持续 7～14 天，每 28 天为 1 个周期，并且需要根据治疗相关性骨髓抑制来减少剂量或中断治疗。

加速期和急变期 CML

虽然新一代 TKI 抑制剂可以暂时诱导加速期或急变期 CML 患者获得血液学和细胞遗传学缓解，但绝大多数患者的维持时间不长。对于这些患者，最佳治疗方式仍然是使用新一代 TKI，联合或不联合额外化疗或临床试验，然后进行 alloSCT。在 8 名加速期 CML 患者中使用新型 BCR-ABL 变构抑制剂阿西米尼进行诱导治疗后，7 名患者达到血液学缓解，中位反应持续时间超过 11 个月。急变期 CML 患者通常需接受急性白血病治疗方案的诱导化疗，并同时使用 TKI。目前唯一能够治愈疾病的方式仍然是 alloSCT。在 TKI 问世之前，若初诊为慢性期 CML 的年轻患者有 HLA 相合供者，通常建议选择 alloSCT，CML 患者接受 alloSCT 后根治率高（50%～75%）的部分原因是移植物抗白血病反应。目前，鉴于 BCR/ABL 抑制剂治疗慢性期 CML 患者的疗效好且毒性低，且 alloSCT 的移植相关死亡率为 20%～30%，因此移植仅适用于加速期或急变期或使用前述治疗失败的慢性期 CML 患者，这是这些患者唯一的治愈方法。目前学界公认在移植后恢复 TKI 维持治疗至少 12 个月，以防止疾病复发。

预后

CML 患者的预后因 TKI 的出现而发生了巨大变化，CML 已经从致死性癌症变成了慢性疾病，TKI 治疗 5 年后有近 90% 的患者可带病生存，10% 患者可永久停药，这是肿瘤治疗的历史性突破。在 TKI 问世前，慢性期 CML 患者的中位总体生存期为数月至数年，接受干扰素治疗者的总体生存期为 6 年。在 TKI 治疗的时代，大多数长期使用 TKI 的患者预期达到正常寿命。多项研究表明，使用 TKI 患者的死亡风险不是由于 CML 相关并发症，而是由于心血管疾病风险增加。因此，当前 CML 临床实践的重点是确定如何最好地平衡 TKI 治疗的长期毒性与获益。虽然获得最佳治疗反应的 CML 患者的标准治疗是持续接受 TKI 治疗，但对 TKI 治疗持续达到分子学缓解至少 3 年的患者可尝试停药（长期成功率可达 40%～50%）。尽管治疗已取得进展，但对于绝大多数患者来说，CML 的真正治愈仍然难以实现。现阶段正在进行的临床研究侧重于通过靶向 CML 干细胞和组合 TKI 方案进一步提高治愈率。

急性白血病

定义和流行病学

急性白血病是由早期造血干细胞恶性转化导致的恶性克隆性疾病。成人白血病的发病率相对较低，为（8～10）/100 000（前列腺癌发病率为 42/100 000，乳腺癌发病率为 62/100 000）。基于形态学、细胞遗传学、免疫分型和分子学研究，急性白血病根据细胞系分为 AML 和 ALL。80%～90% 的成人白血病为 AML（其余为 ALL），而 80%～90% 的儿童白血病是 ALL。

病理学

急性白血病的发病机制复杂，具有高度的生物学异质性。许多急性白血病患者具有可检测到的特征性克隆染色体异常和突变，从而促使带有正常髓系或淋系标志物的造血干细胞发生恶性转化。这些无法进一步分化的未成熟细胞（即原始细胞）不受控制地增殖，导致骨髓被恶性细胞替代、外周血白细胞增多（伴或不伴严重血细胞减少）及快速造血衰竭。已知的白血病危险因素包括高剂量辐射暴露和职业接触苯等化学物质。在既往接受骨髓抑制化疗和（或）放疗的恶性肿瘤患者中，高达 10% 会出现"治疗相关性"AML（tAML）。既往接受过化疗的 t-AML 患者通常使用过烷化剂（如苯丁酸氮芥、美法仑、氮芥）或拓扑异构酶 II 抑制剂（如表鬼臼毒素）。此外，染色体不稳定性疾病（如 21-三体综合征、布卢姆综合征、范科尼贫血和共济失调毛细血管扩张症）患者的白血病发病率升高。

诊断和鉴别诊断

鉴别 AML 和 ALL 对于诊断、治疗和预后十分重要。AML 可通过细胞形态学和发现 Auer 小体（由髓样颗粒聚集形成；急性早幼粒细胞白血病有时可见多个 Auer 小体）与 ALL 区分开来。通过细胞表面抗原、细胞化学和免疫组织化学检查进一步鉴定原始细胞的免疫表型，有助于鉴别髓系或淋系来源。ALL 和 AML 的形态学亚组最初由法国-美国-英国（FAB）分型定义，目前使用 2016 年 WHO 分型，该分型纳入了更新的生物学特性，特别是突变和重现性细胞遗传学异常（表 2.11）。

TABLE 2.11 Classification of Acute Leukemias

FAB Classification of Acute Myeloid Leukemia (AML)
M0: Acute myelocytic leukemia with minimal differentiation
M1: Acute myelocytic leukemia without maturation
M2: Acute myelocytic leukemia with maturation (predominantly myeloblasts and promyelocytes)
M3: Acute promyelocytic leukemia
M4: Acute myelomonocytic leukemia
M5: Acute monocytic leukemia
M6: Erythroleukemia
M7: Megakaryocytic leukemia

FAB Classification of Acute Lymphoblastic Leukemia (ALL)
L1: Predominantly small cells (twice the size of normal lymphocyte), homogeneous population; childhood variant
L2: Larger than L1, more heterogenous population; adult variant
L3: Burkitt-like large cells, vacuolated abundant cytoplasm

WHO 2016 Classification of Acute Leukemia
I. Acute myeloid leukemia (AML)
  A. AML with recurrent genetic abnormalities
    - AML with t(8;21)(q22;q22); *RUNX1-RUNX1T1*
    - AML with inv(16)(p13;q22) or t(16;16)(p13;q22); *CBFB/MYH11*
    - Acute promyelocytic leukemia (AML with t[15;17][q22;q12]; *PML/RARA*
    - AML with t(9;11)(p21.3;q23.3); *MLLT3-KMT2A*
    - AML with t(6;9)(p23;q34.1); *DEK-NUP214*
    - AML with inv(3)(q21.3 q26.2) or t(3;3)(q21.3;q26.2); *GATA2,MECOM*
    - AML (megakaryoblastic) with t(1;22)(p13.3; q13.3); *RBM15-MKL1*
    - AML with *BCR-ABL1*
    - AML with mutant *NPM1*
    - AML with biallelic mutations of *CEBPA*
    - AML with mutated *RUNX1*
  B. AML with myelodysplasia-related changes
  C. Therapy related myeloid neoplasms
  D. AML not otherwise specified
    - AML with minimal differentiation
    - AML without maturation
    - AML with maturation
    - Acute myelomonocytic leukemia
    - Acute monoblastic/monocytic leukemia
    - Pure erythroid leukemia
    - Acute megakaryoblastic leukemia
    - Acute basophilic leukemia
    - Acute panmyelosis with myelofibrosis
  E. Myeloid sarcoma
  F. Myeloid proliferations associated with Down syndrome
  G. Blastic plasmacytoid dendritic cell neoplasm
  H. Acute leukemias of ambiguous lineage
II. Precursor lymphoid neoplasms
  A. B-lymphoblastic leukemia/lymphoblastic lymphoma, not otherwise specified
  B. B-lymphoblastic leukemia/lymphoma with recurrent genetic abnormalities
    - B-lymphoblastic leukemia/lymphoma with t(9;22)(q34.1,q11.2); *BCR-ABL1*
    - B-lymphoblastic leukemia/lymphoma with t(v;11q23.3); *KMT2A*-rearranged
    - B-lymphoblastic leukemia/lymphoma with t(12;21)(p13.2;q22.1); *ETV6-RUNX1*
    - B-lymphoblastic leukemia/lymphoma with hyperdiploidy
    - B-lymphoblastic leukemia/lymphoma with hypodiploidy
    - B-lymphoblastic leukemia/lymphoma with t95;14)(q31.1,q32.1); *IGH/IL3*
    - B-lymphoblastic leukemia/lymphoma with t(;19)(q23,p13.3); *TCF3-PBX1*
    - B-lymphoblastic leukemia/lymphoma, *BCR-ABL1*-like
    - B-lymphoblastic leukemia/lymphoma with iAMP21
  C. T-lymphoblastic leukemia/lymphoblastic lymphoma
    - Early T-cell precursor lymphoblastic leukemia
  D. NK lymphoblastic leukemia/lymphoma

From Swerdlow SH, Campo E, Harris NL, Jaffe ES, Pileri SA, Stein H, Thiele J. WHO Classification of Tumours of Haematopoietic and Lymphoid Tissues (Revised Fourth Edition), IARC, 2016.

CBF, Core binding factor; *ETO*, eight twenty-one; *FAB*, French-American-British; *MDS*, primary myelodysplastic syndrome; *MLL*, mixed-lineage leukemia; *MYH11*, myosin heavy chain gene; *PML*, promyelocytic leukemia; *RARA*, retinoic acid receptor-α; *WHO*, World Health Organization.

表 2.11 急性白血病的分型

急性髓系白血病（AML）的 FAB 分型
M0：急性髓系白血病微分化型
M1：急性髓系白血病未分化型
M2：急性髓系白血病部分分化型（以原始粒细胞和早幼粒细胞为主）
M3：急性早幼粒细胞白血病
M4：急性粒-单核细胞白血病
M5：急性单核细胞白血病
M6：红白血病
M7：巨核细胞白血病

急性淋巴细胞白血病（ALL）的 FAB 分型
L1：原幼淋巴细胞以小细胞（大小是正常淋巴细胞的 2 倍）为主，大小均一；儿童变型
L2：原幼淋巴细胞大于 L1，大小不一；成人变型
L3：原幼淋巴细胞为 Burkitt 样大细胞，胞质内富含空泡

急性白血病的 WHO 2016 分型
I. 急性髓系白血病（AML）
  A. 伴重现性遗传学异常的 AML
- AML 伴 t（8;21）(q22;q22)；*RUNX1-RUNX1T1*
- AML 伴 inv（16）(p13;q22) 或 t（16;16）(p13;q22)；*CBFB/MYH11*
- 急性早幼粒细胞白血病 [AML 伴 t（15;17）(q22;q12)]；*PML/RARA*
- AML 伴 t（9;11）(p21.3;q23.3)；*MLLT3-KMT2A*
- AML 伴 t（6;9）(p23;q34.1)；*DEK-NUP214*
- AML 伴 inv（3）(q21.3 q26.2) 或 t（3;3）(q21.3;q26.2)；*GATA2、MECOM*
- AML（巨核细胞白血病）伴 t（1;22）(p13.3;q13.3)；*RBM15-MKL1*
- AML 伴 *BCR-ABL1*
- AML 伴突变型 *NPM1*
- AML 伴 *CEBPA* 双等位基因突变
- AML 伴 *RUNX1* 突变

  B. AML 伴骨髓增生异常相关改变
  C. 治疗相关髓系肿瘤
  D. AML（非特指型）
- AML 微分化型
- AML 未分化型
- AML 伴部分分化型
- 急性粒-单核细胞白血病
- 急性原始单核细胞/单核细胞白血病
- 红血病
- 急性巨核细胞白血病
- 急性嗜碱性细胞白血病
- 急性全髓细胞增殖症伴骨髓纤维化

  E. 髓系肉瘤
  F. 唐氏综合征相关骨髓增殖症
  G. 母细胞性浆细胞样树突状细胞肿瘤
  H. 系列不明急性白血病

II. 前体淋巴细胞肿瘤
  A. B 淋巴母细胞白血病/淋巴母细胞性淋巴瘤，非特指型
  B. 伴重现性遗传学异常的 B 淋巴母细胞白血病/淋巴瘤
- B 淋巴母细胞白血病/淋巴瘤伴 t（9;22）(q34.1, q11.2)；*BCR-ABL1*
- B 淋巴母细胞白血病/淋巴瘤伴 t（v;11q23.3）；*KMT2A* 重排
- B 淋巴母细胞白血病/淋巴瘤伴 t（12;21）(p13.2;q22.1)；*ETV6-RUNX1*
- B 淋巴细胞白血病/淋巴瘤伴超二倍体
- B 淋巴母细胞白血病/淋巴瘤伴低二倍体
- B 淋巴母细胞白血病/淋巴瘤与 t（95;14）(q31.1, q32.1)；*IGH/IL3*
- B 淋巴母细胞白血病/淋巴瘤伴 t（1;19）(q23, p13.3)；*TCF3-PBX1*
- B 淋巴母细胞白血病/淋巴瘤，*BCR-ABL1* 样
- B 淋巴母细胞白血病/淋巴瘤伴 iAMP21

  C. T 淋巴细胞白血病/淋巴母细胞性淋巴瘤
- 早期前体 T 淋巴母细胞白血病

  D. NK 淋巴母细胞白血病/淋巴瘤

引自 Swerdlow SH，Campo E，Harris NL，Jaffe ES，Pileri SA，Stein H，Thiele J. WHO Classification of Tumours of Haematopoietic and Lymphoid Tissues（Revised Fourth Edition），IARC，2016.

CBF，核结合因子；FAB，法国-美国-英国；MLL，混合谱系白血病；MYH11，肌球蛋白重链基因；PML，早幼粒细胞白血病；RARA，视黄酸受体 α；WHO，世界卫生组织。

Clinical Presentation

Patients exhibit clinical evidence of bone marrow failure similar to other hematopoietic disorders. Complications of disease include anemia, infection, and bleeding from peripheral cytopenias. Proliferating blasts infiltrating the bone marrow may cause bone pain. Blasts may also invade other organs and lead to peripheral, mediastinal, and abdominal lymphadenopathy, hepatosplenomegaly, skin infiltration, and meningeal involvement.

Treatment

Therapy for acute leukemias is divided into several stages. *Induction therapy* is directed at reducing the number of leukemic blasts to an undetectable level and restoring normal hematopoiesis (i.e., complete remission). At complete remission, however, significant subclinical disease persists, requiring further therapy. Subsequent *consolidation therapy* involves continuing chemotherapy with the same agents to induce elimination of additional leukemic cells. With development of a wider range of effective agents, *intensification therapy* has been introduced. It involves the use of high-dose therapy with different non–cross-reactive drugs to eliminate cells with potential primary resistance to the induction regimen. *Maintenance therapy* employs low-dose, intermittent chemotherapy given over a prolonged period to prevent subsequent disease relapse. The goal of therapy is to induce remission (>5% blasts in the bone marrow and recovery of normal peripheral blood counts).

Prognosis

Adverse clinical prognostic factors for AML and ALL are similar despite widely different treatment approaches. In both leukemias, cytogenetic and molecular abnormalities represent the best independent predictors of overall survival (Tables 2.11, 2.12, and 2.13). Clinical factors that predict a poor outcome differ by specific leukemia type but generally include older age (>35 years in ALL, >60 years for AML), secondary or therapy-related disease, antecedent hematologic disorder, high initial leukocyte count (50 to 100 × 10^9/L), poor performance status and comorbidities, extramedullary disease, prolonged time (>4 weeks) or lack of response to initial treatment, and presence of detectable minimal residual disease (MRD) despite morphologic remission.

Acute Myeloid Leukemia

Definition and Epidemiology

AML represents a biologically heterogeneous group of neoplasms with widely divergent clinical outcomes. Long-term cure rates (survival >5 years) range from 5% to 60% after chemotherapy alone, with an overall cure rate of 20% to 30%. AML occurs primarily in older adults, with a median age at diagnosis of 65 years.

Clinical Presentation

Patients most often have complications related to progressively severe cytopenia, such as infection due to leukopenia, shortness of breath or fatigue due to anemia, or bleeding due to thrombocytopenia. AML patients may also have unique acute clinical emergencies requiring immediate stabilization. Leukostasis (i.e., hyperleukocytosis syndrome) caused by high levels of circulating blasts (>80,000 to 100,000) leads to diffuse pulmonary infiltrates and acute respiratory distress. Blast cells may also injure surrounding vasculature, causing life-threatening CNS bleeding and thromboses. High blast cell numbers result in the release of cellular breakdown products (i.e., tumor lysis syndrome), leading to hypokalemia, acidosis, and hyperuricemia with resultant renal failure.

Treatment of leukostasis should be instituted as soon as possible for all patients with white blood cell counts in excess of 100 to 200 × 10^9/L. Treatment consists of leukapheresis, hydroxyurea, and initiation of induction chemotherapy to inhibit further production of circulating tumor cells. Hydration, urine alkalinization to reduce uric acid crystallization, allopurinol, or rasburicase, or a combination, should be initiated as indicated. Red blood cell transfusions are often contraindicated in patients with high numbers of circulating blast cells because of the risk of further increases in blood viscosity. CNS complications such as intracranial bleeding, cranial nerve invasion, and leukemic meningitis are treated with emergency whole brain irradiation or radiation directed to affected sites.

Laboratory evaluation of patients with AML typically shows white blood cell counts ranging from neutropenic levels (<1 × 10^9/L) to extreme leukocytosis (>100,000 × 10^9/L). Severe thrombocytopenia, normocytic anemia, and circulating peripheral blasts are common. Bone marrow aspirate and biopsy typically show a profusion of myeloblasts (20% to 100%) and depressed production of normal mature cells.

Diagnosis

Diagnostic marrow aspirates and/or peripheral blood samples require evaluation by morphology, flow cytometry, cytogenetic, and molecular analyses to distinguish between AML and ALL and to determine biologic subsets of AML disease for prognostic and therapeutic purposes.

In the past, AML subsets were classified based largely on morphologic criteria and immunohistochemical staining as FAB subtypes M0 through M7, largely defined by the stage of cellular differentiation of the abnormal cells (see Table 2.11). Some FAB subsets correlate with specific clinical syndromes, which helps to determine treatment approaches and prognosis. The most common FAB subtype of adult AML is M2. Patients with AML M3 (i.e., acute promyelocytic leukemia) often exhibit spontaneous bleeding from disseminated intravascular coagulation (discussed later). Patients with AML M4 or M5 disease (i.e., acute monocytic-myelomonocytic leukemias) have high levels of circulating white blood cells and may have swollen gums resulting from tissue infiltration with leukemic blasts. Patients with megakaryoblastic leukemia (AML M7) have significant marrow fibrosis and usually exhibit organomegaly and pancytopenia similar to those seen in patients with myelofibrosis and myeloid metaplasia.

Large-scale genomic analyses of AML samples have revealed the vast molecular complexity of this disease and identified myriad gene mutations capable of further refining AML prognosis in conjunction with karyotype. For instance, up to one third of patients with normal-karyotype AML have constitutive activation of the FMS-like tyrosine kinase 3 (FLT3) receptor as a result of point mutations or internal tandem duplications (ITDs) not seen on routine karyotypic testing. *FLT3 ITD* mutations in AML patients predict for lower remission rates, high relapse rates, and shorter overall survival compared with *FLT3*-negative AML patients. Patients with higher *FLT3 ITD* tumor burden (reflected by the ratio of mutant to wild-type *FLT3* or the allelic ratio) have particularly poor prognoses, whereas individuals with low *FLT3 ITD* allelic ratio may have outcomes similar to *FLT3* wild-type patients. Mutations that predict improved overall survival after chemotherapy include biallelic mutations in the transcription factor CCAAT/enhancer binding protein-α *(CEBPA)* and nucleophosmin 1 *(NPM1)* in the absence of *FLT3 ITDs* (see Tables 2.11 and 2.12).

The classification and prognostication of AML was refined in 2016 by the WHO to recognize biologic subtypes with unique genetic abnormalities such as t(8;21), inv(16), t(15;17), and t(9;11) as well as *BCR-ABL1*, biallelic *CEBPA*, and *RUNX1* mutations. Other categories include AML with myelodysplastic-related changes (defined by

临床表现

患者的骨髓衰竭临床表现与其他造血系统疾病相似，包括由外周全血细胞减少所致的贫血、感染和出血。原始细胞增殖浸润骨髓可能引起骨痛。原始细胞可侵袭其他器官，导致外周、纵隔和腹部淋巴结肿大，以及肝脾大、皮肤浸润和脑膜受累。

治疗

急性白血病的治疗分为若干阶段。诱导治疗旨在将白血病细胞数量降至不可检测的水平，并恢复正常造血（即完全缓解）。然而，完全缓解后，亚临床疾病仍然存在，需要进一步治疗。随后的巩固治疗包括用相同的药物继续化疗，以消除残存的白血病细胞。随着更多有效药物的研发，目前已引入强化治疗，包括使用无交叉耐药的药物进行大剂量治疗，以消除对诱导方案可能产生耐药的白血病细胞。维持治疗是指长期给予患者低剂量间歇化疗，以防止疾病复发。治疗的目的是获得缓解（骨髓中原始细胞＞5%，外周血细胞计数恢复正常）。

预后

尽管治疗方法不同，AML 和 ALL 的不良临床预后因素类似。在这两种白血病中，细胞遗传学异常和分子学异常均是总体生存率的最佳独立预测因素（表 2.11 至表 2.13）。提示预后不良的临床因素包括年龄较大（ALL 患者＞35 岁或 AML 患者＞60 岁）、继发性或治疗相关疾病、既往罹患血液疾病、初始白细胞计数升高 [($50 \sim 100) \times 10^9$/L]、一般状况差及合并症、髓外浸润、对初始治疗的反应时间延长（＞4 周）或无反应、虽形态学缓解但仍持续存在可检测到的微量残留病（MRD）。

急性髓系白血病

定义和流行病学

急性髓系白血病（AML）是一种异质性肿瘤。单纯化疗后，长期治愈率（生存期＞5 年）为 5%～60%，总治愈率为 20%～30%。AML 主要见于老年人，诊断时的中位年龄为 65 岁。

临床表现

患者最常见的症状与严重全血细胞减少有关，如白细胞减少引起的感染、贫血引起的气短或乏力、血小板减少引起的出血。AML 患者也可能出现特有的需要紧急处理的临床急症。由外周血原始细胞增多 [＞($80 \sim 100) \times 10^9$/L] 引起的白细胞淤滞症（即高白细胞综合征）可导致弥漫性肺浸润和急性呼吸窘迫。原始细胞也可引起致死性颅内出血和血栓形成。白血病细胞数量增多可引起细胞分解而发生肿瘤溶解综合征，导致低钾血症、酸中毒和高尿酸血症，最终导致肾衰竭。

当患者白细胞计数超过（$100 \sim 200) \times 10^9$/L 时，应尽快对白细胞淤滞症进行治疗。治疗方法包括白细胞去除术、羟基脲和化疗前短期预处理方案，以抑制循环中肿瘤细胞的进一步产生。建议给予水化、碱化尿液，以减少尿酸结晶，可使用别嘌醇和（或）拉布立酶。由于血液黏度有进一步增加的风险，红细胞输注通常禁用于循环中有大量原始细胞的患者。CNS 并发症包括颅内出血、脑神经受侵犯和脑膜白血病，需进行紧急全脑照射或定向辐射治疗。

AML 患者的实验室检查可显示白细胞计数从中性粒细胞减少（＜1×10^9/L）到极端白细胞增多（＞$100\,000 \times 10^9$/L）。常见严重血小板减少、正细胞性贫血和外周血原始细胞。骨髓穿刺和活检通常显示大量原始粒细胞（20%～100%），并抑制正常成熟细胞的产生。

诊断

诊断性骨髓穿刺和（或）外周血样本需要通过形态学、流式细胞术、细胞遗传学和分子学分析以鉴别 AML 和 ALL，并确定 AML 亚型，以利于预后和治疗。

既往主要根据形态学标准和免疫组织化学染色将 AML 按 FAB 分类分为 M0～M7 型，这主要由异常细胞的细胞分化阶段来划分（表 2.11）。一些 FAB 亚型与特定的临床综合征相关，这有助于确定治疗方法和预后。成人 AML 最常见的 FAB 亚型是 M2。AML M3（即急性早幼粒细胞白血病）患者常表现出由弥散性血管内凝血引起的自发性出血（见下文）。AML M4 或 M5（即急性粒-单核细胞白血病或急性单核细胞白血病）患者外周循环中白细胞水平增高，且原始细胞可能浸润组织导致牙龈肿胀。AML M7（即巨核细胞白血病）患者有明显的骨髓纤维化，通常表现出类似于骨髓纤维化的肝脾大和全血细胞减少。

对 AML 样本进行的大规模基因组分析揭示了该病的分子学复杂性，并确定了能够进一步改善 AML 预后的多种基因突变与染色体核型。例如，多达 1/3 的正常核型 AML 患者存在由点突变或内部串联重复（ITD）引起的 FMS 样酪氨酸激酶 3（FLT3）受体的持续激活。与 *FLT3* 突变阴性 AML 患者相比，AML 患者的 *FLT3-ITD* 突变预示着较低的缓解率、较高的复发率和较短的总生存期。*FLT3-ITD* 肿瘤负荷较高的患者（通过突变型与野生型 *FLT3* 的比例或等位基因比例反映）的预后特别差，而 *FLT3-ITD* 等位基因突变比例低的患者可能具有与野生型 *FLT3* 患者相似的预后。提示化疗后预后良好的突变包括转录因子 CCAAT/增强子结合蛋白 α（CEBPA）的双等位基因突变和核仁磷蛋白 1（NPM1）突变（在没有 *FLT3-ITD* 的情况下）（表 2.11 和表 2.12）。

2016 年，WHO 根据遗传学异常 [如 t（8;21）、inv（16）、t（15;17）t（9;11）]、*BCR-ABL*、双等位基因 *CEBPA*、*RUNX1* 基因突变对 AML 进行重新分型，以利于治疗和风险预测。其他分类包括 AML 伴骨髓增

TABLE 2.12 European Leukemia Net (ELN) Classification of Acute Myeloid Leukemia (2017)

Risk Category	Genetic Abnormality
Favorable	t(8;21)(q22;q22.1); *RUNX1-RUNX1T1*
	inv(16)(p13.1q22) or t(16;16)(p13.1;q22): *CBFB-MYH11*
	Mutated *NPM1* without *FLT3-ITD* or with *FLT3-ITD*^{low}
	Biallelic mutated *CEBPA*
Intermediate	Mutated *NPM1* and *FLT-ITD*^{high}
	Wild-type NPM1 without *FLT3-ITD* or with *FLT3* ITD^{low} (without adverse genetic lesions) t(9;11)(p21.3;q23.3): *MLLT3-KMT2A*
	Cytogenetic abnormalities not classified as favorable or adverse)
Adverse	t(6;9)(p23;q34.1); *DEK-NUP214*
	t(v;11q23.3): *KMT2A* rearranged
	t(9;22)(q34.1:q11.2): *BCR-ABL1*
	inv(3)(q21.3q26.2) or t(3;3)(q21.3;q26.2); *GATA2, MECOM (EV11)*
	−5 or del(5q); −7; −17/abn(17p)
	Complex karyotype, monosomal karyotype
	Wild-type *NPM1* and *FLT3-ITD*^{high}
	Mutated *RUNX1*
	Mutated *ASXL1*
	Mutated *TP53*

From Dohner H, Estey EH, Grimwade D, et al. Diagnosis and management of AML in adults: 2017 ELM recommendations from an international expert panel. Blood 129(4): 424-447, 2017.
ITDs, Internal tandem duplications.

TABLE 2.13 Prognostic Factors in Acute Lymphoblastic Leukemia

Factor	Favorable	Unfavorable
Age	2-10 yr	<2 yr or >10 yr
White blood cell count at diagnosis	<30,000/μL	>50,000/μL
Phenotype	Precursor B	Precursor T
Chromosome number	Hyperdiploidy	Pseudo/hypodiploidy, near tetraploidy
Chromosome abnormality	t(12;21)	*MYC* alterations: t(8;14), t(2;8), t(8;22) mixed-lineage leukemia alterations (11q23)
		Philadelphia chromosome: t(9;22), creating *BCR-ABL*
Central nervous system disease at diagnosis	No	Yes
Sex	Women	Men
Ethnicity	White	African American, Hispanic
Time to remission	Short (7-14 days)	Prolonged time to remission or failure to achieve remission

the presence of multilineage dysplasia, prior clinical and pathologic results, and/or characteristic karyotypic aberrations) and therapy-related AML (based on clinical history of prior chemotherapy, irradiation, or other myeloablative therapy preceding AML diagnosis). In the latter case, any marrow dysplasia together with cytopenias is now considered therapy-related AML rather than MDS regardless of blast count (see Table 2.11).

Treatment and Prognosis

Upfront chemotherapy for AML has changed drastically over the last few years due to the advent of multiple new drugs for specific clinical and biological subsets of disease. For decades, it has been known that the clinical factors predictive of poor outcome include advanced age (>60 years old), therapy-related or with antecedent hematologic disorder (termed secondary AML), poor performance status, elevated initial white blood cell counts (>20-30K to >100K), and presence of disease outside the bone marrow. Extramedullary disease includes leukemic involvement in the central nervous system, skin and soft tissues (myeloid or granulocytic sarcoma), and any other organ involvement outside of the bone marrow and peripheral blood. Although these clinical factors are still considered, in this era the most important factors impacting treatment decisions for newly diagnosed patients are (1) overall functionality/comorbidities and (2) AML risk category.

AML is known to be a biologically heterogeneous disease with vast differences in outcomes based on underlying disease. Early AML risk prognostication was based primarily on karyotypic aberrations that have stood the test of time as the most robust independent predictors of response to intensive (cytarabine and anthracycline based) chemotherapy approaches. However, recent advances in genomic and molecular technologies have shed much light on the role of diverse gene mutations to AML pathogenesis. Genes involved in at least eight different biologic processes have been identified in primary AML samples. The most recent AML risk classification proposed by the European Leukemia Net delineates three risk categories (favorable, intermediate, and poor risk) incorporating diagnostic cytogenetic and molecular information (see Table 2.12). Because the presence of certain "actionable" mutations (specifically *CBF, FLT3, NPM1, IDH1,* and *IDH2*) can significantly alter upfront therapy selection, it is recommended that molecular tests evaluating these aberrations be performed in an expedited manner (turnaround time of 3-5 days) in all suspected AML cases (see Table 2.12).

Treatment based on disease subsets

Patients who are younger than 60 years and/or fit for intensive chemotherapy. The "traditional" induction regimens administered in the inpatient setting consist of 7 days of cytosine arabinoside (i.e., cytarabine) and 3 days of high-dose anthracycline (i.e., daunorubicin or idarubicin) and is commonly referred to as "7+3." Once morphologic remission (marrow blasts <5%) and count recovery (WBC >1000, platelets >100,000/mcL) have occurred, an additional two to four cycles of consolidation chemotherapy with high-dose cytarabine with or without anthracycline are administered over 4 to 6 months. Standard 7+3 induction regimens lead to complete remission in 60% to 80% of younger adults with de novo AML. Lower remission rates are achieved for older adults (>60 years) and in patients with antecedent hematologic diseases evolving into AML. After achieving complete remission after induction, patients may be offered additional consolidation chemotherapy or treatment with allogeneic or autologous SCT (see Chapter 1). Decisions about the best time to perform SCT in patients are most often guided by clinical risk factors and prognostic risk category. Although clinical outcomes are improved when patients undergo SCT after initial induction chemotherapy (i.e., during the first complete remission) rather than after disease relapse, chemotherapeutic regimens are also more effective in the first remission than they are after transplantation, and they may be better tolerated than SCT, which carries an overall mortality rate of

表2.12 欧洲白血病网（ELN）AML分型（2017）	
风险类别	遗传学异常
低危	t（8;21）（q22;q22.1）；*RUNX1-RUNX1T1* inv（16）（p13.1q22）或 t（16;16）（p13.1;q22）：*CBFB-MYH11* *NPM1* 突变且 *FLT3-ITD* 阴性或 *FLT3-ITD* 突变低负荷 双等位基因突变 *CEBPA*
中危	*NPM1* 突变且 *FLT3-ITD* 突变高负荷 野生型 *NPM1* 且 *FLT3-ITD* 阴性或 *FLT3-ITD* 突变低负荷（无高危遗传因素）t（9;11）（p21.3;q23.3）：*MLLT3-KMT2A* 不属于低危或高危的细胞遗传学异常
高危	t（6;9）（p23;q34.1）；*DEK-NUP214* t（v;11q23.3）：*KMT2A* 重排 t（9;22）（q34.1;q11.2）：*BCR-ABL1* inv（3）（q21.3q26.2）或 t（3;3）（q21.3;q26.2）：*GATA2*、*MECOM*（*EVI1*） −5 或 del（5q）；−7；−17/abn（17p） 复杂核型、单倍体核型 野生型 *NPM1* 且 *FLT3-ITD* 突变高负荷 *RUNX1* 突变 *ASXL1* 突变 *TP53* 突变

引自 Dohner H, Estey EH, Grimwade D, et al. Diagnosis and management of AML in adults: 2017 ELM recommendations from an international expert panel. Blood 129（4）: 424-447, 2017.
ITD，内部串联重复。

表2.13 ALL的预后因素		
因素	预后良好组	预后不良组
年龄	2～10岁	＜2岁或＞10岁
诊断时的白细胞计数	＜30 000/μl	＞50 000/μl
表型	前体B细胞	前体T细胞
染色体数量	超二倍体	假性/亚二倍体，接近四倍体
染色体异常	t（12;21）	MYC突变：t（8;14）、t（2;8）、t（8;22）混合白血病突变（11q23） 费城染色体：t（9;22），产生 BCR-ABL
诊断时中枢神经系统疾病	无	有
性别	女性	男性
种族	白人	非裔美国人、西班牙裔
缓解时间	短（7～14天）	达到缓解所需的时间长或未能达到缓解

治疗和预后

由于针对特定临床和生物学亚型的多种新药的出现，AML的前期化疗在过去几年中发生了巨大变化。过去几十年，已知预测预后不良的临床因素包括高龄（＞60岁）、治疗相关或既往血液疾病（即继发性AML）、一般状况差、初诊白细胞计数升高［＞（20～30）×10^9/L 至＞100×10^9/L］和髓外病变。髓外病变包括累及中枢神经系统、皮肤和软组织的白血病（髓系肉瘤或粒细胞肉瘤），以及累及除骨髓和外周血以外的任何其他器官。尽管仍应考虑这些临床因素，但当前影响初诊患者治疗决策的最重要因素是整体状况/合并症和AML风险类别。

AML是一组生物学异质性疾病，不同AML亚型预后差异很大。早期的AML风险预测主要基于核型异常，其目前仍是强化化疗方案（基于阿糖胞苷和蒽环类药物）应答最可靠的独立预测因子。基因组和分子技术的新进展揭示了多种基因突变对AML发生机制的影响。现已发现原发性AML中涉及至少8个不同生物学过程的基因。新的AML风险分层由欧洲白血病网结合诊断细胞遗传学和分子信息将AML划分为3个风险类别（低危、中危和高危）（表2.12）。由于某些突变（特别是 CBF、FLT3、NPM1、IDH1 和 IDH2）可显著改变前期治疗选择，因此所有疑诊AML的患者均应尽快（3～5天）检测上述基因（表2.12）。

AML亚组的治疗方案

年龄＜60岁和（或）适合强化化疗的患者 "传统"诱导方案包括7天的阿糖胞苷和3天的蒽环类药物（即柔红霉素或伊达比星）治疗，通常被称为"7+3"。一旦出现形态学缓解（骨髓原始细胞＜5%）和血细胞计数恢复（白细胞计数＞10×10^9/L，血小板＞100×10^9/L），应进行巩固化疗（4～6个月进行2～4个周期），化疗方案为高剂量阿糖胞苷联合或不联合蒽环类药物。标准"7+3"诱导方案可使60%～80%的初诊年轻AML患者获得完全缓解，老年患者（＞60岁）和由其他血液疾病转化而来的AML患者的缓解率较低。达到完全缓解后，患者可接受巩固化疗、alloSCT或自体造血干细胞移植（SCT）（见第1章）。患者进行SCT的最佳时间通常取决于临床危险因素和预后风险分层。虽然在首次完全缓解期间进行SCT的疗效优于疾病复发后行SCT，但首次完全缓解期间化疗的疗效优于移植后化疗，且化疗的耐受性更好，SCT的移

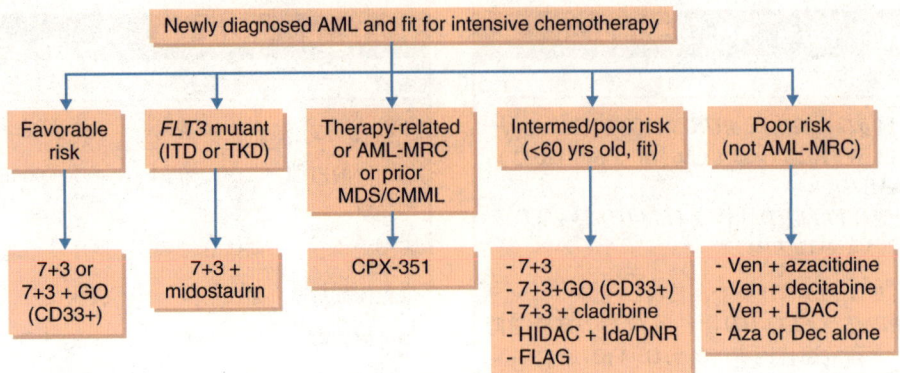

Fig. 2.1 Treatment of patients with newly diagnosed acute myeloid leukemia AML and considered fit for intensive chemotherapy. *7+3,* 7 days of continuous infusional cytarabine 100-200 mg/m2/day plus 3 days of anthracycline (daunorubicin 45-90 mg/m2/day or idarubicin 12 mg/m2/day); *AML,* acute myeloid leukemia; *AML-MRC,* acute myeloid leukemia with myelodysplastic related changes; *CD33+,* expressing CD33 surface antigen; *CMML,* chronic myelomonocytic leukemia (a subtype of MDS); *CPX-351,* liposomal formulation of cytarabine and daunorubicin; *Dec,* decitabine; *DNR,* daunorubicin; *FLAG,* intensive chemotherapy regimen consisting of fludarabine, intermediate-dose cytarabine, and G-CSF; *FLT3,* fms-like tyrosine kinase 3; *GO,* gemtuzumab ozogamicin; *HIDAC,* high-dose cytarabine; *Ida,* idarubicin; *ITD,* internal tandem duplication mutation; *LDAC,* low-dose cytarabine; *MDS,* myelodysplastic syndrome; *TKD,* tyrosine kinase domain mutation; *Ven,* venetoclax.

25% to 30%. Patients whose AML fails to respond to initial induction therapy have a grim overall prognosis and are eligible for treatment with high-dose cytarabine–containing regimens or low-dose therapy incorporating hypomethylating agents (azacitidine, decitabine) and/or experimental agents in order to obtain remission.

Treatment of younger (<60 years old) individuals with AML should be tailored based on specific AML risk classification (Fig. 2.1). Patients with favorable risk AML characterized by t(8;21), inv(16) or del(16q) aberrations are unusually responsive to induction chemotherapy followed by two to four cycles of high-dose cytosine arabinoside consolidation. Long-term 5-year survival rates of 55% to 60% can be obtained. Further improvement in outcomes has been demonstrated with the addition of gemtuzumab ozogamicin (GO), an antibody drug conjugate directed against the CD33+ surface antigen expressed on the majority of myeloid blasts. In a meta-analysis of five randomized controlled clinical trials, the addition of GO to 7+3-based induction and consolidation therapy improved overall survival by 20% over chemotherapy alone. AML patients with favorable disease features potentially responsive to high-dose cytarabine chemotherapy are encouraged to delay SCT until the time of relapse.

Some cytogenetic aberrations confer poor prognosis and are associated with resistance to and/or early relapse following standard chemotherapy regimens. These "poor-risk" cytogenetics include deletions in chromosome 5 or 7, inv(3q), t(3;3), t(6;9), t(9;22) (also known as the Philadelphia chromosome), monosomal karyotype, and three or more karyotypic abnormalities (i.e., complex karyotype). Mutations associated with poor prognosis are *FLT3-ITD, RUNX1, ASXL1,* and *TP53.* Remission rates for these poor-risk cytogenetic and molecular subtypes of AML are low; if remission is achieved, patients remain at high risk for AML relapse within the first 12 months due to presence of chemotherapy-refractory disease. Overall survival rates for poor-prognosis AML are 5% to 15%. AlloSCT is recommended for and represents the best chance for long-term cure of patients with poor-risk AML such as disease associated with unfavorable cytogenetic and molecular features, antecedent hematologic disease, or therapy-related or primary refractory disease. Poor-risk AML patients younger than 60 years undergoing allogeneic bone marrow transplantation from a matched donor have long-term overall survival rates of 40% to 60%, compared with cure rates after conventional chemotherapy of only 5% to 20%. For younger individuals with poor-risk AML appropriate for intensive chemotherapy, the preferred approach is 7+3-based induction (without GO) followed by alloSCT in first remission.

Outcomes of standard cytarabine- and anthracycline-based intensive chemotherapy in patients with therapy-related AML (tAML) or secondary AML (sAML) arising out of antecedent myelodysplastic syndrome (MDS) or with MDS-related changes (AML-MRC) remains dismal. Long-term survival ranges from 10% to 20% regardless of age, and alloSCT is universally considered the only curative approach. Patients 60 years or older with these difficult-to-treat AML subtypes (tAML, sAML, AML, with MRC) achieve improved remission rates and prolonged overall survival, particularly in the context of subsequent alloSCT, following treatment with a liposomal cytarabine and daunorubicin formulation (formerly known as CPX-351) as compared with standard infusion cytarabine and daunorubicin. It has been speculated that the improved drug pharmacokinetics, specifically enhanced marrow drug delivery and retention, may lead to improved eradication of AML blasts in these specific subsets.

FLT3 mutations are the most common gene mutations in AML and constitute an "actionable" mutation because patients with *FLT3-*mutant AML benefit from treatment with oral TKI of mutant FLT3 signaling pathways, similar to BCR/ABL inhibitors in CML. In newly diagnosed patients with *FLT3-*mutant disease, the addition of midostaurin, a first-generation FLT3 TKI, to upfront cytarabine and anthracycline induction and consolidation chemotherapy improved overall survival (but not remission rate) as compared to chemotherapy alone. Of note, these improved outcomes were dependent in part on the majority of patients with *FLT3*-mutant AML undergoing alloSCT at time of remission.

The remaining half of AML patients have intermediate-risk cytogenetics, which is defined as a normal karyotype, trisomy 8, t(9;11), or other cytogenetic abnormalities not included in the other groups. These patients have a 30% to 45% long-term survival rate with standard 7+3 chemotherapy (see Table 2.12). Actionable mutations in *FLT3, NPM-1, IDH1,* and *IDH2* genes occur most frequently in intermediate-risk disease and carry significant therapeutic and prognostic implications. Multiple alternative

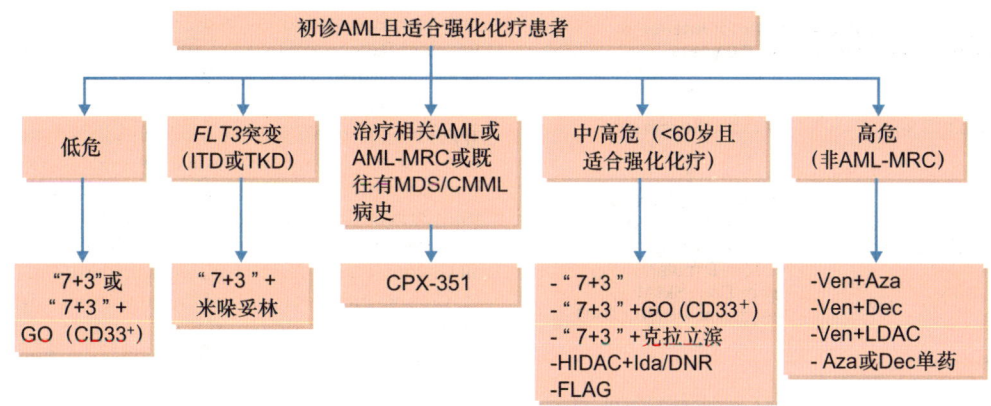

图 2.1 初诊 AML 且适合强化化疗患者的治疗。7+3，连续输注 7 天阿糖胞苷 [100～200 mg/（m²·d）] +3 天蒽环类药物 [柔红霉素 45～90 mg/（m²·d）或伊达比星 12 mg/（m²·d）]；AML，急性髓系白血病；AML-MRC，急性髓系白血病伴骨髓增生异常相关改变；Aza，阿扎胞苷；CD33⁺，表达 CD33 表面抗原；CMML，慢性粒-单核细胞白血病（MDS 的一种亚型）；CPX-351，阿糖胞苷和柔红霉素脂质体制剂；Dec，地西他滨；DNR，柔红霉素；FLAG，包括氟达拉滨、中等剂量阿糖胞苷和 G-CSF 的强化化疗方案；FLT3，FMS 样酪氨酸激酶 3；GO，吉妥珠单抗；HIDAC，高剂量阿糖胞苷；Ida，伊达比星；ITD，内部串联重复突变；LDAC，低剂量阿糖胞苷；MDS，骨髓增生异常综合征；TKD，酪氨酸激酶结构域突变；Ven，维奈克拉

植相关死亡率为 25%～30%。对初始诱导治疗无反应的 AML 患者总体预后很差。为获得缓解，再次诱导治疗方案包括含高剂量阿糖胞苷的化疗方案，低剂量治疗联合去甲基化药物（阿扎胞苷、地西他滨）和（或）进入临床试验。

年轻 AML 患者（<60 岁）的治疗应根据特定的 AML 风险分层进行调整（图 2.1）。伴 t（8;21）、inv（16）或 del（16q）异常的低危 AML 患者通常对诱导化疗随后行 2～4 个疗程的高剂量阿糖胞苷的巩固化疗方案非常敏感。长期 5 年生存率可达 55%～60%。吉妥珠单抗（GO）是一种针对 CD33⁺髓系原始细胞的抗体偶联药物。在纳入 5 项随机对照临床试验的荟萃分析中，与单纯化疗相比，GO 与"7+3"诱导化疗和巩固化疗联合应用可使总生存率提高 20%。高剂量阿糖胞苷化疗对低危 AML 患者的根治率高，SCT 仅作为复发患者的选择。

部分细胞遗传学异常提示预后不良，并与标准化疗方案耐药和（或）早期复发有关。这些遗传学异常包括 5 号或 7 号染色体部分缺失、inv（3q）、t（3;3）、t（6,9）、t（9;22）（即费城染色体）、单体核型和≥3 种核型异常（即复杂核型）。与不良预后相关的突变包括 *FLT3-ITD*、*RUNX1*、*ASXL1* 和 *TP53*。这些预后不良的 AML 亚型的缓解率低；即使缓解，由于存在化疗难治性疾病，患者在治疗后的前 12 个月内仍处于 AML 复发的高风险状态。预后不良的 AML 患者的总生存率为 5%～15%。alloSCT 被推荐作为治愈高危 AML 患者的最佳方法，高危 AML 包括 AML 伴有提示预后不良的细胞遗传学和分子学特征、既往血液病史、治疗相关 AML 或原发性难治性 AML。60 岁以下的高危患者接受传统化疗的治愈率仅为 5%～20%，而行全相合 alloSCT 的长期总体生存率为 40%～60%。对于适合强化化疗的年轻低危 AML 患者，首选"7+3"诱导化疗（无 GO），在首次缓解后进行 alloSCT。

治疗相关 AML（tAML）、由既往 MDS 导致的继发性 AML（sAML）或 AML 伴 MDS 相关改变（AML-MRC）的患者应用基于阿糖胞苷和蒽环类药物的标准强化化疗的临床结局仍然很差。长期生存率仅为 10%～20%，alloSCT 是唯一的治愈性治疗。与阿糖胞苷和柔红霉素的标准方案相比，患有上述难治性 AML 亚型（tAML、sAML、AML-MRC）的 60 岁以上患者接受阿糖胞苷和柔红霉素脂质体制剂（CPX-351）方案化疗并桥接 alloSCT 可提高缓解率，以及延长总生存期。如果可以改进药代动力学使药物在骨髓中浓聚，则有利于这些高危 AML 亚型肿瘤细胞的清除。

FLT3 突变是 AML 中最常见的基因突变，伴有 *FLT3* 突变的患者可获益于针对突变型 FLT3 信号通路的口服 TKI 治疗，这种 TKI 类似于 CML 中的 BCR/ABL 抑制剂。在初诊伴 *FLT3* 突变的 AML 患者中，与单纯化疗相比，在阿糖胞苷和蒽环类药物诱导和巩固化疗中添加米哚妥林（第一代 FLT3 TKI）可改善总生存率（而非缓解率）。需注意，临床结局的改善部分取决于大多数伴 *FLT3* 突变的 AML 患者在获得缓解时接受了 alloSCT。

其余 1/2 的 AML 患者具有中危细胞遗传学因素，包括正常核型、+8、t（9;11）或未列入其他组中的细胞遗传学异常。经过标准化疗，这些患者的长期存活率为 30%～45%（表 2.12）。*FLT3*、*NPM-1*、*IDH1* 和 *IDH2* 基因突变最常见于中危 AML，并能提示疗效和预后。目前正在探索除"7+3"之外的多种替代诱

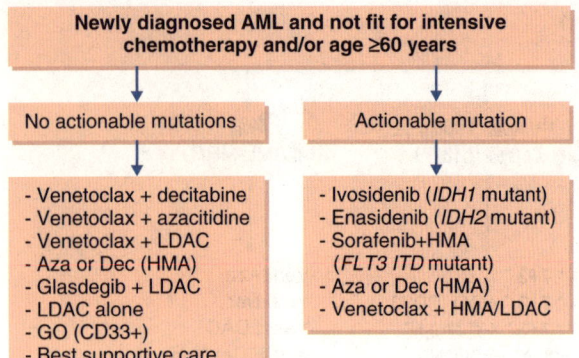

Fig. 2.2 Treatment of patients with newly diagnosed acute myeloid leukemia and considered not fit for intensive chemotherapy and/or age 60 years old or older. *AML*, Acute myeloid leukemia; *Aza,* azacitidine; *CD33+,* expressing CD33 surface antigen; *Dec,* decitabine; *FLT3,* fms-like tyrosine kinase 3; *GO,* gemtuzumab ozogamicin; *HMA,* hypomethylating agents consisting of azacytidine and decitabine; *IDH1,* isocitrate dehydrogenase isoform 1; *IDH2,* isocitrate dehydrogenase isoform 2; *LDAC,* low-dose cytarabine.

induction regimens other than 7+3 have been explored to improve prognosis for intermediate- and poor-risk AML patients. These include substitution of higher-dose intermittent-dosed cytarabine instead of 7-day infusional cytarabine and the addition of other agents (such as cladribine or fludarabine) to cytarabine and anthracycline in attempts to enhance responses. The addition of GO to 7+3 has been shown to improve overall survival in intermediate-risk AML, albeit to a much lesser degree (5.7%) than in favorable-risk patients. Risks of GO include prolonged myelosuppression with associated hemorrhagic complications and increased risk of fatal veno-occlusive disease (VOD), particularly in patients undergoing subsequent alloSCT. Recently, the rate of VOD appears to have been significantly mitigated (4%) by the use of fractionated (i.e., 3 mg/m^2 on days 1, 4, and 7) GO dosing. Intermediate-risk AML patients with unfavorable prognosis (based on clinical or molecular data) ideally should be offered alloSCT, particularly younger individuals with few comorbidities and related family donors. Those patients who are ineligible for allogeneic transplantation because of advanced age, other medical issues, or lack of HLA-compatible donors may be offered chemotherapy or autologous SCT instead. Whether autologous transplantation improves AML outcomes compared with chemotherapy alone is a matter of debate. However, the long-term survival rates after autologous transplantation range from 20% to 40% and are at least equivalent to consolidation chemotherapy regimens for these patients.

Patients 60 years or older and/or not fit for aggressive therapy now have a number of therapeutic options (Fig. 2.2). Because the median age at diagnosis of AML is 65 years, a sizable proportion of AML patients are elderly individuals with major comorbidities or antecedent hematologic or malignant diseases, rendering them poor candidates for intensive induction chemotherapeutic regimens or myeloablative SCT. Infectious complications remain the major cause of morbidity and mortality during intensive inpatient chemotherapy despite advances in prophylactic growth factor support, antibiotics, and antifungal agents. The low expected remission rates (30% to 50%) and high mortality and morbidity rates associated with induction are additional reasons for many patients to decline aggressive therapy. Fortunately, multiple therapeutic options are now available specifically for treatment of these older adults who in the recent past would have been offered only supportive therapy with hydroxyurea, transfusion support alone, and hospice.

Patients older than 75 years old and/or those unfit for and who choose not to receive intensive therapy now have a panoply of low-dose chemotherapy options. Historically, chemotherapy regimens for older patients consisted of either low-dose cytarabine (LDAC) or hypomethylating therapy (HMA) (azacytidine, decitabine). These regimens have been well tolerated, but both are associated with disappointing response rates and median survival duration of less than 6 to 7 months. Low-dose subcutaneous cytarabine resulted in remission rates of about 18%, whereas HMA induced remissions ranging from 20% to 47%. Some individuals treated with HMA also experience hematologic improvement, disease stabilization, and prolonged overall survival, even in absence of complete remission.

Combination regimens adding therapeutic agents to HMA or LDAC backbones now constitute the new standard of care for individuals unable to receive intensive chemotherapy. Venetoclax is a highly potent oral inhibitor of BCL-2, upon which AML cells are dependent for viability. The addition of venetoclax to HMA therapy in older unfit patients resulted in remissions in 67% of patients with a median overall survival of 17.5 months. Of note, almost two thirds of patients with traditionally unfavorable prognostic factors including poor-risk cytogenetics, age 75 years old or older, and secondary AML attained complete remission or complete remission with incomplete count recovery. Venetoclax combined with LDAC resulted in slightly lower overall response rates (54%) and in specific subsets including poor-risk cytogenetics (42%) and secondary AML (35%). Patients who had previously received HMA therapy for MDS prior to venetoclax and LDAC therapy also had lower remission rates (33%) as compared to no prior HMA exposure (62%). Adverse events included significant myelosuppression with risk of infection, sepsis, and pneumonia leading to early death in a proportion of patients. Glasdegib is an oral inhibitor of sonic hedgehog signaling important for leukemia stem cell survival and expansion with minimal single agent activity but improved efficacy when combined with LDAC. Addition of glasdegib to LDAC significantly improved remission rate to 19% and extended overall survival to 8.8 months as compared to LDAC alone (4.9 months). Treatment was well tolerated with relatively little myelosuppression or cytopenia. The excellent tolerability of this regimen with relatively little myelosuppression and the ability to treat patients completely in the outpatient setting makes it an option for select individuals. Gemtuzumab ozogamicin monotherapy represents yet another option for these patients with CD33+ AML with survival duration of less than 6 months.

Treatment decisions may also be altered by the presence of actionable mutations in *FLT3, IDH1,* and *IDH2* genes. Patients with *IDH1-* or *IDH2-*mutant disease are eligible to receive therapy with oral inhibitors of IDH1 (ivosidenib) and IDH2 (enasidenib), respectively. These agents, originally evaluated in the relapsed/refractory setting, result in overall response rates of approximately 40% and are well tolerated without myelosuppression. One unusual toxicity of IDH inhibitors is development of differentiation syndrome, similar to that seen with treatment of acute promyelocytic leukemia (APL), and characterized by elevated white count, fever, edema, and pulmonary infiltrates. Of note, *IDH1/2-*mutant AML patients also experienced very high response rates (80% to 90%) following venetoclax plus HMA/LDAC, making this the preferred regimen over targeted IDH inhibitors for upfront therapy if tolerable in specific patients.

Addition of a first-generation FLT3 TKI (sorafenib) to HMA therapy is recommended for upfront therapy of *FLT3-ITD*–mutant AML in unfit patients. Use of newer-generation TKIs for this indication is currently under investigation. Venetoclax plus HMA or LDAC is also effective in *FLT3*-mutant AML, raising the question of whether FLT3 TKI or venetoclax is the better therapeutic partner to combine with HMA in *FLT3*-mutant AML. However, recent clinical and preclinical data have suggested that *FLT3* mutations may constitute an overall mechanism of resistance to venetoclax based therapy.

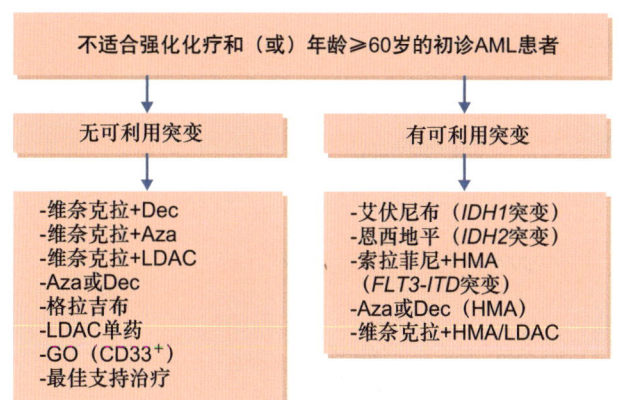

图 2.2 不适合强化化疗和（或）年龄 ≥ 60 岁的初诊 AML 患者的治疗。AML，急性髓系白血病；Aza，阿扎胞苷；CD33$^+$，表达 CD33 表面抗原；Dec，地西他滨；FLT3，FMS 样酪氨酸激酶 3；GO，吉妥珠单抗；HMA，由阿扎胞苷和地西他滨组成的去甲基化药物；IDH1，异柠檬酸脱氢酶亚型 1；IDH2，异柠檬酸脱氢酶亚型 2；LDAC，低剂量阿糖胞苷

导化疗方案，以期改善中高危 AML 患者的预后。这些措施包括用较高剂量阿糖胞苷间歇给药代替 7 天连续输注阿糖胞苷，以及在阿糖胞苷和蒽环类药物中添加其他药物（如克拉立滨或氟达拉滨）以增强疗效。尽管总体生存率比低危患者低 5.7%，但"7 + 3"方案中添加 GO 已被证明可改善中危 AML 患者的总体生存率。GO 可导致骨髓抑制相关的出血并发症和致死性静脉闭塞性疾病（VOD）的风险增加，特别是后续接受 alloSCT 的患者。通过分次给药（即第 1 天、第 4 天和第 7 天给予 3 mg/m^2），GO 治疗后 VOD 的发生率已显著降低（4%）。理想情况下，预后不良（基于临床或分子学检测）的中危 AML 患者应接受 alloSCT，特别是合并症很少的年轻患者和具有同胞全相合供者的患者。由于高龄、其他合并症或缺乏 HLA 相合供者而不适合行 alloSCT（基于临床或细胞遗传学数据）的患者，可选择化疗或自体 SCT。与单纯化疗相比，自体移植能否改善 AML 患者的结局尚存争论。然而，自体移植后的长期生存率为 20% ~ 40%，至少与使用巩固化疗方案的预后类似。

年龄 ≥ 60 岁和（或）不适合行强化化疗的患者目前有多种治疗方案选择（图 2.2）。由于 AML 诊断时的中位年龄为 65 岁，因此相当一部分 AML 患者是具有主要合并症或血液疾病或恶性肿瘤病史的老年人，他们对标准诱导化疗方案或清髓性 SCT 的耐受性较差。尽管会预防性给予生长因子支持，以及使用抗生素和抗真菌药物进行抗感染治疗，但感染并发症仍然是引起住院强化化疗期间发病率和死亡率升高的主要原因。预期缓解率低（30% ~ 50%）、诱导并发症和相关死亡率高导致许多患者拒绝积极治疗。幸运的是，现在有多种治疗方案专门针对这些老年患者，而在不久前，这些老年患者只能接受羟基脲、输血支持治疗和临终关怀。

年龄 > 75 岁和（或）不适合或不愿选择强化治疗的患者越来越多地使用低剂量化疗方案。历史上，老年患者的化疗方案包括低剂量阿糖胞苷（LDAC）或低甲基化治疗（HMA）（阿扎胞苷、地西他滨）。这些方案的耐受性良好，但缓解率不理想，中位生存期少于 6 ~ 7 个月。低剂量皮下注射阿糖胞苷的缓解率约为 18%，而 HMA 的缓解率为 20% ~ 47%。使用 HMA 的患者可获得血液学缓解、病情稳定和总生存期延长，即使没有完全缓解。

在基于 HMA 或 LDAC 的化疗方案中加入其他药物的联合治疗方案已成为无法接受强化化疗患者的新标准治疗。AML 肿瘤细胞的生存依赖于 BCL-2 蛋白，而维奈克拉是一种强效口服 BCL-2 抑制剂。HMA 联合维奈克拉可使 67% 不适合接受强化化疗的老年患者达到缓解，中位总生存期为 17.5 个月。需注意，近 2/3 具有预后不良因素（细胞遗传学异常、年龄 > 75 岁、继发性 AML）的高危患者可达到完全缓解或完全缓解伴血细胞计数不完全恢复。维奈克拉联用 LDAC 的总体反应率略低（54%），其中提示预后不良的细胞遗传学异常组患者的总体反应率为 42%，继发性 AML 患者的总体反应率为 35%。既往因 MDS 接受过 HMA 的患者的缓解率（33%）低于未使用过 HMA 的患者（62%）。该联合治疗的副作用包括显著骨髓抑制导致的感染、感染中毒症和肺炎的风险增加，严重时可致死。格拉吉布是一种口服 sonic hedgehog 信号通路抑制剂，该信号通路对白血病干细胞的生存和扩增至关重要，单药活性极低，但与 LDAC 联用时可提高疗效。LDAC 联合格拉吉布可将缓解率提高至 19%，并将总生存期延长至 8.8 个月，而单用 LDAC 患者的总生存期为 4.9 个月。该方案耐受性良好、骨髓抑制相对较轻，因此患者可在门诊使用，无须住院。对于 CD33$^+$ 且预期寿命不超过 6 个月的 AML 患者，GO 单药也是一种治疗选择。

携带 FLT3、IDH1、IDH2 突变的 AML 患者的治疗方案也因小分子靶向药物的出现而改变。伴有 IDH1 或 IDH2 突变的患者可分别口服 IDH1 抑制剂（艾伏尼布）和 IDH2 抑制剂（恩西地平）治疗。这两种药物（最初用于复发/难治性 AML 患者）的总缓解率约为 40%，且耐受性良好，无骨髓抑制。IDH 抑制剂的罕见副作用是出现分化综合征，类似于急性早幼粒细胞白血病（APL）治疗中出现的分化综合征，其特征是白细胞计数升高、发热、水肿和肺部浸润。需注意，携带 IDH1/2 突变的 AML 患者接受维奈克拉联合 HMA/LDAC 治疗的缓解率高（80% ~ 90%），该方案有望成为优于靶向 IDH 抑制剂的首选诱导化疗方案。

在不适合强化化疗且伴有 FLT3-ITD 突变的 AML 患者中，推荐 HMA 联用第一代 FLT3 TKI（索拉非尼）作为诱导化疗方案。用于治疗这类患者的新一代 TKI 正在研发中。维奈克拉联合 HMA 或 LDAC 也可有效治疗伴有 FLT3 突变的 AML，这就提出了一个问题：对于伴有 FLT3 突变的 AML 患者，HMA 联合 FLT3 TKI 与 HMA 联合维奈克拉哪种疗效更好？然而，近期的基础和临床研究数据表明，FLT3 突变可能是维奈克拉的耐药机制。

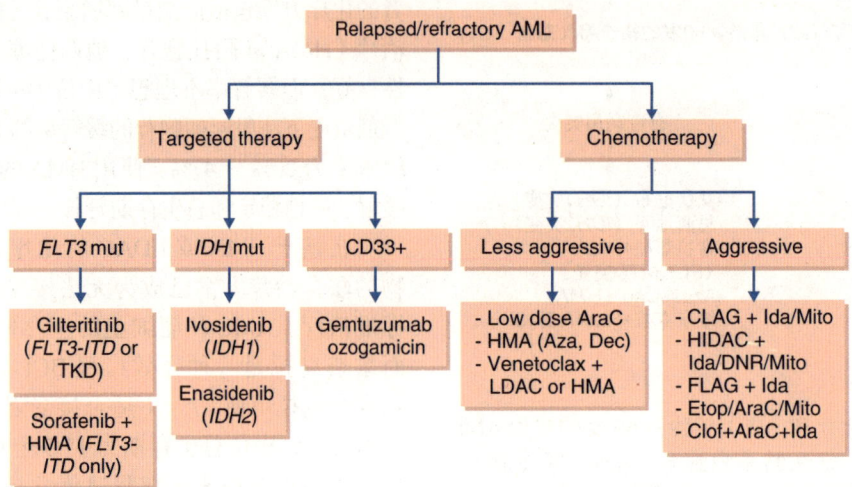

Fig. 2.3 Treatment of patients with relapsed/refractory acute myeloid leukemia. *AML*, Acute myeloid leukemia; *AraC*, cytarabine; *Aza*, azacytidine; *CD33+*, expressing CD33 surface antigen; *CLAG*, intensive chemotherapy regimen including cladribine, intermediate-dose cytarabine, and G-CSF; *Clof*, clofarabine; *Dec*, decitabine; *DNR*, daunorubicin; *Etop/AraC/Mito*, intensive chemotherapy regimen consisting of etoposide, intermediate dose cytarabine, and mitoxantrone; *FLAG*, intensive chemotherapy regimen consisting of fludarabine, intermediate-dose cytarabine, and G-CSF; *FLT3*, fms-like tyrosine kinase 3; *HIDAC*, high-dose cytarabine; *HMA*, hypomethylating agents consisting of azacytidine and decitabine; *Ida*, idarubicin; *IDH*, isocitrate dehydrogenase; *IDH1*, isocitrate dehydrogenase isoform 1; *IDH2*, isocitrate dehydrogenase isoform 2; *ITD*, internal tandem duplication mutation; *LDAC*, low-dose cytarabine; *Mito*, mitoxantrone; *TKD*, tyrosine kinase domain mutation.

Relapsed or refractory disease. Similar to newly diagnosed patients, individuals with AML relapsing following or refractory to standard upfront therapy should be assessed for their overall ability to tolerate aggressive versus less-aggressive therapy and for the presence of actionable mutations (Fig. 2.3).

Next-generation and single cell sequencing technology has demonstrated the importance of repeat molecular testing at the time of AML recurrence. Clonal evolution or emergence as a consequence of prior therapy can lead to a significantly different mutational profile at relapse than at initial AML presentation with significant therapeutic implications. For instance, patients with relapsed/refractory *FLT3*-mutant AML (both ITD and TKD mutations) benefit more from single-agent therapy with a potent next-generation FLT3 TKI, gilteritinib, than from therapy with either intensive or low-dose chemotherapy. Complete remission rate (37% vs. 17%) and overall survival (9.3 vs. 5.6 months) are both improved with FLT3 TKI monotherapy over any non-FLT3 TKI–containing regimen. Patients with relapsed/refractory *IDH1* or *IDH2*-mutant disease can be treated with ivosidenib (IDH1 inhibitor) or enasidenib (IDH2 inhibitor) with complete remission rates of 20% and overall response rates of 40%.

Patients with recurrent AML not characterized by actionable mutations may be treated with aggressive intensive salvage chemotherapy regimens (i.e., cladribine or fludarabine containing programs) or low-dose chemotherapy (i.e., venetoclax plus HMA or LDAC, HMA or LDAC or GO alone). If possible, all patients with relapsed/refractory AML should be considered for alloSCT and clinical trials. Experimental therapies for AML including nontraditional alloSCT have resulted in durable long-term remissions in a proportion of older AML patients and should be pursued based on patient preference, overall health status, and availability of an appropriate HLA-matched donor.

Acute Promyelocytic Leukemia
Definition, Epidemiology, and Pathology

APL, formerly known as the FAB M3 subtype of AML (see Table 2.11), is a rare malignancy that represents 10% to 15% of adult AML. The incidence is increased among younger patients (median age, 40 years). The annual incidence in the United States ranges from 600 to 800 cases. APL is different from other acute leukemias because of its unique disease biology. Morphologically, APL blasts are distinctive immature promyelocytic cells containing large granules and typically high numbers of Auer rods diagnostic of AML. APL is characterized by a chromosomal translocation—t(15;17)(q22;q12)—involving the promyelocytic leukemia gene *(PML)* on chromosome 15 and the retinoic acid receptor-α gene *(RARA)* on chromosome 17. Sequestration of the resulting PML/RARA fusion protein with other proteins produces a complex that represses the gene transcription essential for granulocytic differentiation, effectively arresting differentiation of leukemia cells at the promyelocyte stage.

Clinical Presentation

Clinically, patients with APL often exhibit life-threatening bleeding caused by disseminated intravascular coagulation related to high levels of procoagulant factors released from APL granules. Bleeding complications in the CNS and other sites can be rapidly fatal if the disease is not recognized and treated as a medical emergency. All patients suspected of having APL should be started empirically with all-*trans*-retinoic acid (ATRA) therapy (discussed later) and treated aggressively with transfusions of fresh-frozen plasma, fibrinogen, and platelets until resolution of coagulopathy and disease confirmation. Unlike patients with other AML subsets, APL patients typically have cytopenias rather than leukocytosis. High-risk APL patients are defined as those with white blood cell counts greater than $10 \times 10^9/L$.

Treatment and Prognosis

Treated appropriately, APL is the most curable acute leukemia in adults. The centerpiece of APL treatment is the use of agents that induce the terminal differentiation of leukemic promyelocytes followed by senescence and spontaneous apoptosis. ATRA is an oral derivative of vitamin A shown to overcome growth arrest and permit

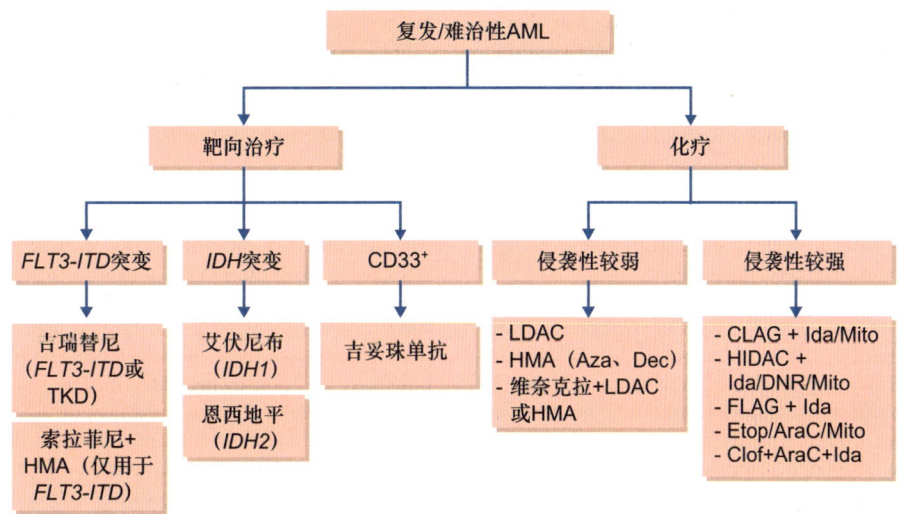

图 2.3 复发 / 难治性 AML 患者的治疗。AML，急性髓系白血病；AraC，阿糖胞苷；Aza，阿扎胞苷；CD33$^+$，表达 CD33 表面抗原；CLAG，包括克拉立滨、中等剂量阿糖胞苷和 G-CSF 的强化化疗方案；Clof，氯法拉滨；Dec，地西他滨；DNR，柔红霉素；Etop/AraC/Mito，包括依托泊苷、中等剂量阿糖胞苷和米托蒽醌的强化化疗方案；FLAG，包括氟达拉滨、中等剂量阿糖胞苷和 G-CSF 的强化化疗方案；FLT3，FMS 样酪氨酸激酶 3；HIDAC，高剂量阿糖胞苷；HMA，包括阿扎胞苷和地西他滨的去甲基化药物；Ida，伊达比星；IDH，异柠檬酸脱氢酶；IDH1，异柠檬酸脱氢酶亚型 1；IDH2，异柠檬酸脱氢酶亚型 2；ITD，内部串联重复突变；LDAC，低剂量阿糖胞苷；Mito，米托蒽醌；TKD，酪氨酸激酶结构域突变

复发 / 难治性 AML 与初诊患者相同，对于诱导化疗后复发或难治性 AML 患者，应评估其对强化化疗和减低强度化疗的耐受性，以及是否具有相关基因突变（图 2.3）。

AML 复发时利用二代测序及单细胞测序技术再次检测相关分子突变至关重要。复发时可检测到与初诊 AML 显著不同的基因突变谱。例如，复发性 / 难治性 *FLT3* 突变型 AML（ITD 和 TKD 突变）患者使用第二代 FLT3 TKI 吉瑞替尼单药治疗的获益大于使用强化化疗或低剂量化疗的获益。FLT3 TKI 单药治疗的完全缓解率（37% *vs.* 17%）和总生存期（9.3 个月 *vs.* 5.6 个月）均优于任何不含 FLT3 TKI 的治疗方案。复发性 / 难治性 *IDH1* 或 *IDH2* 突变患者可接受艾伏尼布（IDH1 抑制剂）或恩西地平（IDH2 抑制剂）治疗，完全缓解率为 20%，总反应率为 40%。

不携带基因突变的复发性 AML 患者可接受强化补救性化疗方案（即包含克拉立滨或氟达拉滨的方案）或低剂量化疗（即维奈克拉＋HMA 或 LDAC，以及 HMA、LDAC 或 GO 单药）。所有复发 / 难治性 AML 患者均应尽可能进行 alloSCT 和参与临床试验。AML 的试验性治疗（如非清髓性 alloSCT）已使部分 AML 老年患者获得持久的长期缓解，因此应根据患者偏好、总体健康状况和 HLA 相合供者情况进行治疗。

急性早幼粒细胞白血病

定义、流行病学和病理学

急性早幼粒细胞白血病（APL）既往被称为 AML 的 FAB M3 型（表 2.11），占成人 AML 的 10%～15%。年轻患者的发病率升高（中位年龄为 40 岁）。美国的年发病人数为 600～800 例。APL 有不同于其他急性白血病的独特生物学特征。从形态学上看，APL 细胞是未成熟的早幼粒细胞，包含大颗粒和大量 Auer 小体。APL 的特征性染色体易位是 t（15,17）(922;912)，涉及 15 号染色体上的早幼粒细胞白血病基因（*PML*）和 17 号染色体上的视黄酸受体 α 基因（*RARA*），形成 *PML/RARA* 融合基因，其翻译产物 PML/RARA 蛋白可与其他蛋白质共同抑制粒细胞分化所必需的基因转录，从而导致白血病细胞分化停滞在早幼粒细胞阶段。

临床表现

临床上，APL 患者常表现为危及生命的出血，这是由于 APL 颗粒释放大量促凝血因子，从而导致弥散性血管内凝血。如果 APL 患者未得到及时诊治，CNS 和其他部位的出血并发症可能迅速致死。疑诊 APL 的所有患者应开始经验性给予全反式维甲酸（ATRA）治疗（见下文），并积极输注新鲜冷冻血浆、纤维蛋白原和血小板，直到解决凝血问题和确诊疾病。与其他 AML 亚型患者不同，APL 患者通常全血细胞减少而非白细胞增多。高危 APL 患者的定义为白细胞计数＞$10×10^9$/L 的患者。

治疗和预后

APL 是目前成人治愈率最高的急性白血病。APL 治疗的关键是用药物诱导早幼粒白血病细胞终末分化，进而衰老和自发凋亡。ATRA 是一种口服维生素 A 衍生物，可通过改变 PML/RARA 的构型来促进正常基因

differentiation of immature APL blast cells into neutrophils by altering the configuration of *PML/RARA* to allow normal gene transcription.

Patients initiated on ATRA must be closely observed for development of retinoic acid or APL differentiation syndrome, which is life-threatening acute cardiopulmonary distress characterized by bilateral pulmonary effusions and infiltrates. This serositis-like disorder is attributed to adhesion of differentiating neoplastic cells to the pulmonary vasculature and carries a 5% to 10% mortality rate. Treatment consists of early initiation of corticosteroids and aggressive diuresis. In severe cases, ATRA should be temporarily withheld.

Although ATRA alone induces clinical remissions in up to 90% of patients with APL, high relapse rates observed after monotherapy led to the practice of combining ATRA with anthracycline with or without cytarabine chemotherapy in initial induction regimens. Using this approach, complete remission rates for APL rose to between 90% and 95%, and more than two thirds of patients with APL treated with standard ATRA-containing induction, consolidation, and maintenance chemotherapy regimens achieved long-term remission.

Relapsed APL patients were treated with arsenic trioxide, a naturally occurring compound used both as a poison and a drug in many countries. Low-dose arsenic therapy promotes APL cell differentiation and apoptosis and induces remission rates in up to 90% of relapsed APL cases. APL differentiation syndrome and prolongation of the QT interval are common side effects of arsenic therapy. Based on its tolerability and non-overlapping cytotoxicities with conventional cytotoxic drugs, arsenic was successfully used for consolidation therapy in APL patients and improved clinical outcomes.

Although highly effective, combination ATRA and chemotherapy regimens for newly diagnosed APL patients are associated with an overall mortality rate of 10% to 20% during the first month of treatment. Most deaths result from uncontrolled hemorrhage, differentiation syndrome, and complications of prolonged myelosuppression after cytotoxic therapy, particularly in older individuals. To address these concerns, a phase III trial randomized lower-risk APL patients to dual-differentiation therapy with ATRA and arsenic only (without cytotoxic chemotherapy) or to standard ATRA and chemotherapy during induction and consolidation. The trial demonstrated that ATRA plus arsenic treatment was not inferior to ATRA plus chemotherapy and was not associated with increased toxicity. Importantly, the trial results led to establishment of differentiation therapy alone without any cytotoxic agents as the standard of care for lower-risk APL patients. Patients with residual *PML/RARA*-positive cells after standard induction and consolidation therapy containing ATRA and arsenic should be considered for autologous or allogeneic SCT. Patients with high-risk APL should continue to receive cytarabine with or without anthracycline drugs in addition to ATRA and arsenic induction, consolidation, and maintenance for curative intent. Given the high cure rates, autologous or allogeneic stem cell transplant is not indicated for APL except for relapsed disease (which often is associated with CNS disease). Newer oral formulations of arsenic are being developed.

Acute Lymphoblastic Leukemia
Definition, Epidemiology, and Pathology

ALL is a neoplasm of immature lymphoblasts expressing markers of B-cell or T-cell lineage. ALL is predominantly a pediatric malignancy, with most cases occurring in children younger than 6 years. In the United States, 5960 new cases were diagnosed in 2018 with 1470 deaths. The median age of onset was 15 years with 27% diagnosed in individuals older than 45 years.

The prior FAB classification system divided ALL into three subtypes (i.e., L1, L2, and L3) based on the morphology of malignant cells. The WHO system reclassified the disease as precursor B-cell or T-cell ALL based on the lineage of specific cell surface antigens found on these cells during normal maturation (see Table 2.11). T-cell ALL represents 15% to 25% of ALL diagnoses. More than 50% of T-cell ALL cases have activating mutations in *NOTCH1*, a key regulator of T-cell fate. One third of adult and 20% of pediatric B-cell ALL cases are associated with detection of the Philadelphia chromosome, t(9;22).

Clinical Presentation

Patients often present with life-threatening cytopenias, or complications of leukostasis. On examination, enlarged lymph nodes, liver, spleen, or testicles are common. Neurologic symptoms including headaches, cranial nerve deficits, or new neuropathies may be indicative of CNS involvement. Several clinical and biologic features at diagnosis have traditionally been identified as poor prognostic factors for survival (see Table 2.13). These include age (in pediatrics <2 years or >10 years, in adults >35 years), elevated white blood cell count at presentation (>100,000/mcL), precursor T phenotype, chromosome number (pseudo/hypodiploidy or near tetraploidy) and specific chromosome abnormalities (such as complex karyotype or Philadelphia chromosome).

Treatment

Newly diagnosed ALL. Progress in the understanding and treatment of this disease over the last few decades has led to cure rates of greater than 90% for children with ALL. Despite this success, only 20% to 40% of adult patients with ALL achieve cure with elderly individuals demonstrating a five-year survival of less than 20%. The poorer outcomes for adults are attributed to differences in the biologic mechanisms of disease in the different age groups and the inability of older patients to tolerate the intensive chemotherapy or transplantation procedures required to achieve long-term responses.

Standard treatment of ALL is lengthy and involves multiple chemotherapeutic agents given over 2 to 3 years. Induction chemotherapy typically includes vincristine, corticosteroids, and L-asparaginase with the addition of an anthracycline, cytarabine, or cyclophosphamide (or a combination) for adult patients. Given the propensity of ALL cells to reside in the CNS and testes (so-called sanctuaries for leukemia cells because standard systemic chemotherapy does not penetrate into these sites), routine administration of intrathecal chemotherapy at the time of diagnosis, followed by multiple additional treatments to prevent leukemia seeding in the CNS is considered a necessary adjunct to systemic chemotherapy for all patients. Younger patients with CD20+, Ph-negative ALL have been shown to have worse outcomes than those with CD20-negative B-ALL. Addition of anti-CD20 antibody (rituximab) directed against B-cell antigens on abnormal lymphoblasts has been shown to enhance outcomes of chemotherapy for these individuals. The benefit of CD20 antibodies in older patients is less certain.

Current complete remission rates following induction chemotherapy range from 97% to 99% for children and 75% to 90% for adults. After normal hematopoiesis returns, patients typically undergo consolidation and intensification therapy with the same drugs, including high-dose methotrexate, cytarabine, and asparaginase to eradicate disease. Thereafter, maintenance chemotherapy given for up to 2 to 3 years after initial remission achievement is usually recommended for all patients. Prolonged treatment is intended to eliminate slow-growing leukemic clones, prevent further transformation, or destroy occult disease in other sites, particularly the CNS.

Although clinical factors (i.e., older age, Philadelphia chromosome–positive disease, high white blood cell count at presentation, or prolonged time to first remission) are important, current ALL therapeutic approaches in both children and adults are primarily guided by measurable (or minimal) residual disease (MRD) status. MRD is defined as the detection of malignant lymphoblasts by highly sensitive

转录，并使 APL 原始细胞分化成熟。

患者开始使用 ATRA 时，必须密切监测视黄酸或 APL 分化综合征的发生，因其会引起致命的急性呼吸衰竭，其特征是双侧肺部渗出和浸润，是由分化的肿瘤细胞黏附于肺血管所致，死亡率为 5%～10%。应尽早使用皮质类固醇激素和利尿治疗。在严重情况下，应暂时停用 ATRA。

尽管单用 ATRA 在 APL 患者中诱导的临床缓解率高达 90%，但持续单用 ATRA 的复发率极高，因此初始诱导治疗采用 ATRA 联合蒽环类化疗药 ± 阿糖胞苷的化疗方案。该方案使 APL 患者的完全缓解率升至 90%～95%，且超过 2/3 的 APL 患者在使用含 ATRA 的标准诱导、巩固和维持化疗方案治疗后实现了根治。

复发性 APL 患者多采用三氧化二砷治疗，它是天然存在的化合物，低剂量砷剂可促进 APL 细胞分化和调亡，对复发性 APL 的缓解率高达 90%。APL 分化综合征和 QT 间期延长是砷剂治疗的常见副作用。基于其耐受性及与常规化疗药物无交叉毒性，砷剂被成功地用于治疗 APL，并极大地改善了患者预后。

虽然有效性较高，但初诊 APL 患者采用 ATRA 联合化疗的第 1 个月的总体死亡率达 10%～20%。大多数死因是致死性出血、分化综合征、长期骨髓抑制导致的并发症，在老年患者中尤为明显。为了解决这些问题，近期一项 III 期随机临床试验将低危 APL 患者随机分为两组，在诱导治疗和巩固治疗期间，一组使用 ATRA＋砷剂（无细胞毒性的化疗药物）的双诱导治疗方案，另一组使用 ATRA＋标准化疗方案。试验结果表明，ATRA＋砷剂的疗效并不劣于 ATRA＋化疗，且不会增加毒性。该临床试验结果使得 ATRA＋砷剂（不化疗）方案成为低危 APL 患者的标准治疗方案。对于经过含 ATRA 和砷剂的标准诱导和巩固治疗后仍有残留 PML/RARA 阳性细胞的患者，应考虑进行自体 SCT 或 alloSCT。高危 APL 患者在使用 ATRA＋砷剂诱导缓解后应继续接受阿糖胞苷联合或不联合蒽环类药物的巩固和维持治疗，以达到治愈目的。鉴于治愈率较高，除复发性 APL（通常伴有中枢神经系统疾病）外，自体 SCT 或 alloSCT 不适用于 APL。现阶段正在研发新型砷口服制剂。

急性淋巴细胞白血病
定义、流行病学和病理学

急性淋巴细胞白血病（ALL）是起源于 B 细胞或 T 细胞的淋巴母细胞肿瘤。ALL 主要见于儿童，大多数病例为 6 岁以下儿童。在美国，2018 年新诊断 5960 例 ALL，1470 例死亡。中位发病年龄为 15 岁，45 岁以上患者占 27%。

FAB 分型根据恶性细胞的形态将 ALL 分为 3 种亚型（即 L1、L2 和 L3）。根据这些细胞在正常成熟过程中发现的特异性表面抗原标志，WHO 分型将该病重新分类为前体 B 细胞或 T 细胞 ALL（表 2.11）。T 细胞 ALL 占所有 ALL 患者的 15%～25%。超过 50% 的 T 细胞 ALL 患者携带 *NOTCH1* 活化突变，NOTCH1 是决定 T 细胞命运的关键调节物。1/3 的成人和 20% 的儿童 B 细胞 ALL 患者具有 t（9;22）。

临床表现

患者通常表现为危及生命的血细胞减少或白细胞瘀滞并发症。体格检查常见淋巴结、肝、脾或睾丸肿大。神经系统症状包括头痛、颅神经损害或可能提示中枢神经系统受累的新发神经病变。诊断时的多种临床和生物学特征被认为是不良预后因素（表 2.13），包括年龄（儿童＜2 岁或＞10 岁，成人＞35 岁）、就诊时白细胞计数升高（＞100×10^9/L）、前体 T 细胞表型、染色体数目（假二倍体/亚二倍体或接近四倍体）和特异性染色体异常（如复杂核型或费城染色体）。

治疗

新诊断 ALL 在过去几十年中，对该病的理解和治疗进展使得 ALL 儿童患者的治愈率达到 90% 以上。尽管取得了这一成功，但仅 20%～40% 的 ALL 成人患者获得治愈，老年患者的 5 年生存率低于 20%。成人的结局较差归因于不同年龄组疾病生物学机制的差异和老年患者无法耐受达到长期缓解所需的强化化疗或移植。

ALL 的标准治疗需 2～3 年，并使用多种化疗药物联合治疗。诱导化疗通常包括长春新碱、皮质类固醇和 L-天冬酰胺酶，成人患者化疗方案中加入蒽环类药物、阿糖胞苷或环磷酰胺（或组合）。由于 ALL 易侵犯 CNS 和睾丸（即白血病细胞的庇护所，因为标准全身化疗不能穿透这些部位），在确诊时应常规鞘内注射化疗药物，随后在全身化疗的同时多次给予鞘内注射，以预防 CNS 白血病。与 CD20$^-$ B 细胞 ALL 患者相比，CD20$^+$、费城染色体阴性（Ph$^-$）的 ALL 年轻患者的预后更差。联用直接针对异常淋巴母细胞 B 细胞抗原的抗 CD20 单抗（利妥昔单抗）可改善这部分患者的化疗效果。抗 CD20 单抗在老年患者中的疗效尚不确定。

接受诱导化疗后，ALL 儿童患者的完全缓解率为 97%～99%，成人患者为 75%～90%。正常造血功能恢复后，患者通常使用相同药物进行巩固和强化治疗，包括高剂量甲氨蝶呤、阿糖胞苷和天冬酰胺酶，以清除肿瘤细胞。因此，建议所有患者在达到诱导缓解后进行 2～3 年的维持化疗。长期治疗旨在消除生长缓慢的白血病细胞克隆，防止其进一步转化或消除隐匿部位（尤其是 CNS）的残留肿瘤细胞。

尽管临床因素（如年龄较大、Ph$^+$、就诊时白细胞计数升高或至首次缓解时间延长）很重要，但目前儿童和成人 ALL 患者治疗方案主要以可测出的微量残留病（MRD）状态为指导。MRD 是指诱导和巩固治疗

PCR or multi-parameter flow cytometry following induction and consolidation therapy at the time of morphologic marrow remission. MRD has been established as an independent predictor of disease relapse and shorter survival with or without subsequent alloSCT. Patients with MRD positive CD19+ B-cell ALL are usually treated with blinatumomab (BiTE), a bispecific single-chain antibody that binds the T-cell receptor CD3 on T cells and the B-cell antigen CD19 expressed by malignant lymphoblasts. Dual binding of CD3 and CD19 by BiTE brings reactive T cells close to tumor cells, redirects T cell lysis, and eliminates disease. Administration of BiTE to ALL patients in clinical remission but with evidence of MRD after standard chemotherapy has been shown to eradicate detectable disease in 76% of patients.

In ALL, as in AML, the worse the prognosis, the earlier transplantation should be offered. Patients with MRD+ disease are considered to have chemoresistant disease, and studies have shown that high-risk ALL patients clearly benefit from alloSCT, preferably from an HLA-matched sibling, during the first remission. Unfortunately, outcomes for high-risk ALL patients without an available HLA-matched donor are poor, and these individuals should pursue alternative transplant options or experimental therapies. No significant benefit has been seen with autologous transplantation over standard chemotherapy for these patients. In contrast, low- and standard-risk ALL patients, particularly pediatric patients, with high rates of long-term remission and survival after conventional chemotherapy and maintenance are recommended to avoid allogeneic SCT unless disease recurs.

In the modern era, ALL therapy is increasingly being tailored for specific patient populations (Table 2.14), including adolescent and young adult (AYA) patients as well as elderly individuals and those with Philadelphia chromosome–positive (Ph+) ALL, Ph-like ALL, and T-cell ALL (T-ALL) subtypes.

Age remains an important determinant of ALL therapy. Historically, adult patients diagnosed with ALL receive treatment regimens with attenuated doses or even omissions (i.e., asparaginase) of the same chemotherapy agents routinely used so successfully in pediatric patients. This is due to significantly higher rates of treatment-related toxicities and death in older individuals with medical comorbidities and decreased tolerance of prolonged chemotherapy. In contrast, multiple retrospective and prospective trials have now demonstrated that AYA patients aged 15 to 39 years of age can benefit from "pediatric-inspired" chemotherapy regimens with dose intensification of corticosteroids, vincristine, asparaginase, and intrathecal chemotherapy. This is reflected in improved overall survival rates of over 70%. In contrast, elderly patients (>60 years old) are increasingly being offered low-intensity regimens designed to preserve outcomes while minimizing toxicity. To further improve responses, recent trials have explored the addition of BiTE and anti-CD20 antibodies to chemotherapy with promising results.

Philadelphia chromosome–expressing (Ph+) ALL is a previously notoriously chemoresistant ALL subtype that occurs much more commonly in adults than children. Treatment has been dramatically altered by the incorporation of newer-generation BCR-ABL1 TKIs into conventional chemotherapy regimens (see Table 2.9). Dasatinib is a second-generation TKI with known CNS penetration that results in superior outcomes over imatinib plus chemotherapy. Ponatinib is a third-generation TKI with activity against ALL cells bearing *BCR-ABL1* tyrosine kinase mutations conferring resistance to other TKIs. Although associated with increased cardiovascular and thrombotic complications, ponatinib and chemotherapy results in very high response rates and 3-year remission rates of over 80%. Five-year overall survival for Ph+ ALL now ranges between 60% and 70%, raising the question of whether alloSCT should be performed for all patients or solely for individuals with persistent MRD+ disease following frontline therapy. Upfront TKI therapy in combination with corticosteroids now leads to almost universal remission rates without requiring cytotoxic agents. Older patients with Ph+ALL are now able to receive much less chemotherapy than previously and continue therapy with sustained responses for months if not years.

Genomic analyses have revealed a biologic subset of ALL with similar gene expression patterns as Ph+ ALL but no evidence of BCR-ABL protein or t(9;22). This so-called "Ph-like" ALL subtype occurs in up to 30% of AYA patients and is associated with Hispanic ethnicity and poor outcomes. Discovery of specific kinase mutations in these patients, such as *JAK1*, *JAK2*, *ABL2*, *CRLF2*, has led to clinical trials incorporating specific TKIs (i.e., ruxolitinib, dasatinib) into treatment regimen to enhance antileukemic efficacy.

T-cell ALL occurs far less frequently than B-cell disease and until recently was believed to confer worse prognosis following treatment with standard ALL chemotherapy regimens. Nelarabine is a purine analogue that is incorporated into malignant lymphoblasts, leading to inhibition of DNA synthesis and apoptosis. This single agent resulted in overall response rates of 20% to 30% in patients with relapsed/refractory T-ALL. This agent is being incorporated into upfront treatment regimens, particularly for high risk patients with ALL, with encouraging results to date.

TABLE 2.14 Treatment of Acute Lymphoblastic Leukemia

Treatment	Patient Population	Clinical Notes
Intensive induction chemotherapy	Newly diagnosed pediatric patients	High remission rates of >90%; long-term survival in pediatric patients >90% vs. 30-40% in adults
Pediatric inspired regimens	Newly diagnosed AYA	Improved 3-year survival of 73%; Dose intensification of steroids, IT chemotherapy, asparaginase and vincristine
Low-intensity chemo regimens	Newly diagnosed older adults	Lower-dose chemotherapy with omission of anthracycline
Rituximab (anti-CD20 ab)	Younger patients with CD20+ disease	Added to standard chemotherapy; not indicated for older patients or CD20-negative disease
BCR-ABL1 inhibitors	Ph-positive ALL	Combined with steroids and standard chemotherapy
Blinatumomab (CD19-CD3 bispecific antibody)	MRD+ and Relapsed refractory CD19+ ALL	Toxicities of cytokine release syndrome and CNS effects. Eliminates MRD+ disease in >70%. Overall survival of 7.7 months in relapsed disease.
Inotuzumab ozogamicin	Relapsed/refractory CD22+ ALL	Risk of veno-occlusive disease (15%) and hepatotoxicity, particularly with prior allogeneic stem cell transplant
Tisagenlecleucel (CD19 chimeric antigen receptor T cells)	Relapsed/refractory CD19+ ALL aged 25 and younger	Response rates of 80%. Toxicities of cytokine release and neurologic symptoms require treatment with steroid and anti-IL-6 antibody

后达到骨髓形态学缓解时通过高灵敏度 PCR 或多参数流式细胞术检测出恶性原始淋巴细胞。MRD 是疾病复发和生存期短（无论是否桥接 alloSCT）的独立预测因子。MRD 阳性的 CD19$^+$ B 细胞 ALL 患者通常接受贝林妥欧单抗（BiTE）治疗，BiTE 是一种双特异性单链抗体，可结合 T 细胞表面的受体 CD3 和白血病细胞上的 B 细胞抗原 CD19。BiTE 与 CD3 和 CD19 的双重结合使反应性 T 细胞接近肿瘤细胞，重新定向 T 细胞裂解，清除肿瘤细胞。在标准化疗后获得临床缓解但具有 MRD 的 ALL 患者中，使用 BiTE 可使 76% 的患者 MRD 转阴。

与 AML 相同，预后越差的 ALL 患者越应及早进行移植。标准诱导化疗和巩固化疗后 MRD 阳性患者可能存在化疗耐药，研究表明，高危 ALL 患者首次诱导缓解后可获益于 alloSCT，尤其是 HLA 全相合同胞供者移植。然而，无 HLA 全相合同胞供者的高危 ALL 患者预后差，这类患者应寻求非亲缘 HLA 全相合 alloSCT 或临床试验。与标准化疗相比，这类患者进行自体移植并没有明显获益。相反，低危和标危 ALL 患者，特别是儿童患者，在常规化疗和维持治疗后长期缓解率高，不需要进行 alloSCT，除非疾病复发。

在现代，ALL 治疗越来越多地针对特定的患者人群进行个体化治疗（表 2.14），包括青少年和年轻成人（AYA）患者及老年患者和费城染色体阳性（Ph$^+$）ALL、Ph 样 ALL 和 T 细胞 ALL（T-ALL）亚型患者。

年龄仍然是 ALL 治疗的重要决定因素。在过去，ALL 成人患者接受的治疗方案与儿童患者相同，但通常将剂量减量甚至减少某些药物（如天冬酰胺酶）。这是由于有内科合并症的老年患者的治疗相关毒性和死亡率显著升高，长期化疗的耐受性下降。相反，多项回顾性和前瞻性试验表明，15～39 岁的患者可从以儿科方案为基础并增加皮质类固醇剂量强化、长春新碱、天冬酰胺酶和鞘内注射化疗的方案中获益，总生存率在 70% 以上。越来越多的老年患者（> 60 岁）接受低强度化疗方案，旨在将化疗药物毒性降至最低，改善临床结局。近期有研究探索了传统化疗方案联合 BiTE 和抗 CD20 抗体，结果令人鼓舞。

Ph$^+$ ALL 的化疗耐药率高，成人化疗的疗效低于儿童。在传统化疗方案中加入新一代 BCR-ABL1 TKI 可显著提高疗效（表 2.9）。达沙替尼是第二代 TKI，可透过血脑屏障，达沙替尼联合化疗的疗效优于伊马替尼联合化疗。普纳替尼是第三代 TKI，对携带 *BCR-ABL1* 酪氨酸激酶突变（这些突变对其他 TKI 耐药）的 ALL 细胞具有强大的杀伤效应。虽然心血管和血栓并发症较其他 TKI 高，但普纳替尼的有效率很高，3 年缓解率超过 80%。在 TKI 治疗时代，Ph$^+$ ALL 患者的 5 年总生存率可达 60%～70%，那么是否应该对所有患者进行 alloSCT，还是仅对在一线治疗后 MRD 持续阳性的患者进行 alloSCT？当前，TKI 联合皮质类固醇作为一线诱导治疗方案的缓解率非常高，已不再需要使用细胞毒性药物。Ph$^+$ ALL 老年患者现已不需要像以前一样接受多次强化化疗也可获得持续数月的缓解状态。

"Ph 样" ALL 是 ALL 的一个生物学亚型，通过基因组分析可发现其基因表达谱与 Ph$^+$ ALL 相似，但无 BCR-ABL 蛋白或 t（9;22）异常。这种 ALL 亚型在青少年和年轻成人中的发生率高达 30%，与西班牙裔和预后不良相关。在这些患者中可发现特异性激酶突变，如 *JAK1*、*JAK2*、*ABL2*、*CRLF2*，这促使当前的探索性临床研究将特异性 TKI（即芦可替尼、达沙替尼）加入传统化疗方案中，以增强抗白血病疗效。

T 细胞 ALL 的发生率远低于 B 细胞 ALL，标准 ALL 化疗方案治疗 T 细胞 ALL 的预后差。奈拉滨是一种嘌呤类似物，可导致恶性原始淋巴细胞的 DNA 合成抑制和细胞凋亡。奈拉滨单药治疗复发 / 难治性 T 细胞 ALL 患者的总反应率为 20%～30%。该药物正在被纳入诱导治疗方案中，特别是对于高危 ALL 患者，目前获得了令人鼓舞的结果。

表 2.14　ALL 的治疗

治疗	患者人群	临床备注
强化诱导化疗	初诊儿童患者	缓解率 > 90%；儿童患者长期生存率 > 90%，成人患者长期生存率为 30%～40%
以儿科方案为基础	初诊青少年和年轻成人患者	3 年生存率为 73%；皮质醇剂量强化、鞘内注射化疗、天冬酰胺酶和长春新碱
低强度化疗方案	初诊老年患者	无蒽环类药物的低剂量化疗
利妥昔单抗（抗 CD20 抗体）	年轻 CD20$^+$ 患者	联合标准化疗；不适用于老年患者或 CD20$^-$ 患者
BCR-ABL1 抑制剂	Ph$^+$ ALL 患者	联合皮质醇和标准化疗
贝林妥欧单抗（CD19-CD3 双特异性抗体）	MRD 阳性和复发 / 难治性 CD19$^+$ ALL 患者	细胞因子释放综合征和 CNS 效应。消除 MRD 阳性疾病的比例 > 70%。复发患者的总生存期为 7.7 个月
奥加伊妥珠单抗	复发 / 难治性 CD22$^+$ ALL 患者	静脉闭塞性疾病（15%）和肝毒性风险，尤其是既往接受过 alloSCT 的患者
Tisagenlecleucel（CD19 嵌合抗原受体 T 细胞）	≥ 25 岁的复发 / 难治性 CD19$^+$ ALL 患者	反应率为 80%。细胞因子释放综合征和神经系统毒性症状需要皮质醇和抗 IL-6 抗体治疗

Relapsed or refractory disease. Although late recurrences can emerge at any time, most ALL relapses arise within 2 years of the initial diagnosis, with recurrence of chemoresistant leukemia cells in the bone marrow, CNS, or testes. All patients with relapsed ALL should be considered for additional therapy followed by alloSCT, which represents the only known cure for disease. Autologous SCT is not routinely recommended. Overall response rates to multiagent salvage chemotherapy incorporating the same agents used in frontline therapy range from 20% to 50% with duration of second remissions lasting less than 6 months. Other chemotherapy agents specifically indicated for relapsed disease include nelarabine for T-ALL, clofarabine for patients younger than 21 years old, and a liposomal formulation of vincristine in patients receiving at least two prior lines of therapy. Each drug induces clinical responses in up to a third of heavily pretreated patients as a single agent with tolerable toxicities.

Perhaps the most exciting strategies for ALL therapy involve technologies specifically exploiting patient host immune responses to induce responses. Numerous immunotherapies targeting the leukemia cell antigens CD19 and CD22 have entered mainstream therapy for ALL as well as other lymphoid malignancies. BiTE results in significantly improved overall survival (7.7 months) as compared with standard chemotherapy (4 months). Patients with lower marrow disease burden and receiving treatment in first relapse benefit most, with 30% of patients proceeding on to alloSCT. Unique side effects of therapy include neurologic symptoms (ranging from change in mental status to seizures to encephalopathy) and cytokine release syndrome characterized by fever, hemodynamic instability, and life-threatening organ damage. Severity of complications is related to extent of tumor burden and is higher than experienced in BiTE therapy of MRD-positive ALL.

Inotuzumab is a CD22-directed antibody conjugated to a DNA damaging agent (calicheamicin). Binding of this antibody drug conjugate to surface CD22 expressed on the ALL surface leads to its internalization, induction of DNA strand breakage, and cell death. In a randomized controlled trial, inotuzumab induced higher overall responses (88%) in patients with first relapsed ALL than standard chemotherapy (32%). Forty percent of patients receiving inotuzumab underwent subsequent alloSCT. However 15% of patients developed VOD, which was largely fatal and occurred primarily in individuals with prior alloSCT who had received multiple doses of therapy.

Cellular immunotherapies that have revolutionized the treatment of all B-cell malignancies were first validated for the treatment of relapsed B-ALL. Chimeric antigen receptor T (CART) cells are autologous T cells collected from patients with relapsed ALL and genetically modified ex vivo to express CD19 chimeric antigen receptors. This effectively reprograms them to recognize and destroy CD19-expressing tumor cells. Infusion of a single dose of CART cells (tisagenlecleucel) following lymphodepleting chemotherapy in individuals (both children and young adults) with multiple relapsed/refractory ALL resulted in the complete eradication of disease in 80% to 90%. Although CART-mediated cytokine release and neurotoxicity can be life-threatening, strategies to mitigate these adverse events with early administration of steroids and the anti-IL-6 antibody (tocilizumab) have allowed CART to be successfully administered at numerous academic centers across the world.

PROSPECTUS FOR THE FUTURE

Insights into the molecular and biologic underpinnings of MPNs and acute leukemia have led to an explosion of novel therapeutic approaches that have transformed the clinical approach to each of these diseases in the past few years.

Myeloproliferative Disease

The importance of the spectacular success of imatinib as targeted therapy for CML cannot be overstated. As the first successful therapy based on an understanding of pathogenesis, imatinib has become emblematic of the translation of an understanding of disease pathogenesis into tangible innovations in clinical care. At present, there are four additional new-generation TKIs for CML therapy in addition to imatinib. The best indicator of how these agents have altered the natural history of disease is the fact that certain patients with sustained undetectable disease for 2 to 3 years are now able to permanently discontinue TKI therapy without disease recurrence.

Similarly, the discovery of *JAK2* mutations in non-CML myeloproliferative diseases opened new avenues for targeted intervention in diseases for which previous therapy was largely supportive. JAK2 inhibition now constitutes standard-of-care therapy for PV and MF independent of *JAK2* mutation status. Newer agents are actively being investigated for MPN therapy including hypomethylating agents, *MDM2* inhibitors, antibody-drug conjugates, and anti-fibrosis agents.

Acute Leukemia

Acute leukemias are clinically aggressive malignancies with survival rates of weeks to a few months if untreated. The availability of multiple targeted and nontargeted agents for distinct biological subsets has changed the therapeutic landscape for these diseases. The first acute leukemia exemplifying this was APL. The discovery of the link between the retinoic acid receptor and the origins of APL provided important insights into the unique sensitivity of this disease to ATRA therapy and paved the road for successful implementation of dual differentiation therapy with ATRA and arsenic. This regimen marks the first time that any acute leukemia was cured without cytotoxic chemotherapy or SCT.

At present, pediatric ALL is now considered a highly curable cancer with long-term remission and survival rates of over 90%. Patients with relapsed disease are eligible to receive the latest advances in novel immunotherapeutic approaches. CART therapy has revolutionized therapy not only for ALL but for all B-cell malignancies such as lymphoma and myeloma. However, durability of response and disease relapse remain major issues. It is uncertain whether patients undergoing CART should also pursue subsequent alloSCT. Antibodies including anti-CD20 antibody (rituximab), the CD19-CD3 bispecific agent (blinatumomab), and the CD22 antibody drug conjugate (inotuzumab) have expanded the armamentarium of strategies for ALL. Incorporation of new-generation oral BCR/ABL kinase inhibitors to routine chemotherapy for Philadelphia chromosome–positive ALL has altered expectations for this subtype.

Tailoring of therapy to disease subtype as well as different age groups (pediatric, AYA, and elderly) has led to true personalized therapy. Future directions include moving agents known to be effective in the relapsed/refractory setting to earlier in the treatment course during induction and/or consolidation. Examples include upfront therapy with BiTe and dasatinib for Ph+ disease or inotuzumab plus mini-hyper CVD or CART cells with MRD testing.

In AML, the "gold standard" (7+3) for induction chemotherapy since the 1970s has finally been replaced, at least in older unfit individuals, by venetoclax-based therapy. The latter results in overall response rates of 60% to 70% and provides a new backbone regimen on which to potentially add novel experimental agents. Single-agent inhibitors of mutant *FLT3*, *IDH1*, and *IDH2* have been shown to be superior to conventional chemotherapy in patients with appropriately mutant disease. Newer clinical trials are exploring combinations of targeted agents (FLT3 and IDH inhibitors) with different chemotherapy backbones (i.e., venetoclax plus HMA) or with each other (i.e., venetoclax and gilteritinib). Development

复发/难治性 ALL　大多数 ALL 复发发生在初次诊断后 2 年内，表现为化疗耐药的白血病细胞出现在骨髓、CNS 或睾丸中。所有复发 ALL 患者均应再次接受化疗，而桥接至 alloSCT（不常规推荐自体移植）是目前唯一的治愈手段。包含与一线诱导化疗相同药物的多药挽救化疗的总缓解率为 20%～50%，且第二次缓解持续时间 < 6 个月。其他用于复发 ALL 的化疗药物包括奈拉滨（适用于 T 细胞 ALL）、氯法拉滨（适用于 21 岁以下患者）和长春新碱脂质体（适用于既往接受过至少 2 线治疗的患者）。以上药物作为单药的临床反应率高达 1/3，且毒性可耐受。

细胞免疫治疗在 ALL 中取得了令人鼓舞的进展。许多针对白血病细胞抗原 CD19 和 CD22 的细胞免疫治疗已成为 ALL 和其他淋系恶性肿瘤的主要治疗策略。与标准化疗相比，BiTE 可显著改善总体生存期（7.7 个月 vs. 4 个月）。骨髓低肿瘤负荷且在首次复发时使用的患者获益最大，30% 的患者后续桥接至 alloSCT。该治疗特有的副作用包括神经系统症状（范围从精神状态改变、癫痫发作到脑病）和以发热、血流动力学不稳定和危及生命的器官损伤为特征的细胞因子释放综合征。并发症的严重程度与肿瘤负荷程度相关，且严重程度较接受 BiTE 治疗的 MRD 阳性 ALL 患者高。

奥加伊妥珠单抗是一种与 DNA 损伤药物（卡奇霉素）结合的靶向 CD22 抗体。该抗体药物偶联物可与 ALL 表面表达的 CD22 结合，导致其内化、诱导 DNA 链断裂和细胞死亡。在一项随机对照试验中，与传统化疗（32%）相比，奥加伊妥珠单抗在首次复发的 ALL 患者中诱导的总体反应率更高（88%）。40% 接受奥加伊妥珠单抗治疗的患者随后桥接至 alloSCT。但是，15% 的患者发生到死性肝小静脉闭塞病，主要发生于既往接受过多次奥加伊妥珠单抗治疗的 alloSCT 患者。

细胞免疫治疗是 B 细胞恶性肿瘤的创新性治疗，其有效性首次在复发 B 细胞 ALL 患者中得到验证。嵌合抗原受体 T（CAR-T）细胞是从复发 ALL 患者中采集的自体 T 细胞，经过基因修饰，可在体外表达 CD19 嵌合抗原受体。CAR-T 细胞可有效识别并破坏表达 CD19 的肿瘤细胞。在复发/难治性 ALL 患者（儿童和年轻成人）中，清淋性化疗后单次输注 CAR-T 细胞（Tisagenlecleucel）的总体缓解率达 80%～90%。尽管 CAR-T 细胞介导的细胞因子释放综合征和神经毒性可能危及生命，但通过早期给予类固醇和抗 IL-6 抗体（托珠单抗）可减轻这些并发症，这使得 CAR-T 细胞治疗目前已在全球广泛应用。

未来展望

人们对 MPN、急性白血病分子和生物学发病机制的深入了解促进了新治疗方法的发展，这些方法有望在未来几年改变这些疾病的临床治疗。

骨髓增生性疾病

伊马替尼作为 CML 的靶向治疗药已取得了巨大成功，其重要性不言而喻。作为第一个利用对发病机制的认识而成功治疗的案例，伊马替尼已成为靶向治疗的典范。除伊马替尼外，目前还有 4 种用于 CML 治疗的新一代 TKI。评估改变病程的最佳指标是 BCR-ABL 基因阴性持续 2～3 年，且永久停用 TKI 而无疾病复发。

类似地，JAK2 突变的发现为非 CML 的骨髓增殖性疾病开辟了靶向治疗的新途径，在此之前，这些患者主要依靠支持治疗。JAK2 抑制剂目前是 PV 和 MF 的一线治疗，无论 JAK2 突变状态如何。用于治疗 MPN 的新型药物正在研究阶段，包括 HMA、MDM2 抑制剂、抗体偶联药物和抗纤维化药物。

急性白血病

急性白血病是侵袭性恶性肿瘤，如果不治疗，生存率仅为数周至数月。针对不同生物学亚型的多种靶向和非靶向药物的出现改变了这些疾病的转归。第一个例子便是 APL。视黄酸受体与 APL 的相关性研究为 ATRA 治疗 APL 提供重要的理论依据，并为 ATRA 联合砷剂的成功奠定了基础，ATRA + 砷剂联合治疗标志着 APL 在不使用细胞毒性化疗或 SCT 的情况下也可以被治愈。

目前，儿童 ALL 被认为是一种可治愈的急性白血病，长期缓解率和生存率超过 90%。复发患者可参与临床试验接受新型免疫治疗。CAR-T 细胞治疗不仅彻底改变了 ALL 的治疗，也改变了所有 B 细胞恶性肿瘤（如淋巴瘤和骨髓瘤）的治疗。然而，缓解时间短和复发仍然是其主要问题。接受 CAR-T 细胞治疗的患者是否应进行后续 alloSCT 目前仍存争议。ALL 的治疗还包括抗 CD20 抗体（利妥昔单抗）、CD19-CD3 双特异性药物（BiTE）和 CD22 抗体药物偶联物（奥加伊妥珠单抗）。常规化疗联合新一代口服 BCR/ABL 激酶抑制剂可使 Ph$^+$ ALL 患者的长期生存期延长。

目前临床医生可根据急性白血病亚型及不同年龄组（儿童、青少年及年轻成人、老年人）进行个体化治疗。未来的发展方向可将临床研究中确认在复发/难治性患者有效的靶向药物应用至诱导和（或）巩固治疗阶段。例如，BiTE 和达沙替尼用于 Ph$^+$ ALL 的诱导治疗，或在 MRD 监测下使用奥加伊妥珠单抗联合 mini-Hyper CVD 或 CAR-T 细胞免疫治疗。

至少对于不适合强化化疗的 AML 老年患者，自 20 世纪 70 年代开始使用的诱导化疗"金标准"（"7 + 3"）已被基于维奈克拉的治疗所取代。维奈克拉的总体反应率为 60%～70%。因此，在维奈克拉的基础上添加其他新型药物是当前的主要治疗方案。携带 FLT3、IDH1 和 IDH2 突变的患者单用上述相应基因抑制剂的疗效优于传统化疗。当前临床研究的方向是探索将靶向药物（FLT3 和 IDH 抑制剂）联用不同化疗基础药物（如维奈克拉 + HMA），或不同靶向药物之间（如维奈

of reduced intensity and haploidentical alloSCT strategies has permitted specific older AML patients the opportunity to be cured of their disease. Similar approaches may soon provide therapeutic entry points into the treatment of other acute leukemias associated with pathognomonic chromosomal translocations and genetic and molecular aberrations.

SUGGESTED READINGS

Arber DA, Orazi A, Hasserjian R, et al: The 2016 revision to the World Health Organization classification of myeloid neoplasms and acute leukemia, Blood 127(20):2391–2405, 2016.

Baxter EJ, Scott LM, Campbell PJ, et al: Acquired mutation of the tyrosine kinase JAK2 in human myeloproliferative disorders, Lancet 365(9464):1054–1061, 2005.

Byrd J, Mrozek K, Dodge R, et al: Pretreatment cytogenetic abnormalities are predictive of induction success, cumulative incidence of relapse, and overall survival in adult patients with de novo acute myeloid leukemia, Blood 100(13):4325–4336, 2002.

Cortes JE, Heidel JH, Hellman A, et al: Randomized comparison of low dose cytarabine with or without glasdegib in patients with newly diagnosed acute myeloid leukemia or high-risk myelodysplastic syndrome, Leukemia 33(2):379–389, 2019.

DiNardo CD, Pratz K, Pullarkat V, et al: Venetoclax combined with decitabine or azacitidine in treatment-naive, elderly patients with acute myeloid leukemia, Blood 133(1):7–17, 2019.

DiNardo CD, Stein EM, de Botton S, et al: Durable remissions with ivosidenib in IDH1-mutated relapsed or refractory AML, N Engl J Med 378(25):2386–2398, 2018.

Dohner H, Estey EH, Grimwade D, et al: Diagnosis and management of AML in adults: 2017 ELM recommendations from an international expert panel, Blood 129(4):424–447, 2017.

Döhner H, Estey EH, Amadori S, et al: Diagnosis and management of acute myeloid leukemia in adults: recommendations from an international expert panel, on behalf of the European LeukemiaNet, Blood 115(3):453–474, 2010.

Harrison CN, Campbell PJ, Buck G, et al: Hydroxyurea compared with anagrelide in high-risk essential thrombocythemia, N Engl J Med 353(1):33–45, 2005.

Harrison CN, Vannucchi AM, Kiladjian JJ, et al: Long-term findings from COMFORT-II, a phase 3 trial of ruxolitinib versus best available therapy for myelofibrosis, Leukemia 30(8):1701–1707, 2016.

Hasford J, Pfirrmann M, Hehlmann R, et al: A new prognostic score for survival of patients with chronic myeloid leukemia treated with interferon alfa. Writing Committee 3 for the Collaborative CML Prognostic Factors Project Group, J Natl Cancer Inst 90(11):850–858, 1998.

Hughes TP, Mauro MJ, Cortes JE, et al: Asciminib in chronic myeloid leukemia after ABL kinase inhibitor failure, N Engl J Med 381(24):2315–2326, 2019.

Kantarjian HM, DeAngelo DJ, Stelljes M, et al: Inotuzumab ozogamicin versus standard therapy for acute lymphoblastic leukemia, N Engl J Med 375(8):740–753, 2016.

Kantarjian H, Stein A, Gokbuget N, et al: Blinatumomab versus chemotherapy for advanced acute lymphoblastic leukemia, N Engl J Med 376(9):836–847, 2017.

Lambert J, Pautas C, Terre C, et al: Gemtuzumab ozogamicin for *de novo* acute myeloid leukemia: final efficacy and safety updates from the open-label, phase III ALFA-0701 trial, Haematologica 104(1):113–119, 2019.

Landolfi R, Marchioli R, Kutti J, et al: Efficacy and safety of low-dose aspirin in polycythemia vera, N Engl J Med 350(2):114–124, 2004.

Maude SL, Laetsch TW, Buechner J, et al: Chimeric antigen receptor T cells for sustained remissions in leukemia, N Engl J Med 378(5):439–448, 2018.

Perl S, Martinelli G, Cortes JE, et al: Gilteritinib or chemotherapy for relapsed or refractory *FLT3*-mutated AML, N Engl J Med 381(18):1728–1740, 2019.

Pfirrman M, Baccarani M, Saussele S, et al: Prognosis of long-term survival considering disease-specific death in patients with chronic myeloid leukemia, Leukemia 30(1):48–56, 2016.

Pullarkat V, Slovak ML, Kopecky KJ, et al: Impact of cytogenetics on the outcome of adult acute lymphocytic leukemia: results of the Southwest Oncology Group 9400 study, Blood 111(5):2563–2572, 2008.

Sokal J, Cox EB, Baccarani M, et al: Prognostic discrimination in "good-risk" chronic granulocytic leukemia, Blood 63(4):789–799, 1984.

Stein EM, DiNardo CD, Pollyea DA, et al: Enasidenib in mutant IDH2 relapsed or refractory acute myeloid leukemia, Blood 130(6):722–731, 2017.

Stock W, Luger SM, Advani AS, et al: A pediatric regimen for older adolescents and young adults with acute lymphoblastic leukemia: results of CALGB 10403, Blood 133(14):1548–1559, 2019.

Stone RM, Mandrekar SJ, Sanford BL, et al: Midostaurin plus chemotherapy for acute myeloid leukemia with a FLT3 mutation, N Engl J Med 377(5):454–464, 2017.

Vannucchi AM, Kiladjian JJ, Greisshammer M, et al: Ruxolitinib versus standard therapy for treatment of polycythemia vera, N Engl J Med 372(5):426–435, 2015.

Wei AH, Strickland SA, Hou JZ, et al: Venetoclax combined with low-Dose cytarabine for previously untreated patients with acute myeloid leukemia: results from a phase Ib/II study, J Clin Oncol 37(15):1277–1284, 2019.

克拉和吉瑞替尼）联用。减低强度和单倍型供者 SCT 方案的开展延长了 AML 老年患者的生存期，并为部分老年患者提供了治愈的机会。类似的方法可能很快能为其他急性白血病（与特异性染色体易位、基因和分子异常相关）的治疗提供切入点。

推荐阅读

Arber DA, Orazi A, Hasserjian R, et al: The 2016 revision to the World Health Organization classification of myeloid neoplasms and acute leukemia, Blood 127(20):2391–2405, 2016.

Baxter EJ, Scott LM, Campbell PJ, et al: Acquired mutation of the tyrosine kinase JAK2 in human myeloproliferative disorders, Lancet 365(9464):1054–1061, 2005.

Byrd J, Mrozek K, Dodge R, et al: Pretreatment cytogenetic abnormalities are predictive of induction success, cumulative incidence of relapse, and overall survival in adult patients with de novo acute myeloid leukemia, Blood 100(13):4325–4336, 2002.

Cortes JE, Heidel JH, Hellman A, et al: Randomized comparison of low dose cytarabine with or without glasdegib in patients with newly diagnosed acute myeloid leukemia or high-risk myelodysplastic syndrome, Leukemia 33(2):379–389, 2019.

DiNardo CD, Pratz K, Pullarkat V, et al: Venetoclax combined with decitabine or azacitidine in treatment-naive, elderly patients with acute myeloid leukemia, Blood 133(1):7–17, 2019.

DiNardo CD, Stein EM, de Botton S, et al: Durable remissions with ivosidenib in IDH1-mutated relapsed or refractory AML, N Engl J Med 378(25):2386–2398, 2018.

Dohner H, Estey EH, Grimwade D, et al: Diagnosis and management of AML in adults: 2017 ELM recommendations from an international expert panel, Blood 129(4):424–447, 2017.

Döhner H, Estey EH, Amadori S, et al: Diagnosis and management of acute myeloid leukemia in adults: recommendations from an international expert panel, on behalf of the European LeukemiaNet, Blood 115(3):453–474, 2010.

Harrison CN, Campbell PJ, Buck G, et al: Hydroxyurea compared with anagrelide in high-risk essential thrombocythemia, N Engl J Med 353(1):33–45, 2005.

Harrison CN, Vannucchi AM, Kiladjian JJ, et al: Long-term findings from COMFORT-II, a phase 3 trial of ruxolitinib versus best available therapy for myelofibrosis, Leukemia 30(8):1701–1707, 2016.

Hasford J, Pfirrmann M, Hehlmann R, et al: A new prognostic score for survival of patients with chronic myeloid leukemia treated with interferon alfa. Writing Committee 3 for the Collaborative CML Prognostic Factors Project Group, J Natl Cancer Inst 90(11):850–858, 1998.

Hughes TP, Mauro MJ, Cortes JE, et al: Asciminib in chronic myeloid leukemia after ABL kinase inhibitor failure, N Engl J Med 381(24):2315–2326, 2019.

Kantarjian HM, DeAngelo DJ, Stelljes M, et al: Inotuzumab ozogamicin versus standard therapy for acute lymphoblastic leukemia, N Engl J Med 375(8):740–753, 2016.

Kantarjian H, Stein A, Gokbuget N, et al: Blinatumomab versus chemotherapy for advanced acute lymphoblastic leukemia, N Engl J Med 376(9):836–847, 2017.

Lambert J, Pautas C, Terre C, et al: Gemtuzumab ozogamicin for *de novo* acute myeloid leukemia: final efficacy and safety updates from the open-label, phase III ALFA-0701 trial, Haematologica 104(1):113–119, 2019.

Landolfi R, Marchioli R, Kutti J, et al: Efficacy and safety of low-dose aspirin in polycythemia vera, N Engl J Med 350(2):114–124, 2004.

Maude SL, Laetsch TW, Buechner J, et al: Chimeric antigen receptor T cells for sustained remissions in leukemia, N Engl J Med 378(5):439–448, 2018.

Perl S, Martinelli G, Cortes JE, et al: Gilteritinib or chemotherapy for relapsed or refractory *FLT3*-mutated AML, N Engl J Med 381(18):1728–1740, 2019.

Pfirrman M, Baccarani M, Saussele S, et al: Prognosis of long-term survival considering disease-specific death in patients with chronic myeloid leukemia, Leukemia 30(1):48–56, 2016.

Pullarkat V, Slovak ML, Kopecky KJ, et al: Impact of cytogenetics on the outcome of adult acute lymphocytic leukemia: results of the Southwest Oncology Group 9400 study, Blood 111(5):2563–2572, 2008.

Sokal J, Cox EB, Baccarani M, et al: Prognostic discrimination in "good-risk" chronic granulocytic leukemia, Blood 63(4):789–799, 1984.

Stein EM, DiNardo CD, Pollyea DA, et al: Enasidenib in mutant IDH2 relapsed or refractory acute myeloid leukemia, Blood 130(6):722–731, 2017.

Stock W, Luger SM, Advani AS, et al: A pediatric regimen for older adolescents and young adults with acute lymphoblastic leukemia: results of CALGB 10403, Blood 133(14):1548–1559, 2019.

Stone RM, Mandrekar SJ, Sanford BL, et al: Midostaurin plus chemotherapy for acute myeloid leukemia with a FLT3 mutation, N Engl J Med 377(5):454–464, 2017.

Vannucchi AM, Kiladjian JJ, Greissshammer M, et al: Ruxolitinib versus standard therapy for treatment of polycythemia vera, N Engl J Med 372(5):426–435, 2015.

Wei AH, Strickland SA, Hou JZ, et al: Venetoclax combined with low-Dose cytarabine for previously untreated patients with acute myeloid leukemia: results from a phase Ib/II study, J Clin Oncol 37(15):1277–1284, 2019.

3

Disorders of Red Blood Cells

Ellice Wong, Michal G. Rose, Nancy Berliner

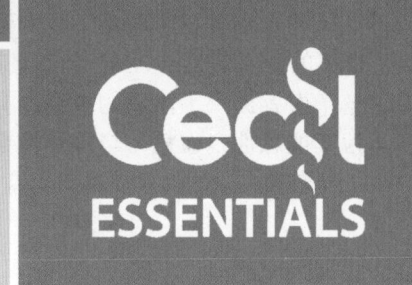

NORMAL RED BLOOD CELL STRUCTURE AND FUNCTION

Erythrocytes, or red blood cells (RBCs), deliver oxygen to all the tissues in the body and carry carbon dioxide back to the lungs for excretion. The erythrocyte is uniquely adapted to these functions. It has a biconcave disk shape that maximizes the membrane surface area for gas exchange, and it has a cytoskeleton and membrane structure that allow it to deform sufficiently to pass through the microvasculature. Passage through capillaries whose diameter may be one fourth the resting diameter of the erythrocyte is made possible by interactions between proteins in the membrane (band 3 and glycophorin) and underlying cytoplasmic proteins that make up the erythrocyte cytoskeleton (spectrin, ankyrin, and protein 4.1).

The mature RBC contains no nucleus and is dependent throughout its life span on proteins synthesized before extrusion of the nucleus and release of the cell from the bone marrow into the peripheral circulation. About 98% of the cytoplasmic protein of the mature erythrocyte is hemoglobin. The remainder is mainly enzymatic proteins, such as those required for anaerobic metabolism and the hexose monophosphate shunt.

Defects in any of the intrinsic structural features of the erythrocyte can result in hemolytic anemia. Abnormalities of the membrane or cytoskeletal proteins are the causes of alterations in erythrocyte shape and flexibility. Inborn defects in the enzymatic pathways for glucose metabolism decrease the resistance to oxidant stress, and inherited abnormalities of hemoglobin structure and synthesis lead to polymerization of abnormal hemoglobin (sickle cell disease) or to the precipitation of unbalanced hemoglobin chains (thalassemia). All of these changes result in decreased erythrocyte survival.

Oxygen is transported by hemoglobin, a tetramer composed of two α chains, two β-like (β, γ, or δ) chains, and four heme molecules, each of which is composed of a protoporphyrin molecule complexed with iron. In fetal life, the main hemoglobin is fetal hemoglobin (HbF: $\alpha_2\gamma_2$); the switch from HbF to adult hemoglobin (HbA: $\alpha_2\beta_2$) occurs in the perinatal period. By 4 to 6 months of age, the level of HbF has fallen to about 1% of total hemoglobin. HbA_2 ($\alpha_2\delta_2$) is a minor adult hemoglobin, representing about 1% of adult hemoglobin (Table 3.1).

CLINICAL PRESENTATION

Anemia, defined as a reduction in RBC mass, is an important sign of disease. It may be caused by decreased production of erythrocytes from nutritional deficiencies, primary hematologic disease, or a response to systemic illness. Alternatively, anemia may be caused by increased blood loss or cellular destruction from hemolysis. Hemolysis may occur as a result of intrinsic abnormalities of the RBC, immune-mediated RBC destruction, or a systemic vascular process. The investigation of anemia is a critical component of the evaluation of the patient and commonly provides valuable insight into systemic illness. Fig. 3.1 provides an overview of the differential diagnosis of anemia.

The symptoms of anemia reflect both the severity and the rapidity with which the reduction in erythrocyte mass has occurred. Patients with acute hemorrhage may exhibit symptoms of hypovolemic shock. Massive hemolysis may result in neurologic impairment or cardiovascular collapse. However, most patients develop anemia more slowly and have few symptoms. Usual complaints are fatigue, decreased exercise tolerance, dyspnea, and palpitations. In patients with coronary artery disease, anemia may precipitate angina. On physical examination, the major sign of anemia is pallor. Patients may be tachycardic and often have significant flow murmurs. Patients with hemolysis often exhibit jaundice and splenomegaly. Patients with iron deficiency may occasionally exhibit signs of pica (i.e., craving for ice or nonfood items such as dirt).

LABORATORY EVALUATION

The key components of the laboratory evaluation of anemia are the reticulocyte count, the peripheral blood smear, erythrocyte indices, nutritional studies, and in some cases the bone marrow aspirate and biopsy.

The *reticulocyte count* allows the critical distinction between anemia arising from a primary failure of RBC production and anemia resulting from increased RBC destruction or bleeding. Erythrocytes newly released from the marrow still contain small amounts of RNA; these cells, termed *reticulocytes,* can be detected with the use of automated counters and fluorescent nucleic acid–binding dyes or manually by staining of the peripheral blood smear with new methylene blue or other supravital stains. In response to anemia, erythropoietin (EPO) production increases, promoting the production and release of increased numbers of reticulocytes. The number of reticulocytes in the peripheral blood therefore reflects the response of the bone marrow to anemia.

The reticulocyte count can be expressed either as a percentage of the total number of RBCs or as an absolute number. In patients without anemia, the normal reticulocyte count is 0.5% to 1.5% of RBCs or 20,000 to 75,000/μL. When the anemia is caused by decreased RBC survival, the appropriate marrow response results in a reticulocyte count greater than 2%, with an absolute count of more than 100,000/μL. If the reticulocyte count is not elevated, a cause of failure of RBC production should be sought. Reticulocyte counts that are expressed as a percentage of total RBCs must be corrected for anemia because decreasing the number of circulating cells increases the reticulocyte percentage without any increase in release from the marrow.

红细胞疾病

马瑞 译 许兰平 唐菲菲 审校 黄晓军 通审

正常红细胞的结构和功能

红细胞（RBC）将氧气输送到全身各组织，再将二氧化碳（CO_2）输送回肺部以排出体外。RBC对这些功能具有独特的适应能力。RBC所具有的双凹圆盘状外形可使其细胞膜面积最大化，从而有利于气体交换，而它特有的细胞骨架及膜结构可使其充分变形以通过毛细血管。RBC的细胞膜蛋白（带3蛋白及血型糖蛋白）与胞质内的细胞骨架蛋白（血影蛋白、锚蛋白及蛋白4.1）相互作用，使RBC可以通过管径仅为静止状态RBC直径1/4的毛细血管。

成熟RBC不含细胞核，在其整个寿命周期中均依赖于脱核前及由骨髓释放入外周血前合成的蛋白质。成熟RBC胞质蛋白中约98%为血红蛋白，其余主要是酶相关蛋白质，包括无氧酵解代谢及磷酸己糖代谢途径中所需的各种酶。

任何RBC的内在结构缺陷均可导致溶血性贫血。细胞膜或骨架蛋白异常可引起RBC形状及变形性改变。葡萄糖代谢途径中酶的先天性缺陷降低了RBC对氧化应激的抵御能力，先天性血红蛋白结构及合成障碍可导致异常血红蛋白多聚化（镰状细胞贫血）或过量血红蛋白链的沉积（地中海贫血）。上述变化均会使RBC寿命缩短。

血液中的氧气通过血红蛋白进行转运，血红蛋白是由2条α链、2条β样（β、γ或δ）链及4个血红素分子构成的四聚体，其中每个血红素分子由原卟啉与铁络合而成。在胎儿期，血红蛋白主要为胎儿型（HbF：$\alpha_2\gamma_2$）；围产期则由胎儿型过渡到成人型（HbA：$\alpha_2\beta_2$）。在4～6月龄时，HbF的水平约降至血红蛋白总量的1%。HbA2（$\alpha_2\delta_2$）是一种次要成人血红蛋白，约占成人血红蛋白的1%（表3.1）。

临床表现

贫血即RBC体量减少，是疾病的一个重要表现。营养不良、原发性血液疾病或其他全身疾病等原因引起的RBC生成减少均可导致贫血。此外，大量失血或溶血引起的RBC破坏亦可导致贫血。溶血的原因包括RBC自身的异常、免疫介导的血细胞破坏或全身血管病变。对贫血原因的研判是患者评估的重要组成部分，常为全身性疾病的诊治提供重要线索。图3.1概述了贫血的鉴别诊断。

贫血的症状既反映了RBC体量减少的程度，也反映了RBC体量减少的速度。急性出血患者可表现为低血容量性休克。大量溶血可导致神经系统功能障碍或心血管系统崩溃。但是，多数患者的贫血发展缓慢，几乎没有症状；常见主诉包括乏力、活动耐量降低、呼吸困难和心悸。在冠状动脉疾病患者中，贫血可能会引发心绞痛。体格检查主要可见面色苍白。患者可出现心动过速，且常可闻及明显心脏杂音。溶血性贫血患者常出现黄疸和脾大。部分缺铁性贫血患者可出现异食癖（如喜食冰或土等非可食用物品）。

实验室检查

贫血的实验室检查主要包括网织红细胞计数、外周血涂片、红细胞指数和营养评估，部分病例还需进行骨髓穿刺和活检。

网织红细胞计数可用于鉴别原发性RBC生成障碍所致的贫血与RBC破坏增加或失血所致的贫血。骨髓释放的RBC在短期内仍含有少量RNA，此类细胞即网织红细胞，可在荧光核酸染色后使用自动计数仪计数，也可在使用亚甲蓝或其他活体染料对外周血涂片染色后进行人工计数。贫血时，促红细胞生成素（EPO）生成增加，促进产生和释放更多的网织红细胞。因此，外周血中网织红细胞的数量反映了骨髓对贫血的反应。

网织红细胞计数可用其占RBC总数的百分比来表示，亦可用其绝对值来表示。在非贫血患者中，网织红细胞的正常占比为0.5%～1.5%，绝对值为20 000～75 000/μl。当贫血由RBC寿命缩短所致时，骨髓的代偿反应可使网织红细胞占比升至>2%，绝对值增至>100 000/μl。若网织红细胞计数未出现相应增多，则应考虑是否存在RBC生成减少所致的贫血。对贫血患者而言，循环中血细胞减少可导致网织红细胞比例的相对升高，但骨髓释放的网织红细胞可能并无增加，故此时以百分比表示的网织红细胞计数需进行校正。校

The *corrected reticulocyte count* is calculated by multiplying the reticulocyte count by the ratio of the patient's hematocrit to a normal hematocrit. An additional calculation, the reticulocyte index or reticulocyte production index (RPI), determines whether the reticulocyte count is appropriate for the degree of anemia. The RPI corrects for both the degree of anemia and release of reticulocytes from the marrow by multiplying the ratio of the patient's hematocrit to a normal hematocrit by the reticulocyte percentage divided by a maturation term. The maturation term signifies the time in days for RBCs to mature (ranging from 1 for a hematocrit ≥40% to 2.5 for a hematocrit <20%). An RPI greater than 3 is considered an appropriate marrow response (e.g., from increased RBC destruction or bleeding) and an RPI less than 2 is an inappropriate marrow response (e.g., a RBC production problem).

Evaluation of the *peripheral blood smear* may provide important clues to the cause of anemia. Erythrocyte morphologic examination is especially critical in the evaluation of anemia associated with reticulocytosis, wherein an examination of the smear is essential to distinguish between immune hemolysis (which results in spherocytes) and microangiopathic hemolysis (which causes schistocytes or erythrocyte fragmentation). Changes associated with other causes of anemia include sickle and target cells that are characteristic of hemoglobinopathies, teardrop cells and nucleated RBCs associated with myelofibrosis and marrow infiltration, intracorpuscular parasites in malaria and babesiosis, and pencil-shaped deformities associated with severe iron deficiency. Examination of myeloid cells and platelets may also be helpful. Hypersegmented neutrophils and large platelets support the diagnosis of megaloblastic anemia, and the presence of immature blast forms may be diagnostic of leukemia. Fig. 3.2 presents some common peripheral blood smear findings in patients with anemia.

In patients with anemia and an elevated reticulocyte count, the vigorous production of new erythroid cells suggests that marrow function is normal and is responding appropriately to the stress of the anemia. Bone marrow examination in this situation is rarely indicated because the marrow will simply show erythroid hyperplasia, usually without revealing any primary pathologic anomaly of the marrow. Evaluation in these cases should be focused on determining whether the cause of RBC consumption is bleeding or hemolysis. In contrast, bone marrow examination is more often required for the evaluation of hypoproliferative anemia. After common abnormalities such as iron deficiency and other nutritional deficiencies have been ruled out, marrow aspiration and biopsy are indicated to search for abnormalities such as marrow infiltration, marrow involvement with granulomatous disease, marrow aplasia, or myelodysplasia.

The *mean corpuscular volume* (MCV) is an extremely helpful tool in the diagnosis of anemia with a low reticulocyte count (hypoproliferative

TABLE 3.1 Structure and Distribution of Human Hemoglobins

Name of Hemoglobin (Hb)	Distribution	Structure
A	95-98% of adult Hb	$\alpha_2\beta_2$
A_2	1.5-3.5% of adult Hb	$\alpha_2\delta_2$
F	Fetal, 0.5-1.0% of adult Hb	$\alpha_2\gamma_2$
Gower 1	Embryonic	$\zeta_2\varepsilon_2$
Gower 2	Embryonic	$\alpha_2\varepsilon_2$
Portland	Embryonic	$\zeta_2\gamma_2$

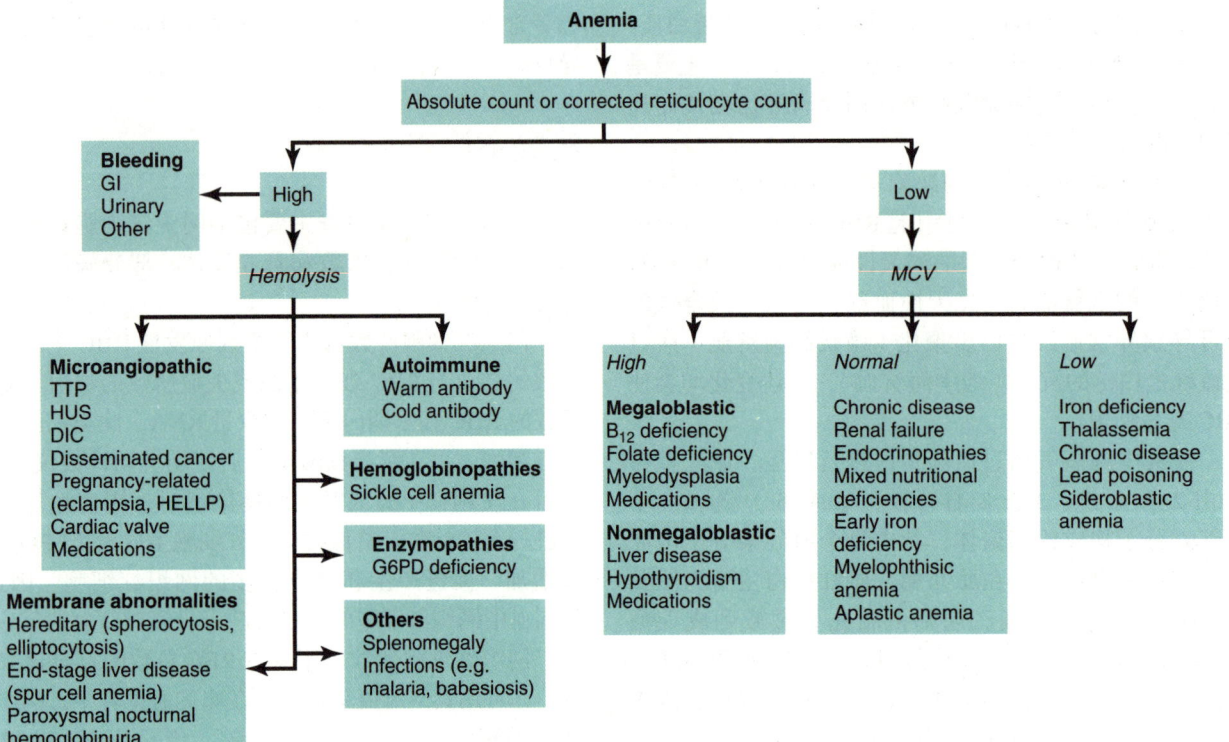

Fig. 3.1 Overview of the differential diagnosis of anemia. *DIC,* Disseminated intravascular coagulation; *G6PD,* glucose-6-phosphate dehydrogenase; *GI,* gastrointestinal; *HELLP,* hemolysis, elevated liver enzyme levels, and low platelet count; *HUS,* hemolytic-uremic syndrome; *MCV,* mean corpuscular volume; *TTP,* thrombotic thrombocytopenic purpura.

正的网织红细胞计数的计算方法是患者网织红细胞计数乘以患者血细胞比容与正常血细胞比容的比值。另一种计算方法为网织红细胞指数或网织红细胞生成指数（RPI），其可反映网织红细胞计数是否与贫血程度相符。RPI 通过患者血细胞比容与正常血细胞比容的比值乘以网织红细胞百分比，再除以患者网织红细胞成熟时间而计算得出，其同时校正了贫血程度和骨髓释放网织红细胞的状态。其中，成熟时间是指 RBC 成熟的时间（天）[范围从 1（血细胞比容 ≥ 40% 时）到 2.5（血细胞比容 < 20% 时）]。RPI > 3 时，认为骨髓对 RBC 破坏或出血等的反应适当；RPI < 2 时，认为骨髓反应不佳（如存在 RBC 生成障碍）。

外周血涂片可为贫血的病因诊断提供重要线索。

表 3.1 人血红蛋白的结构和分布

血红蛋白(Hb) 名称	分布	结构
A	占成人血红蛋白的 95%～98%	$\alpha_2\beta_2$
A_2	占成人血红蛋白的 1.5%～3.5%	$\alpha_2\delta_2$
F	胎儿，占成人血红蛋白的 0.5%～1.0%	$\alpha_2\gamma_2$
Gower 1	胚胎	$\zeta_2\varepsilon_2$
Gower 2	胚胎	$\alpha_2\varepsilon_2$
Portland	胚胎	$\zeta_2\gamma_2$

在伴有网织红细胞增多的贫血中，RBC 的形态学检查非常关键，其中血涂片对于鉴别免疫性溶血（可出现球形红细胞）和微血管病性溶血（可出现破碎红细胞）非常重要。其他与贫血病因相关的形态学改变包括镰状细胞和靶形红细胞（血红蛋白病的特征性改变），泪滴状细胞，有核红细胞（与骨髓纤维化和骨髓浸润、疟疾和巴贝虫病中的细胞内寄生虫有关），铅笔状改变（与严重缺铁相关）等。评估髓系细胞和血小板也有助于贫血的鉴别诊断。中性粒细胞分叶过多及大血小板支持巨幼细胞贫血的诊断，而原始细胞的出现则提示白血病。图 3.2 展示了贫血患者中常见的外周血涂片表现。

在伴有网织红细胞计数增多的贫血患者中，新的 RBC 大量生成提示骨髓造血功能正常，对贫血应激的反应适当。此种情况下很少需要进行骨髓穿刺检查，因为此时的骨髓穿刺结果可能仅表现为红系增生，通常不会发现源于骨髓的病变。此时评估的重点应集中于鉴别 RBC 消耗的原因是出血还是溶血。相比之下，低增生性贫血通常需行骨髓穿刺进行鉴别诊断。在排除贫血常见的原因（如铁缺乏和其他营养缺乏）后，骨髓穿刺及活检可为骨髓浸润、肉芽肿病累及骨髓、骨髓发育异常、骨髓增生异常等诊断提供依据。

平均红细胞体积（MCV）在诊断网织红细胞计数减低的贫血（低增生性贫血）中非常重要。根据 RBC

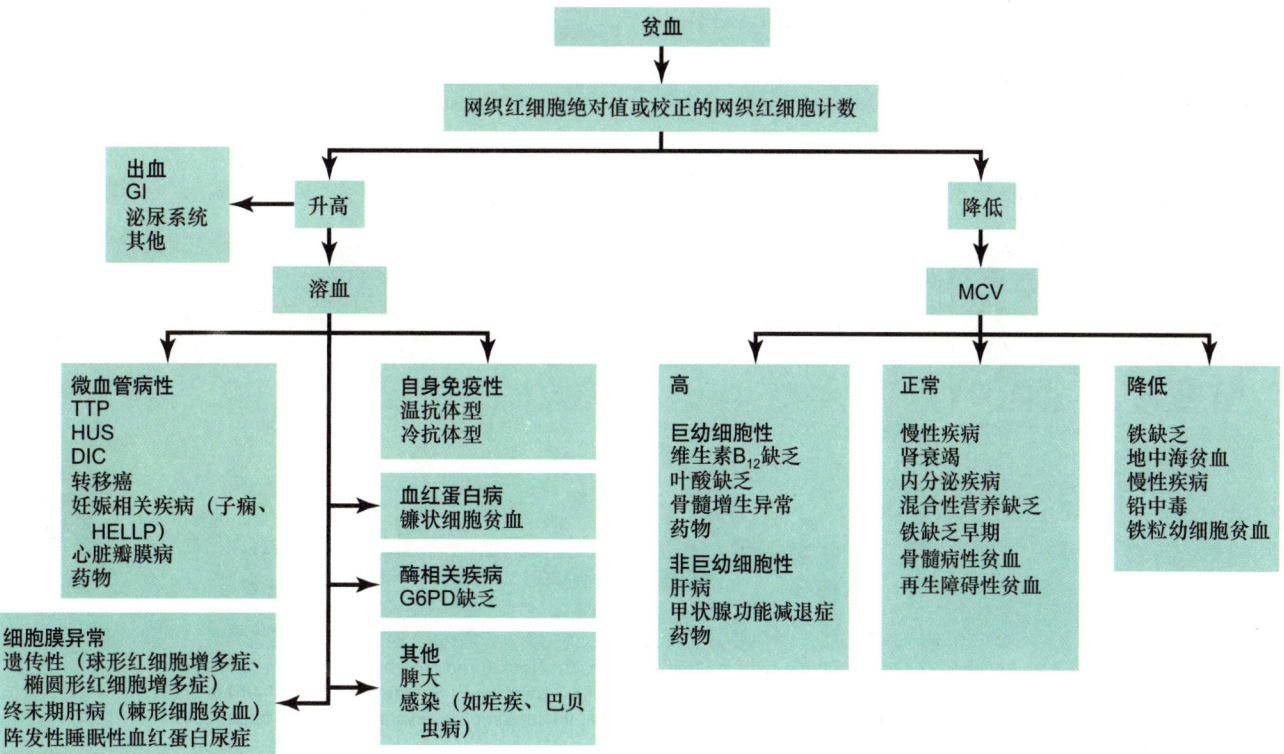

图 3.1　贫血的鉴别诊断。DIC，弥散性血管内凝血；G6PD，葡萄糖 -6- 磷酸脱氢酶；GI，胃肠道；HELLP，溶血、肝酶水平升高和血小板计数减低；HUS，溶血性尿毒综合征；MCV，平均红细胞体积；TTP，血栓性血小板减少性紫癜

anemia). The size of the RBCs (measured in femtoliters per cell) is used to characterize the anemia as microcytic (MCV <80), normocytic (MCV 80 to 96), or macrocytic (MCV >96).

EVALUATION OF HYPOPROLIFERATIVE ANEMIAS

Microcytic Anemias

The differential diagnosis of microcytic anemia is outlined in Table 3.2. Microcytosis and hypochromia are the hallmarks of anemias caused by defects in hemoglobin synthesis, which can reflect either failure of heme synthesis or abnormalities in globin production. The leading cause of microcytic anemia is iron deficiency, in which lack of heme synthesis results from the absence of iron to incorporate into the porphyrin ring (see later discussion). Up to 30% of patients with anemia of chronic inflammation have microcytosis. Lead poisoning blocks the incorporation of iron into heme, also resulting in a microcytic anemia.

Sideroblastic anemias arise from failure to synthesize the porphyrin ring, usually as a result of inhibition of the heme synthetic pathway enzymes. Congenital sideroblastic anemia may respond to pyridoxine, a cofactor for several of the heme synthetic pathway enzymes. A more common cause of acquired sideroblastic anemia is alcohol use; ethanol inhibits most of the enzymes in the heme synthetic pathway. Failure of globin synthesis occurs in thalassemic syndromes (see "Hemoglobinopathies"). All these disorders lead to decreased mean corpuscular hemoglobin concentration, resulting in hypochromia and a decrease in RBC size (i.e., low MCV).

Iron Deficiency Anemia

Iron deficiency is the leading cause of anemia worldwide. Although the presentation of classic iron deficiency anemia is linked with a microcytic anemia, early iron deficiency is associated with a normocytic anemia. Consequently, iron deficiency should be considered in all patients with anemia, and iron indices should be a part of the evaluation of any patient with hypoproductive anemia, regardless of the MCV.

Iron is acquired in the diet from heme sources (i.e., meat) and from nonheme sources (e.g., vegetables such as spinach). Iron from heme is better absorbed than nonheme iron. Iron absorption is increased in iron deficiency, hypoxia, ineffective erythropoiesis, and hereditary hemochromatosis (most commonly caused by mutations in the *HFE* gene). Iron is absorbed from the proximal small intestine; it is transported in the cell bound to ferroportin and through the plasma bound to transferrin. Its uptake into the RBC precursors is mediated through the transferrin receptor. Iron absorption from the intestine is further regulated by hepcidin (see "Anemia of Inflammation"). Iron outside hemoglobin-producing cells is stored in ferritin. Men and women have

TABLE 3.2 Differential Diagnosis of Anemia With Low Reticulocyte Count

Microcytic Anemia (MCV <80 fL/cell)
Iron deficiency
Thalassemia minor
Anemia of chronic inflammation
Sideroblastic anemia
Lead poisoning

Macrocytic Anemia (MCV >100 fL/cell)
Megaloblastic anemias
Folate deficiency
Vitamin B_{12} deficiency
Drug-induced megaloblastic anemia
Myelodysplasia
Nonmegaloblastic macrocytosis
Liver disease
Hypothyroidism
Reticulocytosis

Normocytic Anemia (MCV 80-100 fL/cell)
Early iron deficiency
Aplastic anemia
Myelophthisic disorders
Endocrinopathies
Anemia of chronic inflammation
Anemia of renal failure
Mixed nutritional deficiency

MCV, Mean corpuscular volume.

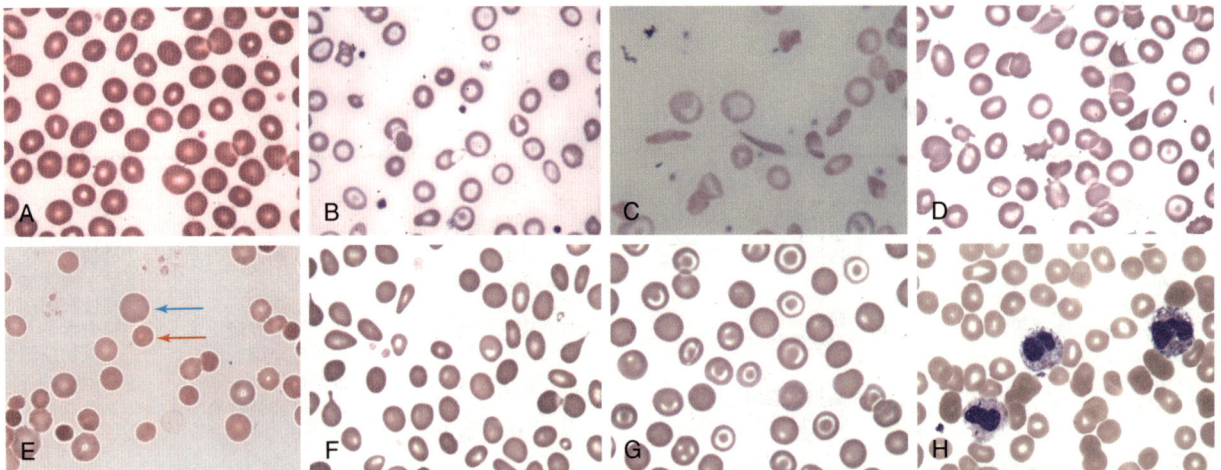

Fig. 3.2 Peripheral blood smears in patients with anemia. (A) Normal red blood cells. (B) Iron deficiency anemia. (C) Sickle cell anemia. (D) Microangiopathic hemolytic anemia. (E) Spherocytosis *(blue arrow)* and reticulocytosis *(red arrow)* in autoimmune hemolytic anemia. (F) Teardrops in myelofibrosis. (G) Target cells. (H) Pseudo-Pelger-Huet anomaly in myelodysplasia.

的大小（以 fl 为单位）可将贫血分为小细胞性（MCV < 80 fl）、正细胞性（MCV 80～96 fl）及大细胞性（MCV > 96 fl）。

低增生性贫血的评估

小细胞性贫血

小细胞性贫血的鉴别诊断见表 3.2。小细胞和低色素表明贫血由血红蛋白合成不足引起，反映了血红素合成或珠蛋白生成异常。小细胞性贫血的主要原因是铁缺乏，在缺铁性贫血中，铁含量不足导致无法与卟啉环结合而生成血红素（见下文）。高达 30% 的慢性炎症性贫血呈小细胞性。铅中毒可阻碍铁参与形成血红素，也可引起小细胞性贫血。

铁粒幼细胞贫血源自卟啉环合成障碍，通常由血红素合成通路中的酶受到抑制所致。吡哆醇是血红素合成通路中多种酶的辅因子，可能对先天性铁粒幼细胞贫血有效。乙醇可抑制血红素合成通路中的大多数酶，故酒精使用是获得性铁粒幼细胞贫血的常见原因。珠蛋白合成障碍常见于地中海贫血（见下文"血红蛋白病"）。上述疾病均可引起平均红细胞血红蛋白浓度降低，导致低色素及 RBC 体积减小（即低 MCV）。

缺铁性贫血

铁缺乏是全球范围内贫血的首要病因。尽管典型缺铁性贫血表现为小细胞性贫血，但在疾病早期常表现为正细胞性贫血。因此，所有贫血患者均应考虑缺铁因素，无论 MCV 正常与否，铁相关检验均应作为低增生性贫血患者的常规检查。

铁主要来源于饮食，包括血红素来源（如肉类）和非血红素来源（如菠菜等蔬菜类）。血红素来源的铁较非血红素来源的铁更易吸收。在铁缺乏、缺氧、无效红细胞生成和遗传性血色病（通常由 *HFE* 基因突变引起）等情况下，铁吸收增加。铁由近端小肠吸收，通过膜铁转运蛋白进入细胞，在血浆中与转铁蛋白结合进行输送，再通过转铁蛋白受体介导进入前体 RBC。铁经肠道吸收的过程由铁调素进一步调节（见下文"炎症性贫血"）。RBC 外的铁储存于铁蛋白中。男性

表 3.2　伴有网织红细胞计数减低的贫血的鉴别诊断

小细胞性贫血（MCV < 80 fl）
缺铁性贫血
轻型地中海贫血
慢性炎症性贫血
铁粒幼细胞贫血
铅中毒

大细胞性贫血（MCV > 100 fl）
巨幼细胞贫血
叶酸缺乏
维生素 B_{12} 缺乏
药物诱发的巨幼细胞贫血
骨髓增生异常
非巨幼细胞性巨红细胞症
肝病
甲状腺功能减退症
网织红细胞增多症

正细胞性贫血（MCV 80～100 fl）
缺铁性贫血早期
再生障碍性贫血
骨髓病性贫血
内分泌疾病
慢性炎症性贫血
肾衰竭所致的贫血
混合性营养缺乏

MCV，平均红细胞体积。

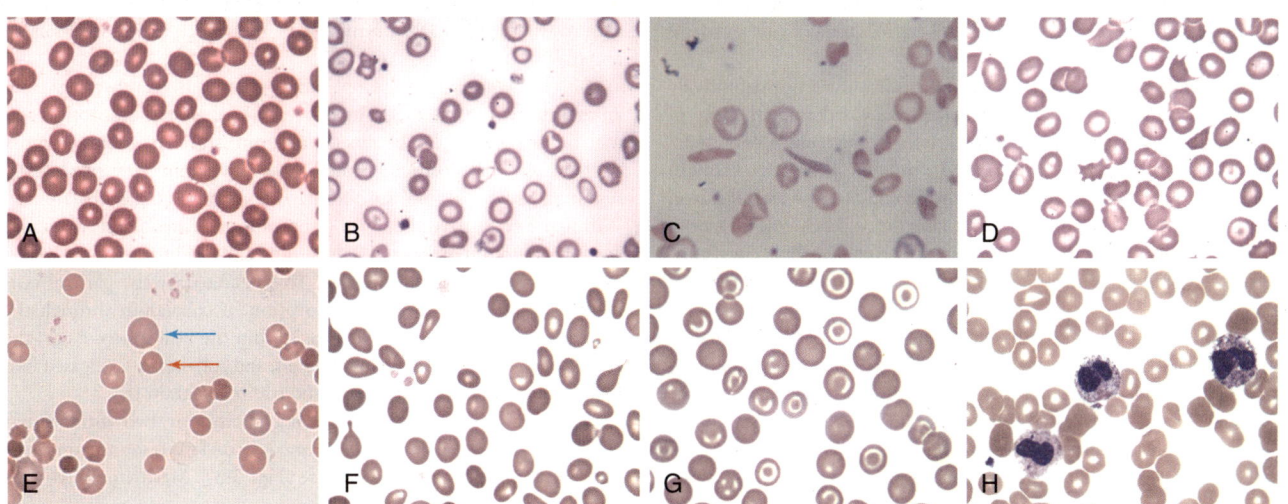

图 3.2　贫血患者的外周血涂片。**A**. 正常红细胞。**B**. 缺铁性贫血。**C**. 镰状细胞贫血。**D**. 微血管病性溶血性贫血。**E**. 自身免疫性溶血性贫血中的球形红细胞（蓝色箭头）和网织红细胞（红色箭头）。**F**. 骨髓纤维化中的泪滴状细胞。**G**. 靶形红细胞。**H**. 骨髓增生异常综合征中的假性 Pelger-Huët 畸形

total-body iron concentrations of 50 mg/kg and 40 mg/kg, respectively. Between 60% and 75% of the iron is found in hemoglobin. A small amount (2 mg/kg) is found in heme and nonheme enzymes, and 5 mg/kg is found in myoglobin. The remainder is stored in ferritin, which resides primarily in liver, bone marrow, spleen, and muscle. The capacity for excreting iron is limited, and iron overload occurs in patients with excessive absorption from the gastrointestinal tract (as a result of ineffective erythropoiesis or congenital hemochromatosis) and in those receiving chronic transfusions. Iron overload leads to increased iron deposition in these tissues and secondary deposition in endocrine and other organs, resulting in liver dysfunction, heart failure, diabetes, and other endocrine abnormalities.

The most frequent cause of iron deficiency is occult blood loss. All men and postmenopausal women who are found to be iron deficient should have an evaluation for a source of gastrointestinal blood loss and malignancy, regardless of the detection of occult blood. In premenopausal women, iron deficiency is most frequently related to loss of iron with menstruation (about 15 mg per month) and during pregnancy (about 900 mg per pregnancy). *Helicobacter pylori* infection can cause iron deficiency even in the absence of intestinal bleeding. Dietary deficiency of iron is most commonly seen in multiparous women of childbearing age, in young children whose growth outstrips their intake of iron, and in babies who drink mostly milk at the expense of an intake of iron-containing foods.

Laboratory evaluation. As previously stated, early iron deficiency does not exhibit the hallmark microcytosis and hypochromia that characterize classic iron deficiency. Evaluation of the blood smear in advanced iron deficiency often demonstrates hypochromic RBCs, target cells, and pencil-shaped elongated cells. Iron deficiency is frequently associated with reactive thrombocytosis.

The mainstay of the diagnosis of iron deficiency is the peripheral blood iron indices. These include iron concentration, total iron-binding capacity (TIBC), transferrin saturation, and ferritin concentration. The transferrin saturation is the ratio of serum iron to transferrin concentration; it is normally at least 20%. Iron deficiency results in a decrease in serum iron and an increase in iron-binding capacity, decreasing this ratio to less than 10%. Chronic inflammatory conditions (e.g., infection, inflammation, malignancy) often decrease both iron and TIBC, but the transferrin saturation usually remains above 20%. The ferritin level is a reflection of total-body iron stores. The liver synthesizes ferritin in proportion to total-body iron, and a level of less than 12 ng/mL strongly supports a diagnosis of iron deficiency. Unfortunately, ferritin is an acute phase reactant, and levels rise in the setting of fever, inflammatory disease, infection, or other stresses. However, ferritin levels in response to stress do not often rise above 100 ng/mL, and levels higher than 100 ng/mL usually rule out iron deficiency.

If the indirect measurement of iron indices does not definitively confirm or refute a diagnosis of iron deficiency, a therapeutic trial of iron supplementation may be considered. Alternatively, a bone marrow examination can be performed to provide a direct assessment of marrow iron stores. Presence of iron in the marrow excludes iron deficiency anemia because marrow iron stores will be depleted before there is any fall in RBC production resulting from iron deficiency; conversely, complete absence of marrow iron confirms the diagnosis of iron deficiency.

Treatment. Oral iron supplementation (e.g., ferrous sulfate or ferrous gluconate two or three times daily) has been the standard treatment for uncomplicated iron deficiency, but patient compliance is often limited by gastrointestinal side effects, notably dose-dependent constipation or diarrhea. However, emerging data suggest that standard iron dosing may be counterproductive. A recent study demonstrated that a large oral dose of iron stimulates an increase in hepcidin (regulator of iron balance), which in turn suppresses further iron absorption up to 48 hours later, supporting an every-other-day dosing strategy. In iron-deficient women without anemia, cumulative iron absorption was superior in those receiving an alternate-day dosing over daily dosing and better tolerated. Larger prospective studies in patients with iron deficiency anemia are needed to confirm these findings. Overall, iron should be administered for several months after resolution of anemia to allow for the reconstitution of iron stores.

In patients with malabsorption, a complete inability to tolerate oral iron, or iron demands that outstrip replacement with oral supplements, parenteral iron may be administered. Historically, intravenous iron, specifically high-molecular-weight iron dextran, has been associated with anaphylaxis and was subsequently removed from markets globally. The newer parenteral iron formulations are safe and effective, including low-molecular-weight iron dextran, ferric gluconate, iron sucrose, ferumoxytol, iron isomaltoside, and ferric carboxymaltose. As previously stated, all male patients and postmenopausal women with iron deficiency require evaluation for a source of gastrointestinal bleeding.

Macrocytic Anemias

Two categories of hypoproductive macrocytic anemias exist: megaloblastic anemias and nonmegaloblastic macrocytic anemias. Megaloblastic anemias arise from a failure of DNA synthesis and result in lack of synchrony between the maturation of the nucleus and the cytoplasm of hematopoietic cells. Nonmegaloblastic macrocytic anemias usually reflect membrane abnormalities resulting from defects in cholesterol metabolism and are most commonly found in patients with advanced liver disease or severe hypothyroidism. Reticulocytosis greater than 10% causes an elevated MCV on automated blood counts because reticulocytes are larger than mature RBCs.

Megaloblastic Anemias

Megaloblastic anemias result from a block in the synthesis of critical nucleotide precursors of DNA, which leads to a cell cycle arrest in S phase. Cytoplasmic maturation occurs, but maturation of the nucleus is arrested. Cells take on a bizarre appearance, with large immature nuclei surrounded by more mature-appearing cytoplasm. Interference with DNA synthesis affects all rapidly dividing cells, so patients with megaloblastic syndromes often have pancytopenia and gastrointestinal symptoms such as diarrhea and malabsorption. In women, megaloblastic changes of the cervical mucosa occur and may cause abnormal results on Papanicolaou smears. The most common causes of megaloblastic anemia are deficiencies of vitamin B_{12} or folate, medications that inhibit DNA synthesis or that block folate metabolism, and myelodysplasia.

Cobalamin deficiency. Cobalamin (vitamin B_{12}) is absorbed from animal protein in the diet. The process of cobalamin absorption and metabolism is complex because cobalamin is always bound to other proteins. In the stomach, protein-bound vitamins are released by digestion with pepsin and are bound to haptocorrin (transcobalamin I). Within the proximal duodenum, pancreatic proteases digest cobalamin away from haptocorrin, and cobalamin binds to intrinsic factor (IF), also known as transcobalamin III. IF is secreted by the parietal cells of the stomach and mediates absorption of cobalamin through the cubam receptor in the distal ileum. Within the ileal mucosal cell, the IF-cobalamin complex is again digested, and cobalamin is released into the plasma bound to haptocorrin and transcobalamin II.

Within the cell, cobalamin is a cofactor for two intracellular enzymes, L-methylmalonyl–coenzyme A (CoA) mutase and homocysteine-methionine methyltransferase (Fig. 3.3). Methylmalonyl-CoA

和女性体内的总铁浓度分别为 50 mg/kg 和 40 mg/kg。其中，60%～75% 的铁存在于血红蛋白中，少量（2 mg/kg）存在于血红素及非血红素酶中，5 mg/kg 存在于肌红蛋白中。剩余部分储存在铁蛋白中，其主要分布于肝、骨髓、脾和肌肉。人体排出铁的能力是有限的，胃肠道吸收铁过多（红系无效造血或遗传性血色病）或慢性输血的患者常存在铁过载。铁过载可导致组织中铁沉积增加，继发内分泌器官及其他脏器中的次生沉积，导致肝功能异常、心力衰竭、糖尿病及其他内分泌功能异常。

铁缺乏的最常见原因是隐性失血。所有存在铁缺乏的男性及绝经后女性均应评估是否存在胃肠道失血和恶性疾病，无论粪便潜血是否呈阳性。在绝经前女性中，铁缺乏常与月经（每月约丢失 15 mg）和妊娠期（每次约丢失 900 mg）铁丢失相关。即使没有胃肠道出血，幽门螺杆菌感染也可能引起铁缺乏。膳食原因导致的铁缺乏常见于育龄期多胎孕产的女性、生长期铁摄入相对不足的儿童，以及以牛奶为主要食物、较少摄取其他含铁辅食的婴儿。

实验室检查 如前所述，铁缺乏早期可能并无小细胞、低色素等缺铁性贫血的典型表现。严重铁缺乏患者血涂片中常可见红细胞淡染、靶形红细胞和铅笔状长细胞。铁缺乏还常引起反应性血小板增多。

诊断缺铁性贫血的关键指标是外周血的铁相关指标，包括铁浓度、总铁结合力（TIBC）、转铁蛋白饱和度及铁蛋白浓度。转铁蛋白饱和度是血清铁与转铁蛋白浓度的比值，正常情况下不低于 20%。铁缺乏可导致血清铁减少及铁结合力增加，使该比值降至 10% 以下。在慢性炎症情况下（如感染、炎症、恶性肿瘤），血清铁和 TIBC 同时降低，但转铁蛋白饱和度通常保持在 20% 以上。铁蛋白水平反映了体内贮存的总铁含量。肝合成的铁蛋白总量与总铁含量成正比，铁蛋白 < 12 ng/ml 是缺铁性贫血的有力证据。然而，铁蛋白同时也是一种急性时相反应蛋白，在发热、炎症性疾病、感染或其他应激反应中水平也可升高。但是，应激反应时通常铁蛋白 ≤ 100 ng/ml，且铁蛋白 > 100 ng/ml 时通常可排除铁缺乏。

如果铁相关指标测定未能确诊铁缺乏，则可考虑试验性补铁治疗。此外，亦可行骨髓穿刺以直接检测骨髓中的铁含量。缺铁性贫血时，在出现 RBC 生成减少之前，骨髓中的铁即已耗竭，故骨髓中检测到铁即可排除缺铁性贫血；反之，骨髓中未检测到铁，则支持缺铁性贫血的诊断。

治疗 口服补充铁剂（如硫酸亚铁或葡萄糖酸亚铁，2～3 次 / 日）是单纯铁缺乏的标准治疗，但常因胃肠道副作用（尤其是与剂量相关的便秘或腹泻）而影响患者的用药依从性。然而，越来越多的证据表明，铁剂的标准剂量可能存在争议。近期研究发现，单次口服大剂量铁剂可刺激铁调素（铁代谢平衡的调节分子）分泌增加，在长达 48 h 内可反射性抑制铁吸收，提示隔日口服的用药方式可能更为合理。在存在铁缺乏但尚未出现贫血表现的女性患者中，隔日用药较每日用药者表现出更高的吸收效率和更好的耐受性。未来尚需大规模前瞻性研究以进一步证实上述发现。总体上，铁剂应坚持应用至贫血纠正后数月，以便补足体内的贮存铁。

对于铁吸收不良、口服铁剂完全不耐受和口服铁剂无法满足需求量的患者，可给予肠外补铁治疗。既往应用的静脉注射铁剂（特别是高分子量右旋糖酐铁）常引起过敏反应，随后已撤出全球市场。较新的静脉制剂（如低分子量右旋糖酐铁、葡萄糖醛酸铁、蔗糖铁、异麦芽糖苷铁和羧甲基麦芽糖铁）更为安全有效。如前所述，所有存在铁缺乏的男性患者及绝经后女性患者均要求评估是否存在胃肠道出血。

大细胞性贫血

低增生性大细胞性贫血共分为两类：巨幼细胞贫血和非巨幼细胞性大细胞性贫血。巨幼细胞贫血由造血细胞不能合成 DNA 导致核-质发育不平衡所致。非巨幼细胞性大细胞性贫血通常反映了因胆固醇代谢缺陷引起的细胞膜异常，常见于晚期肝病或严重甲状腺功能减退症患者。此外，由于网织红细胞的体积较成熟 RBC 大，因此在使用自动血细胞分析仪测定时，网织红细胞计数 > 10% 也可引起 MCV 升高。

巨幼细胞贫血

巨幼细胞贫血是由于某些关键核苷酸前体合成中断，干扰 DNA 形成，导致细胞周期停滞于 S 期。RBC 的胞质发育成熟，而细胞核的发育则停滞。巨幼细胞形态特异，表现为相对成熟的胞质环绕着体积偏大的未成熟细胞核。DNA 合成障碍可影响所有处于快速分裂期的细胞，因此巨幼细胞贫血患者常出现全血细胞减少和胃肠道症状，如腹泻和消化不良。在女性中，可出现宫颈黏膜细胞的巨幼样变，导致宫颈涂片结果异常。巨幼细胞贫血最常见的病因包括维生素 B_{12} 或叶酸缺乏、应用抑制 DNA 合成或阻断叶酸代谢的药物及骨髓增生异常。

维生素 B_{12} 缺乏 维生素 B_{12}（钴胺素）来源于膳食中的动物蛋白。维生素 B_{12} 通常与其他蛋白结合，其吸收和代谢的过程非常复杂。在胃中，经过胃蛋白酶的酶解，维生素 B_{12} 与蛋白质解离，继而与钴胺素转运蛋白 I 结合。在近端十二指肠，胰蛋白酶使维生素 B_{12} 与钴胺素转运蛋白 I 解离，并与内因子（IF；又称钴胺素转运蛋白 III）结合。IF 由胃壁细胞分泌，通过回肠末端的 cubam 受体介导维生素 B_{12} 的吸收。在回肠黏膜细胞内，IF-维生素 B_{12} 复合物被再次酶解，维生素 B_{12} 与钴胺素转运蛋白 I 及钴胺素转运蛋白 II 结合，并释放入血浆。

在细胞内，维生素 B_{12} 是两种细胞内酶［即 L-甲基丙二酰辅酶 A（CoA）变位酶和同型半胱氨酸-甲硫氨酸甲基转移酶］的辅因子（图 3.3）。甲基丙二酰

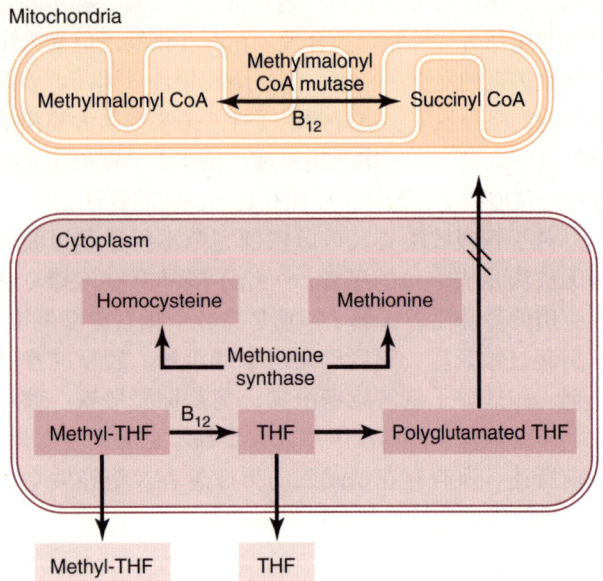

Fig. 3.3 Metabolic pathways of folic acid and cobalamin. *CoA*, Coenzyme A; *THF*, tetrahydrofolate.

TABLE 3.3 Causes of Cobalamin Deficiency

Malabsorption of vitamin B_{12}
Pernicious anemia
Partial or total gastrectomy
Pancreatic insufficiency
Bacterial overgrowth
Diseases of the terminal ileum
Tapeworm infection
Nutritional (vegans)
Congenital deficiency of intrinsic factor or haptocorrin

TABLE 3.4 Causes of Folate Deficiency

Dietary Insufficiency
Increased Folate Requirements
Pregnancy
Lactation
Hemolysis
Exfoliative dermatitis
Malignancy

Malabsorption
Sprue
Crohn's disease
Short bowel syndrome

Antifolate Medications
Chemotherapy agents (e.g., methotrexate, pemetrexed)
Sulfa drugs

---

mutase is a mitochondrial enzyme that functions in the citric acid cycle to convert methylmalonyl-CoA to succinyl-CoA. The cytoplasmic enzyme homocysteine-methionine methyltransferase is necessary for the transfer of methyl groups from *N*-methyltetrahydrofolate to homocysteine to form methionine. Demethylated tetrahydrofolate is necessary as a carbon donor in the conversion of deoxyuridine to deoxythymidine. Absence of cobalamin results in a *trapping* of tetrahydrofolate in its methylated form, which blocks the synthesis of thymidine 5′-triphosphate for incorporation into DNA. The megaloblastic changes induced by cobalamin deficiency are mediated through this functional folate deficiency, which explains the similarity in the hematologic abnormalities induced by cobalamin and folate deficiency.

Causes of cobalamin deficiency. The most common cause of cobalamin deficiency is pernicious anemia, an autoimmune disease associated with gastric parietal cell atrophy, defective gastric acid secretion, and absence of IF. Anti–parietal cell and anti-IF antibodies are frequently found in patients with pernicious anemia and other autoimmune conditions such as type 1 diabetes, vitiligo, Graves' disease, Addison's disease, and hypoparathyroidism. Many other lesions in the gastrointestinal tract can interfere with absorption of cobalamin (Table 3.3). Gastrectomy causes loss of parietal cell function and IF secretion. Pancreatic insufficiency interferes with digestion of the haptocorrin-cobalamin complex, thus hindering the binding of cobalamin to IF and ileal absorption. Resection of the terminal ileum prevents vitamin B_{12} absorption, as do diseases that affect ileal mucosal function, such as Crohn's disease, sprue, intestinal tuberculosis, and lymphoma. Because the body stores of cobalamin are large and daily loss of cobalamin is low, the stores of cobalamin are adequate for 3 to 4 years if intake stops abruptly; signs of cobalamin deficiency do not develop until defective absorption has occurred for several years. Nutritional cobalamin deficiency is rare and is seen only in individuals who have been on strict vegan diets that exclude all animal products for many years. Infants born to vegan mothers who are breastfed are also at risk for development of cobalamin deficiency.

Folate deficiency. Folate is widely present in foods such as leafy vegetables, fruits, and animal protein. However, because it is destroyed by prolonged cooking, fresh fruits and vegetables are the most reliable sources of folate. Consequently, nutritional folate deficiency is common in malnourished individuals who eat very little fresh fruits and vegetables. Folate deficiency can also be caused by increased demand, as occurs with pregnancy, hemolysis, or exfoliative dermatitis, and by increased losses, which occur with dialysis (Table 3.4). Folate is absorbed in the proximal small intestine, and malabsorption of folate can also lead to folate deficiency.

Other causes of megaloblastic anemia. Drugs and toxins are common causes of megaloblastic anemia. Some drugs, such as methotrexate and sulfa drugs, act as direct folate antagonists and mimic folate deficiency. Purine and pyrimidine analogue chemotherapeutic agents (e.g., azathioprine, 5-fluorouracil) are direct DNA-synthesis inhibitors. Antiviral agents cause megaloblastic changes by unclear mechanisms. Alcohol interferes with folate metabolism, increasing the effect of frequent concomitant nutritional folate deficiency. Myelodysplastic syndrome commonly appears as a macrocytic anemia, with megaloblastic changes primarily in the erythroid series.

Clinical manifestations of megaloblastic anemia. The development of megaloblastic anemia is usually gradual, allowing adequate time for concomitant plasma expansion to prevent hypovolemia. Consequently, patients are frequently severely anemic at presentation. They may have yellowish skin as the result of a combination of pallor from reduced red cell mass and jaundice from ineffective erythropoiesis and intramedullary hemolysis. Some patients have glossitis and cheilosis. With severe anemia, patients usually have an MCV greater than 110 fL/cell, although concomitant iron deficiency, caused by malabsorption secondary to megaloblastic

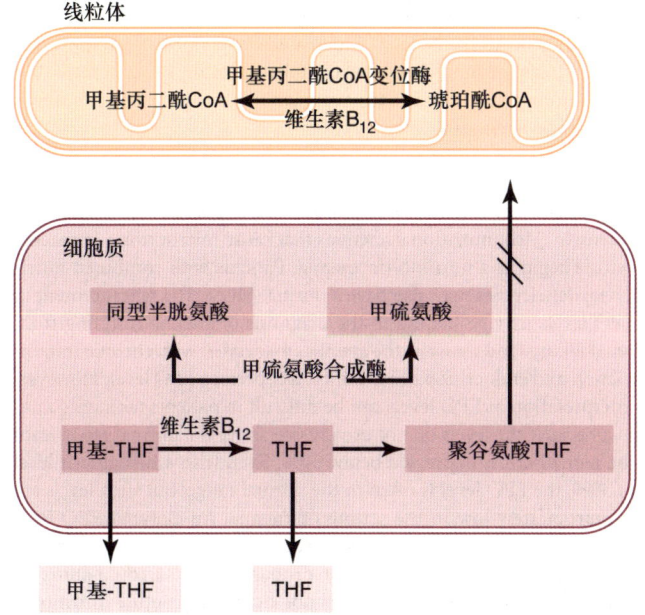

图 3.3 叶酸和钴胺素（维生素 B_{12}）的代谢途径。CoA，辅酶 A；THF，四氢叶酸

表 3.3　维生素 B_{12} 缺乏的原因
维生素 B_{12} 吸收不良
恶性贫血
部分或全胃切除术
胰腺功能不全
细菌过度生长
末端回肠疾病
绦虫感染
营养不良（素食者）
先天性内因子或钴胺素转运蛋白 I 缺乏

CoA 变位酶是一种线粒体酶，在柠檬酸循环中可将甲基丙二酰 CoA 转化为琥珀酰 CoA。同型半胱氨酸-甲硫氨酸甲基转移酶是一种胞质酶，可将甲基从 N-甲基四氢叶酸转移至同型半胱氨酸，以形成甲硫氨酸。去甲基四氢叶酸是脱氧尿嘧啶向脱氧胸腺嘧啶转化过程中必要的一碳单位供体。维生素 B_{12} 缺乏使四氢叶酸持续甲基化，继而阻止胸苷 5′-三磷酸的生成，使其无法参与 DNA 合成。因此，维生素 B_{12} 缺乏引起的巨幼样改变实际上是通过功能性叶酸缺乏来介导的，这也正是维生素 B_{12} 缺乏与叶酸缺乏所导致的血液学异常非常相似的原因。

维生素 B_{12} 缺乏的原因　维生素 B_{12} 缺乏最常见的原因是恶性贫血，恶性贫血是一种自身免疫病，表现为胃壁细胞萎缩、胃酸分泌缺陷和 IF 缺乏。抗胃壁细胞及抗 IF 抗体常见于恶性贫血和其他自身免疫病（如 1 型糖尿病、白癜风、Graves 病、Addison 病和甲状旁腺功能减退症）患者。其他胃肠疾病也可干扰维生素 B_{12} 的吸收（表 3.3）。胃切除术可导致胃壁细胞功能障碍和 IF 分泌缺陷。胰腺功能不全可干扰钴胺素转运蛋

表 3.4　叶酸缺乏的原因
膳食摄入不足
叶酸需求增加
妊娠
哺乳
溶血
剥脱性皮炎
恶性肿瘤
吸收不良
口炎性腹泻
克罗恩病
短肠综合征
抗叶酸药物
化疗药物（如甲氨蝶呤、培美曲塞）
磺胺类药物

白 I-维生素 B_{12} 复合物的解离，阻碍维生素 B_{12} 与 IF 结合及在回肠部位的吸收。末端回肠切除术和其他累及回肠黏膜的疾病（包括克罗恩病、口炎性腹泻、肠结核、淋巴瘤等）均会阻碍维生素 B_{12} 的吸收。维生素 B_{12} 体内贮存量较大，且日常消耗较少，因而在禁食情况下，体内的维生素 B_{12} 贮存量可维持 3～4 年，直到吸收障碍存在数年后才会出现相应症状。膳食性维生素 B_{12} 缺乏症非常罕见，仅见于长期严格素食者。若母亲为素食者，其婴儿在母乳喂养的情况下也可能发生维生素 B_{12} 缺乏。

叶酸缺乏　叶酸广泛存在于绿叶蔬菜、水果和动物蛋白中。但是，由于长时间烹饪会破坏叶酸，故新鲜水果和蔬菜是叶酸最主要的来源。因此，膳食叶酸缺乏常见于摄入新鲜蔬果较少的个体。在妊娠、溶血、剥脱性皮炎等情况下，叶酸的需求增加；血液透析时叶酸丢失增加，也是导致叶酸缺乏的原因（表 3.4）。叶酸在近端小肠吸收，吸收障碍也可导致叶酸缺乏。

巨幼细胞贫血的其他病因　药物及毒物也是巨幼细胞贫血的常见原因。某些药物（如甲氨蝶呤和磺胺类药物）作为直接针对叶酸的拮抗剂可引起类似叶酸缺乏的症状。嘌呤和嘧啶类似物（如硫唑嘌呤、5-氟尿嘧啶）可直接抑制 DNA 合成。抗病毒药物也可引起细胞巨幼样变，其机制不明。酒精可干扰叶酸代谢，加重其使用者经常合并的膳食性叶酸缺乏的表现。骨髓增生异常综合征通常表现为巨幼细胞贫血，其巨幼样变以红系为主。

巨幼细胞贫血的临床表现　巨幼细胞贫血通常呈慢性病程，在此期间血浆已充分代偿，从而不会表现为低血容量。因此，患者在就诊时通常已发生重度贫血。由于贫血引发的苍白及无效造血和骨髓内原位溶血导致的黄疸，患者面色可呈黄白色。部分患者会出现舌炎和唇炎。重度贫血患者通常 MCV ＞ 110 fl，但同期存在的铁缺乏（继发于胃肠道细胞巨幼样变引起的铁吸收障碍）可能使巨幼细胞的体积减小。患者常

changes in the intestinal tract, may decrease the macrocytosis. Patients frequently have pancytopenia.

A peripheral blood smear demonstrates large, oval cells (macro-ovalocytes), hypersegmented neutrophils, and large platelets. The bone marrow is hypercellular, with megaloblastic changes and abnormally large erythroid series precursors. In addition, intramedullary destruction of erythrocytes (ineffective hematopoiesis) causes elevated concentrations of bilirubin (hence the jaundice described earlier) and lactate dehydrogenase.

Cobalamin deficiency is associated with neurologic abnormalities that are not seen with other causes of megaloblastic anemia. The neurologic signs may range widely, from a subtle loss of vibratory sensation and position sense caused by demyelination of the dorsal columns to frank dementia and neuropsychiatric disease. The neurologic changes may be present without anemia, especially if a patient with cobalamin deficiency is treated with folate, which may correct the hematologic manifestations of megaloblastic anemia but does not treat the neurologic abnormalities. The neurologic manifestations of cobalamin deficiency are thought to be secondary to loss of function of the mitochondrial enzyme methylmalonyl-CoA mutase. One proposed explanation is that the failure to metabolize odd-chain fatty acids, which results in their improper incorporation into myelin, causes the neurologic dysfunction. This explains why these findings are uniquely seen in patients with cobalamin deficiency and are not seen in those with the megaloblastic anemias caused by abnormalities in the folate pathway.

Serum levels of both cobalamin and folate should be measured in patients with megaloblastic anemia because megaloblastic changes in the gut mucosa can cause concomitant malabsorption of folate in the presence of cobalamin deficiency and vice versa. RBC folate levels better reflect the body folate stores and should be measured if a deficiency is clinically suggested but the serum folate levels are normal. Recent studies have shown, however, that many patients with pernicious anemia may have normal serum cobalamin levels. Homocysteine levels are elevated in cobalamin and folate deficiency, and methylmalonic acid levels are elevated in cobalamin deficiency. These levels should be measured if cobalamin deficiency is suggested but serum cobalamin levels are in the normal range. Anti-IF and anti–parietal cell antibodies may help determine the cause of cobalamin deficiency.

Treatment of megaloblastic anemia. For patients with cobalamin deficiency, both high-dose oral and parenteral cobalamin administration have been shown to be effective. The oral dose should be at least 1000 µg daily. Patients with neurologic abnormalities or medication noncompliance and those who have not responded to oral therapy should receive parenteral therapy with 1000 µg subcutaneously or intramuscularly several times per week for four to eight doses. Maintenance therapy should then be instituted with 1000 µg parenterally monthly. Therapy with cobalamin should be accompanied by folate therapy because concomitant secondary folate deficiency may develop when RBC production increases with the availability of cobalamin. Treatment of pernicious anemia should be continued for life.

Patients with folate deficiency should receive replacement with 1 to 5 mg per day of oral folate. As previously stated, it is critical to be certain that patients are not cobalamin deficient: Replacement of folate may correct the hematologic parameters in patients with cobalamin deficiency, but it will not improve the neurologic sequelae.

After treatment of megaloblastic anemia, a rapid response usually occurs. Reticulocytosis is seen as early as 2 days after therapy and peaks within 7 to 10 days. Despite rapid resolution of neutropenia, hypersegmentation of neutrophils may persist for several days. During this period, rapid cellular proliferation and turnover occur, which may precipitate hypokalemia, hyperuricemia, or hypophosphatemia. Patients should also be monitored for the development of iron deficiency, which may occur in the face of increased hematopoiesis. Anemia and other cytopenias should respond completely within 1 to 2 months, but the neurologic manifestations of cobalamin deficiency improve slowly and may be irreversible.

Normocytic Anemias

The differential diagnosis of a normocytic hypoproductive anemia is extensive. Most nutritional anemias that cause microcytosis or macrocytosis begin as a normocytic anemia. Patients with combined nutritional deficiencies may also have a normal MCV. The measurement of EPO levels may be helpful in the diagnosis of anemia resulting from renal failure, and many of the anemias associated with chronic inflammation and endocrinopathies exhibit a depressed EPO level. However, interpretation of EPO levels can be difficult in patients with mild anemia because the levels do not usually rise above the normal range until the hematocrit is depressed below 30%. Even with a hematocrit level of 30%, the EPO level is often in the normal range, but such levels are inappropriately low in the setting of anemia. An elevated EPO level suggests an inadequate marrow response to anemia and increases the likelihood of myelophthisis or primary bone marrow failure. In patients for whom the diagnosis is not clear after routine nutritional and endocrine studies, a bone marrow examination is indicated to rule out primary pathologic conditions of the marrow.

Anemia of Inflammation

The anemia of inflammation (previously called anemia of chronic disease) occurs in patients with chronic inflammatory, infectious, malignant, or autoimmune disorders. Patients have low-serum iron levels, but in contrast to the iron indices in iron deficiency anemia, the iron-binding capacity is also reduced, and the transferrin saturation is usually greater than 10%. Ferritin levels are often elevated, both as an acute phase reactant and as a reflection of decreased iron incorporation. These patients have inappropriately high levels of hepcidin, an acute phase reactant that facilitates the metabolism of ferroportin and reduces both intestinal iron absorption and iron mobilization from macrophages. Cytokines, including tumor necrosis factor, the interleukins, and interferon, also play a role in the anemia of inflammation, both by inducing hepcidin and by directly increasing EPO resistance in erythroid progenitors. Patients have an absolute or relative EPO deficiency, poor iron incorporation into developing erythrocytes, and shortened erythrocyte survival time. The prevalence of anemia of inflammation increases with age; most likely, this is related to age-related comorbidities and mediated through an increase in inflammatory cytokines and a relative EPO resistance.

Treatment of normocytic anemias. The mainstay of therapy for the anemia of chronic inflammation is treatment of the underlying condition and correction of nutritional deficiencies. Iron supplementation should be offered to all patients with a ferritin level lower than 100 ng/mL. Erythroid-stimulating agents (ESAs) have been shown to reduce transfusion needs in many of these patients. However, randomized studies and meta-analyses have shown that their use is associated with an increased incidence of arterial and venous thromboembolic events, an increased risk of mortality from cancer, and a reduced survival time. ESA should be avoided in cancer patients if they are being treated with curative intent, and in all other patients with cancer they should be offered only after a careful discussion of the risks and benefits (grade 1B recommendation).

Anemia of Chronic Kidney Disease

Most patients who have a glomerular filtration rate of less than 30 mL/min have anemia primarily reflecting low EPO levels. ESAs can

表现为全血细胞减少。

外周血涂片可见大的椭圆形细胞（大卵圆形红细胞）、中性粒细胞分叶过多和大血小板。骨髓增生活跃，细胞呈巨幼样变，红系祖细胞体积异常增大。此外，骨髓原位溶血（无效造血）可导致胆红素水平（导致前文所述的黄疸）和乳酸脱氢酶水平升高。

维生素 B_{12} 缺乏可导致神经系统异常，而其他原因所致的巨幼细胞贫血则不会引起神经系统症状。维生素 B_{12} 缺乏所致的神经系统症状表现多样，轻者可表现为由脊髓背侧段脱髓鞘引起的振动觉及位置觉减弱，重者可表现为痴呆或神经精神疾病。患者有时可仅表现为神经系统症状而无贫血，特别是使用叶酸治疗维生素 B_{12} 缺乏的患者，叶酸可纠正血液系统的巨幼细胞贫血，但不能治疗神经系统异常症状。目前认为，维生素 B_{12} 缺乏时的神经系统表现继发于甲基丙二酰 CoA 变位酶的功能缺失。一个可能的解释是该酶的功能缺失使奇数链脂肪酸代谢发生障碍，导致其异常整合入神经髓鞘，从而引起神经功能异常。这解释了为什么神经系统异常仅见于维生素 B_{12} 缺乏引起的巨幼细胞贫血，而不出现在叶酸缺乏引起的贫血中。

当维生素 B_{12} 缺乏时，肠黏膜细胞的巨幼样变可引起叶酸吸收不良，导致叶酸水平降低，反之亦然，故巨幼细胞贫血患者应同时检测维生素 B_{12} 和叶酸水平。RBC 中的叶酸水平可以更准确地反映体内叶酸储备，因此若临床表现提示叶酸缺乏但血清叶酸水平正常时，应检测 RBC 中的叶酸水平。但是，近期研究表明，许多恶性贫血患者血清维生素 B_{12} 水平可能是正常的。维生素 B_{12} 缺乏或叶酸缺乏时，同型半胱氨酸水平升高，但甲基丙二酸水平仅在维生素 B_{12} 缺乏时升高。因此，如果怀疑维生素 B_{12} 缺乏，但血清维生素 B_{12} 水平在正常范围时，应对上述指标进行检测。检测抗 IF 抗体和抗壁细胞抗体有助于明确维生素 B_{12} 缺乏的病因。

巨幼细胞贫血的治疗　对于维生素 B_{12} 缺乏的患者，高剂量口服和肠外维生素 B_{12} 给药均有效。口服剂量应至少达到 1000 μg/d。伴有神经系统异常、口服给药依从性差或无效的患者，应予 1000 μg 皮下或肌内注射治疗，每周可多次给药，共给药 4～8 次。维持治疗为每月 1000 μg，肠外给药。补充维生素 B_{12} 后，RBC 生成增加可引起叶酸相对缺乏，故给予维生素 B_{12} 治疗的同时应予叶酸治疗。恶性贫血应终身维持治疗。

叶酸缺乏的患者应接受口服叶酸治疗，剂量为 1～5 mg/d。如前所述，确认患者无维生素 B_{12} 缺乏非常重要，因为补充叶酸可改善维生素 B_{12} 缺乏患者的血液学指标，但无法改善其神经系统症状。

巨幼细胞贫血患者通常对治疗反应迅速。治疗后 2 天即可观察到网织红细胞增多，并在 7～10 天内达到峰值。尽管中性粒细胞计数迅速回升，其分叶过多的现象可能持续数日。在此期间，细胞增殖迅速，可能导致低钾血症、高尿酸血症或低磷血症。同时，应注意监测患者是否出现继发于造血增加的铁缺乏。贫血及其他血细胞减少将在 1～2 个月内完全缓解，但维生素 B_{12} 缺乏导致的神经症状则改善缓慢，甚至是不可逆的。

正细胞性贫血

正细胞性低增生性贫血的鉴别诊断非常多。营养物质缺乏所致的小细胞性或大细胞性贫血在初期均可表现为正细胞性贫血。混合性营养缺乏的患者也可具有正常 MCV。EPO 水平测定有助于诊断由肾衰竭引起的贫血，但慢性炎症和内分泌疾病相关的贫血也可导致 EPO 水平下降。在轻度贫血患者中测定 EPO 并无很大意义，因为只有当血细胞比容降至 30% 以下时，EPO 水平才可能高于正常值。即使血细胞比容降至 30%，EPO 水平通常仍在正常范围内，但对于贫血患者则显得相对低下。EPO 水平升高表明骨髓对贫血的反应不足，提示骨髓痨或原发性骨髓衰竭的可能性。当常规营养评估及内分泌科检查仍不能确诊疾病时，需行骨髓穿刺以除外骨髓原发性疾病。

炎症性贫血

炎症性贫血（既往被称为慢性病贫血）发生于患有慢性炎症、感染性疾病、恶性肿瘤或自身免疫病的患者中。患者血清铁水平降低，但与缺铁性贫血的铁相关指标相反，患者铁结合力降低，通常转铁蛋白饱和度 > 10%。铁蛋白水平通常升高，既因为铁蛋白是一种急性时相反应蛋白，也因为铁利用减低。铁调素水平明显升高，其作为一种急性时相反应蛋白，可促进转铁蛋白的代谢，减少肠内铁吸收及巨噬细胞对铁的动员。肿瘤坏死因子、白介素和干扰素等细胞因子可诱导铁调素生成，并增加红系祖细胞对 EPO 的抵抗，在炎症性贫血中发挥一定作用。患者 EPO 水平绝对或相对降低，铁利用不良，RBC 寿命缩短。炎症性贫血的发生率随年龄而升高，这可能与年龄相关合并症增加有关，其机制可能包括炎性细胞因子增加和 EPO 抵抗增加。

正细胞性贫血的治疗　慢性炎症性贫血的主要治疗方法是治疗原发病和纠正营养缺乏。所有铁蛋白 < 100 ng/ml 的患者均应行补铁治疗。促红细胞生成剂（ESA）已被证实可减少这类患者的输血需求。然而，随机试验和荟萃分析显示，ESA 的使用与动静脉血栓栓塞事件增加、癌症死亡风险增加及生存期缩短相关。因此，癌症患者在治疗肿瘤期间应避免使用 ESA；所有癌症患者必须在慎重评估风险和获益后才可应用 ESA（推荐类别Ⅰ B 类）。

慢性肾脏病性贫血

当肾小球滤过率 < 30 ml/min 时，多数患者会出现贫血，其主要与低 EPO 水平相关。ESA 有助于减少

TABLE 3.5 Differential Diagnosis of Hemolytic Anemia

Immune Hemolytic Anemia
Immunoglobulin G (warm antibody)–mediated hemolysis
Immunoglobulin M (cold antibody)–mediated hemolysis

Hemolysis From Causes Extrinsic to the Erythrocyte
Microangiopathic hemolysis
Disseminated intravascular coagulation
Thrombotic thrombocytopenic purpura
Preeclampsia, eclampsia, HELLP syndrome
Drugs (mitomycin, cyclosporine, gemcitabine)
Valvular hemolysis
Splenomegaly
Infection (e.g., malaria, babesiosis)

Hemolytic Anemia Caused by Disorders of the Erythrocyte Membrane
Inherited membrane abnormalities
Hereditary spherocytosis
Hereditary elliptocytosis
Hereditary pyropoikilocytosis
Hereditary stomatocytosis

Acquired Membrane Abnormalities
Paroxysmal nocturnal hemoglobinuria
Spur cell anemia

Hemolysis Caused by Erythrocyte Enzymopathies
Glucose-6-phosphate dehydrogenase deficiency
Other enzyme deficiencies

Hemoglobinopathies
Sickle cell disease
Other sickle syndromes
Thalassemia

HELLP, Hemolysis, elevated liver enzymes, and low-platelet count in association with preeclampsia.

help prevent transfusions in this population; however, their use has been associated with an increased risk of stroke, access thrombosis, hypertension, and even mortality in some studies, especially when the hemoglobin levels were normalized. Therefore, most guidelines recommend a target hemoglobin concentration of 10 to 11.5 g/dL when using ESA in patients with chronic kidney disease (grade IB). As in the management of anemia of chronic inflammation, nutritional deficiencies should be corrected before the use of ESAs. The evaluation and treatment of primary marrow failure syndromes and hematologic malignancies are discussed in Chapters 1 and 2 respectively.

EVALUATION OF ANEMIA WITH RETICULOCYTOSIS

An elevated reticulocyte count in the setting of anemia signals a compensatory response by a normal marrow to premature loss of erythrocytes. Hemolysis is the premature destruction of RBCs in the reticuloendothelial system (extrinsic hemolysis) or in blood vessels (intrinsic or intravascular hemolysis). The only other condition that causes anemia with reticulocytosis is acute bleeding. The differential diagnosis of hemolytic anemia is outlined in Table 3.5.

Whereas examination of the peripheral blood smear is helpful in characterizing any anemia, it is absolutely critical in the evaluation of hemolytic anemia. Morphologic examination of the erythrocytes is helpful in distinguishing immune hemolysis from microangiopathic hemolytic anemia. In addition, other RBC morphologic abnormalities are characteristic for specific diseases such as sickle cell disease (sickled cells), enzyme defects (*bite* cells), and erythrocyte membrane abnormalities (spherocytes, elliptocytes, stomatocytes).

Immune Hemolytic Anemia

Immune-mediated hemolysis results from coating of the erythrocyte membrane with antibodies or complement, or both. It may be mediated by immunoglobulin G (IgG) antibodies (*warm* antibody) or by IgM antibodies (*cold* antibody). The designations *warm* and *cold* denote the temperature at which maximal antibody binding takes place and the clinical syndromes caused by the two types of antibodies are distinct.

The diagnosis of hemolytic anemia is based on the direct and indirect antiglobulin (Coombs) tests. To perform a direct Coombs test, the patient's erythrocytes are mixed with antisera or monoclonal antibodies directed against human immunoglobulins and human complement. The cells are then monitored for agglutination, the presence of which confirms the presence of antibody or complement on the patient's RBCs. The indirect Coombs test is performed by mixing the patient's serum with ABO-compatible erythrocytes and then combining this mixture with antisera against IgG; the indirect Coombs tests allows for the evaluation of antibody in the patient's serum.

IgG-Mediated (Warm) Hemolytic Anemia

Classic autoimmune hemolytic anemia (AIHA) is caused by IgG antibody directed against erythrocyte antigens. Warm type hemolysis may be primary (idiopathic) or associated with autoimmune disease, lymphoproliferative disorders, or drugs. Patients exhibit acute anemia, jaundice, and an elevated reticulocyte count. Some patients have splenomegaly. The peripheral blood smear demonstrates spherocytes (see Fig. 3.2E). Laboratory analysis confirms the presence of IgG on the erythrocyte membrane, as demonstrated by a positive Coombs test; in some patients, the erythrocytes are also coated with complement. Some patients do not have reticulocytosis; in them, the antibody may be destroying both reticulocytes and mature erythrocytes.

The mainstay of therapy for AIHA is corticosteroids. Patients are usually treated with 1 to 2 mg/kg of prednisone, and in responding patients, doses are tapered slowly over several months. Patients who fail to respond to prednisone or cannot be tapered off the prednisone can be treated with other immunosuppressive agents, such as cyclophosphamide, azathioprine, chlorambucil, or rituximab. Some patients respond to intravenous immunoglobulin. Splenectomy is effective in many patients who are corticosteroid refractory or corticosteroid resistant, and it is associated with greater sustained response rates than other immunosuppressive therapies in corticosteroid-resistant patients. However, patients who do not respond and who have ongoing hemolysis after splenectomy are at high risk for secondary thromboembolic events.

Warm antibodies mediate *drug-induced hemolysis.* Several mechanisms exist through which drugs may induce AIHA (Table 3.6). Penicillin produces hemolysis by binding to erythrocytes and acting as a hapten; the antibody is directed against the drug, and hemolysis occurs only in the presence of the drug. Type 2 hemolysis is caused by the formation of an antibody-drug complex that binds to the erythrocyte membrane and activates complement. Drugs associated with this type of hemolysis include quinidine, quinine, and rifampin. Still other drugs, including methyldopa and procainamide, cause hemolysis by inducing the production of *true* antierythrocyte antibodies

表 3.5 溶血性贫血的鉴别诊断
免疫性溶血性贫血 IgG（温抗体）介导的溶血 IgM（冷抗体）介导的溶血
红细胞外部因素引起的溶血 微血管病变 弥散性血管内凝血 血栓性血小板减少性紫癜 先兆子痫、子痫、HELLP 综合征 药物（丝裂霉素、环孢素、吉西他滨） 心脏瓣膜溶血 脾大 感染（如疟疾、巴贝虫病）
红细胞膜缺陷引起的溶血 遗传性红细胞膜异常 遗传性球形红细胞增多症 遗传性椭圆形红细胞增多症 遗传性嗜派洛宁异形红细胞症 遗传性口形红细胞增多症
获得性红细胞膜异常 阵发性睡眠性血红蛋白尿症 棘细胞性贫血
红细胞酶缺陷引起的溶血 葡萄糖-6-磷酸脱氢酶缺乏症 其他酶缺陷
血红蛋白病 镰状细胞贫血 其他镰状细胞综合征 地中海贫血

HELLP，溶血、肝酶升高、与先兆子痫相关的血小板减少。

这些患者的输血需求，但一些研究提示，ESA 的使用与卒中、血栓形成、高血压甚至死亡率升高相关，特别是在血红蛋白水平正常时。因此，多数指南推荐，慢性肾脏病患者使用 ESA 时的目标血红蛋白水平为 10～11.5 g/dl（推荐类别ⅠB类）。治疗慢性炎症性贫血时，应在使用 ESA 前纠正营养缺乏。原发性骨髓衰竭综合征和血液系统恶性肿瘤的评估和治疗见第1章及第2章。

伴有网织红细胞增多的贫血的评估

在贫血情况下，网织红细胞计数增多提示正常骨髓对 RBC 异常消耗的代偿反应。溶血是指 RBC 在网状内皮系统（血管外溶血）或血管中（血管内溶血）的过早破坏。除溶血外，急性失血是唯一一种会导致网织红细胞增多的贫血的情况。溶血性贫血的鉴别诊断见表 3.5。

外周血涂片在各类贫血的鉴别中非常重要，在溶血性贫血中尤为关键。RBC 形态检测有助于区分免疫性溶血与微血管病性溶血。此外，RBC 形态的其他异常是特定疾病［如镰状细胞贫血（镰状细胞）、酶缺陷（咬损细胞）和 RBC 膜异常（球形红细胞、椭圆形红细胞、口形红细胞）］的特征性表现。

免疫性溶血性贫血

免疫介导的溶血是由于 RBC 膜表面结合了抗体和（或）补体，包括免疫球蛋白 G（IgG）抗体（温抗体）和 IgM 抗体（冷抗体）。"温抗体"和"冷抗体"的命名来源于该抗体发挥最大活性时的最适温度，而由这两类抗体引发的溶血在临床表现上也不尽相同。

溶血性贫血的诊断基于直接及间接抗球蛋白（Coombs）试验。直接 Coombs 试验是将患者 RBC 与针对免疫球蛋白和补体的抗血清或单克隆抗体相混合，然后监测细胞凝集，以证实患者 RBC 上存在抗体或补体。间接 Coombs 试验则是将患者的血清与其 ABO 血型相容的 RBC 混合，然后将该混合物与抗 IgG 的抗血清混合。间接 Coombs 试验可检测出患者血清中的抗体。

IgG 介导的（温抗体型）溶血性贫血

经典的自身免疫性溶血性贫血（AIHA）由针对 RBC 抗原的 IgG 抗体引起。温抗体型溶血可为原发性（特发性），或与自身免疫病、淋巴增殖性疾病或药物相关。患者表现为急性贫血、黄疸及网织红细胞计数增多。部分患者可出现脾大。外周血涂片可见球形红细胞。Coombs 试验阳性，提示 RBC 膜上存在 IgG 抗体；部分患者 RBC 表面同时存在补体。由于抗体可同时破坏网织红细胞及成熟 RBC，因此部分患者可能不出现网织红细胞增多。

皮质类固醇是 AIHA 的主要治疗手段。常用治疗为泼尼松 1～2 mg/kg，激素治疗有效的患者可在数月内缓慢减量。泼尼松治疗无效或激素依赖的患者可应用其他免疫抑制剂治疗，包括环磷酰胺、硫唑嘌呤、苯丁酸氮芥或利妥昔单抗等。静脉注射免疫球蛋白对部分患者有效。脾切除术可用于治疗激素无效或抵抗的患者；在激素抵抗患者中，脾切除术较其他免疫抑制治疗具有更好的长期疗效。然而，脾切除术无效或术后持续溶血的患者出现继发性血栓栓塞事件的风险相当高。

温抗体可介导药物诱导的溶血。药物诱发的 AIHA 存在多种机制（表 3.6）。青霉素可与 RBC 结合，并作为半抗原诱发溶血，在这种情况下，抗体直接针对药物，且溶血仅在用药时发生。在 2 型溶血中，抗体与药物形成复合物结合于 RBC 膜表面，并激活补体。可引发 2 型溶血的药物包括奎尼丁、奎宁和利福平。其他药物（包括甲基多巴和普鲁卡因胺）则通过诱导直

TABLE 3.6 Drug-Induced Autoimmune Hemolytic Anemia

Type	Mechanism	Common Drugs Implicated	Direct Coombs Test	Indirect Coombs Test
1	Hapten mediated	Penicillin Cephalothin	IgG positive Complement positive or negative	Positive only in the presence of drug
2	Immune complex mediated	Quinine Quinidine Phenacetin Rifampin	IgG negative Complement positive	Positive only in the presence of drug
3	True anti-RBC antibody	Isoniazid Tetracycline Chlorpromazine Methyldopa Levodopa Procainamide Ibuprofen Interferon-α	IgG positive Complement negative	Positive also in absence of drug

IgG, Immunoglobulin G; *RBC,* red blood cell.

directed against Rh and other RBC antigens. Antibody may persist in the absence of the drug, but not all patients with a positive Coombs test have evidence of hemolysis.

IgM-Mediated (Cold) Hemolytic Anemia

Cold-type immune hemolysis is usually postinfectious. The most common associated infectious agents are *Mycoplasma pneumoniae* and Epstein-Barr virus (EBV). IgM antibodies are produced that are directed against the RBC antigen I *(Mycoplasma)* or i (EBV). The antibodies bind at lower temperatures, present in fingers and toes, and bind complement. During the return to the central circulation, the IgM falls off the RBC, leaving complement bound. The Coombs test is negative for IgG and IgM but positive for complement. Hemolysis is self-limited, is rarely severe, and resolves with supportive therapy. In cases of severe hemolysis requiring transfusion, the patient should be kept warm, and blood should be administered through a blood warmer to minimize further hemolysis.

Cold agglutinin disease is a chronic IgM antibody–mediated hemolysis that is usually seen in association with lymphoproliferative diseases. Hemolysis is usually low grade; if severe, it responds poorly to steroids and splenectomy. Acute severe IgM-mediated hemolysis may respond to plasmapheresis, rituximab, and treatment directed against the lymphoproliferative disorder when present. Supportive therapy includes avoidance of exposure to the cold.

Hemolysis From Causes Extrinsic to the Erythrocyte
Microangiopathic Hemolysis

Microangiopathic hemolytic anemia (MAHA) is caused by traumatic destruction of RBCs as they pass through small vessels. The leading causes of MAHA include thrombotic thrombocytopenic purpura and hemolytic-uremic syndrome (TTP/HUS) (see Table 3.5 and Fig. 3.1). Other causes include pregnancy-related syndromes such as preeclampsia, eclampsia, and the HELLP syndrome (*h*emolysis, *e*levated *l*iver enzyme levels, and *l*ow *p*latelet count); drugs; and metastatic cancers. A similar hemolytic picture can be seen in traumatic hemolysis on a damaged cardiac valve (native or prosthetic).

The finding of schistocytes (fragmented erythrocytes) on the peripheral blood smear confirms the diagnosis of MAHA (see Fig. 3.2D). The presence of normal prothrombin and partial thromboplastin times supports a diagnosis of TTP/HUS over that of disseminated intravascular coagulation. Diagnosis and management are described further in Chapter 7.

TABLE 3.7 Congenital Red Blood Cell Membrane Abnormalities

Condition	Abnormal Membrane Proteins	Inheritance
Spherocytosis	Spectrin, ankyrin, band 3, protein 4.2	Autosomal dominant Recessive (rare)
Elliptocytosis	Spectrin, protein 4.1	Autosomal dominant Recessive (rare)
Pyropoikilocytosis	Spectrin	Recessive
Stomatocytosis	Sodium channel permeability defect	Autosomal dominant

Infection

Hemolysis can be caused by direct infection of RBCs by parasites, as seen in malaria, babesiosis, and bartonellosis. Severe, overwhelming hemolysis can be seen in clostridial sepsis, in which bacterial toxins directly damage the membrane.

Hemolytic Anemias Caused by Disorders of the Erythrocyte Membrane
Inherited Membrane Abnormalities

Hereditary spherocytosis (HS) is caused by heterogeneous congenital abnormalities in proteins of the erythrocyte cytoskeleton (Table 3.7). Most patients with HS have dominantly inherited mutations in spectrin or ankyrin. HS is characterized by hemolytic anemia, splenomegaly, and the presence of prominent spherocytes in the peripheral blood. Spherocytes are the result of *conditioning* of the erythrocytes in the spleen, during which venous sinus endothelial cells and reticuloendothelial cells remove portions of the abnormal membrane that are caused by the disordered cytoskeleton. Spherocytes reflect membrane loss that decreases the membrane-to-cytoplasm ratio. Because a high membrane-to-cytoplasm ratio is responsible for the flexible, biconcave shape of the normal erythrocyte, the erythrocyte loses its biconcave morphologic characteristics and assumes a spherocytic shape with loss of membrane. Spherocytes

表 3.6　药物诱导的自身免疫性溶血性贫血

类型	机制	常见药物	直接 Coombs 试验	间接 Coombs 试验
1 型	半抗原介导	青霉素 头孢噻吩	IgG 阳性 补体阳性或阴性	仅用药时阳性
2 型	免疫复合物介导	奎宁 奎尼丁 非那西丁 利福平 异烟肼 四环素 氯丙嗪	IgG 阴性 补体阳性	仅用药时阳性
3 型	真正的红细胞抗体	甲基多巴 左旋多巴 普鲁卡因胺 布洛芬 干扰素 α	IgG 阳性 补体阴性	未用药时也阳性

IgG，免疫球蛋白 G；RBC，红细胞。

接针对 RBC 表面 Rh 及其他 RBC 抗原的抗体引发溶血。抗体可不依赖于药物而存在，但并非所有 Coombs 试验阳性的患者均会发生溶血。

IgM 介导的（冷抗体型）溶血性贫血

冷抗体型溶血常发生于感染后。最常见的感染包括肺炎支原体和 EB 病毒（EBV）。IgM 抗体可直接针对 RBC 抗原 I（支原体）或 RBC 抗原 i（EBV）。在患者的手指和足趾中，抗体在较低温度下与 RBC 结合，继而结合补体。血液由肢端返回中央循环的过程中，IgM 从 RBC 表面脱落，但补体仍结合于 RBC 表面。Coombs 试验呈 IgG 和 IgM 阴性，补体阳性。溶血常为自限性，较少出现严重溶血，通过支持治疗即可缓解。在需要输血的严重溶血中，患者应注意保暖，且输血前应将血液置于加热器中加热，以避免发生进一步溶血。

冷凝集素病是由 IgM 抗体介导的慢性溶血，通常与淋巴细胞增殖性疾病相关。溶血通常较轻；但一旦发生严重溶血，患者对激素和脾切除术的反应较差。IgM 介导的急性重症溶血可采用血浆置换、利妥昔单抗等治疗；若存在淋巴细胞增殖性疾病，可采用针对性治疗。支持治疗包括避免接触寒冷环境等。

红细胞外部因素引起的溶血

微血管病性溶血

微血管病性溶血性贫血（MAHA）由 RBC 通过微小血管时的机械性破坏引起。MAHA 的主要原因包括血栓性血小板减少性紫癜和溶血性尿毒综合征（TTP/HUS）（表 3.5 和图 3.1）。其他原因包括妊娠相关综合征［如先兆子痫、子痫和 HELLP 综合征（溶血、肝酶升高、血小板减少）］，药物及转移癌。类似的溶血现象可见于心脏瓣膜（包括自体或人工瓣膜）损伤引起的机械性溶血。

外周血涂片出现破碎红细胞（红细胞碎片）可证

表 3.7　遗传性红细胞膜异常

表型	异常膜蛋白	遗传方式
遗传性球形红细胞增多症	血影蛋白、锚蛋白、带 3 蛋白、蛋白质 4.2	常染色体显性遗传 隐性遗传（罕见）
遗传性椭圆形红细胞增多症	血影蛋白、蛋白质 4.1	常染色体显性遗传 隐性遗传（罕见）
遗传性嗜派洛宁异形红细胞症	血影蛋白	隐性遗传
遗传性口形红细胞增多症	钠通道通透性缺陷	常染色体显性遗传

实 MAHA 的诊断（图 3.2D）。凝血酶原时间及部分凝血活酶时间正常支持 TTP/HUS 的诊断，有助于与弥散性血管内凝血进行鉴别。该病的诊断和治疗详见第 7 章。

感染

寄生虫可直接感染 RBC 而引起溶血，可见于疟疾、巴贝虫病和巴尔通体病。致死性溶血可见于梭菌感染中毒症，在这类疾病中，细菌毒素可直接损伤细胞膜。

红细胞膜缺陷引起的溶血性贫血

遗传性红细胞膜异常

遗传性球形红细胞增多症（HS）是 RBC 骨架蛋白先天性缺陷引起的溶血性贫血（表 3.7）。多数 HS 患者具有血影蛋白或锚蛋白突变，呈常染色体显性遗传。HS 的特征表现包括溶血性贫血、脾大及外周血中出现球形红细胞。球形红细胞是 RBC 经脾"处理"的产物；在脾中，静脉窦内皮细胞及网状内皮细胞会移除异常细胞骨架造成的异常细胞膜。球形红细胞的细胞膜面积减小，细胞膜与胞质比例降低；由于正常 RBC 的变形性及双凹圆盘状外形与细胞膜-胞质比例高相关，因此细胞膜面积减小使球形红细胞无法保持双凹圆盘状外形，而呈现球形外观。球形红细胞的变形性差，在微血

are less flexible and may be destroyed in the microvasculature. The laboratory finding characteristic of HS is increased osmotic fragility, which is caused by the loss of distensibility associated with a decrease in surface membrane. HS is usually a mild disorder with well-compensated hemolysis. Patients typically have exacerbations during infections or when given marrow-suppressing medication. Patients with significant hemolysis should receive folate supplementation. Many patients require cholecystectomy for pigment stones. Severe, symptomatic anemia is treated with partial or total splenectomy.

Hereditary elliptocytosis (HE) is caused by dominantly inherited mutations affecting the interactions between membrane proteins and underlying cytoplasmic proteins. The most common abnormalities affect the interactions with spectrin and protein 4.1, which causes the RBCs to assume an elliptical shape. As in HS, patients usually have mild hemolysis and splenomegaly.

Hereditary pyropoikilocytosis (HPP) is a rare recessive disorder that is frequently caused by the inheritance of two different membrane disorders (e.g., one allele for HS and one for HE). Patients have severe hemolysis with microspherocytes and elliptocytes on the peripheral blood smear. As with HS, treatment for symptomatic anemia in HE and HPP is splenectomy.

Hereditary stomatocytosis is caused by autosomal dominant mutations leading to abnormalities in RBC permeability and volume, either in an overhydrated form (OHS), dehydrated form (DHS) or near normal form. These rare membranopathies are heterogeneous in presentation with syndromic and nonsyndromic forms with varying degrees of hemolytic anemia and are confirmed with genetic testing. Treatment is supportive but splenectomy should be avoided due to increased risk of thrombosis in certain types and care should be made to distinguish from hereditary spherocytosis for which splenectomy is the indicated therapy.

More information on hemolytic anemias caused by inherited membrane disorders can be found in Chapter 152, "Hemolytic Anemias: Red Cell Membrane and Metabolic Defects," in *Goldman-Cecil Medicine*, 26th Edition.

Acquired Membrane Abnormalities

Paroxysmal nocturnal hemoglobinuria. Paroxysmal nocturnal hemoglobinuria (PNH) is an acquired clonal disease that is associated with an abnormality of complement regulation. Normal erythrocytes are protected from complement-mediated cell lysis by the presence of membrane proteins, including delay-accelerating factor (DAF or CD55) and membrane inhibitor of reactive lysis (MIRL or CD59). Both these proteins are members of a family of proteins that are anchored to the membrane by a glycosyl phosphatidylinositol (GPI) anchor. Patients with PNH have clonal mutations in phosphatidyl inositol glycan A (PIG-A), the enzyme required for synthesis of GPI. These mutations arise in the hematopoietic stem cell, and subsequently all hematopoietic cells lack GPI-anchored proteins. Absence of GPI-anchored proteins from erythrocytes renders them susceptible to complement-mediated lysis. The diagnosis can be made by flow cytometric documentation of the absence of CD55 or CD59 on the surface of RBCs or leukocytes.

PNH is a clonal stem cell disorder with several unique characteristics. Patients suffer from episodic acute intravascular hemolysis with a release of free hemoglobin that results in the hemoglobinuria for which the disease is named. The dark, hemoglobin-pigmented urine is most prominent in the morning after concentrating overnight during sleep. Patients are also susceptible to venous thrombotic complications, including Budd-Chiari syndrome, portal vein thrombosis, cerebrovascular thrombosis, and peripheral veins. The disease is associated with a risk for development of myelodysplasia, myelofibrosis, acute

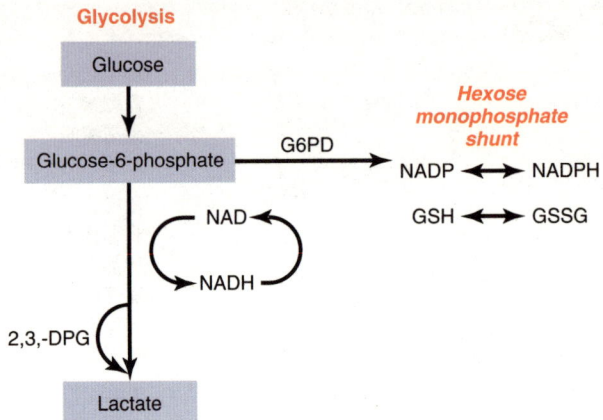

Fig. 3.4 Metabolism of the red blood cell. *2,3-DPG*, 2,3-Diphosphoglycerate; *G6PD*, glucose-6-phosphate dehydrogenase; *GSH*, reduced glutathione; *GSSG*, reduced and oxidized glutathione; *NAD*, nicotinamide adenine dinucleotide; *NADH*, reduced form of NAD; *NADP*, nicotinamide adenine dinucleotide phosphate; *NADPH*, reduced form of NADP.

leukemia, or aplastic anemia. Furthermore, patients with aplastic anemia who respond to immunosuppressive therapy frequently develop PNH-like clones. In the past, treatment has been largely supportive. However, treatment with eculizumab and ravulizumab, monoclonal antibodies that bind to the C5 component of complement, have been shown to reduce hemolysis and transfusion requirements in this disease. Eculizumab also reduces thromboembolic events; this end point has not yet been addressed in the more recently approved ravulizumab. Young patients should be considered for allogeneic stem cell transplantation.

Spur cell anemia. Spur cells (acanthocytes) are cells with abnormal membrane morphology found in patients with advanced liver disease, severe malnutrition, malabsorption, or asplenia. The membrane acquires protrusions as a result of the presence of abnormal lipids. The changes may be associated with mild hemolysis, although in patients with advanced liver disease, it is difficult to distinguish hemolysis from hypersplenism. Similar changes may be observed in patients with abetalipoproteinemia.

Hemolytic Anemias Caused by Disorders of Erythrocyte Enzymes

Glucose-6 Phosphate Dehydrogenase Deficiency

Glucose-6-phosphate dehydrogenase (G6PD) is a critical enzyme in the hexose monophosphate shunt pathway. By maintaining intracellular stores of reduced glutathione, it protects erythrocytes from membrane and hemoglobin oxidation (Fig. 3.4). The gene for G6PD resides on the X chromosome, and therefore almost all patients with G6PD deficiency are male. Most G6PD mutations are found in African and Mediterranean populations, most likely because they confer resistance to malaria. The African form of G6PD deficiency is relatively mild, whereas the Mediterranean form is severe.

Absence of G6PD renders erythrocytes sensitive to oxidative stress. In the setting of infection, inflammation acidosis, or oxidant drugs, hemoglobin may precipitate within the cells, causing hemolysis. Many drugs are associated with hemolysis in the setting of G6PD deficiency, including sulfonamides, antimalarials, dapsone, aspirin, and phenacetin. The diagnosis should be considered in male patients of African or Mediterranean extraction who have evidence of hemolysis in the

管系统中易被破坏。HS 的特征性实验室检查主要包括与细胞膜表面积减小、变形性差相关的渗透脆性增加。HS 通常症状轻微，机体可充分代偿。感染或使用骨髓抑制药物可导致溶血加重。有明显溶血表现的患者应接受叶酸治疗。许多患者需行胆囊切除术以预防胆色素结石。严重症状性患者可行脾部分或全部切除术。

遗传性椭圆形红细胞增多症（HE）是一种常染色体显性遗传病，其基因突变影响膜蛋白与胞质蛋白的相互作用。最常见的突变可影响血影蛋白与蛋白质 4.1 的相互作用，导致红细胞呈椭圆形。与 HS 患者的症状相似，HE 患者通常表现为轻度溶血和脾大。

遗传性嗜派洛宁异形红细胞症（HPP）是一种罕见的常染色体隐性遗传病，通常是因为患者遗传了两种不同的红细胞膜疾病（如 HS 的一个等位基因和 HE 的一个等位基因）。患者可表现为严重溶血，外周血涂片可见微球形细胞和椭圆形细胞。与 HS 相同，出现贫血症状的 HE 及 HPP 患者可行脾切除术。

遗传性口形红细胞增多症由常染色体显性遗传突变引起，导致 RBC 通透性和体积异常，分为过度水化型（OHS）、脱水型（DHS）或接近正常型。这类罕见的红细胞膜疾病可表现为不同程度的溶血性贫血，可为系统性表现或单一表现，需经基因检测证实。治疗以支持治疗为主；由于特定分型患者切脾后血栓风险增加，故应避免行脾切除术，但应注意与 HS 进行鉴别，因为后者建议行脾切除术治疗。

遗传性红细胞膜异常引起的溶血性贫血的其他内容详见第 26 版 Goldman-Cecil Medicine 第 152 章 "溶血性贫血：红细胞膜和代谢缺陷"。

获得性红细胞膜异常

阵发性睡眠性血红蛋白尿症（PNH） PNH 是一种由补体调控异常所致的获得性克隆性疾病。在 RBC 膜上，某些膜蛋白［包括衰变加速因子（DAF；又称 CD55）和反应性细胞裂解的膜抑制因子（MIRL；又称 CD59）］可保护正常 RBC 免受补体攻击而引发细胞裂解。这两种蛋白质均属于膜锚连蛋白，通过糖基磷脂酰肌醇（GPI）锚定于细胞膜上。磷脂酰肌醇聚糖 A（PIG-A）是合成 GPI 所必需的酶，PNH 患者存在该酶的克隆性突变。这些突变发生于造血干细胞水平，故所有后代造血细胞均缺乏 GPI 锚定蛋白。GPI 锚定蛋白的缺乏使得 RBC 易受补体的攻击。流式细胞术可检测 RBC 或白细胞表面上 CD55 或 CD59 的缺失，有助于 PNH 的诊断。

PNH 是一种克隆性造血干细胞疾病，具有多种独特的临床表现。患者可表现为阵发性急性血管内溶血，使游离血红蛋白增多，导致血红蛋白尿，该病亦由此得名。患者尿液经浓缩过夜后，深色血红蛋白色素尿在早晨最为明显。患者还易出现血栓栓塞性疾病，包括布-加综合征、门静脉血栓形成、脑血栓和外周静脉血栓。该病还可进展为骨髓增生异常、骨髓纤维化、

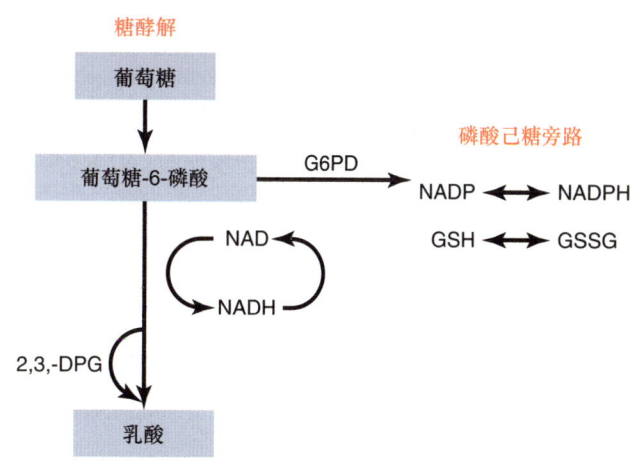

图 3.4 红细胞代谢。2,3-DPG，2,3-二磷酸甘油酸；G6PD，葡萄糖-6-磷酸脱氢酶；GSH，还原型谷胱甘肽；GSSG，还原型和氧化型谷胱甘肽；NAD，烟酰胺腺嘌呤二核苷酸；NADH，NAD 的还原形式；NADP，烟酰胺腺嘌呤二核苷酸磷酸；NADPH，NADP 的还原形式

急性白血病或再生障碍性贫血等。接受免疫抑制治疗的再生障碍性贫血患者常出现 PNH 样克隆。该病的传统治疗以支持治疗为主。目前证实依库珠单抗和瑞武丽珠单抗（均为单克隆抗体，可与补体中的 C5 组分结合）可改善溶血，减少输血需求。此外，依库珠单抗还可减少血栓栓塞事件，目前尚未证实瑞武丽珠单抗具有该作用。年轻患者应考虑 alloSCT。

棘形细胞贫血 棘形红细胞表现为异常的细胞形态，可见于进展期肝病、严重营养不良、吸收不良或脾缺如患者。细胞膜由于异常脂质的存在而呈棘形。这种异常可引起轻度溶血，即使是在晚期肝病患者中，因此溶血和脾功能亢进很难鉴别。类似异常也可见于先天性 β-脂蛋白缺乏症患者。

红细胞酶缺陷引起的溶血性贫血

葡萄糖-6-磷酸脱氢酶缺乏症

葡萄糖-6-磷酸脱氢酶（G6PD）是磷酸己糖旁路途径中的关键酶。通过维持细胞内还原型谷胱甘肽的含量，保护 RBC 膜及血红蛋白免于氧化损伤（图 3.4）。G6PD 基因位于 X 染色体上，因此几乎所有患者均为男性。多数 G6PD 突变见于非洲和地中海地区人群，可能与该基因对疟疾的抗性有关。非洲型 G6PD 缺乏症通常病情较轻，而地中海型则更为严重。

G6PD 缺乏使得 RBC 对氧化应激更为敏感。在感染、酸中毒或应用氧化剂等情况下，血红蛋白可在细胞内沉淀而引发溶血。多种药物在 G6PD 缺乏症患者中可引发溶血，包括磺胺类药物、抗疟药、氨苯砜、阿司匹林和非那西丁。如果患者为来自非洲或地中海地区的男性，且在感染、应用氧化剂后发生溶血，则需警惕该诊断。地中海型 G6PD 缺乏症患者可在接触蚕豆后发生溶血。患者的 RBC 内含有海因茨小体

setting of acute infection or recent exposure to oxidant drugs. Patients with the Mediterranean variant of G6PD deficiency may develop hemolysis on exposure to fava beans (favism). Cells with precipitated hemoglobin contain Heinz bodies that can be visualized with crystal violet staining of the peripheral blood smear. These inclusions are removed in the spleen, resulting in the additional finding of bite cells in the blood smear. The diagnosis can be confirmed with measurement of G6PD levels in the peripheral blood. However, reticulocytes and young RBCs in patients with G6PD deficiency have a higher enzyme level; consequently, if the diagnosis is probable, the patients with a normal G6PD level should be retested at a time removed from the acute episode, when the percentage of young RBCs is high. The mainstay of preventing hemolysis in these patients is avoidance of oxidative stress, especially drugs implicated in causing hemolysis. Splenectomy is recommended only for patients with severe episodic or chronic hemolysis.

Other Enzyme Deficiencies

Enzyme deficiencies as rare causes of hemolytic anemia have been reported involving almost all of the enzymes of the glycolytic pathway. The most common of these is pyruvate kinase deficiency. Autosomal genes encode these enzymes, and the pattern of inheritance is therefore autosomal recessive.

More information on hemolytic anemias caused by inherited enzyme deficiencies can be found in Chapter 152, "Hemolytic Anemias: Red Cell Membrane and Metabolic Defects," in *Goldman-Cecil Medicine*, 26th Edition.

Hemoglobinopathies

Hemoglobinopathies are disorders caused by mutations that result in the synthesis of quantitatively or qualitatively abnormal hemoglobins. The most common of these are the sickle syndromes and the thalassemias, which, like G6PD deficiency, arose in areas of the world with endemic malaria.

Sickle Cell Disease

Sickle cell disease, the most common of the sickle syndromes, arises from a point mutation that causes a substitution of valine for glutamic acid in the sixth amino acid of the β-globin gene. It has arisen as an independent mutation in diverse populations in Africa, India, the Mediterranean, and the Middle East. The substitution of a hydrophobic for a hydrophilic residue renders the deoxygenated sickle hemoglobin (HbS) less soluble and therefore susceptible to polymerization and precipitation. The rate of precipitation of HbS is exquisitely sensitive to the intracorpuscular concentration of deoxygenated hemoglobin. Sickling is therefore increased in settings in which that concentration is increased, either by changes in cellular hydration (dehydration) or by changes in the oxygen dissociation curve (e.g., hypoxia, acidosis, high altitude).

Acute manifestations. Most of the acute complications of sickle cell disease are related to vaso-occlusion (Table 3.8). Painful crises, secondary to occlusions of the microvasculature and ischemia of organs and tissues, can occur anywhere, with pain most commonly experienced in the extremities, chest, abdomen, and back. Painful crises are commonly precipitated by infections, dehydration, rapid changes in temperature, and pregnancy. Often, however, no obvious precipitating cause is found for an acute painful crisis.

Vaso-occlusion in the pulmonary circulation can be a particularly ominous complication of sickle cell disease. It results in the *acute chest syndrome*, which is characterized by chest pain, hypoxemia, and pulmonary infiltrates. The roles of infection, infarction, and in situ thrombosis in the acute chest syndrome are indistinguishable, but all patients should receive antibiotics for presumed pneumonia. Because hypoxemia predisposes to further sickling and increasing respiratory compromise, the acute chest syndrome is life-threatening and is an indication for emergent exchange transfusion.

Neurologic events are a major cause of morbidity in patients with sickle cell disease. Acute large-vessel occlusions occur in children, with a recurrence rate of 70% if untreated; such strokes are an indication for long-term exchange transfusion, which has been shown to decrease the rate of repeated occlusions. For reasons that are poorly understood, such large-vessel occlusions rarely occur in adults. Adults may suffer hemorrhagic strokes as a result of aneurysmal dilation of proliferative vessels that form in response to repeated micro-occlusions in the cerebral vessels.

Any toxic or infectious insult that transiently suppresses bone marrow activity can cause an *aplastic crisis*. The shortened survival time of the RBC in sickle cell disease renders patients highly dependent on vigorous ongoing marrow activity, and short intervals of decreased reticulocyte formation can cause profound anemia. Most dramatic are infections associated with parvovirus B19, which directly infects erythroid precursors. Supportive care is usually all that is required. However, some patients go on to develop bone marrow necrosis, with a leukoerythroblastic picture; this development may be further complicated by bone marrow embolization to the lungs.

Certain vascular beds are especially prone to complications of sickle cell disease. The renal medulla is highly susceptible to damage by vaso-occlusion because its high tonicity and low oxygen tension both significantly increase the concentration of HbS. All patients with sickle cell disease develop defects in the ability to concentrate urine, and by adulthood, they are uniformly isosthenuric. Acute episodes of hematuria secondary to papillary necrosis are common.

The spleen is another site in which recurrent sickling uniformly occurs. Although in childhood the spleen can sequester blood cells, by adulthood all patients have become functionally asplenic from repeated infarctions of the microvasculature. This contributing factor increases the susceptibility of patients with sickle cell disease to infections with encapsulated organisms. Acute infection remains a significant cause of death. For unclear reasons, patients with sickle cell disease are particularly prone to osteomyelitis, and there is an unusually high incidence of *Salmonella* as the responsible organism.

Chronic manifestations. Sickle cell disease used to be a disease of childhood. As more patients survive to adulthood, it has become clear that repeated episodes of vaso-occlusion lead to damage to almost every end organ (see Table 3.8). Renal failure and pulmonary failure are leading causes of death in adult patients with sickle cell disease. Other long-term complications include chronic skin ulcers, retinopathy, and liver dysfunction. In addition, most patients require cholecystectomy for pigment stones.

TABLE 3.8 Clinical Manifestations of Sickle Cell Disease

Acute Manifestations	Chronic Manifestations
Vaso-occlusive crisis	Chronic renal disease
Painful crisis	Isosthenuria
Acute chest syndrome	Chronic renal failure
Priapism	Chronic pulmonary disease
Cerebrovascular events	Sickle hepatopathy
Thrombotic stroke	Proliferative retinopathy
Hemorrhagic stroke	Avascular necrosis
Aplastic crisis	Skin ulcers
Splenic sequestration	
Osteomyelitis	

（Heinz 小体），其由沉积的血红蛋白形成，可通过对外周血涂片行结晶紫染色进行检测。这些包涵体可被脾吞噬，因此在血涂片中还可出现咬损细胞。外周血 G6PD 水平测定可确诊该病。然而，由于急性溶血时幼稚红细胞增多，而网织红细胞及幼稚红细胞含有较多 G6PD，因此对于 G6PD 水平正常但仍怀疑 G6PD 缺乏症的患者，应在急性溶血恢复后重新检测 G6PD 水平。在这些患者中，预防溶血的主要方法是避免氧化应激，特别是避免应用可引起溶血的药物。脾切除术仅推荐用于严重发作性溶血或慢性溶血患者。

其他酶缺陷

目前研究表明，尽管由酶缺陷导致的溶血较少见，但几乎涉及糖酵解途径中的所有酶。其中丙酮酸激酶缺乏最常见。这类酶通常由常染色体基因编码，因此呈常染色体隐性遗传。

遗传性酶缺陷所致溶血性贫血详见 *Goldman-Cecil Medicine* 第 26 版第 152 章"溶血性贫血：红细胞膜和代谢缺陷"。

血红蛋白病

血红蛋白病相关的基因突变可引起血红蛋白合成质量或数量的异常，其中最常见的是镰状综合征和地中海贫血。与 G6PD 缺乏症类似，该病多见于地方性疟疾流行区。

镰状细胞贫血

镰状细胞贫血是最常见的镰状综合征，是由于 β-珠蛋白基因的点突变导致其蛋白的第 6 个氨基酸谷氨酸被缬氨酸取代。该突变广泛存在于非洲、印度、地中海和中东地区的不同人群中。由于疏水性氨基酸残基取代了亲水性残基，未携带氧气的镰状血红蛋白（HbS）溶解性较差，易于聚集和沉淀。HbS 的沉淀速率取决于细胞内未携氧血红蛋白的浓度。因此，当细胞水合（或脱水）状态或氧解离曲线（如缺氧、酸中毒、高海拔）变化时，未携氧血红蛋白浓度增加，镰状改变更为明显。

急性表现 多数镰状细胞贫血的急性并发症与血管闭塞相关（表 3.8）。疼痛危象继发于微血管系统闭塞及组织器官缺血，可出现于全身各部位，最常见的部位包括四肢、胸部、腹部和背部。疼痛危象的诱因包括感染、脱水、温度快速变化和妊娠等。但是，急性疼痛危象通常无明显诱因。

肺循环血管闭塞是镰状细胞贫血的严重并发症，可导致急性胸部综合征，主要表现为胸痛、低氧血症和肺浸润。在急性胸部综合征中，感染、梗死和原位血栓栓塞常难以区分，但所有患者均应接受抗生素治

表 3.8 镰状细胞贫血的临床表现	
急性表现	**慢性表现**
血管闭塞危象	慢性肾脏病
疼痛危象	等渗尿
急性胸部综合征	慢性肾衰竭
阴茎异常勃起	慢性肺病
脑血管事件	镰状肝病
缺血性卒中	增殖性视网膜病
出血性卒中	血管坏死
再生障碍危象	皮肤溃疡
脾隔离症	
骨髓炎	

疗，以预防肺炎。由于低氧血症可进一步引起镰状改变，加重呼吸窘迫，故急性胸部综合征是紧急换血的指征。

神经系统事件是镰状细胞贫血患者的主要并发症。急性大血管闭塞主要见于儿童，如果未经治疗，复发率为 70%。这类卒中是长期换血的指征，该治疗可降低反复栓塞的发生率。类似的大血管栓塞很少见于成人，其原因未明。在成人中，由于颅内血管反复发生微小闭塞，血管增生并呈动脉瘤样扩张，故更易发生出血性卒中。

抑制骨髓造血功能的中毒性或感染性损伤均可导致再生障碍危象。在镰状细胞贫血中，RBC 寿命缩短，导致患者高度依赖于骨髓当下的造血活性，短时间内网织红细胞生成减少即可引发严重贫血。细小病毒 B19 可直接感染红系祖细胞，导致严重贫血。发生再生障碍危象时，通常仅需给予支持治疗。然而，部分患者可持续进展为骨髓坏死，出现幼粒幼红细胞，且骨髓栓子可循环至肺部引发肺栓塞。

某些部位的血管床更易受到镰状细胞贫血的影响。肾髓质极易受到血管闭塞的损伤，因为其高张力和低氧张力均可显著增加 HbS 的浓度。所有镰状细胞贫血患者均存在尿液浓缩功能障碍，在成年后均表现为等渗尿。急性阵发性血尿亦常见，一般继发于肾乳头坏死。

脾是镰状细胞贫血累及的另一重要器官。尽管儿童患者的脾尚存在吞噬血细胞的功能，但成年时，由于微血管反复梗死，脾均呈无功能状态。这导致镰状细胞贫血患者更易发生包膜病原体感染。急性感染仍是镰状细胞贫血致死的主要病因。镰状细胞贫血患者更易患骨髓炎，且多以沙门菌属为致病菌，其机制不明。

慢性表现 镰状细胞贫血曾经是一种儿童疾病。随着越来越多的患者存活至成年，反复发生的血管闭塞可导致几乎所有器官损伤（表 3.8）。肾衰竭和肺衰竭是成人患者的主要死亡原因。其他长期并发症包括慢性皮肤溃疡、视网膜病变和肝功能障碍。此外，大多数患者需行胆囊切除术以预防胆色素结石。

TABLE 3.9 Thalassemic Syndromes

Disorder	Genotypic Abnormality	Clinical Phenotype
β-Thalassemia		
Thalassemia major (Cooley's anemia)	Homozygous β^0-thalassemia	Severe hemolysis, ineffective erythropoiesis, transfusion dependency, iron overload
Thalassemia intermedia	Compound heterozygous β^0- and β^+-thalassemia	Moderate hemolysis, severe anemia, but not transfusion dependent; iron overload
Thalassemia minor	Heterozygous β^0- or β^+-thalassemia	Microcytosis, mild anemia
α-Thalassemia		
Hydrops fetalis	—/—	Severe anemia, intrauterine anasarca from congestive heart failure; death in utero or at birth
Hemoglobin H	α–/—	Microcytic anemia and mild hemolysis; not transfusion dependent
α-Thalassemia trait	$\alpha\alpha$/— (α-thalassemia 1) or $-\alpha/-\alpha$ (α-thalassemia 2)	Mild microcytic anemia
Silent carrier	$-\alpha/\alpha\alpha$	Normal complete blood count

Treatment. Treatment of sickle cell disease remains largely supportive. Painful crises are treated with fluid, oxygen supplementation, and analgesics. Patients with any indication of infection should receive antibiotics. Patients with symptomatic anemia should be transfused. Exchange transfusion is indicated for chest syndrome, stroke, bone marrow necrosis, and priapism. More controversial indications for exchange transfusion include intractable pain and slow response to other supportive measures. The goal of exchange transfusion is to achieve a level of 30% to 40% HbS. As previously mentioned, patients who have sustained a thrombotic large-vessel stroke should undergo chronic exchange transfusion.

Hydroxyurea has been the main disease-modifying agent for patients with sickle cell disease. Treatment with hydroxyurea, an agent that increases the concentration of HbF in patients with sickle cell disease, reduces the incidence of vaso-occlusive crises. The efficacy of hydroxyurea in patients with recurrent crises has been demonstrated in a randomized study, and follow-up studies have revealed a survival advantage for patients treated with hydroxyurea. More recently, three additional agents have been approved; two further reduced sickle cell crises (L-glutamine and crizanlizumab) and the last increased hemoglobin levels (voxelotor). In a randomized study, L-glutamine therapy demonstrated significantly fewer sickle cell crises with most patients on both arms already receiving hydroxyurea. L-glutamine is hypothesized to reduce oxidative stress and potential pain crises by increasing reduced nicotinamide adenine dinucleotide in sickle cells. In another randomized trial, crizanlizumab, a P-selectin inhibitor, also significantly reduced sickle cell crises. P-selectin initiates the process of leukocyte adhesion to vascular endothelium during inflammation that leads to vaso-occlusion. Most recently, voxelotor, an agent that inhibits HbS polymerization by stabilizing the oxygenated hemoglobin state, has led to decreased hemolysis and improved anemia and is now an approved therapy.

The only curative treatment for sickle cell disease is allogeneic stem cell transplant although lack of donor matches remains a barrier.

Other Sickle Syndromes

Hemoglobin C. Hemoglobin C (HbC) is caused by another substitution, glutamic acid to lysine, in the sixth position of the β-globin chain. Homozygous HbC causes very mild symptoms of anemia and is usually clinically silent. Patients with hemoglobin S-C (HbSC) are compound heterozygotes for HbS and HbC. These patients are symptomatic, although the clinical manifestations are milder than in patients with homozygous HbS (HbSS). They have a higher hematocrit, but the higher viscosity increases the degree of retinopathy. They do not sustain splenic infarctions; unlike patients with HbSS, they usually have splenomegaly. Consequently, they occasionally have episodes of acute splenomegaly associated with profound decreases in hemoglobin concentration and hematocrit (splenic sequestration crisis). Although such crises also occur in children with HbSS, functional asplenia prevents this complication in adults with HbSS.

Sickle cell β-thalassemia. Patients who are double heterozygotes for HbS and β-thalassemia have a spectrum of disease dependent on the level of β-globin that they produce. Sickle cell β^+-thalassemia is a milder disease than HbSS, probably because of the decreased intracorpuscular concentration of HbS. Patients with sickle cell β^0-thalassemia (see discussion that follows) produce no normal β chains and have essentially the same phenotype as patients with HbSS.

Thalassemia

The thalassemic syndromes (Table 3.9) are a heterogeneous group of disorders associated with decreased or absent synthesis of either α- or β-globin chains. Severe thalassemic syndromes are associated with severe hemolytic anemia and are diagnosed in early childhood. However, mild forms of thalassemia minor frequently cause mild microcytic anemia with little or no evidence of hemolysis. These syndromes are often confused with iron deficiency because of the decreased MCV.

β-Thalassemia. Over 100 mutations have been described that lead to β-thalassemia, causing a decrease or absence of expression from the β-globin locus. The decreased expression of β-globin can be caused by structural mutations in the coding region of the gene, which result in nonsense mutations, truncated messenger RNA (mRNA), and no expression of intact globin from the affected allele (β^0-thalassemia). However, a large number of mutations that result in decreased transcription or translation or altered splicing of the β-globin mRNA result in reduction but not elimination of globin-chain expression from the affected allele (β^+-thalassemia).

Defective globin-chain synthesis in β-thalassemia causes both decreased normal hemoglobin production and the production of a relative excess of α chains. The decrease in normal hemoglobin synthesis results in a hypochromic anemia, and the excess α chains form insoluble α-chain complexes and cause hemolysis. In mild thalassemic syndromes, the excess α chains are insufficient to cause significant hemolysis, and the primary finding is a microcytic anemia. In severe

表 3.9 地中海贫血综合征

疾病	基因异常	临床表型
β-地中海贫血		
重型地中海贫血（Cooley 贫血）	β^0-地中海贫血基因纯合子	严重溶血、无效红细胞生成、输血依赖、铁过载
中间型地中海贫血	β^0-地中海贫血和 β^+-地中海贫血基因杂合子	中度溶血、严重贫血、铁过载，但非输血依赖
轻型地中海贫血	β^0-地中海贫血或 β^+-地中海贫血基因杂合子	轻度小细胞性贫血
α-地中海贫血		
胎儿水肿综合征	−/−	严重贫血、充血性心力衰竭和胎儿宫内全身水肿；在妊娠期间或出生时死亡
血红蛋白 H 病	α-地中海贫血/−	小细胞性贫血和轻度溶血；非输血依赖
α-地中海贫血轻型	αα/−−（α-thal 1）或 −α/−α（α-thal 2）	轻度小细胞性贫血
无症状携带者	−α/αα	血常规正常

治疗 支持治疗仍是镰状细胞贫血的主要治疗。疼痛危象的治疗包括补液、吸氧、镇痛等。有感染表现的患者需接受抗生素治疗。有贫血症状的患者需给予输血。换血疗法适用于出现急性胸部综合征、卒中、骨髓坏死及阴茎异常勃起的患者。对于顽固性疼痛和其他支持治疗效果不佳者，采用换血疗法是有争议的。换血疗法的目标是使 HbS 水平降至 30%～40%。如前所述，反复出现血栓性大血管卒中的患者应接受长期换血疗法。

羟基脲是镰状细胞贫血患者的主要治疗药物。羟基脲可增加 RBC 中 HbF 的浓度，并降低血管闭塞性危象的发生率。一项随机研究证实了羟基脲在复发性危象患者中的疗效，且随访研究显示使用羟基脲治疗的患者具有较长的生存期。近期，另有 3 种药物获得批准：其中 2 种（左旋谷氨酰胺和立赞利珠单抗）可进一步减少镰状细胞危象，另一种（沃塞洛托）可升高血红蛋白水平。在随机试验中，左旋谷氨酰胺治疗显著降低了镰状细胞危象的发生率，尽管治疗组和对照组的多数患者正在接受羟基脲治疗。左旋谷氨酰胺可能通过增加镰状细胞中还原的烟酰胺腺嘌呤二核苷酸（NAD）来减少氧化应激和可能的疼痛危象。在另一项随机试验中，立赞利珠单抗（一种 P 选择素抑制剂）也可显著减少镰状细胞危象。在炎症状态下，P 选择素可介导白细胞对血管内皮的黏附，导致血管栓塞。沃塞洛托通过稳定含氧血红蛋白的状态以抑制 HbS 多聚化，从而减轻溶血、改善贫血，目前已获批用于治疗镰状细胞贫血。

alloSCT 是镰状细胞贫血的唯一根治方法，但其应用受限于缺乏匹配供者。

其他镰状综合征

血红蛋白 C 在血红蛋白 C（HbC）中，β 链的第 6 个氨基酸由谷氨酸突变为赖氨酸。纯合子 HbC 患者呈轻度贫血，通常无临床症状。血红蛋白 S-C（HbSC）患者是 HbS 和 HbC 的杂合子，通常有临床症状，但较纯合子 HbS（HbSS）患者轻微。HbSC 患者具有较高的血细胞比容，但血液黏度较高会加重视网膜病变。患者通常脾大，但一般不像 HbSS 患者那样出现脾梗死。患者可间断出现急性脾大，继而引起血红蛋白浓度和血细胞比容的显著降低（脾隔离危象）。脾隔离危象也可发生于 HbSS 儿童，但对 HbSS 成人而言，由于脾功能丧失，几乎不会发生此种危象。

镰状细胞 β-地中海贫血 对于 HbS 和 β-地中海贫血的杂合子患者，其疾病严重程度取决于 β-珠蛋白的水平。镰状细胞 β^+-地中海贫血患者的症状较 HbSS 轻微，这可能是由于 HbS 的细胞内浓度降低。镰状细胞 β^0-地中海贫血患者无法产生正常的 β 链（见下文），具有与 HbSS 患者基本相同的表型。

地中海贫血

地中海贫血综合征（表 3.9）是一组异质性疾病，由 α-珠蛋白或 β-珠蛋白链合成减少或缺失所致。重型地中海贫血综合征可引起严重的溶血性贫血，一般在幼年期即可诊断。然而，轻型地中海贫血常仅引起轻微的小细胞性贫血，少见或不出现溶血。由于 MCV 降低，这些疾病常与铁缺乏混淆。

β-地中海贫血 目前发现，可导致 β-地中海贫血的基因突变超过 100 个，这些突变可导致 β-珠蛋白减少或缺如。基因编码区的结构性突变可引起无义突变、信使 RNA（mRNA）中断及受累等位基因不表达（β^0-地中海贫血）。然而，多数突变虽可引起转录、翻译减少或 mRNA 剪接异常，从而导致珠蛋白链产生减少，但一般不会完全阻断 β-珠蛋白的生成（β^+-地中海贫血）。

在 β-地中海贫血中，球蛋白链合成异常导致 β 链生成减少和 α 链相对过量。正常血红蛋白合成的减少导致低色素性贫血，过量的 α 链则形成不可溶的 α 链聚合物，并引发溶血。在轻型地中海贫血综合征中，过量的 α 链不足以引起显著溶血，所以临床主要表现为小细胞性贫血。在重型地中海贫血中，溶血可发生

forms of thalassemia, hemolysis occurs both in the peripheral blood and in the marrow, with intense secondary expansion of the marrow production of RBCs. The expansion of the marrow space causes severe skeletal abnormalities, and the ineffective erythropoiesis also provides a powerful stimulus to absorb iron from the intestine.

The clinical spectrum of β-thalassemia reflects the heterogeneity of the molecular lesions causing the disease (see Table 3.9). β-Thalassemia major results from homozygous $β^0$-thalassemia, leading to severe hemolytic anemia; such patients are diagnosed in infancy and are transfusion dependent from birth. Patients with β-thalassemia intermedia also have two β-thalassemia alleles, but at least one of them is a mild $β^+$ mutation. These patients have severe chronic hemolytic anemia but do not require transfusions. Because of ineffective erythropoiesis, the patients chronically hyperabsorb iron and may develop iron overload in the absence of transfusions. β-Thalassemia minor is usually caused by heterozygous β-thalassemia, although it may reflect the inheritance of two mild thalassemic mutations. These are the patients in whom iron deficiency is often misdiagnosed. Iron studies show normal to increased iron with normal iron saturation. Documentation of a compensatory increase in HbA_2 and HbF on hemoglobin electrophoresis confirms the diagnosis.

α-Thalassemia. α-Thalassemia is almost always caused by mutations that delete one or more of the α-chain loci on chromosome 16. Four α-chain loci exist with two, almost identical, copies of the α-globin gene on each chromosome. The spectrum of α-thalassemia therefore reflects the lack of one, two, three, or all four α-globin genes (see Table 3.9). In general, the clinical manifestations of α-thalassemia are milder than those of β-thalassemia for two reasons. First, the presence of four α-chain genes allows for adequate α-chain synthesis unless three or four loci are deleted. Second, β-chain tetramers are more soluble than their α-chain counterparts and do not cause hemolysis. Patients with the loss of a single α-chain gene are silent carriers and have a normal hematocrit and MCV. Patients with deletion of two α chains, either on the same chromosome (−−/αα, called α-thal 1) or on different chromosomes (−α/−α; α-thal 2), are microcytic and mildly anemic. Patients who inherit one α-thal 1 allele and one α-thal 2 allele (−−/−α) have hemoglobin H disease. Hemoglobin H is the product of excess β-chain production, specifically $β_4$; it causes mild hemolytic anemia and minimal or no intramedullary erythrocyte destruction. Inheritance of the homozygous α-thal 2 allele results in no functional α-chain loci and is incompatible with life. The fetus is unable to make any functional hemoglobin beyond embryonic development because HbF also requires α chains. Free γ chains form tetramers, termed *hemoglobin Barts*. Hemoglobin Barts have an extremely high oxygen affinity, and failure to release oxygen in peripheral tissues results in severe congestive heart failure and anasarca, a clinical picture termed *hydrops fetalis*. Affected fetuses are stillborn or die soon after birth.

Treatment. Though management of patients with thalassemia is mainly supportive (transfusion therapy, folic acid supplementation, iron chelation as needed), a disease-modifying erythroid maturation agent, luspatercept, has recently been approved. Luspatercept binds to specific TGFβ ligands that inhibit aberrant Smad2/3 signaling and results in improved erythropoiesis. A randomized trial of luspatercept demonstrated lowered transfusion burden in adults primarily with β-thalassemia.

More information on the thalassemias, sickle cell disease, and other hemoglobinopathies can be found in Chapter 153, "The Thalassemias," and Chapter 154, "Sickle Cell Disease and Other Hemoglobinopathies," ❖ in *Goldman-Cecil Medicine*, 26th Edition.

PROSPECTUS FOR THE FUTURE

Anemia is increasingly recognized as a marker of increased morbidity and mortality in adults with a wide range of medical conditions, including renal failure, malignancy, cardiac disease, inflammatory conditions, and other chronic diseases. Advances in understanding the pathophysiology of anemia of chronic inflammation are contributing to knowledge of iron metabolism and the roles cytokines play in hematopoiesis. These developments are paving the way for the development of new therapies for patients with anemia and iron overload. Ongoing progress in stem cell transplantation will contribute to the ability to treat and potentially cure various hemoglobinopathies, and gene therapy approaches are also being piloted.

SUGGESTED READINGS

Andrews NC: Forging a field: the golden age of iron biology, Blood 112:219–230, 2008.

Auerbach M, Macdougall I: The available intravenous iron formulations: History, efficacy, and toxicology, Hemodial Int 21:S83–S92, 2017.

Bain BJ: Diagnosis from the blood smear, N Engl J Med 353:498–507, 2005.

Bennett CL, Silver SM, Djulbegovic B, et al: Venous thromboembolism and mortality associated with recombinant erythropoietin and darbepoetin administration for the treatment of cancer-associated anemia, J Am Med Assoc 299:914–924, 2008.

Cappellini MD, et al: The Believe trial: results of a phase 3, randomized, double-blind, placebo-controlled study of luspatercept in adult beta-thalassemia patients who require regular red blood cell (RBC) transfusions. Abstract #164, ASH Annual Meeting, December 1, 2018; San Diego, CA.

Finberg KE: Unraveling mechanisms regulating systemic iron homeostasis, Hematology Am Soc Hematol Educ Program 2011:532–537, 2011.

Ganz T: Anemia of inflammation, N Engl J Med 381:1148–1157, 2019.

Kenneth AI, Kutlar A, Kanter J, et al: Crizanlizumab for the prevention of pain crises in sickle cell disease, N Engl J Med 376:429–439, 2017.

Kidney Disease: Improving Global Outcomes (KDIGO): Anemia Work Group: KDIGO clinical practice guidelines for anemia in chronic kidney disease, Kidney Int Suppl 2:279–335, 2012.

Lee JW, Sicre de Fontbrune F, Wong Lee Lee L, et al: Ravulizumab (ALXN1210) vs eculizumab in adult patients with PNH naïve to complete inhibitors: the 301 study, Blood 133:530–539, 2019.

Lin JC: Approach to anemia in the adult and child. In Hoffman R, Benz EJ, Silberstein LE, et al, editors: Hoffman: hematology—basic principles and practice, ed 7, Philadelphia, 2018, Elsevier, pp 458–467.

Moretti D, Goede JS, Zeder C, et al: Oral iron supplements increase hepcidin and decrease iron absorption from daily or twice-daily doses in iron-depleted young women, Blood 126:1981–1989, 2015.

Niihara Y, et al: A phase 3 trial of L-glutamine in sickle cell disease, N Engl J Med 379:226–235, 2018.

Stabler SP: Vitamin B12 deficiency, N Engl J Med 368:149–160, 2013.

Stoffel NU, Cercamondi CI, Brittenham G, et al: Iron absorption from oral iron supplements given on consecutive versus alternative days and as single morning doses versus twice-daily split in iron-depleted women: two open-label, randomized controlled trials, Lancet Haematol 4:PE524–E533, 2017.

Thompson A, Walters MC, Kwiatkowski J, et al: Gene therapy in patients with transfusion-dependent β-thalassemia, N Engl J Med 378:1479–1493, 2018.

Vichinsky E, Hoppe CC, Ataga KI, et al: A phase 3 randomized trial of voxelotor in sickle cell disease, N Engl J Med 381:509–519, 2019.

Yutaka N, Miller ST, Kanter J, et al: A phase 3 trial of L-glutamine in sickle cell disease, N Engl J Med 379:226–235, 2018.

于外周血和骨髓，骨髓中可继发显著的红系增生。骨髓腔扩张可导致严重的骨骼病变，且无效 RBC 生成也强烈刺激了肠道对铁的吸收。

在 β-地中海贫血中，临床表现的严重程度反映了其分子学异常的异质性（表3.9）。重型 β-地中海贫血由 β^0 纯合子所致，导致严重的溶血性贫血；这类患者在婴儿期即可诊断并终身依赖输血。中间型地中海贫血患者也有2个 β-地中海贫血等位基因，但其中至少包含1个 β^+ 突变。这类患者表现为严重的慢性溶血性贫血，但一般不需要输血。由于无效 RBC 生成，患者长期过度吸收铁，可能在未输血的情况下出现铁过载。轻型 β-地中海贫血通常由杂合子 β-地中海贫血基因引起，也可由2个轻型地中海贫血基因突变所致。轻型患者常被误诊为缺铁性贫血。在这些患者中，铁相关化验可显示血清铁正常或增加，铁饱和度正常。血红蛋白电泳提示 HbA_2 和 HbF 代偿性增加有助于诊断。

α-地中海贫血

α-地中海贫血几乎均由基因突变引起，这些突变导致16号染色体上的1个或多个 α-链基因座缺失。每条16号染色体上均有2个几乎相同的 α-珠蛋白基因，共4个 α-链基因座。α-地中海贫血的严重程度反映了 α-珠蛋白基因缺失的数目（1个、2个、3个或4个）（表3.9）。总体而言，α-地中海贫血的临床表现较 β-地中海贫血轻，原因有二：第一，4个 α-链基因的存在保证了足够的 α-链合成，除非有3个或4个基因座缺失；第二，β-链四聚体较 α-链四聚体溶解性更好，故不引起溶血。单个 α-链基因缺失的患者为无症状携带者，具有正常的血细胞比容和 MCV。在同一染色体（$--/\alpha\alpha$，即 α-thal 1）或不同染色体（$-\alpha/-\alpha$，即 α-thal 2）上缺失两条 α 链的患者表现为轻度小细胞性贫血。同时具有1个 α-thal 1 等位基因和1个 α-thal 2 等位基因（$--/-\alpha$）的患者表现为血红蛋白 H 病。血红蛋白 H 是 β-链过量的产物，特别是 β_4；该病可引起轻度溶血性贫血，几乎不出现原位溶血。α-thal 2 纯合子无法合成 α-链，患者一般不能存活。由于 HbF 的形成也需要 α-链，因此在胚胎发育过程中，胎儿无法合成任何功能性血红蛋白。游离 γ 链形成四聚体，即血红蛋白巴特。血红蛋白巴特对氧气具有极高的亲和力，在外周组织中无法释放氧气，导致严重充血性心力衰竭和全身水肿，临床上称为胎儿水肿综合征。患病胎儿一般为死产，或在出生后不久死亡。

治疗

支持治疗（输血、补充叶酸，必要时祛铁）是地中海贫血患者的主要治疗方法，目前罗特西普（一种改善病情的红细胞成熟促进剂）已获批上市。罗特西普可与特定的 TGFβ 配体结合，抑制异常的 Smad2/3 信号通路，促进红系造血。随机临床试验提示，在成人 β-地中海贫血患者中，罗特西普可有效减少输血。

地中海贫血、镰状细胞贫血和其他血红蛋白病的详细内容见 *Goldman-Cecil Medicine* 第26版第153章"地中海贫血"和第154章"镰状细胞贫血和其他血红蛋白病"。

未来展望

越来越多的研究认为，贫血与多种疾病的并发症发生率及死亡率升高相关，包括肾衰竭、恶性肿瘤、心脏病、炎症性疾病及其他慢性疾病。深入理解慢性炎症性贫血的病理生理学机制有助于研究铁代谢及细胞因子在造血中的作用。这些发展为贫血和铁过载新治疗的研发铺平了道路。干细胞移植技术的持续进展将有助于治疗及治愈多种血红蛋白病，而基因治疗的应用也正在不断拓展。

推荐阅读

Andrews NC: Forging a field: the golden age of iron biology, Blood 112:219–230, 2008.

Auerbach M, Macdougall I: The available intravenous iron formulations: History, efficacy, and toxicology, Hemodial Int 21:S83–S92, 2017.

Bain BJ: Diagnosis from the blood smear, N Engl J Med 353:498–507, 2005.

Bennett CL, Silver SM, Djulbegovic B, et al: Venous thromboembolism and mortality associated with recombinant erythropoietin and darbepoetin administration for the treatment of cancer-associated anemia, J Am Med Assoc 299:914–924, 2008.

Cappellini MD, et al: The Believe trial: results of a phase 3, randomized, double-blind, placebo-controlled study of luspatercept in adult beta-thalassemia patients who require regular red blood cell (RBC) transfusions. Abstract #164, ASH Annual Meeting, December 1, 2018; San Diego, CA.

Finberg KE: Unraveling mechanisms regulating systemic iron homeostasis, Hematology Am Soc Hematol Educ Program 2011:532–537, 2011.

Ganz T: Anemia of inflammation, N Engl J Med 381:1148–1157, 2019.

Kenneth AI, Kutlar A, Kanter J, et al: Crizanlizumab for the prevention of pain crises in sickle cell disease, N Engl J Med 376:429–439, 2017.

Kidney Disease: Improving Global Outcomes (KDIGO): Anemia Work Group: KDIGO clinical practice guidelines for anemia in chronic kidney disease, Kidney Int Suppl 2:279–335, 2012.

Lee JW, Sicre de Fontbrune F, Wong Lee Lee L, et al: Ravulizumab (ALXN1210) vs eculizumab in adult patients with PNH naïve to complete inhibitors: the 301 study, Blood 133:530–539, 2019.

Lin JC: Approach to anemia in the adult and child. In Hoffman R, Benz EJ, Silberstein LE, et al, editors: Hoffman: hematology—basic principles and practice, ed 7, Philadelphia, 2018, Elsevier, pp 458–467.

Moretti D, Goede JS, Zeder C, et al: Oral iron supplements increase hepcidin and decrease iron absorption from daily or twice-daily doses in iron-depleted young women, Blood 126:1981–1989, 2015.

Niihara Y, et al: A phase 3 trial of L-glutamine in sickle cell disease, N Engl J Med 379:226–235, 2018.

Stabler SP: Vitamin B12 deficiency, N Engl J Med 368:149–160, 2013.

Stoffel NU, Cercamondi CI, Brittenham G, et al: Iron absorption from oral iron supplements given on consecutive versus alternative days and as single morning doses versus twice-daily split in iron-depleted women: two open-label, randomized controlled trials, Lancet Haematol 4:PE524–E533, 2017.

Thompson A, Walters MC, Kwiatkowski J, et al: Gene therapy in patients with transfusion-dependent β-thalassemia, N Engl J Med 378:1479–1493, 2018.

Vichinsky E, Hoppe CC, Ataga KI, et al: A phase 3 randomized trial of voxelotor in sickle cell disease, N Engl J Med 381:509–519, 2019.

Yutaka N, Miller ST, Kanter J, et al: A phase 3 trial of L-glutamine in sickle cell disease, N Engl J Med 379:226–235, 2018.

Clinical Disorders of Granulocytes and Monocytes

Ellice Wong, Michal G. Rose, Nancy Berliner

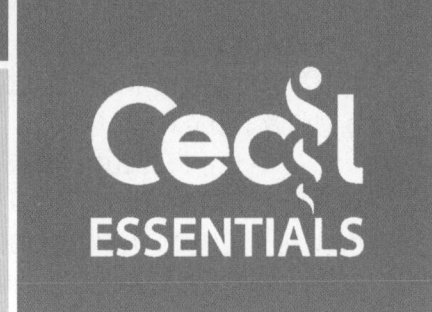

INTRODUCTION

Leukocytes, or white blood cells (WBCs), provide the main defense against bacterial infection. Granulocytes (primarily neutrophils) and monocytes are phagocytic cells that can kill ingested bacteria through the generation of reactive intermediates. Monocytes also release inflammatory mediators that increase the activity of lymphocytes. Lymphocyte function is discussed in Chapter 5.

NORMAL GRANULOCYTE DEVELOPMENT, STRUCTURE, AND FUNCTION

Neutrophils

Neutrophils (i.e., polymorphonuclear leukocytes) are the predominant WBC in the peripheral blood. They are morphologically recognizable by their characteristic segmented nucleus and cytoplasmic granules that are functionally important (Fig. 4.1).

Neutrophils achieve intracellular killing of bacteria through chemotaxis, margination, adhesion, and phagocytosis (Fig. 4.2). *Chemotaxis* is the ordered movement of the cell toward an attracting stimulus, such as bacterial formyl peptides or complement fragments (i.e., C3b and C5a). In *margination,* neutrophils move toward endothelial cells lining the blood vessel walls. Neutrophils attach to endothelial cells by interaction of neutrophil surface glycoproteins (i.e., CD11b/CD18) with endothelial adhesion molecules (i.e., intercellular adhesion molecule 1 and endothelial leukocyte adhesion molecule 1) in a process called *adhesion*. In response to a chemotactic stimulus, the adherent neutrophils move toward the target along the endothelial surface.

The leukocyte adhesion deficiency (LAD) syndromes are associated with impaired migration of leukocytes (particularly neutrophils) from the vasculature into tissues resulting in neutrophilia, inability to form pus, impaired wound healing, and recurrent bacterial infections. This rare group of congenital diseases is characterized by beta integrin defects, selectin receptor abnormalities, as well as loss of the C3b receptor (which mediates opsonin-induced phagocytosis). Disease therefore results both from failure of adhesion and from failure to phagocytose opsonized bacteria.

Phagocytosis requires recognition of target bacteria or debris by the neutrophil. Targets are opsonized by the surface binding of immunoglobulin or complement factor C3b. The neutrophil has surface receptors for C3b and the Fc portion of immunoglobulin G, which allows recognition and binding to the opsonized target. The target then becomes engulfed in a phagocytic vacuole, which fuses with neutrophil granules inside the cell.

Intracellular killing occurs by oxygen-dependent and oxygen-independent mechanisms. Contents of the primary granules, including cathepsin G, defensins, and lysozyme, break down the bacterial cell wall and kill the target organism. However, the major mechanism of bacterial killing is the *respiratory burst.* Stimulation of the neutrophil activates a membrane-bound oxidase complex, which generates superoxide through the transfer of an electron from reduced nicotinamide-adenine dinucleotide phosphate (NADPH). The interaction of superoxide with water generates hydroxyl ions. Myeloperoxidase catalyzes the formation of hypochlorite ion from hydrogen peroxide and chloride. The NADPH oxidase is a multisubunit enzyme. Absence or decreased activity of any one subunit impairs bacterial killing and results in chronic granulomatous disease, a congenital illness in which patients are predisposed to life-threatening bacterial infections.

More recently, *neutrophil extracellular traps (NETS)* have been proposed as an extracellular mechanism for neutrophil-induced antimicrobial activity. Activated neutrophils have been shown to release nucleic acids with histones and granule proteins extracellularly to trap and kill bacteria.

Neutrophil granules give neutrophils their characteristic appearance and have important functions in neutrophil-mediated activation and killing. *Primary granules* arise early in myeloid differentiation and are found in neutrophils and monocytes. They contain a large number of proteins, including myeloperoxidase, acid hydrolases, and neutral proteases. These granules fuse with the phagocytic vacuole and aid in the digestion of ingested bacteria. *Secondary granules* arise later in the differentiation pathway and give the neutrophil its characteristic granular (electron-dense) appearance. These granules contain lactoferrin, transcobalamin, and the matrix-modifying enzymes collagenase and gelatinase. On neutrophil stimulation, the granules are released into the extracellular space. Lactoferrin and transcobalamin act as antibacterial proteins by sequestering iron and vitamin B_{12} away from bacteria, and collagenase and gelatinase break down connective tissue at the site of inflammation.

Abnormalities in neutrophil granules have been described in rare clinical syndromes. Absence of myeloperoxidase produces surprisingly mild symptoms and may be associated with defects in control of fungal infections. Secondary granule deficiency is rare and is associated with a slight increase in the risk of bacterial infections.

Eosinophils and Basophils

In addition to neutrophils, eosinophils and basophils are granulocytes that arise from myeloid precursors in the bone marrow. They transit rapidly from the marrow to the blood and into the peripheral tissues, where they play a role in allergic and inflammatory reactions. Like neutrophils, they have secondary granules that give them a characteristic appearance and are functionally important. Both cell types occur in small numbers under normal conditions.

Although eosinophils are capable of phagocytosis, most of the activity of these cells is mediated through the release of granule

中性粒细胞和单核细胞相关疾病

高海涛 译 唐菲菲 许兰平 审校 黄晓军 通审

引言

白细胞（WBC）在对抗细菌感染时发挥主要作用。粒细胞（主要是中性粒细胞）和单核细胞是吞噬细胞，可以通过产生反应性介质杀死细菌。单核细胞也可以释放炎症介质，增强淋巴细胞的活性。淋巴细胞功能的相关讨论见第 5 章。

正常粒细胞的发育、结构和功能

中性粒细胞

中性粒细胞（即多形核白细胞）是外周血中主要的 WBC，其形态学特点为特征性的分叶核和具有重要功能的胞质颗粒（图 4.1）。

中性粒细胞通过趋化、边集、黏附和吞噬作用杀死胞内细菌（图 4.2）。趋化是指细胞向刺激物 [如细菌甲酰基肽或补体片段（即 C3b 和 C5a）] 有序地移动。边集是指中性粒细胞向血管内皮细胞移动。中性粒细胞通过其表面糖蛋白（即 CD11b/CD18）和内皮黏附分子（即胞内黏附分子 1 和内皮白细胞黏附分子 1）的相互作用黏附在内皮细胞上，该过程被称为黏附。黏附的中性粒细胞遇到趋化刺激后，沿着内皮表面向目标移动。

白细胞黏附缺陷症（LAD）综合征与 WBC（尤其是中性粒细胞）从脉管系统进入组织的迁移受损有关，导致中性粒细胞增多、无法形成脓液、伤口愈合受损和反复细菌感染。这种罕见的先天性疾病的特征是 β 整合素缺陷、选择素受体异常及 C3b 受体（介导调理素诱导的吞噬作用）缺失。因此，疾病既源于黏附失败，也源于未能吞噬调理细菌。

吞噬作用需要中性粒细胞识别目标细菌或碎片。目标细菌通过表面结合免疫球蛋白或补体因子 C3b 而得到调理。中性粒细胞表面存在 C3b 和免疫球蛋白 G 的 Fc 段受体，后者可以识别和结合调理后的细菌。随后，细菌被吞噬至吞噬泡中，后者在胞内与中性粒细胞颗粒融合。

细胞内杀伤通过氧气依赖和非氧气依赖机制进行。初级颗粒的内容物（包括组织蛋白酶 G、防御素和溶菌酶）可以分解细菌细胞壁并杀死目标微生物。然而，杀菌的主要机制为呼吸爆发。中性粒细胞被刺激后可激活膜结合氧化酶复合体，后者可通过还原型烟酰胺腺嘌呤二核苷酸磷酸（NADPH）的电子转移产生超氧化物。超氧化物与水相互作用可产生氢氧离子。髓过氧化物酶催化过氧化氢和氯化氢生成次氯酸离子。NADPH 氧化酶是一种多亚基酶，任何一个亚基的缺失或减少都会降低杀菌活性，并导致慢性肉芽肿病，后者是一种先天性疾病，患者易发生致死性细菌感染。

近年来，中性粒细胞胞外诱捕网（NETS）被认为是中性粒细胞介导抗菌活性的细胞外机制。研究证实，活化的中性粒细胞能释放含有组蛋白的核酸及颗粒蛋白至胞外，用以捕获并杀灭细菌。

中性粒细胞颗粒使中性粒细胞具有特征性形态，并在中性粒细胞介导的激活和杀菌作用中发挥重要功能。初级颗粒在早期髓系分化时出现，可见于中性粒细胞和单核细胞。初级颗粒含有大量蛋白质，包括髓过氧化物酶、酸性水解酶和中性蛋白酶。这些颗粒与吞噬泡融合，有助于对吞噬细菌的消化。次级颗粒在分化过程中较晚出现，使中性粒细胞具有特征性的颗粒状（电子致密）外观。这些颗粒包括乳铁蛋白、钴胺素转运蛋白、基质改良胶原酶和明胶酶。中性粒细胞受到刺激后，颗粒释放至胞外。乳铁蛋白和钴胺素转运蛋白可以螯合铁和维生素 B_{12}，从而发挥抗菌作用，胶原酶和明胶酶则可以分解炎症部位的结缔组织。

中性粒细胞颗粒异常可见于一些罕见的临床综合征。髓过氧化物酶缺失仅会造成轻微的症状，并可能与真菌感染抑制缺陷相关。次级颗粒缺乏很罕见，可导致细菌感染风险的轻微上升。

嗜酸性粒细胞和嗜碱性粒细胞

除中性粒细胞外，嗜酸性粒细胞和嗜碱性粒细胞也起源于骨髓的髓系前体细胞，它们可以很快地从骨髓进入血液及外周组织，参与过敏反应及炎症性反应。与中性粒细胞一样，嗜酸性粒细胞和嗜碱性粒细胞的特征性外观也源自其次级颗粒，后者对细胞功能具有重要意义。正常情况下，嗜酸性粒细胞和嗜碱性粒细胞的数目均较少。

虽然嗜酸性粒细胞具有吞噬作用，但这些细胞的大部分活性通过释放颗粒内容物来调控。寄生虫和螨

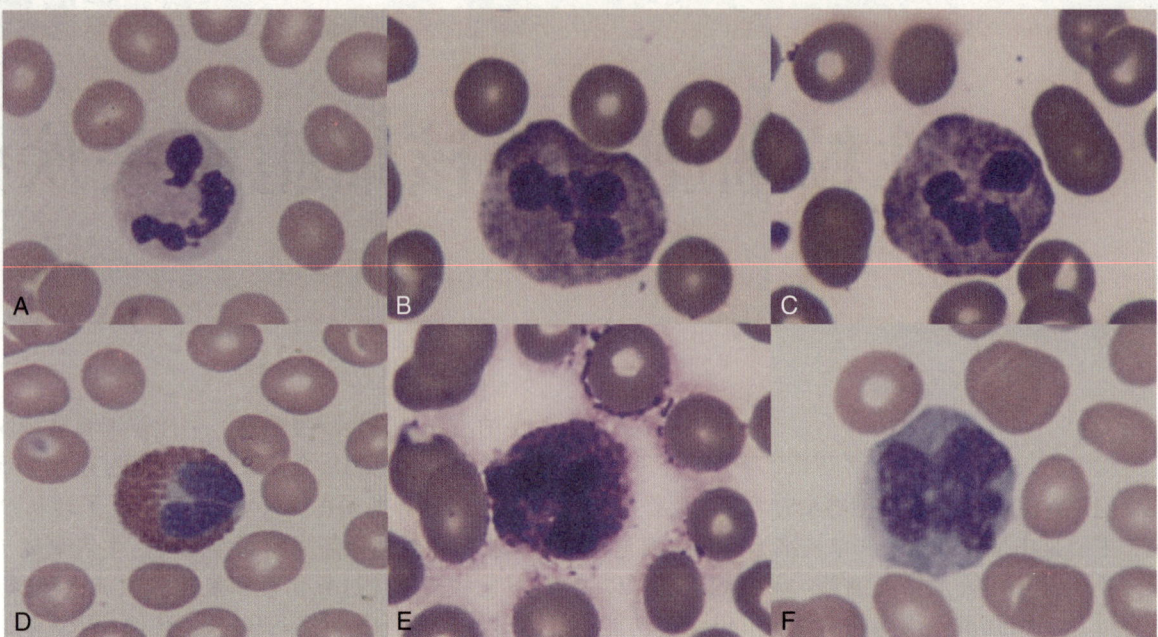

Fig. 4.1 Normal granulocytes and monocytes in peripheral blood. (A to C) Neutrophils (i.e., polymorphonuclear cells). (D) Eosinophils. (E) Basophils. (F) Monocytes. (Courtesy Robert J. Homer, MD, PhD, Yale School of Medicine, New Haven, Conn.)

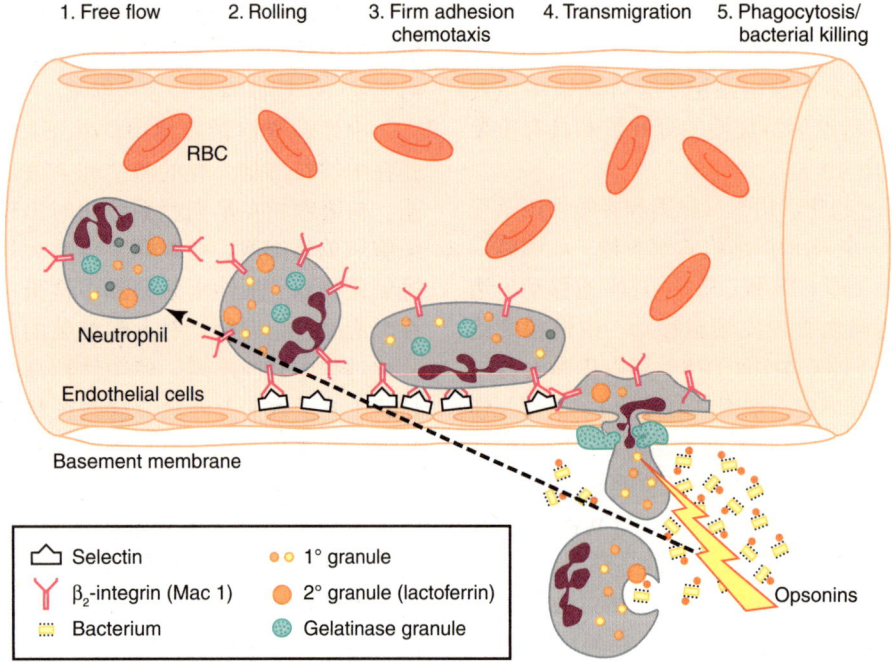

Fig. 4.2 Sequence of neutrophil activation shows the process of rolling, engagement with the vessel wall, attachment, diapedesis, and phagocytosis. *Mac 1*, Macrophage antigen 1 (CD1 lb/CD18); *RBC*, red blood cell.

contents. The eosinophil numbers are elevated in parasitic and helminthic infections, in which these cells are thought to play a role in the allergic response to those organisms. Cell numbers are also elevated in allergic reactions and in collagen vascular diseases, linking their function to immunomodulation. Hypereosinophilic syndromes, in which extremely high levels of eosinophils can be seen, are rare, and hypereosinophilia can be associated with damage to the lung, peripheral nervous system, and endocardial tissues. The differential diagnosis of eosinophilia is outlined in Table 4.1.

Basophils play a role in immediate hypersensitivity reactions and chronic inflammatory conditions including tuberculosis, ulcerative colitis, and rheumatoid arthritis. Their numbers are also notably increased in chronic myeloid leukemia.

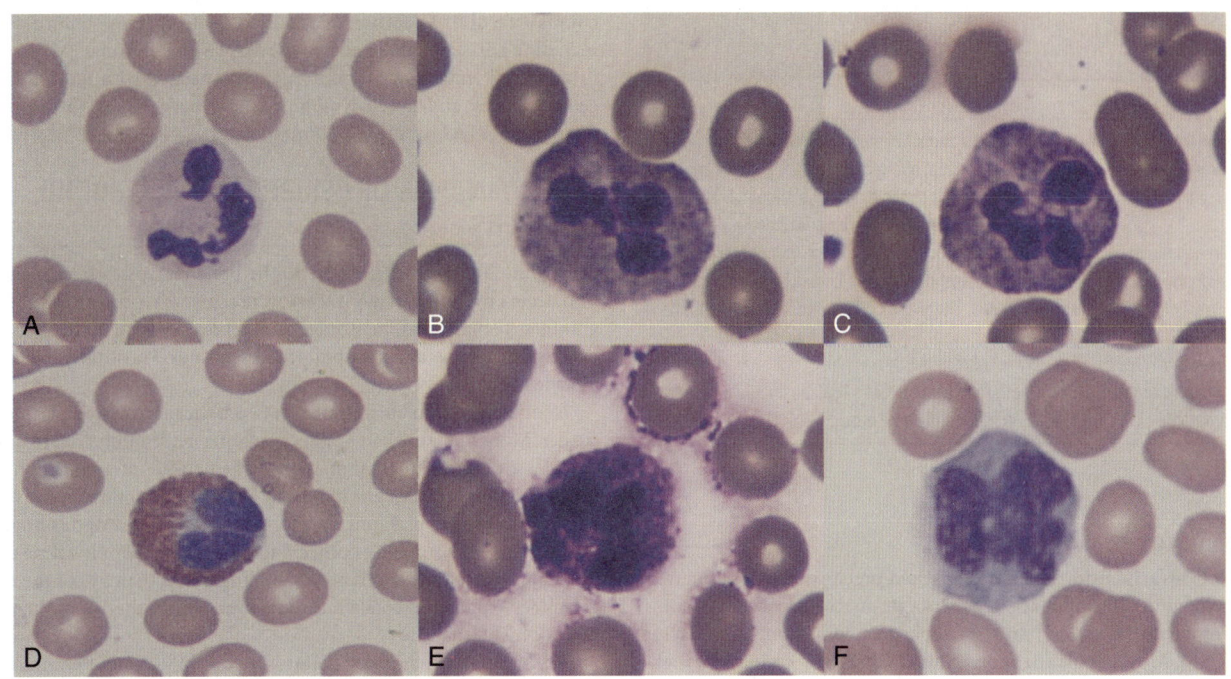

图4.1 外周血中正常的粒细胞和单核细胞。A～C. 中性粒细胞（即多形核白细胞）。D. 嗜酸性粒细胞。E. 嗜碱性粒细胞。F. 单核细胞（经 Robert J. Homer，MD，PhD，Yale School of Medicine，New Haven，Conn. 授权）

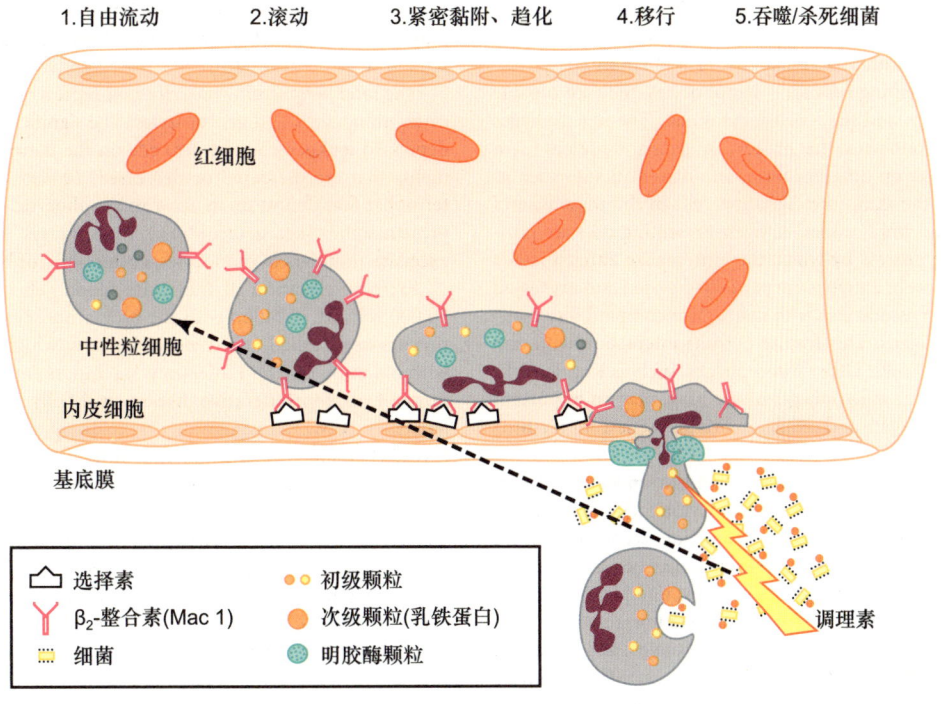

图4.2 中性粒细胞激活顺序：滚动、结合于细胞壁、附着、渗出和吞噬。Mac 1，巨噬细胞抗原-1（CD11b/CD18）；RBC，红细胞

虫感染时嗜酸性粒细胞数量增多，从而参与对这些微生物的过敏反应。出现过敏反应和胶原血管病时，嗜酸性粒细胞也会增多，这与其免疫调节功能相关。高嗜酸性粒细胞增多综合征是一种罕见疾病，患者嗜酸性粒细胞水平极度升高，可对肺、周围神经系统和心内膜组织造成损害。表4.1列出了嗜酸性粒细胞增多症的鉴别诊断。

嗜碱性粒细胞介导速发型超敏反应和慢性炎症性疾病，包括结核、溃疡性结肠炎和类风湿关节炎。在慢性髓系白血病中，嗜碱性粒细胞水平显著升高。

TABLE 4.1 Differential Diagnosis of Eosinophilia

Causes	Comments
Infection[a]	Especially parasites; less commonly mycobacteria
Allergic diseases[a]	Drugs, asthma, allergic rhinitis, atopy, urticaria
Pulmonary diseases[a]	Churg-Strauss disease, Löffler's pneumonia, pulmonary infiltrates with eosinophilia
Drug reactions[a]	Usually disappears when drug discontinued
Malignancy[a]	Paraneoplastic, angioimmunoblastic T-cell lymphoma, Hodgkin's and non-Hodgkin's lymphoma
Connective tissue diseases[a]	Rheumatoid arthritis, eosinophilic fasciitis, vasculitis
Primary hypereosinophilic syndrome	More than 6 months of >1500 eosinophils/μL with no other apparent cause

[a]Reactive forms.

Monocytes

Monocytes arise from a common myeloid precursor along with granulocytes under the influence of granulocyte-macrophage colony-stimulating factor (GM-CSF) and macrophage colony-stimulating factor (M-CSF). Most circulating monocytes are marginated along the walls of blood vessels. They migrate from the vessels into tissues, where they develop into macrophages.

The monocyte-macrophage lineage has many diverse functions. These phagocytic cells perform chemotaxis, phagocytosis, and intracellular killing in much the same manner as neutrophils. They are especially important in killing infectious mycobacterial, fungal, and protozoal species.

Monocytes interact with other components of the immune system. They are antigen-presenting cells for T lymphocytes, they are capable of cellular cytotoxicity, and they secrete cytokines. The macrophages (i.e., differentiated monocytes) that process antigens and present them to T lymphocytes take on different forms in different tissues such as Langerhans cells in the skin, interdigitating cells in the thymus, and dendritic cells in the lymph nodes. Antigen-presenting cells are nonphagocytic, and the process by which they internalize antigen is not fully understood. Protein antigens are partially digested and expressed on the cell surface in association with major histocompatibility complex class II (Ia) antigens. This feature permits interaction with and activation of helper T cells. Other macrophages, such as Kupffer cells of the liver and alveolar macrophages of the lung, play an important role in removing particulate and cellular debris and senescent erythrocytes from the circulation.

Monocytes are capable of antibody-dependent and antibody-independent cytotoxicity against tumor cells. Cytotoxicity is increased by tumor necrosis factor, interleukin-1, and interferon, which are secreted by monocytes. Monocytes secrete large numbers of immunomodulatory proteins (e.g., tumor necrosis factor, interleukin-1, interferon), cytokines (e.g., granulocyte colony-stimulating factor [G-CSF], GM-CSF), coagulation proteins, cell adhesion proteins, and proteases.

Monocytosis can be present in inflammatory as well as primary hematologic conditions. Infections such as tuberculosis, endocarditis, and syphilis are commonly associated with a reactive monocytosis. Hematologic malignancies such as chronic myelomonocytic leukemia, juvenile myelomonocytic leukemia, and some types of acute myeloid leukemia have clonal monocytosis as a hallmark feature. A reactive monocytosis has also been observed in some lymphomas.

Monocytopenia is observed in stress states including severe sepsis and as a result of myelosuppressive chemotherapy. Low monocyte counts can also be found in acquired bone marrow failure states including aplastic anemia and myelodysplastic syndrome (MDS) and in hairy cell leukemia. Monocytopenia associated with natural killer cell deficiency and B-cell lymphoma have been linked to disorders involving GATA2 or SAMD9L mutations.

DETERMINANTS OF PERIPHERAL NEUTROPHIL NUMBERS

Most granulocyte precursors are in the bone marrow, where maturation occurs over 6 to 10 days. Marrow precursors represent 20% of the granulocyte mass, and the storage pool represents 75% of the granulocyte mass. Peripheral neutrophils represent only 5% of the total granulocyte mass.

Neutrophils circulate in transit between the marrow and peripheral tissues. More than one half of the circulating neutrophils adhere to the vascular endothelium (margination). The half-life of a neutrophil in the circulation was thought to be 6 to 12 hours, but more recent studies suggest it may be as long as 3 to 4 days. After neutrophils migrate into tissues, they survive another 1 to 4 days. The peripheral neutrophil count therefore represents a sampling of less than 5% of the total granulocyte pool and is taken during a very short interval of the total neutrophil lifespan.

The peripheral white cell count is a poor reflection of granulocyte kinetics. Abnormalities in neutrophil number can occur rapidly and may reflect a change in marrow granulocyte production or a shift among various cellular compartments. An elevated peripheral white cell count may result from increased marrow production, or it may reflect mobilization of neutrophils from the marginated pool or release from the marrow storage pool. Similarly, a low granulocyte count may reflect decreased marrow production, increased margination or sequestration in the spleen, or increased destruction of peripheral cells.

The *total peripheral white cell count* represents the sum of lymphocytes, monocytes, and granulocytes. The significance of an elevated or depressed leukocyte count depends on the nature of the cellular elements that are increased or decreased. *Leukocytosis* is a nonspecific term that may denote an increase in lymphocytes (i.e., lymphocytosis) or neutrophils (i.e., neutrophilia). In rare cases, increases may reflect excessive numbers of monocytes, eosinophils, or basophils.

Extreme elevation of the white blood cell count to more than 50,000 cells/μL of blood with the premature release of early myeloid precursors is called a *leukemoid reaction*, which may be associated with inflammation and infection. It requires consideration of a diagnosis of myeloproliferative disease, especially chronic myelogenous leukemia (CML). Evaluation of the peripheral blood smear may reveal characteristic changes that provide clues to the underlying disorder. A leukoerythroblastic smear shows immature granulocytes, teardrop-shaped erythrocytes, nucleated erythrocytes, and increased platelets. These changes reflect marrow infiltration (i.e., myelophthisis) by fibrous tissue, granulomas, or neoplasm. As with leukocytosis, leukopenia may reflect lymphopenia or neutropenia. Neutropenia is generally defined by an absolute neutrophil count of less than 1500 cells/μL, although institutional laboratory reference ranges may vary slightly.

NEUTROPHILIA

Neutrophilia usually results from other processes, and it rarely indicates a primary hematologic disorder (Table 4.2). However, patients with a persistently elevated neutrophil count, especially when associated with an elevated hematocrit or platelet count, should be evaluated to rule out a primary myeloproliferative neoplasm. Peripheral blood evaluation for

表 4.1 嗜酸性粒细胞增多症的鉴别诊断

病因	备注
感染[a]	尤其见于寄生虫感染；其次可见于分枝杆菌感染
过敏性疾病[a]	药物、哮喘、过敏性鼻炎、特应性、荨麻疹
肺部疾病[a]	Chrug-Strauss 综合征、Löffler 肺炎、嗜酸性粒细胞肺浸润
药物反应[a]	常在停药后缓解
恶性肿瘤[a]	副肿瘤性、血管免疫母细胞性 T 细胞淋巴瘤、霍奇金淋巴瘤和非霍奇金淋巴瘤
结缔组织病[a]	类风湿关节炎、嗜酸细胞性筋膜炎、血管炎
原发性高嗜酸性粒细胞增多综合征	嗜酸性粒细胞 > 1500/μl，持续 6 个月，除外其他原因

[a] 反应性升高。

单核细胞

单核细胞与粒细胞来自共同的髓系前体细胞，前者受粒细胞-巨噬细胞集落刺激因子（GM-CSF）和巨噬细胞集落刺激因子（M-CSF）的影响，大部分循环的单核细胞沿血管壁边集，从血管迁移至组织中，发育为巨噬细胞。

单核-巨噬细胞系具有多种功能。这些吞噬细胞和中性粒细胞一样，都可以进行趋化、吞噬和细胞内杀伤。这些细胞在杀灭传染性分枝杆菌、真菌和原虫时尤为重要。

单核细胞与免疫系统的其他成分相互作用。它是 T 淋巴细胞的抗原提呈细胞，可以产生细胞毒性，并能分泌特定的细胞因子。巨噬细胞（即已分化的单核细胞）处理抗原并向 T 淋巴细胞提呈，它在不同组织中以不同形式存在：在皮肤中为朗格汉斯细胞，在胸腺中为交错突细胞，在淋巴结中为树突状细胞。抗原提呈细胞为非吞噬性，它们内化抗原的过程尚未完全明确。蛋白质抗原被部分消化，并与 Ⅱ（Ⅰa）型主要组织相容性复合体抗原共同在细胞表面表达。该特点使其可与辅助性 T 细胞相互作用，并激活辅助性 T 细胞。其他巨噬细胞（如肝内的库普弗细胞和肺内的肺泡巨噬细胞）在清除微粒、细胞碎片及循环中衰老的红细胞中发挥着重要作用。

单核细胞可以针对肿瘤细胞产生抗体依赖和非抗体依赖的细胞毒性作用。单核细胞分泌的肿瘤坏死因子、白介素-1 和干扰素可增强细胞毒性。单核细胞可分泌大量免疫调节蛋白（如肿瘤坏死因子、白介素-1、干扰素），细胞因子［如粒细胞集落刺激因子（G-CSF）、GM-CSF］，凝血蛋白，细胞黏附蛋白和蛋白酶。

单核细胞增多症可见于炎症性疾病和原发性血液疾病。结核、心内膜炎及梅毒等常伴有反应性单核细胞增多。血液系统恶性肿瘤（如慢性粒-单核细胞白血病、幼年型粒-单核细胞白血病及某些类型的急性髓系白血病）的特征之一即克隆性单核细胞增多。此外，部分淋巴瘤中亦可观察到反应性单核细胞增多现象。

单核细胞减少症可见于应激状态（包括严重感染中毒症）和骨髓抑制性化疗后。单核细胞计数减少亦可见于获得性骨髓衰竭状态，如再生障碍性贫血、骨髓增生异常综合征（MDS）和毛细胞白血病。与自然杀伤细胞缺乏和 B 细胞淋巴瘤相关的单核细胞减少症已被发现与涉及 GATA2 或 SAMD9L 基因突变的疾病有关。

外周中性粒细胞计数的决定因素

大多数粒细胞前体细胞存在于骨髓中，成熟过程需要 6～10 天。骨髓前体细胞占所有粒细胞的 20%，贮存池占所有粒细胞的 75%。外周血中性粒细胞仅占全部粒细胞的 5%。

中性粒细胞在骨髓和外周组织中转换循环，超过 50% 的循环中性粒细胞黏附于血管内皮（边集）。循环中性粒细胞的半衰期为 6～12 h，但近期研究表明，其半衰期可长达 3～4 天。中性粒细胞迁移至组织后，可以继续存活 1～4 天。因此，外周血中性粒细胞计数占全部粒细胞池的 5% 以下，并仅存在于中性粒细胞寿命中非常短的时间内。

外周血 WBC 计数很难反映粒细胞动力学。中性粒细胞计数异常可快速出现，并可能反映了骨髓粒细胞生成的变化或不同细胞池之间的转换。外周血 WBC 计数减少可源于骨髓生成增多，或反映边缘池中性粒细胞的动员，或来自骨髓贮存池的释放。同理，粒细胞计数减少可反映骨髓生成减少、边集或脾扣留增多，以及外周血细胞破坏增多。

外周血 WBC 总数为淋巴细胞、单核细胞和粒细胞的总和，WBC 计数增多或减少的意义取决于增多或减少的细胞组分的性质。白细胞增多症是一个非特指的术语，可指淋巴细胞增多（即淋巴细胞增多症）或中性粒细胞增多（即中性粒细胞增多症）。有时会出现单核细胞、嗜酸性粒细胞或嗜碱性粒细胞数量同时增多的罕见情况。

血液中 WBC 计数极端升高（> 50 000/μl）并出现早期髓系前体细胞过早释放被称为类白血病反应，可能与炎症和感染相关。当出现类白血病反应时，需考虑骨髓增生性疾病的诊断，尤其是慢性粒细胞白血病（CML）。外周血涂片可反映特征性改变，从而为疾病诊断提供线索。血涂片可见未成熟粒细胞、泪滴状红细胞、有核红细胞及血小板增多。这些改变反映了骨髓被纤维组织、肉芽肿或肿瘤浸润（即脊髓痨）。与白细胞增多症相同，白细胞减少症可指淋巴细胞减少症或中性粒细胞减少症。尽管各机构实验室参考值范围可能略有不同，但中性粒细胞减少症通常被定义为中性粒细胞绝对值 < 1500/μl。

中性粒细胞增多症

中性粒细胞增多症通常继发于其他疾病，很少为原发性血液疾病（表 4.2）。然而，对于中性粒细胞计数持续增多的患者，尤其是血细胞比容或血小板计数也升

TABLE 4.2 Differential Diagnosis of Neutrophilia

Primary Hematologic Disease
Congenital neutrophilia
Leukocyte adhesion deficiency
Myeloproliferative disorders

Due to Other Disease Processes
Infection (acute or chronic)
Acute stress
Drugs (e.g., steroids, lithium)
Cytokine stimulation (e.g., granulocyte colony-stimulating factor)
Chronic inflammation
Malignancy
Myelophthisis
Marrow hyperstimulation
Chronic hemolysis, immune thrombocytopenia
Recovery from marrow suppression
Asplenia
Smoking
Metabolic and endocrine disorders (e.g., pregnancy, eclampsia, thyroid storm, Cushing disease)

TABLE 4.3 Differential Diagnosis of Neutropenia

Decreased Production of Neutrophils	Increased Peripheral Destruction
Congenital and/or constitutional cause	Sepsis
Constitutional neutropenia	Immune destruction
Benign chronic neutropenia	Drug related
Kostmann syndrome	Associated with collagen vascular disease
Cyclic neutropenia	Isoimmune (in newborns)
Postinfectious cause	Large granular lymphocyte leukemia
Nutritional deficiency (B_{12}, folate, copper)	Hypersplenism and/or sequestration
Drug-induced cause	
Primary marrow failure	
Aplastic anemia	
Myelodysplastic syndromes	
Acute leukemias	

the BCR/ABL fusion product can be performed to consider CML, and assays for JAK2 V617F, JAK2 exon 12, calreticulin, and MPL mutations can help to consider non-CML myeloproliferative neoplasms.

Neutrophilia related to acute infection, stress, toxic exposures like smoking, or corticosteroid administration primarily reflects demargination and is usually transient. Persistent neutrophilia usually reflects chronic bone marrow stimulation. Nevertheless, a bone marrow aspirate and biopsy are rarely indicated in the work-up of neutrophilia. The exception is for patients who demonstrate leukoerythroblastic changes, for which a bone marrow examination and culture may be indicated to consider tuberculosis or fungal infection, marrow infiltration with tumor, or marrow fibrosis. Cytogenetic and molecular studies should be performed to help eliminate the diagnosis of marrow malignancies, and the marrow should be cultured for mycobacteria and fungi.

NEUTROPENIA

Differential Diagnosis

Neutropenia may reflect decreased production, increased sequestration, or peripheral destruction of neutrophils (Table 4.3). Patients should first be evaluated for splenomegaly to consider the possibility of sequestration.

For patients who are asymptomatic and for whom previous studies are unavailable, the possibility of constitutional or cyclic neutropenia should be entertained and can be evaluated by serial peripheral blood counts. The normal neutrophil count varies among ethnic groups and is most commonly lower in individuals with African ancestry as compared to white individuals (i.e., constitutional or benign ethnic neutropenia [BEN]). The absence of the red blood cell Duffy antigen has been demonstrated to be associated with BEN. As the Duffy antigen is utilized by the parasite *Plasmodium vivax* to enter the red blood cell, it is believed that positive selection for the null allele enabled individuals in West Africa to be protected against malaria and have a survival advantage. Cyclic neutropenia is a relatively benign disorder, in which cyclical changes occur in all hematopoietic cell lines but are most dramatic in the neutrophil lineage. At the nadir of the neutrophil counts, patients may have infections, but the condition is often clinically silent.

In contrast, patients with congenital agranulocytosis or severe congenital neutropenia (SCN) exhibit profound neutropenia and infections in the perinatal period. Kostmann syndrome is a subset of SCN that was described more than 50 years ago as an autosomal recessive disorder; later studies demonstrated that SCN can reflect autosomal dominant, autosomal recessive, X-linked, or sporadic mutations.

About 50% of autosomal dominant SCN and almost 100% of cyclic neutropenia cases are associated with inherited mutations in the neutrophil elastase gene. The mutations are thought to produce a misfolded neutrophil elastase protein, which accumulates in the endoplasmic reticulum and activates the unfolded protein response. This complex cellular stress response coordinates the degradation of misfolded protein in the endoplasmic reticulum and can trigger cellular apoptosis if the stress is severe. Later studies have established that autosomal recessive SCN (i.e., Kostmann syndrome) is caused by mutations in the *HAX1* gene, which encodes a mitochondrial protein that is required for stabilization of the mitochondrial membrane. Absence of HAX1 results in loss of the mitochondrial membrane potential and induction of apoptosis.

Until G-CSF became available, most patients with SCN died in early childhood, but the availability of cytokine therapy has prolonged survival. However, SCN is also associated with a significantly increased incidence of acute leukemia, a complication that has become apparent as patients survive longer. Up to 30% of patients with SCN develop acute myelogenous leukemia over 10 years. Acute myelogenous leukemia in these patients is often associated with truncation mutations in the G-CSF receptor. These acquired somatic mutations may contribute to the pathogenesis of leukemia but do not contribute to the congenital neutropenia. The role of the G-CSF receptor mutations in the pathogenesis of leukemic transformation is controversial, as is the relationship between G-CSF therapy and the acquisition of these mutations.

Neutropenia may occur during or after viral, bacterial, or mycobacterial infections. Postviral neutropenia is especially common in children and probably reflects increased neutrophil consumption and a viral suppression of marrow neutrophil production. Neutropenia may be seen as a complication of overwhelming sepsis and is associated with a poor prognosis.

Drug-induced neutropenia may reflect dose-dependent marrow suppression or an idiosyncratic immune response. The former is one of the most common complications of chemotherapeutic drugs and is also common with antibiotics such as sulfamethoxazole-trimethoprim.

表 4.2　中性粒细胞增多症的鉴别诊断
原发性血液疾病
先天性中性粒细胞增多症
白细胞黏附缺陷症
骨髓增生性疾病
继发于其他疾病
感染（急性或慢性）
急性应激
药物（如类固醇、锂剂）
细胞因子刺激（如粒细胞集落刺激因子）
慢性炎症
恶性肿瘤
脊髓痨
骨髓刺激过度
慢性溶血、免疫性血小板减少症
骨髓抑制恢复
脾切除术后
吸烟
代谢性疾病和内分泌疾病（如妊娠、子痫、甲状腺危象、库欣病）

表 4.3　中性粒细胞减少症的鉴别诊断	
中性粒细胞生成减少	外周破坏增多
先天性和（或）体质性病因	感染中毒症
体质性中性粒细胞减少症	免疫性破坏
良性慢性中性粒细胞减少症	药物相关
Kostmann 综合征	与胶原血管病相关
周期性中性粒细胞减少症	同种免疫（新生儿）
感染后	大颗粒淋巴细胞白血病
营养缺乏（维生素 B_{12}、叶酸、铜）	脾功能亢进和（或）脾扣留
药物诱导	
原发性骨髓衰竭	
再生障碍性贫血	
骨髓增生异常综合征	
急性白血病	

高的患者，应进行评估，以除外原发性骨髓增殖性肿瘤（MPN）。评估外周血 *BCR/ABL* 融合基因可排除 CML，而 *JAK2 V617F*、JAK2 第 12 号外显子、钙网蛋白和 *MPL* 突变检测有助于排除非 CML 骨髓增殖性肿瘤。

与急性感染、应激、有毒物质暴露（吸烟等）或应用皮质类固醇相关的中性粒细胞增多症主要由贮存池向边缘池释放所致，常为一过性。持续性中性粒细胞增多通常反映慢性骨髓刺激。然而，中性粒细胞增多症的病因筛查很少需要进行骨髓穿刺和活检，但对于出现幼粒幼红细胞增多者，需要进行骨髓检查和培养，以排除结核或真菌感染、肿瘤骨髓浸润或骨髓纤维化。应进行骨髓细胞遗传学和分子生物学检查，以排除骨髓恶性肿瘤，并进行骨髓分枝杆菌和真菌培养。

中性粒细胞减少症

鉴别诊断

中性粒细胞减少反映了中性粒细胞生成减少、脾扣留增多或外周破坏增多（表 4.3）。患者应先评估脾大，以排除扣留的可能性。

对于无症状和无既往检查结果的患者，应考虑体质性或周期性中性粒细胞减少症的可能性，并通过连续外周血计数进行评估。不同人种中性粒细胞计数的正常值各异，与白人相比，非裔人群的中性粒细胞水平通常较低［即体质性或良性种族性中性粒细胞减少症（BEN）］。红细胞 Duffy 抗原缺失已被证实与 BEN 相关。由于 Duffy 抗原是疟原虫进入红细胞的媒介，因此，人们认为对缺失等位基因的自然选择使得西非人群能够得到保护，免受疟疾的侵害并获得了生存优势。周期性中性粒细胞减少症是一种相对良性的疾病，患者的所有造血细胞系均会出现周期性改变，但中性粒细胞系的变化最为显著。患者的中性粒细胞计数处于谷值时可能发生感染，但临床上通常较为隐匿。相反，先天性粒细胞缺乏症或严重先天性中性粒细胞减少症（SCN）患者的中性粒细胞显著减少，围生期即可出现感染。Kostmann 综合征是 SCN 的一个亚类，这是 50 多年前发现的一种常染色体隐性遗传病，后续研究发现 SCN 可呈常染色体显性遗传、常染色体隐性遗传、X 连锁遗传或由散发性突变导致。

约 50% 由常染色体显性遗传的 SCN 和几乎 100% 的周期性中性粒细胞减少症患者与中性粒细胞弹性蛋白酶基因遗传性突变相关。这些突变生成一种错误折叠的中性粒细胞弹性蛋白酶蛋白，后者在内质网积累并激活未折叠蛋白应答。该复杂的细胞应激反应协调内质网中错误折叠蛋白的降解，严重应激时可触发细胞凋亡。后期研究发现，常染色体隐性遗传的 SCN（即 Kostmann 综合征）由 *HAX1* 基因突变引起，该基因编码一种用于稳定线粒体膜的线粒体蛋白。HAX1 缺乏可引起线粒体膜电位的丢失，并诱导细胞凋亡。

在 G-CSF 上市之前，大部分 SCN 患者在童年早期即死亡，细胞因子治疗的出现延长了这些患者的生存期。然而，SCN 也与急性白血病的发病率显著上升相关，后者会随患者存活时间的延长而明显增加。30% 的 SCN 患者会在 10 年内出现急性髓系白血病。这些急性髓系白血病常与 G-CSF 受体的截短突变相关，这些获得性突变可能是白血病的致病机制，但不会引起先天性中性粒细胞减少症。G-CSF 受体突变在白血病转化的发病机制中的作用尚存争议，且 G-CSF 治疗与获得以上突变的关系也存在争议。

病毒感染、细菌感染或分枝杆菌感染期间或感染后会出现中性粒细胞减少。病毒感染后中性粒细胞减少在儿童中尤为常见，这可能反映了中性粒细胞消耗增加和病毒感染抑制骨髓生成中性粒细胞。中性粒细胞减少症也可能是严重感染中毒症的一种并发症，预后很差。

药物诱导的中性粒细胞减少症可由剂量依赖性骨髓抑制和体质性免疫反应所致，前者是化疗药物最常见的并发症，也常见于抗生素使用后，如磺胺甲噁唑-甲氧苄啶。氯霉素可导致体质性再生障碍性贫血，也

Chloramphenicol causes dose-dependent marrow suppression, although its more ominous complication is the rare idiosyncratic reaction that gives rise to marrow aplasia. Drugs that are most commonly associated with neutropenia include clozapine, sulfasalazine, ticlopidine, and the thionamide antithyroid agents. Most drug-induced neutropenias respond rapidly to discontinuation of the offending agent. The administration of G-CSF may speed recovery.

Autoimmune neutropenia may be seen as a primary disease or as a secondary manifestation of systemic autoimmune disease or lymphoproliferative disease. Primary autoimmune neutropenia is a disorder of infants and young children that resolves spontaneously in more than 90% of patients within 2 years. Secondary autoimmune neutropenia is a common accompaniment to systemic lupus erythematosus. Although not usually clinically severe, neutropenia is often a marker of disease activity.

Neutropenia in rheumatoid arthritis may be associated with splenomegaly (i.e., Felty syndrome) and is part of the spectrum of large granular lymphocyte (LGL) leukemia. LGL leukemia is a clonal expansion of suppressor T cells. Patients who develop LGL leukemia in association with rheumatoid arthritis share a common HLA-DR4 haplotype with patients with Felty syndrome, suggesting that they are in a common spectrum of disease. LGL leukemia is also a relatively common cause of acquired neutropenia in elderly patients in the absence of rheumatoid arthritis. Recent data have linked LGL leukemia to mutations in the *STAT3* gene.

Laboratory Evaluation

Unless the diagnosis of benign ethnic or cyclic neutropenia is likely, the evaluation of the patient with neutropenia should include stopping all potentially offending drugs and performing serologic studies to rule out collagen vascular disease. Unlike the evaluation of patients with leukocytosis, bone marrow examination is indicated early for those with neutropenia and is frequently diagnostic. Neutropenia often reflects primary hematologic disease, and bone marrow examination enables the physician to diagnose marrow failure syndromes, leukemia, and MDS. In the absence of bone marrow failure, other causes of neutropenia may give a characteristic bone marrow picture. All patients undergoing bone marrow examination should have cytogenetic and molecular studies performed to aid in the diagnosis of MDS.

Sudden onset of agranulocytosis that does not affect platelets or erythrocytes typically is attributable to drug or toxin exposure. Bone marrow examination is rarely necessary. If performed, drug-induced neutropenia produces a characteristic maturation arrest of myeloid cells. Rather than actual inhibition of neutrophil maturation, this feature reflects the immune destruction of myeloid precursors that leaves only the earliest cells behind.

Treatment

The therapeutic approach to patients with neutropenia depends on the degree of depression of the neutrophil count. Neutrophil counts between 1000 and 1500 cells/µL are not usually associated with significant impairment of the host response to bacterial infection and require no intervention beyond that demanded for diagnosis and treatment of the underlying cause. Patients with neutrophil counts between 500 and 1000 cells/µL should be alerted to their slightly increased risk of infection, although serious problems are rarely encountered in patients with functional neutrophils and counts higher than 500 cells/µL.

Patients with neutrophil counts lower than 500 cells/µL are at significant risk for infection, although this is especially true of patients with acute or chemotherapy-induced neutropenia. In contrast, patients with chronic idiopathic neutropenia may be asymptomatic with absolute neutrophil counts below 100. All patients with neutrophil counts below 500 cells/µL should be instructed to notify the physician at the first sign of infection or fever, and they must be managed aggressively with intravenous antibiotics regardless of the documentation of a source or infecting organism. Patients with a significantly depressed neutrophil count may exhibit few signs of infection because much of the inflammatory response at the site of infection is generated by the neutrophils themselves.

In patients with severe immune-mediated neutropenia, corticosteroids and intravenous immunoglobulin may be helpful in elevating the neutrophil count and in preventing infectious complications. G-CSF may increase the peripheral white cell count and may help resolve infections in neutropenia induced by drugs, including chemotherapy. It has been efficacious for some patients with immune-mediated neutropenia and those with MDS.

For a deeper discussion of these topics, please see Chapter 158, "Leukocytosis and Leukopenia" in *Goldman-Cecil Medicine*, 26th Edition.

PROSPECTUS FOR THE FUTURE

Significant progress has been made in elucidating the molecular pathogenesis of severe congenital neutropenia and cyclic neutropenia. Compounds that modulate the unfolded protein response may play a role in the treatment of these disorders. Other studies of the molecular basis of myeloid differentiation are establishing the importance of transcription factor function in neutrophil maturation and are providing insights into the pathogenesis of leukemia and myelodysplasia. Their findings may delineate pathways with entry points for therapeutic intervention in myeloid malignancies.

SUGGESTED READINGS

Aktari M, Curtis B, Waller EK: Autoimmune neutropenia in adults, Autoimmun Rev 9:62–68, 2009.

Andres E, Maloisel F: Idiosyncratic drug-induced agranulocytosis and acute neutropenia, Curr Opin Hematol 15:15–21, 2008.

Beekman R: Touw IP: G-CSF and its receptor in myeloid malignancy, Blood 115:5131–5136, 2010.

Berliner N: Lessons from congenital neutropenia: 50 years of progress in understanding myelopoiesis, Blood 111:5427–5432, 2008.

Berliner N: Leukocytosis and leukopenia. In Goldman L, Schafer AI, editors: Goldman-Cecil Medicine, ed 26, Philadelphia, 2019, Elsevier Saunders.

Brinkmann V, Reichard U, Goosmann C, et al: Neutrophil extracellular traps kill bacteria, Science 303:1532–1535, 2004.

Dinauer MC, Coates TD: Disorders of phagocyte function. In Hoffman R, Benz EJ, Heslop H, Weitz J, editors: Hematology: basic principles and practice, ed 7, Philadelphia, 2018, Elsevier, pp 691–709.

Glogauer M: Disorders of phagocyte function. In Goldman L, Schafer AI, editors: Goldman-Cecil Medicine, Philadelphia, 2011, Elsevier Saunders, p 24.

Mortaz E, Alipoor SD, Adcock IM, Mumby S, Koenderman L: Update on Neutrophil Function in Severe Inflammation, Front Immunol 9:1–14, 2018.

Nauseef WM, Borregaard N: Neutrophils at work, Nature Immunology 15:602–611, 2014.

Pillay J, den Braber I, Vrisekoop N, et al: In vivo labeling with 2H$_2$O reveals a human neutrophil lifespan of 5.4 days, Blood 116:625–627, 2010.

Rappoport N, Simon AJ, Amariglio N, Rechavi G: The Duffy antigen receptor for chemokines, ACKR1,- 'Jeanne DARC' of benign neutropenia, Br J Haematol 184:497–507, 2019.

Xia J, Link DC: Severe congenital neutropenia and the unfolded protein response, Curr Opin Hematol 15:1–7, 2008.

Yipp BG, Paul K: NETosis: how vital is it? Blood 122:2784–2794, 2013.

Zhang R, Shah MV, Loughran Jr TP: The root of many evils: indolent large granular lymphocyte leukaemia and associated disorders, Hematol Oncol 28:105–117, 2010.

可引起剂量依赖性骨髓抑制。最常引起中性粒细胞减少症的药物包括氯氮平、柳氮磺吡啶、噻氯匹定和硫酰胺类抗甲状腺药物。停用相关药物后大多数中性粒细胞减少症可快速缓解。应用 G-CSF 可加速缓解。

自身免疫性中性粒细胞减少症分为原发性或继发性（继发于系统性自身免疫病或淋巴细胞增生性疾病）。原发性自身免疫性中性粒细胞减少症见于婴幼儿，90% 以上的患者可在 2 年内自发缓解。继发性自身免疫性中性粒细胞减少症通常是系统性红斑狼疮的合并症，虽然在临床上通常不严重，但常可以反映疾病活动度。

类风湿关节炎出现中性粒细胞减少与脾大（即 Felty 综合征）相关，是大颗粒淋巴细胞（LGL）白血病谱系的一部分。LGL 白血病是抑制性 T 细胞的克隆性扩增。类风湿关节炎伴有 LGL 白血病的患者与 Felty 综合征患者具有相同的 HLA-DR4 单体型，提示两者属于相同的疾病谱系。对于无类风湿关节炎的老年患者，LGL 白血病也是获得性中性粒细胞减少症的一种相对常见的病因。近期数据发现，LGL 白血病与 STAT3 基因突变有关。

实验室评估

除非疑诊良性种族性或周期性中性粒细胞减少症，否则中性粒细胞减少症患者的评估应包括停用所有可能致病的药物和进行血清学检查，以除外胶原血管病。与评估白细胞增多症患者不同，中性粒细胞减少症患者应早期进行骨髓检查，以协助诊断。中性粒细胞减少常反映原发性血液疾病，骨髓检查有助于诊断骨髓衰竭综合征、白血病和 MDS。如果不存在骨髓衰竭，其他病因引起的中性粒细胞减少症可能会有特征性骨髓图像。所有进行骨髓检查的患者均应进行细胞遗传学和分子学检查，这有助于诊断 MDS。

不影响血小板或红细胞且突然起病的粒细胞缺乏症通常由药物或毒素暴露引起，一般不需要进行骨髓检查。如果对药物诱导的中性粒细胞减少症患者进行骨髓检查，其典型形态为髓系细胞成熟停滞，该特征反映了髓系前体细胞遭到免疫系统破坏，仅剩最早期的细胞，而不是对中性粒细胞成熟产生抑制。

治疗

中性粒细胞减少症患者的治疗取决于中性粒细胞计数减少的程度。中性粒细胞计数为 1000～1500/μl 通常不会严重损害宿主对细菌感染的应答，因此除了诊断和治疗基础疾病外，无须其他干预。尽管中性粒细胞功能正常及计数 > 500/μl 的患者很少出现严重的问题，但中性粒细胞计数为 500～1000/μl 的患者应注意感染风险的轻度增加。

中性粒细胞计数 < 500/μl 的患者感染风险显著增加，尤其是急性出现的或化疗所致的中性粒细胞减少症。相比之下，慢性特发性中性粒细胞减少症患者可能无症状，即使其中性粒细胞绝对值 < 100/μl。对于所有中性粒细胞计数 < 500/μl 的患者，当出现感染或发热时应第一时间就诊，无论是否明确病原体或感染灶，均应积极给予静脉输注抗生素。中性粒细胞计数显著减少的患者很少会出现感染征象，因为感染灶内大部分炎症反应是由中性粒细胞本身产生的。

对于严重的免疫介导的中性粒细胞减少症患者，糖皮质激素和静脉免疫球蛋白可能有助于增加中性粒细胞计数和预防感染并发症。G-CSF 可增加外周血 WBC 计数，有助于治疗药物（包括化疗）诱导的中性粒细胞减少症患者的感染。G-CSF 对于部分免疫介导的中性粒细胞减少症和 MDS 患者也有效。

有关此专题的深入讨论，请参阅 Goldman-Cecil Medicine 第 26 版第 158 章"白细胞增多症和白细胞减少症"。

未来展望

人们在阐明严重先天性中性粒细胞减少症和周期性中性粒细胞减少症的分子机制方面已取得重大进展，调控未折叠蛋白应答的药物可能对上述疾病有效。对髓系分化的分子机制研究确立了中性粒细胞成熟过程中转录因子功能的重要性，为白血病和骨髓增生异常的发病机制提供了理论基础。以上发现为髓系恶性肿瘤的治疗提供了切入点。

推荐阅读

Aktari M, Curtis B, Waller EK: Autoimmune neutropenia in adults, Autoimmun Rev 9:62–68, 2009.

Andres E, Maloisel F: Idiosyncratic drug-induced agranulocytosis and acute neutropenia, Curr Opin Hematol 15:15–21, 2008.

Beekman R: Touw IP: G-CSF and its receptor in myeloid malignancy, Blood 115:5131–5136, 2010.

Berliner N: Lessons from congenital neutropenia: 50 years of progress in understanding myelopoiesis, Blood 111:5427–5432, 2008.

Berliner N: Leukocytosis and leukopenia. In Goldman L, Schafer AI, editors: Goldman-Cecil Medicine, ed 26, Philadelphia, 2019, Elsevier Saunders.

Brinkmann V, Reichard U, Goosmann C, et al: Neutrophil extracellular traps kill bacteria, Science 303:1532–1535, 2004.

Dinauer MC, Coates TD: Disorders of phagocyte function. In Hoffman R, Benz EJ, Heslop H, Weitz J, editors: Hematology: basic principles and practice, ed 7, Philadelphia, 2018, Elsevier, pp 691–709.

Glogauer M: Disorders of phagocyte function. In Goldman L, Schafer AI, editors: Goldman-Cecil Medicine, Philadelphia, 2011, Elsevier Saunders, p 24.

Mortaz E, Alipoor SD, Adcock IM, Mumby S, Koenderman L: Update on Neutrophil Function in Severe Inflammation, Front Immunol 9:1–14, 2018.

Nauseef WM, Borregaard N: Neutrophils at work, Nature Immunology 15:602–611, 2014.

Pillay J, den Braber I, Vrisekoop N, et al: In vivo labeling with $2H_2O$ reveals a human neutrophil lifespan of 5.4 days, Blood 116:625–627, 2010.

Rappoport N, Simon AJ, Amariglio N, Rechavi G: The Duffy antigen receptor for chemokines, ACKR1,- 'Jeanne DARC' of benign neutropenia, Br J Haematol 184:497–507, 2019.

Xia J, Link DC: Severe congenital neutropenia and the unfolded protein response, Curr Opin Hematol 15:1–7, 2008.

Yipp BG, Paul K: NETosis: how vital is it? Blood 122:2784–2794, 2013.

Zhang R, Shah MV, Loughran Jr TP: The root of many evils: indolent large granular lymphocyte leukaemia and associated disorders, Hematol Oncol 28:105–117, 2010.

5

Disorders of Lymphocytes

Iris Isufi, Stuart Seropian

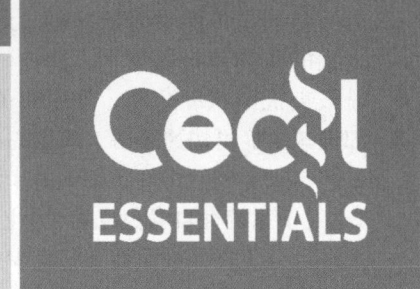

INTRODUCTION

The central cell of the immune system is the lymphocyte. Lymphocytes mediate the adaptive immune response, providing specificity to the immune system by responding to specific pathogens and conferring long-lasting immunity to reinfection. Lymphocytes are derived from hematopoietic stem cells that reside in the bone marrow and give rise to all of the cellular elements of the blood. The two major functional classes of lymphocytes—B lymphocytes (B cells) and T lymphocytes (T cells)—are distinguished by their site of development, antigenic receptors, and function.

The major disorders of lymphocytes include neoplastic transformations of specific subsets of lymphocytes that result in an array of lymphomas or leukemias, congenital or acquired defects in lymphocyte development or function with resultant immunodeficiency, and physiologic responses to infection or antigenic stimulation that lead to lymphadenopathy, lymphocytosis, or lymphocytopenia.

LYMPHOCYTE DEVELOPMENT, FUNCTION, AND LOCALIZATION

B Cells

B cells are characterized by surface immunoglobulins (i.e., antibodies). Their major function is to mount a humoral immune response to antigens by producing antigen-specific antibodies.

B cells develop in the bone marrow in a series of highly coordinated steps that involve sequential rearrangement of the heavy- and light-chain immunoglobulin genes and expression of B-cell–specific cell surface proteins (Fig. 5.1). Rearrangement of the immunoglobulin genes results in generation of a large repertoire of B cells that are each characterized by an immunoglobulin molecule with unique antigenic specificity. Mature B cells migrate from the bone marrow to lymphoid tissue throughout the body and are readily identified by cell surface immunoglobulin and antigens that are B cell specific, including CD19, CD20, and CD21.

In response to antigen binding to cell surface immunoglobulin, mature B cells are activated to proliferate and undergo differentiation to end-stage plasma cells, which lose most of their B-cell surface markers and produce large quantities of soluble antibodies. Neoplastic disorders of B cells arise from B cells at different stages of development, and B-cell lymphomas can have highly varied morphology and cell surface expression of B-cell antigens (i.e., immunophenotype).

T Cells

T cells perform an array of functions in the immune response, including those that are regarded as classic cellular immune responses. T-cell precursors migrate from the bone marrow to the thymus, where they differentiate into mature T-cell subsets and undergo selection to eliminate autoreactive T cells that respond to self-peptides. In the thymus, T-cell precursors undergo a coordinated process of differentiation that involves rearrangement and expression of the T-cell receptor (TCR) genes and acquisition of cell surface proteins that are unique to T cells, including CD3, CD4, and CD8.

As T cells mature in the thymus, they ultimately lose the CD4 or CD8 protein. Mature T cells are composed of two major groups: $CD4^+$ and $CD8^+$ cells. After T-cell maturation and selection in the thymus, mature $CD4^+$ and $CD8^+$ T cells migrate to lymph nodes, spleen, and other sites in the peripheral immune system. Mature T cells constitute about 80% of peripheral blood lymphocytes, 40% of lymph node cells, and 25% of splenic lymphoid cells.

Mature $CD4^+$ and $CD8^+$ T-cell subsets mediate distinct immune functions. $CD8^+$ cells *(cytotoxic T cells)* kill virus-infected or foreign cells and suppress immune functions. $CD4^+$ cells *(helper T cells)* activate other immune cells such as B cells and macrophages by producing cytokines and through direct cell contact.

Similar to B cells, T cells express unique TCR molecules that recognize specific peptide antigens. In contrast to B cells, T cells respond only to peptides that are processed intracellularly and bound to (or presented by) specialized cell surface antigen-presenting proteins, designated major histocompatibility complex (MHC) molecules. $CD4^+$ and $CD8^+$ T cells are MHC class restricted in their response to peptide-MHC complexes. $CD4^+$ cells recognize antigenic peptide fragments when they are presented by MHC class II molecules, and $CD8^+$ cells recognize antigenic peptide fragments when they are presented by MHC class I molecules. Binding of the TCR by a specific peptide-MHC complex triggers activation signals that lead to the expression of gene products that mediate the wide diversity of helper functions of $CD4^+$ cells or cytotoxic effector functions of $CD8^+$ cells.

Lymphoid System

Lymphocytes localize to peripheral lymphoid tissue, which is the site of antigen-lymphocyte interaction and lymphocyte activation. The peripheral lymphoid tissue is composed of lymph nodes, the spleen, and mucosal lymphoid tissue. Lymphocytes circulate continuously through these tissues through the vascular and lymphatic systems.

Lymph nodes are highly organized lymphoid tissues that are sites of convergence of the lymphatic drainage system, which carries antigens from draining lymph to the nodes, where they are trapped. A lymph node consists of an outer cortex and an inner medulla (Fig. 5.2). The cortex is organized into lymphoid follicles composed predominantly of B cells. Some of the follicles contain central areas or germinal centers, where activated B cells proliferate after encountering a specific antigen, that are surrounded by a mantle zone. The T cells are distributed more diffusely in paracortical areas surrounding follicles.

淋巴细胞疾病

阎禹廷 译 易树华 邱录贵 审校 王建祥 通审

引言

淋巴细胞是免疫系统的核心细胞。淋巴细胞介导适应性免疫反应，通过响应特定病原体为免疫系统提供特异性，并对再次感染产生长期免疫力。淋巴细胞来源于骨髓中的造血干细胞，后者能够生成血液中的所有细胞成分。淋巴细胞主要分为两大功能性类别：B淋巴细胞（B细胞）和T淋巴细胞（T细胞），两者在发育部位、抗原受体和功能上有所不同。

淋巴细胞疾病主要包括：①特定淋巴细胞亚群的肿瘤学转变，导致一系列淋巴瘤或白血病的发生；②先天性或获得性淋巴细胞发育或功能缺陷，导致免疫缺陷；③对感染或抗原刺激的生理反应，导致淋巴结肿大（淋巴结病）、淋巴细胞增多或淋巴细胞减少。

淋巴细胞的发育、功能和定位

B细胞

B细胞的特征在于其表面携带免疫球蛋白（即抗体）。它们的主要功能是通过产生抗原特异性抗体，从而激发体液免疫反应。

B细胞在骨髓中的发育需经过一系列高度协调的步骤，包括重链和轻链免疫球蛋白基因的有序重排，以及B细胞特异性细胞表面蛋白的表达（图5.1）。免疫球蛋白基因的重排可产生大量B细胞库，每个B细胞都具有独特的抗原特异性免疫球蛋白分子。成熟B细胞从骨髓迁移到全身淋巴组织，并可通过细胞表面免疫球蛋白和B细胞特异性抗原（如CD19、CD20和CD21）进行识别。

抗原与细胞表面免疫球蛋白结合后，成熟B细胞被激活，开始增殖并分化为终末期浆细胞，这些浆细胞失去大部分B细胞表面标志物，并产生大量可溶性抗体。B细胞的肿瘤性疾病源于不同发育阶段的B细胞，B细胞淋巴瘤的肿瘤细胞形态和抗原表达（即免疫表型）差异很大。

T细胞

T细胞在免疫反应中发挥多种功能，包括经典的细胞免疫反应。前体T细胞从骨髓迁移到胸腺，然后分化为成熟的T细胞亚群，并经过选择，从而清除对自身肽段产生反应的自身反应性T细胞。在胸腺中，前体T细胞会经历协调的分化过程，包括重排和表达T细胞受体（TCR）基因，并获得T细胞特有的表面蛋白，包括CD3、CD4和CD8。

随着T细胞在胸腺中成熟，它们最终会失去CD4或CD8蛋白。成熟T细胞由两个主要亚群组成：$CD4^+$细胞和$CD8^+$细胞。在胸腺中经历成熟和选择后，成熟$CD4^+$细胞和$CD8^+$ T细胞迁移到淋巴结、脾和外周免疫系统的其他部位。成熟T细胞约占外周血淋巴细胞的80%、淋巴结细胞的40%和脾淋巴细胞的25%。

成熟$CD4^+$ T细胞和$CD8^+$ T细胞亚群执行不同的免疫功能。$CD8^+$细胞（细胞毒性T细胞）负责杀死感染的病毒或外源细胞，并抑制免疫功能。$CD4^+$细胞（辅助性T细胞）的功能是通过产生细胞因子和直接接触细胞来激活其他免疫细胞，如B细胞和巨噬细胞。

与B细胞相似，T细胞表达特有的TCR分子，这些分子可用于识别特定的肽抗原。与B细胞不同，T细胞仅对细胞内处理并与特定细胞表面抗原提呈蛋白[即主要组织相容性复合体（MHC）分子]结合或呈递的肽段做出反应。$CD4^+$ T细胞和$CD8^+$ T细胞对肽-MHC复合物的反应受MHC类别的限制。$CD4^+$细胞识别由MHC II类分子呈现的抗原性肽段，而$CD8^+$细胞识别由MHC I类分子呈现的抗原性肽段。TCR与特定的肽-MHC复合物结合会触发激活信号，从而导致基因产物的表达，介导$CD4^+$细胞的各种辅助功能或$CD8^+$细胞的细胞毒性效应功能。

淋巴系统

淋巴细胞定位于外周淋巴组织，即抗原-淋巴细胞相互作用和淋巴细胞激活的场所。外周淋巴组织由淋巴结、脾和黏膜淋巴组织组成。淋巴细胞通过血管和淋巴系统持续在这些组织中循环。

淋巴结是高度组织化的淋巴组织，是淋巴引流系统的汇聚点，该系统将抗原从引流的淋巴液中带到淋巴结，并在其中被捕获。淋巴结由外部的皮质和内部的髓质组成（图5.2）。皮质由以B细胞为主的淋巴滤泡组成。部分淋巴滤泡含有中心区或生发中心，在遇到特定抗原后，活化的B细胞在此增殖，并被淋巴结外套层包绕。T细胞则在滤泡周围的副皮质区弥漫分布。

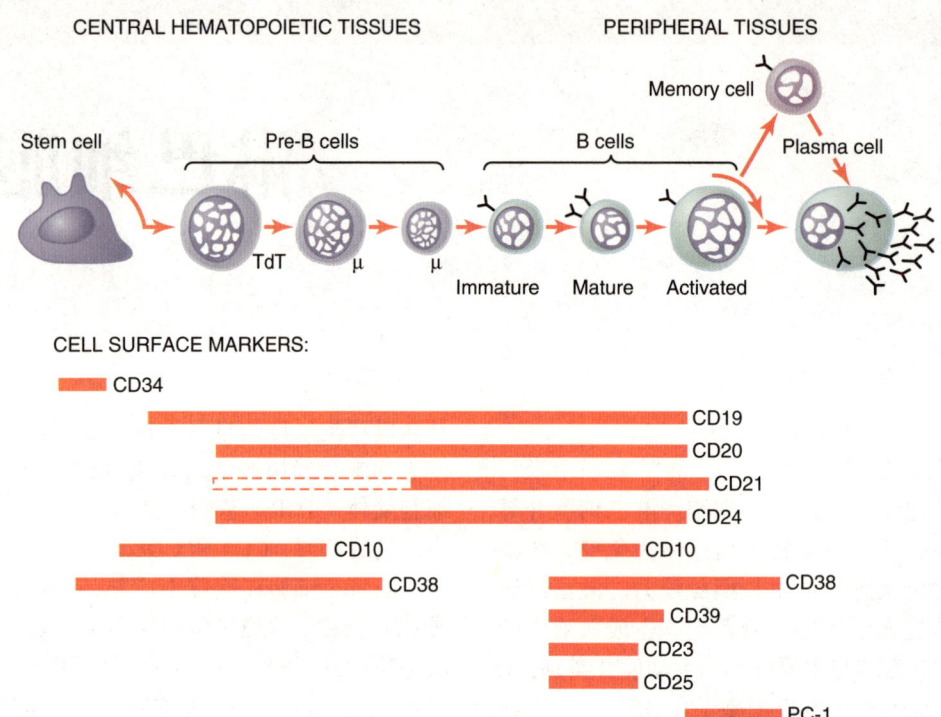

Fig. 5.1 The maturation of B lymphocytes. *Top*, The changes in immunoglobulin production and maturation. *Bottom*, The appearance and disappearance of surface markers. *TdT*, Terminal deoxynucleotidyl transferase. (Modified from Ferrarini M, Grossi CE, Cooper MD: Cellular and molecular biology of lymphoid cells. In Handin RI, Lux SE, Stossel TP, editors: *Blood: Principles and Practice of Hematology*, Philadelphia, 1995, JB Lippincott, p 643.)

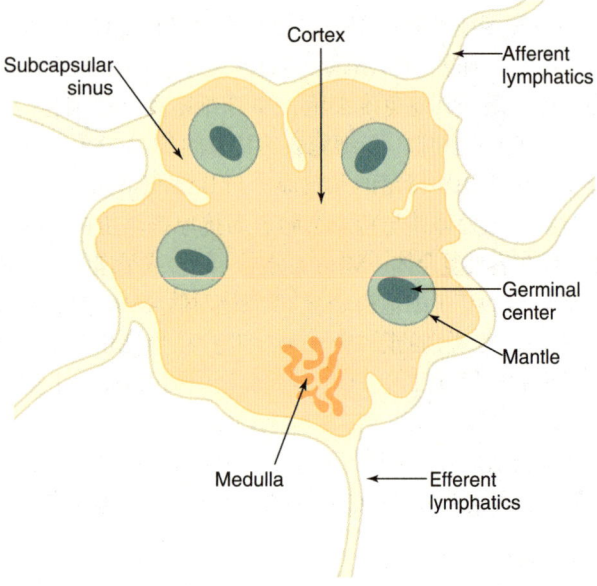

Fig. 5.2 Structure of the normal lymph node. The cortical area contains the follicles, which consist of a germinal center and a mantle zone. The medulla contains a complex of channels that lead to the efferent lymphatics.

The spleen traps antigens from blood rather than from the lymphatic system and is the site of disposal of senescent red cells. Lymphocytes in the spleen reside in the areas described as white pulp, which surround the arterioles entering the organ. As in lymph nodes, the B and T cells are segregated into a periarteriolar lymphoid sheath that is composed of T cells and flanking follicles composed of B cells.

The mucosa-associated lymphoid tissues (MALTs) collect antigen from epithelial surfaces and include the gut-associated lymphoid tissue (i.e., tonsils, adenoids, appendix, and Peyer patches of the small intestine) and more diffusely organized aggregates of lymphocytes at other mucosal sites.

Lymphocytes circulate in the blood and represent 20% to 40% of peripheral blood leukocytes in adults; the proportion is higher in newborns and children. The majority of peripheral blood lymphocytes are T cells, and the remaining lymphocytes are largely B cells. A small percentage of peripheral blood lymphoid cells represents a third category of lymphoid cells referred to as natural killer (NK) cells. These cells do not bear the characteristic cell surface molecules of B or T cells, and their immunoglobulin or TCR genes have not undergone rearrangement. Morphologically, the cells are large, with abundant cytoplasm containing azurophilic granules, and they are often called *large granular lymphocytes*. Functionally, they are part of the innate immune system, responding nonspecifically to a wide range of pathogens without requiring prior antigenic exposure.

NEOPLASIA OF LYMPHOID ORIGIN

Malignant transformation of lymphocytes leads to a diverse array of lymphoid cancers, including tumors that arise from T cells, B cells, or NK cells. Lymphoid malignancies usually involve lymphoid tissues, but they can arise in or spread to any site. The major clinical groupings of lymphoid malignancies include non-Hodgkin's lymphomas (NHLs), Hodgkin's lymphoma, lymphoid leukemias, and plasma cell dyscrasias.

Non-Hodgkin's Lymphomas
Definition and Epidemiology
The NHLs comprise a heterogeneous group of lymphoid malignancies that have different histologic appearances, cells of origin and

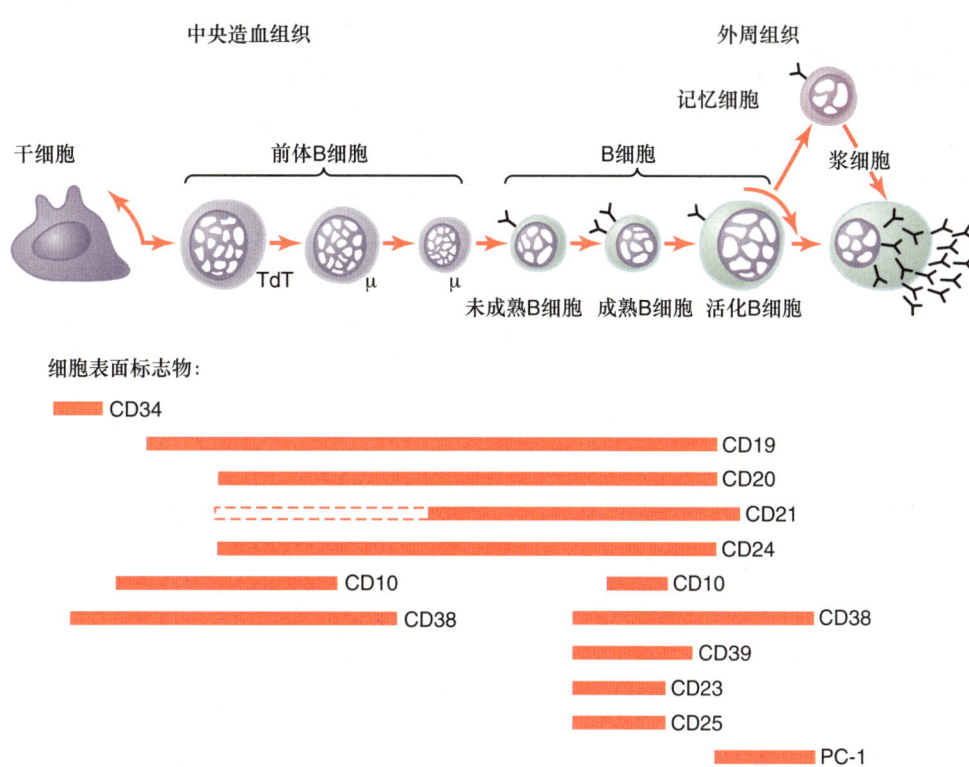

图5.1　B淋巴细胞的成熟过程。上图：免疫球蛋白生成和成熟过程中的改变。下图：表面标志物的出现和消失。TdT，末端脱氧核苷酸转移酶（改编自 Ferrarini M, Grossi CE, Cooper MD: Cellular and molecular biology of lymphoid cells. In Handin RI, Lux SE, Stossel TP, editors: Blood: Principles and Practice of Hematology, Philadelphia, 1995, JB Lippincott, p 643.）

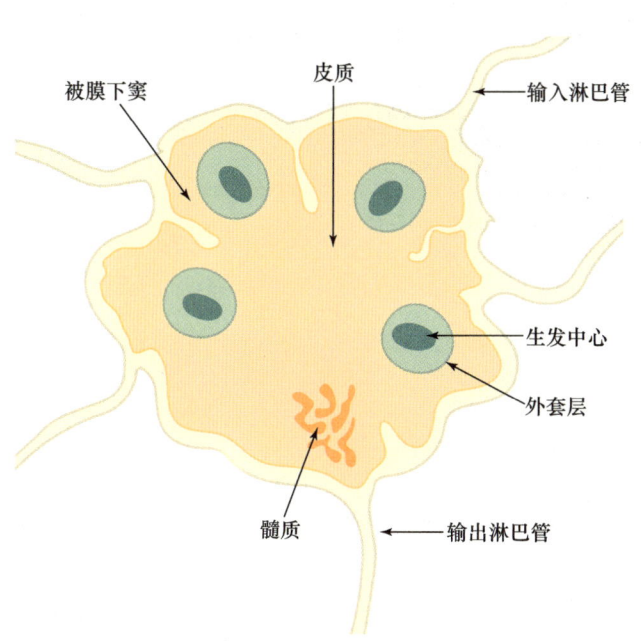

图5.2　正常淋巴结的结构。皮质含有由生发中心和外套层组成的滤泡。髓质包含一系列通向输出淋巴管的复杂通道

体、阑尾和小肠派尔集合淋巴结）及位于其他黏膜部位的更分散的淋巴细胞聚集体。

淋巴细胞在血液中循环，占成人外周血白细胞的20%~40%，新生儿和儿童的比例更高。绝大多数外周血淋巴细胞为T细胞，其余主要是B细胞。外周血中少量的淋巴细胞属于第三类淋巴细胞，即自然杀伤细胞（NK细胞）。这些细胞不具有B细胞或T细胞的特征性细胞表面分子，且其免疫球蛋白或TCR基因未发生重排。从形态上看，这些细胞较大，胞质丰富，含嗜天青颗粒，通常被称为大颗粒淋巴细胞。从功能上讲，它们是先天性免疫系统的一部分，不需要先接触抗原即可对多种病原体产生非特异性反应。

淋巴细胞起源的肿瘤

淋巴细胞的恶性转化可导致多种不同类型的淋巴系统恶性肿瘤，包括起源于T细胞、B细胞或NK细胞的肿瘤。淋巴系统恶性肿瘤通常累及淋巴组织，但它们可起源于或扩散至任何部位。淋巴系统恶性肿瘤主要分为非霍奇金淋巴瘤（NHL）、霍奇金淋巴瘤、淋巴细胞白血病和浆细胞疾病。

非霍奇金淋巴瘤

定义和流行病学

NHL包括一组异质性淋巴系统恶性肿瘤，它们具有不同的组织学表现、细胞起源、免疫表型、分子生

脾从血液（而非淋巴系统）中捕获抗原，并作为清除衰老红细胞的场所。脾内的淋巴细胞位于白髓区域，该区域环绕着进入脾的小动脉。与在淋巴结中类似，B细胞和T细胞在脾中被分隔成由T细胞组成的围动脉淋巴鞘和由B细胞组成的相邻滤泡。

黏膜相关淋巴组织（MALT）可从上皮表面收集抗原，MALT包括肠道相关淋巴组织（即扁桃体、腺样

TABLE 5.1   2016 WHO Classification of Mature Lymphoid, Histiocytic, and Dendritic Neoplasms

Mature B-Cell Neoplasms
Chronic lymphocytic leukemia/small lymphocytic lymphoma
Monoclonal B-cell lymphocytosis[a]
B-cell prolymphocytic leukemia
Splenic marginal zone lymphoma
Hairy cell leukemia
Lymphoplasmacytic lymphoma
    Waldenström's macroglobulinemia
Monoclonal gammopathy of undetermined significance (MGUS), IgM[a]
μ Heavy-chain disease
γ Heavy-chain disease
α Heavy-chain disease
Monoclonal gammopathy of undetermined significance (MGUS), IgG/A[a]
Plasma cell myeloma
Solitary plasmacytoma of bone
Extraosseous plasmacytoma
Monoclonal immunoglobulin deposition diseases[a]
Extranodal marginal zone lymphoma of mucosa-associated lymphoid tissue (MALT lymphoma)
Nodal marginal zone lymphoma
Follicular lymphoma
    In situ follicular neoplasia[a]
    Duodenal-type follicular lymphoma[a]
Pediatric-type follicular lymphoma[a]
Primary cutaneous follicle center lymphoma
Mantle cell lymphoma
    In situ mantle cell neoplasia[a]
Diffuse large B-cell lymphoma (DLBCL), NOS
    Germinal center B-cell type[a]
    Activated B-cell type[a]
T-cell/histiocyte-rich large B-cell lymphoma
Primary DLBCL of the central nervous system (CNS)
Primary cutaneous DLBCL, leg type
EBV+ DLBCL, NOS[a]
DLBCL associated with chronic inflammation
Lymphomatoid granulomatosis
Primary mediastinal (thymic) large B-cell lymphoma
Intravascular large B-cell lymphoma
ALK+ large B-cell lymphoma
Plasmablastic lymphoma
Primary effusion lymphoma
Burkitt lymphoma
High-grade B-cell lymphoma, with MYC and BCL2 and/or BCL6 rearrangements[a]
High-grade B-cell lymphoma, NOS[a]
B-cell lymphoma, unclassifiable, with features intermediate between DLBCL and classical Hodgkin lymphoma

Mature T and NK Neoplasms
T-cell prolymphocytic leukemia
T-cell large granular lymphocytic leukemia
Aggressive NK-cell leukemia
Systemic EBV+ T-cell lymphoma of childhood[a]
Hydroa vacciniforme–like lymphoproliferative disorder[a]
Adult T-cell leukemia/lymphoma
Extranodal NK-/T-cell lymphoma, nasal type
Enteropathy-associated T-cell lymphoma
Monomorphic epitheliotropic intestinal T-cell lymphoma[a]
Hepatosplenic T-cell lymphoma
Subcutaneous panniculitis-like T-cell lymphoma
Mycosis fungoides
Sézary syndrome
Primary cutaneous CD30+ T-cell lymphoproliferative disorders
    Lymphomatoid papulosis
    Primary cutaneous anaplastic large cell lymphoma
Primary cutaneous γδ T-cell lymphoma
Peripheral T-cell lymphoma, NOS
Angioimmunoblastic T-cell lymphoma
Anaplastic large-cell lymphoma, ALK+
Anaplastic large-cell lymphoma, ALK−[a]

Hodgkin's Lymphoma
Nodular lymphocyte predominant Hodgkin's lymphoma
Classical Hodgkin's lymphoma
    Nodular sclerosis classical Hodgkin's lymphoma
    Lymphocyte-rich classical Hodgkin's lymphoma
    Mixed cellularity classical Hodgkin's lymphoma
    Lymphocyte-depleted classical Hodgkin's lymphoma

Posttransplant Lymphoproliferative Disorders (PTLD)
Plasmacytic hyperplasia PTLD
Infectious mononucleosis PTLD
Florid follicular hyperplasia PTLD[a]
Polymorphic PTLD
Monomorphic PTLD (B- and T-/NK-cell types)
Classical Hodgkin's lymphoma PTLD

Provisional entities, histiocytic and dendritic cell entities are not included.
[a]Denotes new entities.

immunophenotypes, molecular biologic factors, clinical features, prognoses, and outcomes with therapy. According to the Surveillance, Epidemiology, and End Results (SEER) database, the NHLs are the seventh most common cancer type, with an estimated 74,200 cases occurring in 2019 and 19,970 patients succumbing to these diseases. The NHLs occur at a median age of 67 and are more common in men and in white individuals. The rate of NHLs increased slowly between 2000 and 2010 but has been decreasing slowly since that time. The annual death rate has fallen an average of 2.2% from 2007 to 2016.

Pathology

In view of the heterogeneity of NHLs, classification systems have been devised to identify specific pathologic subtypes that correlate with distinct clinical entities. These systems have evolved steadily over the past 50 years as correlations between histopathologic and biologic behavior have emerged. Pathologic classification schemes have attempted to correlate malignant NHL subtypes with normal cellular counterparts. The World Health Organization (WHO) classification (Table 5.1) is the most current and incorporates morphologic features, immunophenotype, genetic features, and molecular features, with an emphasis on biologic

表 5.1 2016 WHO 成熟淋巴细胞肿瘤、组织细胞肿瘤和树突状细胞肿瘤分类

成熟 B 细胞肿瘤
慢性淋巴细胞白血病/小淋巴细胞淋巴瘤
单克隆 B 细胞淋巴细胞增多症 [a]
B 细胞幼淋巴细胞白血病
脾边缘区淋巴瘤
毛细胞白血病
淋巴浆细胞性淋巴瘤
　瓦尔登斯特伦巨球蛋白血症
意义未明单克隆丙种球蛋白血症（MGUS）IgM 型 [a]
　μ 重链病
　γ 重链病
　α 重链病
意义未明单克隆丙种球蛋白血症（MGUS）IgG/A 型 [a]
多发性骨髓瘤
骨孤立性浆细胞瘤
骨外浆细胞瘤
单克隆免疫球蛋白沉积病 [a]
结外边缘区黏膜相关淋巴组织淋巴瘤（MALT 淋巴瘤）
结内边缘区淋巴瘤
滤泡性淋巴瘤
　原位滤泡性肿瘤 [a]
　原发性肠道滤泡性淋巴瘤 [a]
儿童滤泡性淋巴瘤
原发性皮肤滤泡中心淋巴瘤
套细胞淋巴瘤
　原位套细胞肿瘤 [a]
弥漫大 B 细胞淋巴瘤（DLBCL），非特指型
　生发中心 B 细胞型 [a]
　活化 B 细胞型 [a]
富于 T 细胞/组织细胞的大 B 细胞淋巴瘤
中枢神经系统（CNS）原发性 DLBCL
原发性皮肤 DLBCL，腿型
EBV+ DLBCL，非特指型 [a]
慢性炎症相关性 DLBCL
淋巴瘤样肉芽肿病
原发性纵隔（胸腺）大 B 细胞淋巴瘤
血管内大 B 细胞淋巴瘤
ALK+ 大 B 细胞淋巴瘤
浆母细胞淋巴瘤
原发性渗出性淋巴瘤
伯基特淋巴瘤
高级别 B 细胞淋巴瘤伴有 MYC 和 BCL2 和（或）BCL6 重排 [a]
高级别 B 细胞淋巴瘤，非特指型 [a]
B 细胞淋巴瘤，未分类型，具有 DLBCL 和经典型霍奇金淋巴瘤特征的中间型

成熟 T 细胞和 NK 细胞肿瘤
T 细胞幼淋巴细胞白血病
T 细胞性大颗粒淋巴细胞白血病
侵袭性 NK 细胞白血病
儿童系统性 EBV+ T 细胞淋巴瘤 [a]
种痘水疱病样淋巴增殖性疾病 [a]
成人 T 细胞白血病/淋巴瘤
结外 NK 细胞/T 细胞淋巴瘤，鼻型
肠病相关性 T 细胞淋巴瘤
单形性嗜上皮性肠 T 细胞淋巴瘤 [a]
肝脾 T 细胞淋巴瘤
皮下脂膜炎样 T 细胞淋巴瘤
蕈样肉芽肿病
塞扎里综合征（Sézary 综合征）
原发性皮肤 CD30+ T 细胞淋巴增殖性疾病
　淋巴瘤样丘疹病
　原发性皮肤间变性大细胞淋巴瘤
原发性皮肤 γδ T 细胞淋巴瘤
外周 T 细胞淋巴瘤，非特指型
血管免疫母细胞性 T 细胞淋巴瘤
间变性大细胞淋巴瘤，ALK+
间变性大细胞淋巴瘤，ALK−

霍奇金淋巴瘤
结节性淋巴细胞为主型霍奇金淋巴瘤
经典型霍奇金淋巴瘤
　结节硬化型经典型霍奇金淋巴瘤
　富于淋巴细胞的经典型霍奇金淋巴瘤
　混合细胞型经典型霍奇金淋巴瘤
　淋巴细胞消减型经典型霍奇金淋巴瘤

移植后淋巴增殖性疾病（PTLD）
浆细胞性增生 PTLD
传染性单核细胞增多症 PTLD
滤泡性增生 PTLD [a]
多形性 PTLD
单形性 PTLD（B 细胞和 T 细胞/NK 细胞型）
经典型霍奇金淋巴瘤 PTLD

本表中不包含暂定亚型、组织细胞和树突状细胞亚型。
[a] 新亚型。

物学因素、临床特征、预后及治疗转归。根据美国国立癌症研究所监测、流行病学和最终结果（SEER）数据库，NHL 是第七大癌症类型，2019 年美国估计有 74 200 例新发病例，并有 19 970 例患者因该病去世。NHL 的中位发病年龄为 67 岁，男性和白人群体中更为常见。NHL 的发病率在 2000—2010 年缓慢升高，随后持续缓慢下降。2007—2016 年，NHL 的年死亡率平均下降了 2.2%。

病理学

鉴于 NHL 的异质性，目前已经制定了病理分类系统，以明确临床诊疗不同的特定病理亚型。在过去 50 年中，随着对组织病理学与生物学行为之间相关性的逐步认识，这些分类系统也在不断更新。病理分类方案尝试将恶性 NHL 亚型与正常细胞联系起来。世界卫生组织（WHO）分类（表 5.1）是当前最新的分类，其结合了形态学特征、免疫表型、遗传特征和分子特

TABLE 5.2 Causes of Lymphadenopathy

Infectious Diseases
Viral: infectious mononucleosis syndromes (cytomegalovirus, Epstein-Barr virus), acquired immunodeficiency syndrome, rubella, herpes simplex, infectious hepatitis
Bacterial: localized infection with regional adenopathy (streptococci, staphylococci), cat-scratch disease *(Bartonella henselae)*, brucellosis, tularemia, listeriosis, bubonic plague *(Yersinia pestis)*, chancroid *(Haemophilus ducreyi)*
Fungal: coccidioidomycosis, histoplasmosis
Chlamydial: lymphogranuloma venereum, trachoma
Mycobacterial: scrofula, tuberculosis, leprosy
Protozoan: toxoplasmosis, trypanosomiasis
Spirochetal: Lyme disease, syphilis, leptospirosis

Immunologic Diseases
Rheumatoid arthritis
Systemic lupus erythematosus
Mixed connective tissue disease
Sjögren's syndrome
Dermatomyositis
Serum sickness
Drug reactions: phenytoin, hydralazine, allopurinol

Malignant Diseases
Lymphomas
Solid tumors metastatic to lymph nodes: melanoma, lung, breast, head and neck, gastrointestinal tract, Kaposi's sarcoma, unknown primary tumor, renal, prostate

Atypical Lymphoid Proliferations
Giant follicular lymph node hyperplasia
Transformation of germinal centers
Castleman disease

Miscellaneous Diseases and Diseases of Unknown Cause
Dermatopathic lymphadenitis
Sarcoidosis
Immunoglobulin G4 (IgG4) lymphadenopathy
Amyloidosis
Mucocutaneous lymph node syndrome (Kawasaki disease)
Sinus histiocytosis (Rosai-Dorfman syndrome)
Multifocal Langerhans cell (eosinophilic) granulomatosis
Lipid storage diseases: Gaucher's and Niemann-Pick diseases

Epstein-Barr virus (EBV) is associated with several biologically aggressive NHLs, including acquired immunodeficiency syndrome (AIDS)–related diffuse, aggressive lymphomas, the lymphoproliferative disorders that arise in immunosuppressed patients after organ transplantation, and the form of Burkitt lymphoma that is endemic in Africa. Human T-cell lymphotropic virus type 1 (HTLV-1) is causally linked with adult T-cell leukemia/lymphoma, which is endemic in areas of Japan and the Caribbean basin. The human herpesvirus 8 (HHV-8) of Kaposi's sarcoma has been implicated in a variant of diffuse, aggressive NHL that arises in serosal cavities and is encountered almost exclusively in patients infected with human immunodeficiency virus (HIV).

Several indolent lymphomas have been linked to infectious agents that appear to indirectly promote lymphomagenesis through chronic antigen stimulation, resulting in B-lymphocyte proliferation. *Helicobacter pylori* infection is linked to gastric MALT lymphomas in this manner; eradication of infection with antibiotics is often associated with regression of the lymphoma.

Clinical Presentation

Although numerous subtypes of NHL are recognized, most disease entities may be viewed conceptually as clinically indolent (i.e., low grade) or aggressive (i.e., high grade). Indolent lymphomas typically grow slowly, do not always require therapy, and have a long natural history. A clinical history of recurring and regressing adenopathy may be elicited. Constitutional symptoms such as fever, weight loss, or night sweats occur in about 20% of patients with NHL at the time of onset. These symptoms are more common in patients with aggressive subtypes of NHL. Aggressive lymphomas are associated with limited survival in the absence of therapy.

Most patients with NHL exhibit painless lymphadenopathy involving one or more peripheral nodal sites. NHL can involve extranodal sites, and patients can exhibit a variety of symptoms that reflect the site of involvement. Common sites of extranodal disease include the gastrointestinal tract, bone marrow or focal bone lesions, liver, skin, and Waldeyer ring in the nasopharynx and oropharynx, although virtually any site can be involved. Aggressive subtypes of NHL are more likely than indolent lymphomas to involve extranodal sites.

Central nervous system involvement, including leptomeningeal spread, rarely occurs with the indolent subtypes but does occur with the aggressive variants. The most aggressive NHLs (i.e., Burkitt and lymphoblastic lymphomas) have a particular propensity to spread to the leptomeninges.

Diagnosis and Differential Diagnosis

Many causes of lymphadenopathy exist in addition to lymphoid malignancies (Table 5.2). A thorough history and careful physical examination are important before performing a lymph node biopsy. The investigation of lymphadenopathy can be organized according to the location of the enlarged nodes (i.e., localized or generalized) and clinical symptoms.

Cervical lymphadenopathy is most often caused by infections of the upper respiratory tract, including infectious mononucleosis syndromes, viral syndromes, and bacterial pharyngitis. Unilateral axillary, inguinal, or femoral adenopathy may be caused by skin infections involving the extremity, including cat-scratch fever. Generalized lymphadenopathy may be caused by systemic infections (e.g., HIV, cytomegalovirus), drug reactions, autoimmune diseases, or one of the systemic lymphadenopathy syndromes. If the cause of persistent lymphadenopathy is not apparent after a thorough evaluation, an excisional lymph node biopsy should be undertaken. An enlarged supraclavicular lymph node strongly suggests malignancy and should always be sampled.

The accurate diagnosis of lymphoma requires excisional biopsy of a lymph node or generous biopsy of involved lymph tissue. Fine-needle aspiration or needle biopsy is rarely sufficient. Analysis of the

and therapeutic implications. The most common NHLs encountered in the United States are diffuse large B-cell lymphoma (DLBCL), follicular lymphoma, small lymphocytic lymphoma or leukemia (i.e., chronic lymphocytic leukemia [CLL]), and mantle cell lymphoma.

Etiology

The cause of most NHLs is unknown. In most patients no apparent genetic predisposition or epidemiologic or environmental factor can be identified. Many of the NHL subtypes carry pathognomonic chromosomal translocations that often involve an immunoglobulin locus (or TCR locus in T-cell NHLs) and an oncogene or growth regulatory gene. The cause of these aberrant chromosomal rearrangements is unknown.

Patients with congenital immunodeficiency syndromes or autoimmune disorders are at increased risk for NHL. Oncogenic human viruses play a causal role in some of the less common NHL variants.

表 5.2　引起淋巴结肿大的原因
传染性疾病
病毒性：传染性单核细胞增多综合征（巨细胞病毒、EB 病毒）、获得性免疫缺陷综合征、风疹、单纯疱疹、传染性肝炎
细菌性：局部感染伴区域淋巴结肿大（链球菌、葡萄球菌）、猫抓病（汉赛巴尔通体）、布鲁氏菌病、兔热病、李斯特菌病、腺鼠疫（鼠疫耶尔森菌）、软下疳（杜克雷嗜血杆菌）
真菌性：球孢子菌病、组织胞浆菌病
衣原体性：性病性淋巴肉芽肿、沙眼
分枝杆菌性：淋巴结结核、结核病、麻风
原虫性：弓形虫病、锥虫病
螺旋体性：莱姆病、梅毒、钩端螺旋体病
免疫系统疾病
类风湿关节炎
系统性红斑狼疮
混合性结缔组织病
干燥综合征
皮肌炎
血清病
药物反应：苯妥英、肼屈嗪、别嘌醇
恶性疾病
淋巴瘤
转移至淋巴结的实体瘤：黑色素瘤、肺癌、乳腺癌、头颈癌、胃肠道癌、卡波西肉瘤、原发位不明的肿瘤、肾癌、前列腺癌
非典型淋巴增殖
巨大淋巴结增生症
生发中心转化
卡斯尔曼病
其他疾病及病因不明的疾病
皮病性淋巴结炎
结节病
免疫球蛋白 G4（IgG4）相关淋巴结肿大
淀粉样变性
黏膜皮肤淋巴结综合征（川崎病）
窦组织细胞增生（Rosai-Dorfman 综合征）
多灶性朗格汉斯细胞（嗜酸性）肉芽肿病
脂质贮积病：戈谢病和尼曼-皮克病

征，并强调了生物学和治疗的意义。在美国，最常见的 NHL 类型是弥漫大 B 细胞淋巴瘤（DLBCL）、滤泡性淋巴瘤、小淋巴细胞淋巴瘤或白血病［即慢性淋巴细胞白血病（CLL）］和套细胞淋巴瘤。

病因

大多数 NHL 的病因不明。在大多数患者中，无法确定明显的遗传倾向或流行病学因素或环境因素。许多 NHL 亚型携带特征性染色体易位，通常涉及免疫球蛋白基因位点（或 T 细胞淋巴瘤涉及 TCR 基因位点）、癌基因或生长调节基因。这些异常染色体重排的原因尚不清楚。

先天性免疫缺陷综合征或自身免疫病患者罹患 NHL 的风险增加。一些少见的 NHL 亚型与人类致癌病毒密切相关。EB 病毒（EBV）与多种生物学上具有侵袭性的 NHL 有关，包括获得性免疫缺陷综合征（AIDS）相关性弥漫侵袭性淋巴瘤、器官移植后免疫抑制患者出现的淋巴增殖性疾病，以及在非洲地区流行的伯基特淋巴瘤。人类嗜 T 淋巴细胞病毒-1（HTLV-1）与成人 T 细胞白血病/淋巴瘤有关，该病在日本和加勒比地区流行。卡波西肉瘤中的人类疱疹病毒 8（HHV-8）已被证明与一种弥漫侵袭性 NHL 亚型有关，该亚型发生在浆膜腔中，且几乎仅见于人类免疫缺陷病毒（HIV）感染者。

多种惰性淋巴瘤与感染性病原体有关，这些病原体似乎可通过慢性抗原刺激而间接导致 B 淋巴细胞增殖，促进淋巴瘤发生。幽门螺杆菌感染就是以这种方式导致胃 MALT 淋巴瘤；使用抗生素根除感染通常可使淋巴瘤消退。

临床表现

虽然 NHL 的亚型众多，但大多数亚型在概念上可分为临床惰性淋巴瘤（即低级别）或侵袭性淋巴瘤（即高级别）。惰性淋巴瘤通常生长缓慢，不一定需要治疗，且自然病程较长，可能出现反复淋巴结肿大和消退的临床病史。约 20% 的 NHL 患者在发病时会出现发热、体重减轻或盗汗等全身症状。这些症状在侵袭性 NHL 亚型患者中更为常见。如果不及时治疗，侵袭性淋巴瘤患者的生存期较短。

大多数 NHL 患者表现为无痛性淋巴结肿大，涉及 1 个或多个外周淋巴结区域。NHL 可累及结外部位，患者可表现为相应病变部位的各种症状。常见的结外病变部位包括胃肠道、骨髓或局灶性骨病变、肝、皮肤，以及鼻咽部和口咽部的 Waldeyer 环，但实际上任何部位均可受累。与惰性淋巴瘤相比，侵袭性 NHL 亚型更可能累及结外部位。

中枢神经系统受累（包括软脑膜播散）在惰性淋巴瘤亚型中极少发生，但在侵袭性淋巴瘤中较常见。最具侵袭性的 NHL 亚型（如伯基特淋巴瘤和淋巴母细胞淋巴瘤）非常容易播散至软脑膜。

诊断和鉴别诊断

除淋巴系统恶性肿瘤外，还有许多可引起淋巴结肿大的原因（表 5.2）。在进行淋巴结活检前，详细询问病史和仔细的体格检查非常重要。淋巴结肿大的检查可根据肿大淋巴结的部位（即局部或全身）和临床症状来选择。

颈部淋巴结肿大最常由上呼吸道感染引起，包括传染性单核细胞增多综合征、病毒感染和细菌性咽炎。单侧腋窝淋巴结、腹股沟淋巴结或股部淋巴结肿大可能由累及四肢的皮肤感染引起，包括猫抓病。全身性淋巴结肿大可能由全身性感染（如 HIV、巨细胞病毒）、药物反应、自身免疫病或系统性淋巴结病综合征引起。若经全面评估后仍不能明确持续性淋巴结肿大的原因，则应进行淋巴结切除活检。锁骨上淋巴结肿大强烈提示恶性肿瘤，应及时进行病理学活检。

淋巴瘤的准确诊断需要对淋巴结进行切除活检或对受累淋巴组织进行充分活检，细针穿刺或针吸活检

TABLE 5.3 Staging Evaluation for Lymphomas

Required Evaluation Procedures
Biopsy of lesion with review by an experienced hematopathologist
History with attention to the presence or absence of B symptoms
Physical examination with attention to node-bearing areas (including Waldeyer ring) and size of liver and spleen
Standard blood work:
  Complete blood count
  Lactate dehydrogenase and β_2-microglobulin
  Evaluation of renal function
  Liver function tests
  Calcium, uric acid
Bone marrow aspirate and biopsy
Radiologic studies, including:
  Chest radiograph (posteroanterior and lateral)
  Chest, abdomen, and pelvic CT scans
  PET scan (in Hodgkin's and aggressive lymphomas)

Procedures Required Under Certain Circumstances
Plain bone radiographs of symptomatic sites or abnormal areas on bone scan
Brain or spinal CT or MRI if neurologic signs or symptoms
Serum and urine protein electrophoresis
Lumbar puncture with cerebrospinal fluid cytology (Burkitt and lymphoblastic lymphoma)

B symptoms, Fever, sweats, and weight loss >10% of body weight; *CT,* computed tomography; *MRI,* magnetic resonance imaging; *PET,* positron emission tomography.

TABLE 5.4 Staging System for Hodgkin and Non-Hodgkin's Lymphoma

Stage[a]	Involvement	Extranodal E Status
I	One node or a group of adjacent nodes	Single extranodal lesions without nodal involvement
II	Two or more nodal groups on the same side of the diaphragm	Stage I or II by nodal extent with limited contiguous extranodal involvement
II bulky	As above with bulky disease[b]	
III	Nodes on both sides of the diaphragm; nodes above the diaphragm with spleen involvement	
IV	Additional noncontiguous extralymphatic involvement	

[a]Staging systems for Hodgkin's and non-Hodgkin's lymphomas are similar. For Hodgkin's lymphoma, the presence or absence of symptoms should be documented with each stage designation: A (asymptomatic) or B (fever, sweats, and weight loss >10% of body weight).
[b]For Hodgkin's lymphoma bulky disease includes nodal mass >10 cm or >⅓ of the transthoracic diameter

pathologic specimen should include routine histologic examination and immunophenotyping, immunohistochemistry, chromosome analysis, fluorescence in situ hybridization (FISH) testing, and molecular studies. Immunophenotyping can determine the cell of origin (i.e., B cell, T cell, NK cell, or nonlymphoid cell), and the pattern of cell surface antigens aids subclassification. In the case of B-cell NHLs, immunophenotyping can also reveal whether the process is monoclonal in origin (i.e., neoplastic) by determining if surface immunoglobulin is restricted to κ or λ light chain. Immunohistochemistry utilizing stains to assess expression levels of proteins such as MYC and BCL-2 provides prognostic information. In some cases, cytogenetic analysis or molecular studies of immunoglobulin or TCR gene rearrangement may be required to determine the pathologic subtype of lymphoma or to establish a monoclonal process. Chromosome analysis may reveal a complex karyotype often associated with worse prognosis, or deletion of chromosome 17p where the tumor suppressor gene p53 locus is found. FISH probes can identify translocations such as t(8;14) leading to high MYC expression in Burkitt lymphoma, t(14;18) leading to deregulated expression of the BCL-2 gene in follicular B-cell lymphoma, or t(11;14) leading to cyclin D1 (a regulator of the G1-S transition) overexpression in mantle cell lymphoma, among other abnormalities. If a lymph node biopsy is nondiagnostic and unexplained lymph node enlargement persists, biopsy should be repeated.

For patients with bone marrow and peripheral blood involvement, such as in small lymphocytic lymphoma or CLL, the diagnosis may be made based on immunophenotyping of peripheral blood lymphocytes by flow cytometry. Care must be taken to exclude the possibility of aggressive lymphoma with involved lymph nodes or extranodal sites in a patient harboring a low-grade or indolent lymphoma such as small lymphocytic lymphoma that is confined to the blood or bone marrow.

Treatment

After a lymphoma has been diagnosed, patients should undergo complete staging evaluation (Table 5.3). Staging determines the extent of involvement, provides prognostic information, and may influence the choice of therapy. The Lugano modification of the Ann Arbor staging classification is used to stage patients with NHL and Hodgkin's lymphoma (Table 5.4).

A variety of ancillary tests may be performed in specific situations. For example, a test for HTLV-1 and HIV should be performed if adult T-cell leukemia/lymphoma is suspected. Patients with a clinical history suggesting immunodeficiency or behavioral risk factors should be tested for HIV. A gastrointestinal series or endoscopy may be warranted for patients with gastrointestinal symptoms or patients at risk for gastrointestinal involvement (i.e., mantle cell and other lymphomas involving the Waldeyer ring). The choice of therapy is guided by stage, specific subtype, and clinical considerations such as age and the medical condition of the patient. Multiple novel agents are available for therapy of lymphoid neoplasms (Table 5.5). Such agents may be combined or used with traditional chemotherapy.

Lymphoma Subtypes

Indolent non-Hodgkin's lymphomas. The common low-grade or indolent conditions include follicular lymphoma, small lymphocytic lymphoma (which is identical to CLL), and marginal zone lymphomas.

Follicular lymphoma (FL) accounts for 20% of adult lymphomas and is the most common indolent lymphoma. It is a mature clonal B-cell neoplasm that histologically retains nodular architecture in the lymph node, which is infiltrated by small, mature-appearing lymphocytes. The immunophenotype is positive for surface markers (CD10, CD19, CD20, CD21) and negative for CD5. Follicular lymphomas are characterized by the t(14;18) translocation that juxtaposes the immunoglobulin heavy chain *(IGH)* locus with the antiapoptotic B-cell CLL/lymphoma 2 gene *(BCL2);* the BCL2 protein is uniformly overexpressed in follicular lymphomas, immortalizing affected cells. Additional gain of function mutations and altered T-cell function in the malignant microenvironment are thought to play a role in pathogenesis.

表 5.3 淋巴瘤的分期评估
必需的评估步骤
对病灶进行活检，并由经验丰富的血液病理学家进行诊断
病史询问，特别注意是否存在 B 症状
体格检查，特别注意淋巴结分布区域（包括 Waldeyer 环）及肝和脾的大小
常规血液检查：
全血细胞计数
乳酸脱氢酶和 β_2-微球蛋白
肾功能检查
肝功能检查
钙、尿酸
骨髓穿刺和活检
影像学检查，包括：
胸部 X 线检查（后前位和侧位片）
胸部、腹部和盆腔 CT
PET（用于霍奇金淋巴瘤和侵袭性淋巴瘤）
特定情况下需要做的检查：
症状部位或骨扫描异常区域的骨 X 线平片
如果有神经系统体征或症状，进行脑或脊柱 CT 或 MRI
血清和尿蛋白电泳
腰椎穿刺并进行脑脊液细胞学检查（用于伯基特淋巴瘤和淋巴母细胞性淋巴瘤）

B 症状，发热、盗汗和体重减轻超过体重的 10%；CT，计算机断层成像；MRI，磁共振成像；PET，正电子发射断层成像。

表 5.4 霍奇金淋巴瘤和非霍奇金淋巴瘤的分期系统		
分期[a]	累及范围	结外器官状态
I	1 个淋巴结或 1 组相邻的淋巴结	单个结外病变，无淋巴结受累
II II 巨块型	同侧膈肌的 2 个或更多淋巴结群 同 II 期，伴有巨块病变[b]	I 期或 II 期淋巴结侵犯伴有连续的结外器官受累
III	双侧膈肌的淋巴结；膈肌上方的淋巴结伴有脾受累	
IV	额外的非连续性结外受累	

[a] 霍奇金淋巴瘤和非霍奇金淋巴瘤的分期系统类似。对于霍奇金淋巴瘤，每个分期应记录是否存在症状：A（无症状）或 B（发热、盗汗和体重减轻超过体重的 10%）。
[b] 对于霍奇金淋巴瘤，巨块病变包括淋巴结肿块 > 10 cm 或 > 胸腔直径的 1/3。

治疗

在确诊淋巴瘤后，患者应进行完整的分期评估（表 5.3）。分期可确定受累范围，提供预后信息，并可能影响治疗选择。Lugano 修订版 Ann Arbor 分期系统可用于 NHL 和霍奇金淋巴瘤的分期（表 5.4）。

在特定情况下，可能需要进行一系列辅助检查。例如，疑诊成人 T 细胞白血病/淋巴瘤时应进行 HTLV-1 和 HIV 检测；临床病史提示免疫缺陷或有行为危险因素的患者，应进行 HIV 检测；对于有胃肠道症状或有胃肠道受累风险的患者（如套细胞淋巴瘤和其他累及 Waldeyer 环的淋巴瘤），可能需要进行胃肠道相关检查或内镜检查。治疗方案的选择需依据分期、特定亚型及临床因素（如患者年龄和身体状况）综合考虑。多种新型药物可用于治疗淋巴肿瘤（表 5.5）。这些药物可以相互联合或与传统化疗联合使用。

淋巴瘤亚型

惰性非霍奇金淋巴瘤 常见的低级别或惰性 NHL 包括滤泡性淋巴瘤、小淋巴细胞淋巴瘤（即 CLL）和边缘区淋巴瘤。

滤泡性淋巴瘤（FL）占成人淋巴瘤的 20%，是最常见的惰性淋巴瘤。它是一种成熟的克隆性 B 细胞肿瘤，在组织学上淋巴结保持结节样结构，且被小的、外观成熟的淋巴细胞浸润。其免疫表型为表面标志物（CD10、CD19、CD20、CD21）阳性，CD5 阴性。FL 的特征是存在 t（14;18）易位，使免疫球蛋白重链（IGH）位点与抗凋亡的 B 细胞 CLL/淋巴瘤 2 基因（*BCL2*）并列；BCL2 蛋白在 FL 中均呈过表达，使受累细胞永生化。额外的功能获得突变和肿瘤微环境中的 T 细胞功能改变在 FL 的发生发展中发挥重要作用。

通常无法明确诊断。对病理标本的分析应包括常规组织学检查和免疫表型分析、免疫组织化学染色、染色体分析、荧光原位杂交（FISH）检测和分子检测。免疫表型分析可确定细胞起源（即 B 细胞、T 细胞、NK 细胞或非淋巴细胞），且细胞表面抗原的表达模式有助于进一步区分亚型。对于 B 细胞 NHL，免疫表型分析还可通过确定表面免疫球蛋白是否仅限于 κ 或 λ 轻链来判断是否为单克隆起源（即肿瘤性）。免疫组织化学染色评估 MYC 和 BCL-2 等蛋白质表达水平可提供预后信息。在某些情况下，可能需要进行细胞遗传学分析或免疫球蛋白分子检测或 TCR 基因重排检测，以确定淋巴瘤的病理亚型或确定是否为单克隆。染色体分析可显示复杂核型（通常与预后较差相关）或发现染色体 17p（肿瘤抑制基因 p53 位点）缺失。FISH 探针可识别染色体易位，如伯基特淋巴瘤伴有 t（8;14）导致 MYC 高表达，滤泡性淋巴瘤伴有 t（14;18）导致 *BCL-2* 基因表达失调，以及套细胞淋巴瘤伴有 t（11;14）导致周期蛋白 D1（调节细胞周期各时期的转换）过表达。若淋巴结活检结果无诊断意义，但持续存在无法解释的淋巴结肿大，应重复进行组织活检进一步明确诊断。

对于骨髓和外周血受累的患者（如小淋巴细胞淋巴瘤），可通过流式细胞术对外周血淋巴细胞进行免疫分型来做出诊断。但对于血液或骨髓的低级别或惰性淋巴瘤（如小淋巴细胞淋巴瘤），必须注意排除淋巴结或结外病灶已经转化为侵袭性淋巴瘤的可能性。

TABLE 5.5 New Therapeutic Agents in Use for Lymphoma and Plasmacytic Disorders

Class	Agents	Target	Mechanism of Action	Indications
Monoclonal Antibodies	Rituximab Obinutuzumab	CD20	Complement-mediated and antibody-dependent cytotoxicity. Apoptosis of tumor cells	Most B-cell lymphomas
	Daratumumab	CD 38		Multiple myeloma
Antibody-Drug Conjugates	Brentuximab	CD 30	Antibody bound tubulin inhibitor delivered to tumor cell	Hodgkin's lymphoma and CD30+ lymphomas
	Polatuzumab	CD79a		DLBCL
Imids	Thalidomide Lenalidomide Pomalidomide	Cereblon, immune-modulation	Bind cereblon, activating E3 ubiquitin ligase complex	Multiple myeloma NHL subtypes (lenalidomide)
Kinase Inhibitors				
BTK Inhibitors	Ibrutinib Acalabrutinib Zanubrutinib	Bruton tyrosine kinase	Blocks B-cell receptor signaling	CLL, MCL, MZL, WM
Pi3k Inhibitors	Idelalisib Copanlisib	Phosphatidylinositol-3-kinase	Blocks B-cell receptor signaling	CLL, FL
BCL-2 Inhibitor	Venetoclax	BCL-2	Blocks antiapoptotic protein BCL-2 leading to programmed cell death	CLL
Proteosome Inhibitors	Bortezomib Carfilzomib Ixazomib	Proteasome	Inhibition of toxic protein degradation in malignant cells	Multiple myeloma MCL
CAR-T Cells	Axicabtagene ciloleucel Tisagenlecleucel	CD19	Direct binding of genetically engineered T cell to malignant B cells	DLBCL ALL

ALL, Acute lymphocytic leukemia; *BTK*, Bruton tyrosine kinase; *CLL*, chronic lymphocytic leukemia; *DLBCL*, diffuse large B-cell lymphoma; *FL*, follicular lymphoma; *IMIDS*, Immunomodulatory agents; *MCL*, mantle cell lymphoma; *MZL*, marginal aone lymphoma; *WM*, Waldenström's macroglobulinemia.

Follicular lymphoma is a low-grade, indolent neoplasm with a long natural history (median survival approaches 10 years), but 70% of patients have advanced-stage (III/IV) disease at diagnosis, often with bone marrow involvement, and cure is not considered feasible with standard treatment modalities for most patients. Follicular NHL may eventually transform to a more aggressive lymphoma, characterized pathologically by diffuse large cell infiltrates and clinically by rapidly expanding lymph nodes or tumor masses, rising lactate dehydrogenase (LDH) levels, and the onset of disease-related symptoms.

Management of follicular lymphomas is influenced by the stage. For the rare patient with early-stage (I/some non-bulky II) disease after clinical staging, the appropriate treatment is radiation therapy. With the use of locoregional lymphoid irradiation, more than one half of patients with early-stage disease achieve a durable remission or cure.

For patients with advanced-stage disease, management is more controversial. Although advanced-stage indolent NHL is responsive to a variety of treatments, incurability and long natural history have led to the practice of deferring treatment until symptoms develop. This strategy is referred to as the *watch and wait approach*. A prospective study of early intervention compared observation to the anti-CD20 monoclonal antibody rituximab alone and to rituximab followed by maintenance but found no difference in overall survival or histologic transformation rates. Indications for treatment include cosmetic or mechanical problems caused by enlarging lymph nodes, high tumor burden, constitutional symptoms, and evidence of marrow compromise.

Multiple treatment options are available, including monoclonal antibody therapies, targeted agents, immunomodulatory agents, chemotherapeutic agents, and radiolabeled antibodies. For most patients appropriate treatment includes the chimeric anti–B-cell monoclonal antibody rituximab, with or without systemic chemotherapy. The addition of rituximab to chemotherapy has increased response rates, duration of remission, and in some studies, overall survival (level I evidence obtained from at least one properly designed, randomized controlled trial).

The choice of chemotherapy to employ in combination with rituximab may be influenced by patient age and medical condition. Multiple options are available, and no regimen has proved superior with regard to overall survival. The combination of bendamustine, a unique agent with properties similar to alkylating agents and purine analogues, plus rituximab appeared advantageous compared with the CHOP regimen (i.e., cyclophosphamide, hydroxydaunorubicin [doxorubicin], Oncovin [vincristine], and prednisone) plus rituximab in a randomized trial with regard to toxicity, response rate, and progression-free survival (level I evidence).

Most patients respond to treatment, and at least one third achieve a clinical complete remission. The combination of bendamustine-rituximab results in median time to progression of 5 to 6 years. Treatment with cytotoxic agents is typically discontinued when the maximum response has been achieved, but rituximab may be continued on an intermittent schedule to maintain remission. It has been shown to prolong remission times in randomized studies (level 1 evidence). Risk of recurrence and cost considerations may influence the use of this therapy because rituximab may also be used at the time of recurrence with similar outcomes.

After a patient relapses, subsequent remissions may be achieved but are often less durable compared to first remission. Therapeutic options for patients who relapse include retreatment with chemotherapy, often with a different drug or combination than that used initially. Patients in relapse can also be treated with rituximab as a single agent. For patients who are refractory to rituximab, several humanized anti-CD20 antibodies have been developed. Obinutuzumab is a humanized glycoengineered anti-CD20 antibody with enhanced antibody-dependent cellular cytotoxicity function. It has single agent activity in relapsed FL and has shown high response rates in combination with chemotherapy. Immunomodulators such as lenalidomide also have strong activity in combination with anti-CD20 antibodies in the relapsed setting. PI3 kinase inhibitors idelalisib and copanlisib have an overall

表 5.5 淋巴瘤和浆细胞疾病的新治疗药物

分类	药物	靶点	作用机制	适应证
单克隆抗体	利妥昔单抗 奥妥珠单抗	CD20	补体介导的和抗体依赖的细胞毒性、肿瘤细胞凋亡	大多数 B 细胞淋巴瘤
	达雷妥尤单抗	CD38		多发性骨髓瘤
抗体-药物偶联物	维布妥昔单抗 泊洛妥珠单抗	CD30 CD79a	抗体结合微管蛋白抑制剂被递送到肿瘤细胞	霍奇金淋巴瘤和 CD30[+] 淋巴瘤 DLBCL
免疫调节剂	沙利度胺 来那度胺 泊马度胺	cereblon、免疫调节	结合 cereblon、激活 E3 泛素连接酶复合物	多发性骨髓瘤 NHL 亚型（来那度胺）
激酶抑制剂 BTK 抑制剂	伊布替尼 阿卡替尼 泽布替尼	Bruton 酪氨酸激酶	阻断 B 细胞受体信号	CLL、MCL、MZL、WM
Pi3k 抑制剂	艾代拉里斯 可泮利塞	磷脂酰肌醇 3 激酶	阻断 B 细胞受体信号	CLL、FL
BCL-2 抑制剂	维奈妥拉	BCL-2	阻断抗凋亡蛋白 BCL-2，导致程序性细胞死亡	CLL
蛋白酶体抑制剂	硼替佐米 卡非佐米 伊沙佐米	蛋白酶体	抑制肿瘤细胞中的毒性蛋白质降解	多发性骨髓瘤 MCL
CAR-T 细胞	阿基仑赛 替沙来塞	CD19	基因工程改造的 T 细胞与恶性 B 细胞直接结合	DLBCL ALL

ALL，急性淋巴细胞白血病；BTK，Bruton 酪氨酸激酶；CLL，慢性淋巴细胞白血病；DLBCL，弥漫大 B 细胞淋巴瘤；FL，滤泡性淋巴瘤；MCL，套细胞淋巴瘤；MZL，边缘区淋巴瘤；WM，瓦尔登斯特伦巨球蛋白血症。

FL 是一种低度恶性的惰性肿瘤，其自然病程较长（中位生存期接近 10 年），但 70% 的患者在诊断时已处于晚期（Ⅲ期/Ⅳ期），且常伴有骨髓受累，对于大多数患者，标准治疗模式难以实现治愈。滤泡性 NHL 最终可能转变为更具侵袭性的淋巴瘤，其病理特征为弥漫大细胞浸润，临床表现为淋巴结或肿块迅速扩大、乳酸脱氢酶（LDH）水平升高、出现与疾病相关的症状。

FL 的管理受疾病分期的影响。对于临床分期为早期（Ⅰ期/部分Ⅱ期非巨块型）的罕见患者，适当的治疗方法是放疗。通过局部区域照射，超过 1/2 的早期患者能够实现持久缓解或治愈。

对于晚期患者，管理策略目前仍存在争议。尽管晚期惰性 NHL 对多种治疗反应良好，但由于其不可治愈性和较长的自然病程，通常采取推迟治疗，直至出现症状才启动治疗。这种方法被称为"观察等待策略"。在一项比较早期干预和观察等待策略的前瞻性试验中，一组患者采用观察等待策略，另一组患者接受抗 CD20 单克隆抗体利妥昔单抗单药进行早期干预，并使用利妥昔单抗进行维持治疗，结果发现，这两组患者的总体生存率或组织学转化率并无差异。治疗的指征包括淋巴结肿大引起外观问题或压迫症状、高肿瘤负荷、全身症状及有骨髓衰竭的证据。

对于需要启动治疗的晚期患者，目前有多种治疗手段可供选择，包括单克隆抗体、靶向药物、免疫调节剂、化疗药物和放射性标记抗体。大多数患者可选择 B 细胞单克隆抗体利妥昔单抗单药使用，或与全身化疗联合使用。在化疗中加入利妥昔单抗可提高反应率、延长缓解期，并在一些研究中提高了总体生存率（Ⅰ级证据；即数据来自至少 1 项设计合理的随机对照试验）。

与利妥昔单抗联用的化疗药物选择可能受患者年龄和身体状况的影响。多种化疗方案可供使用，且没有任何一种方案在总体生存率方面优于其他方案。在一项随机试验中，与 CHOP 方案（即环磷酰胺、多柔比星、长春新碱和泼尼松）+ 利妥昔单抗相比，苯达莫司汀（一种具有与烷化剂和嘌呤类似物相似特性的药物）+ 利妥昔单抗的组合在毒性、反应率和无进展生存期方面均表现出优势（Ⅰ级证据）。

大多数 FL 患者对治疗有反应，且至少 1/3 的患者可实现临床完全缓解。苯达莫司汀-利妥昔单抗联合治疗的中位进展时间为 5～6 年。当达到完全缓解时，通常会停用细胞毒性药物，但利妥昔单抗可间歇使用，以维持缓解状态。随机对照试验表明，这种维持治疗可延长缓解时间（Ⅰ级证据）。复发风险和成本因素可能影响维持治疗的使用，因为利妥昔单抗也可在复发时使用，且效果相似。

患者复发后，虽然可能再次实现缓解，但与首次缓解相比，通常持续时间较短。复发患者的治疗选择包括再次化疗，通常选用与初次治疗不同的药物或联用初次治疗的药物。复发患者也可单用利妥昔单抗。对于利妥昔单抗难治性患者，目前已开发了多种人源化抗 CD20 抗体。奥妥珠单抗是一种人源化糖基化抗 CD20 抗体，具有增强的抗体依赖性细胞毒性功能。它在复发性 FL 中表现出较好的单药活性，且与化疗联用时显示出较高的反应率。免疫调节剂（如来那度胺）与抗 CD20 抗体联用也在复发患者中表现出较好的治疗效果。PI3 激酶抑制剂艾代拉里斯和可泮利塞的总体反应率为 56%，中位缓解持

response rate of 56% with median response duration of 12 months. Radioactively labeled anti-CD20 antibodies such as ibritumomab tiuxetan (yttrium labeled) have also been used for patients with relapsed or refractory follicular lymphoma and have been associated with high response rates. Administration of radiolabelled antibodies requires treatment in a specialized center with nuclear medicine expertise and has limited the use of these agents. For patients who have clinical or pathologic evidence of transformation to a higher grade of lymphoma, treatment that is appropriate for a diffuse, aggressive histology should be offered (discussed later).

High-dose chemotherapy with autologous or allogeneic stem cell transplantation for follicular NHLs may be appropriate for selected patients with recurrent or refractory disease. Long-term follow-up of patients undergoing allogeneic transplantation suggests that some patients are cured with this modality, but the morbidity associated with allogeneic transplantation has limited its widespread use for indolent lymphomas.

In addition to the follicular NHLs, the MALT lymphomas and closely related marginal zone lymphomas are considered low-grade, indolent subtypes. Given the excellent prognosis, localized nature, and long natural history of the MALT lymphomas, they are usually managed conservatively with local treatment modalities (i.e., radiation or surgery) and avoidance of systemic chemotherapy. The monoclonal antibody rituximab has activity against MALT lymphomas and may be used when systemic therapy is desired. The gastric MALT lymphomas are highly associated with *H. pylori* infection, and remissions may be achieved with eradication of the infection. Antibiotic therapy is therefore first-line treatment for early *H. pylori*–positive gastric MALT lymphoma.

Aggressive non-Hodgkin's lymphomas. Aggressive NHLs include DLBCL, high-grade lymphoma with C-MYC and BCL-2 and/or BCL-6 rearrangements, B-cell lymphoma unclassifiable with features intermediate between DLBCL and classical Hodgkin's lymphoma, Burkitt lymphoma, lymphoblastic lymphoma, anaplastic large cell lymphoma, and peripheral T-cell lymphomas. Most of the aggressive lymphomas are B cell in origin; aggressive T-cell lymphomas are managed similarly but have an overall worse prognosis compared with their B-cell counterparts.

DLBCL is the most common subtype of NHL, constituting up to 30% of adult NHL in Western countries. Patients present with rapidly enlarged nodal masses; about 30% will have fevers, night sweats or weight loss, and 40% may have involvement of organs outside of lymph nodes. In contrast to patients with low-grade NHLs, all patients with aggressive histology should be offered immediate therapy because these lymphomas are life-threatening and potentially curable. The standard initial therapy for all patients with diffuse, aggressive NHL, regardless of stage, is a multidrug chemotherapy regimen that includes an anthracycline in combination with rituximab.

For DLBCL, CHOP plus rituximab (R-CHOP) is the most widely used treatment regimen. Patients with early-stage disease (I/nonbulky II) may be treated with local radiation therapy after a minimum of three cycles of R-CHOP if there is a need to limit exposure to chemotherapy. Patients with advanced-stage disease require six cycles of R-CHOP; the role of local radiation to sites of bulky disease in the setting of advanced-stage disease is not well established. Complete remissions can be achieved with R-CHOP or similar regimens, and more than 50% of patients are cured. Identifying prognostic biomarkers for the subset of patients who respond less well or who suffer early disease relapse is a priority.

In the early 2000s, gene expression profiling (GEP) using microarrays shed significant light into the biologic heterogeneity of DLBCL. Three distinct signatures were identified corresponding to potential cells of origin (COO): germinal center B-cell–like (GCB), activated B-cell–like (ABC), and primary mediastinal large B-cell lymphoma (PMBL), with approximately 15% of cases remaining unclassifiable. The GCB subtype arises from centroblasts, whereas the ABC subtype arises from a plasmablastic cell just prior to germinal center exit. These gene signatures have prognostic implications, with GCB-DLBCLs having a more favorable overall survival than ABC cases. PMBL displays a GEP profile that resembles that of Hodgkin's lymphoma and has a more favorable prognosis than either DLBCL subtype.

In addition to the COO, molecular subtypes of DLBCL have prognostic impact. Up to 15% of DLBCL cases contain translocations involving the MYC gene on chromosome 8q24 in combination with BCL-2 and/or BCL-6 translocations (referred to as "double or triple hit" NHL). C-MYC is a pro-oncogene that encodes a transcription factor that when dysregulated leads to uncontrolled cellular proliferation and survival. BCL-2 is an oncogene on chromosome 8q21 that when translocated leads to dysregulation of the antiapoptotic protein BCL-2. BCL-6 is a master regulator of the germinal center reaction and a transcriptional repressor. Double or triple hit NHL has the worst clinical outcome and is insufficiently treated with R-CHOP. Most patients have advanced stage disease, elevated LDH, bone marrow and CNS involvement. In general, more intensive regimens such as dose-adjusted EPOCH-R (etoposide, prednisone vincristine [Oncovin], cyclophosphamide, hydroxydaunorubicin [doxorubicin]-rituximab) or HyperCVAD-R (hyperfractionated doses of cyclophosphamide, vincristine, doxorubicin [Adriamycin], dexamethasone-rituximab) are used.

MYC and BCL-2 proteins can be overexpressed in DLBCL in the absence of gene translocation. Such "double-expressor" lymphomas have an intermediate prognosis. Most cases of double-hit lymphoma are of GCB origin whereas most cases of double-expresser lymphomas are of ABC origin.

Many studies have examined alternatives to R-CHOP therapy, including study of more intensive chemotherapy combinations or with addition of new agents such as ibrutinib or lenalidomide. To date, these approaches have largely failed to show improvements in disease control and survival for standard-risk patients and, therefore, R-CHOP remains the default standard of care for initial treatment of most patients.

Published studies of consolidation with high-dose chemotherapy and autologous stem cell transplantation (ASCT) following R-CHOP induction have also been largely negative. In particular, ASCT does not abrogate the negative prognostic impact of C-MYC translocations. In retrospective study, no difference in relapse-free and overall survival with ASCT has been identified in double hit patients who received intensified upfront treatment regimens such as DA-EPOCH-R (dose adjusted EPOCH-R) or HyperCVAD-R. However, a survival benefit for ASCT has been noted in double hit patients treated with R-CHOP, emphasizing the inferior outcomes with R-CHOP in this specific patient population.

Patients who relapse after achieving a remission may be cured with high-dose chemotherapy and ASCT, which is standard therapy if relapsed disease remains responsive to regular doses of chemotherapy. In the pre-rituximab era, cure rates with salvage chemotherapy and ASCT approached 50%. However, the large lymphoma CORAL study showed that patients who received rituximab with CHOP as part of upfront therapy had poor PFS (progression-free survival) of 21%. Patients who relapsed within a year of treatment with R-CHOP had very poor outcomes as well.

This high-risk relapsed patient population is now the target of clinical trials with chimeric antigen receptor T-cell (CAR-T) therapy. In this type of cellular immunotherapy, patients' autologous T cells are

续时间为 12 个月。放射性核素标记的抗 CD20 抗体［如替伊莫单抗（标记钇）］也被用于治疗复发或难治性 FL，且具有较高的反应率。放射性标记抗体的给药需要在具有核医学专业资质的中心进行，这限制了这些药物的使用。对于临床或病理学证据显示已经转化为侵袭性淋巴瘤的患者，应给予侵袭性淋巴瘤的相关治疗（见下文）。

对于复发或难治性滤泡性 NHL，大剂量化疗联合自体造血干细胞移植（SCT）或异基因造血干细胞移植（alloSCT）可能是合适的选择。长期随访发现，部分患者通过 alloSCT 可获得治愈，但相关死亡率也限制了其在惰性淋巴瘤中的广泛应用。

除滤泡性 NHL 外，MALT 淋巴瘤等边缘区淋巴瘤也被视为低级别惰性淋巴瘤亚型。鉴于 MALT 淋巴瘤预后良好、呈局灶性生长及自然病程长的特点，通常采用保守局部治疗（即放疗或手术），并避免进行全身化疗。单克隆抗体利妥昔单抗对 MALT 淋巴瘤有效，当患者需要全身治疗时可选用。胃 MALT 淋巴瘤与幽门螺杆菌感染高度相关，根除感染可实现缓解。因此，对于早期幽门螺杆菌阳性的胃 MALT 淋巴瘤，抗生素治疗是一线治疗方案。

侵袭性非霍奇金淋巴瘤 侵袭性 NHL 包括 DLBCL、伴有 *C-MYC* 和 *BCL-2* 和（或）*BCL-6* 重排的高级别淋巴瘤、兼具 DLBCL 和经典型霍奇金淋巴瘤特征的未分类型 B 细胞淋巴瘤、伯基特淋巴瘤、淋巴母细胞性淋巴瘤、间变性大细胞淋巴瘤和外周 T 细胞淋巴瘤。大多数侵袭性淋巴瘤起源于 B 细胞；侵袭性 T 细胞淋巴瘤的管理与 B 细胞淋巴瘤类似，但总体预后较差。

DLBCL 是最常见的 NHL 亚型，占西方国家成人 NHL 的约 30%。患者临床表现为迅速增大的淋巴结肿块；约 30% 的患者会出现发热、盗汗或体重减轻，40% 的患者可能有淋巴结外器官受累。与低级别 NHL 患者不同，所有侵袭性淋巴瘤患者均应立即接受治疗，因为这些淋巴瘤可能危及生命且可能被治愈。无论疾病分期如何，所有弥漫性侵袭性 NHL 患者的标准初始治疗方案均为包含蒽环类药物的多药化疗联合利妥昔单抗。

对于 DLBCL，CHOP 方案联合利妥昔单抗（R-CHOP）是最广泛使用的治疗方案。早期（Ⅰ期/Ⅱ期非巨块型）患者在接受至少 3 个周期的 R-CHOP 治疗后，如有必要降低化疗暴露，则可加用局部放疗。晚期患者需要进行 6 个周期的 R-CHOP 治疗；局部放疗对于晚期患者巨块型病灶的作用尚未明确。R-CHOP 或类似方案可实现完全缓解，超过 50% 的患者可被治愈。当务之急是明确能识别缓解效果不佳或早期疾病复发的高危患者的预后生物标志物。

21 世纪初，基于微阵列的基因表达谱（GEP）揭示了 DLBCL 的生物异质性。目前已识别出 3 种分别对应于潜在细胞起源（COO）的亚型：生发中心 B 细胞样（GCB）型、活化 B 细胞样（ABC）型和原发纵隔大 B 细胞淋巴瘤（PMBL），其中约有 15% 的病例仍无法分类。GCB 型起源于中心母细胞，而 ABC 型起源于生发中心退出前的浆母细胞。这些基因特征具有预后意义，GCB-DLBCL 的总体生存率高于 ABC 型。PMBL 的 GEP 特征与霍奇金淋巴瘤相似，且预后优于其他 DLBCL 亚型。

除 COO 分型外，DLBCL 的分子亚型也具有预后意义。多达 15% 的 DLBCL 患者伴有位于 8 号染色体 q24 位点的 *MYC* 基因易位，同时伴有 *BCL-2* 和（或）*BCL-6* 易位（即"双打击"或"三打击"NHL）。*C-MYC* 是一种原癌基因，编码一种转录因子，这种转录因子失调会导致细胞增殖和存活失控。*BCL-2* 是位于 8 号染色体 q21 位点的癌基因，当其易位时会导致抗凋亡蛋白 BCL-2 失调。BCL-6 是生发中心反应的主要调节因子和转录抑制因子。"双打击"或"三打击"NHL 患者的临床结局最差，且 R-CHOP 方案的治疗效果不佳。大多数患者处于疾病晚期，LDH 水平升高，骨髓和中枢神经系统受累。通常情况下，临床上会选择更激进的治疗方案，如剂量调整的 EPOCH-R（DA-EPOCH-R；包括依托泊苷、泼尼松、长春新碱、环磷酰胺、多柔比星、利妥昔单抗）或 HyperCVAD-R（大剂量环磷酰胺、长春新碱、多柔比星、地塞米松、利妥昔单抗）。

在 DLBCL 中，MYC 和 BCL-2 蛋白可在无基因易位的情况下过表达，此类"双表达"淋巴瘤的预后中等。大多数"双打击"淋巴瘤起源于 GCB 型，而大多数"双表达"淋巴瘤起源于 ABC 型。

许多研究探讨了 R-CHOP 治疗的替代方案，包括更激进的化疗组合或添加新药物（如伊布替尼或来那度胺）。迄今为止，这些替代方案大多未能明显改善疾病缓解率和患者生存率，因此对于大多数患者，R-CHOP 仍然是公认的一线标准治疗方案。

关于 R-CHOP 诱导治疗后使用大剂量化疗和自体 SCT 巩固治疗的研究大多呈阴性结果，尤其是自体 SCT 并不能消除 *C-MYC* 易位带来的不良预后影响。在回顾性研究中，对于接受前期强化治疗方案（如 DA-EPOCH-R 或 HyperCVAD-R）的"双打击"NHL 患者，自体 SCT 在无复发生存期和总生存期方面并没有表现出优势。然而，在接受 R-CHOP 治疗的"双打击"NHL 患者中，自体 SCT 显示出生存获益，这强调了 R-CHOP 治疗在这一特定患者群体中的治疗效果较差。

缓解后复发的患者可能通过大剂量化疗和自体 SCT 实现治愈，如果复发患者仍对常规剂量化疗敏感，则其可作为标准治疗手段。在利妥昔单抗上市之前，挽救性化疗和自体 SCT 的治愈率接近 50%。然而，大型淋巴瘤 CORAL 研究表明，前期治疗为 R-CHOP 方案的患者，其大剂量化疗的无进展生存期（PFS）仅为 21%。接受 R-CHOP 治疗后 1 年内复发的患者，其预后非常差。

这些高复发风险患者群体目前正成为嵌合抗原受体 T（CAR-T）细胞治疗临床试验的目标群体。在这种

collected and genetically modified to express a chimeric T-cell receptor that recognizes one or more surface antigens, such as CD19, on the lymphoma cell. There are two FDA-approved CAR-T products for patients whose disease does not respond adequately to salvage chemotherapy, tisagenlecleucel and axicabtagene ciloleucel. Complete remission rates are in the order of 40% for a group of patients with otherwise poor outcomes. These therapies are being compared to ASCT in randomized trials. Despite promising efficacy, CAR-T cell therapy can result in considerable toxicities, including cytokine release syndrome, neurotoxicity, cytopenias, hypogammaglobulinemia, and infections. Patients are carefully monitored by a multidisciplinary team of physicians with experience in delivering cellular therapies.

Mantle cell lymphoma. Mantle cell lymphoma (MCL) accounts for 3% to 10% of adult NHL in Western countries and is most common in older male patients. Caucasians have a higher incidence compared to other ethnicities. The median age at presentation is 68. Mantle cell lymphomas are mature B-cell neoplasms that appear to arise in the mantle zone of the lymphoid follicle and display a highly characteristic immunophenotype, expressing the CD5 antigen and other B-cell markers, but CD23 expression is absent, in contrast to CLL. Mantle cell lymphomas are characterized by a pathognomonic t(11;14) chromosomal translocation that juxtaposes the immunoglobulin heavy chain gene (14q32 locus) with the *BCL1* gene, which encodes the growth-promoting protein cyclin D1. Demonstration of the translocation or expression of cyclin D1 protein by immunohistochemistry allows a definitive diagnosis in most cases. Pathologic classification as a blastoid or pleomorphic subtype and a high proliferation rate are features associated with more aggressive behavior and a poor outcome. TP53, Notch-1, and Notch-2 mutations are also associated with an aggressive clinical course. Two MCL subtypes are recognized in the WHO 2016 classification with different clinical manifestations and molecular pathways: Nodal MCL, the most common variant with an aggressive clinical course and multiple oncogenic mutations, and a leukemic, non-nodal subtype of MCL seen in 10% to 20% of patients, who have an indolent clinical course. These latter patients present with lymphocytosis, splenomegaly, and bone marrow involvement.

Patients are usually treated with systemic chemotherapy combined with rituximab, but durable remissions are difficult to achieve. High-dose chemotherapy with autologous stem cell transplantation is often applied during first remission for younger patients and has been associated with more durable remissions (level II-1 evidence, which is evidence obtained from well-designed controlled trials without randomization). Patients with TP53 mutations do not benefit from high-dose chemotherapy and are preferentially enrolled in clinical trials of new agents. Multiple agents and regimens are available for those who are not candidates for transplantation and patients with recurrent disease.

The Bruton tyrosine kinase (BTK) inhibitors ibrutinib and acalabrutinib and the BCL-2 inhibitor venetoclax have shown remarkable activity in relapsed MCL in combination with anti-CD20 antibodies. They are also being investigated as frontline treatment in combination with immunochemotherapy or in chemotherapy-free combinations. CAR-T cell therapy trials are ongoing in MCL and provide hope for patients who have progressed on the BTK inhibitors. Allogeneic SCT can provide a cure in 30% of patients with MCL and is a considered in relapsed patients and those with TP53 mutations.

High-grade non-Hodgkin's lymphomas. The two high-grade subtypes, Burkitt lymphoma (BL) and lymphoblastic lymphoma, are rare in the adult population. Nonetheless, these subtypes are important because they are potentially curable with appropriate therapy and often require urgent, inpatient treatment at the time of diagnosis due to their highly aggressive nature, rapid growth, and tendency to develop tumor lysis on initiation of therapy.

Lymphoblastic lymphoma in adults is an aggressive lymphoma that is considered the lymphomatous counterpart of acute T-cell lymphocytic leukemia. B-cell lymphoblastic lymphoma is less common. Lymphoblastic lymphoma usually afflicts young adult men and involves the mediastinum and bone marrow, with a propensity to relapse in the leptomeninges.

Burkitt lymphoma is a rare B-cell lymphoma in adults that is highly aggressive with a propensity to involve the bone marrow and central nervous system. Burkitt lymphoma is characterized cytogenetically by the pathognomonic t(8;14) translocation that moves the *MYC* oncogene from chromosome 8 to a location close to the enhancers of the antibody heavy-chain genes (*IGH* locus) on chromosome 14. In central Africa, where Burkitt lymphoma is endemic in children, it is usually associated with EBV. However, in the United States, it is uncommon for sporadic Burkitt lymphoma to be EBV positive. Recently, Burkitt-like lymphoma with 11q aberrations has been included in the WHO classification as a provisional entry. The 11q aberrations are particularly frequent in immunocompromised hosts, such as patients after organ transplantation. Recurrent ID3 mutations are found in about 30% of cases of BL, and ID3 has been recently implicated as a tumor suppressor gene with a role in pathogenesis.

Burkitt lymphoma and lymphoblastic lymphomas require treatment with intensive multiagent chemotherapy, including intrathecal chemotherapy to prevent leptomeningeal relapse. These lymphomas undergo rapid tumor lysis on initiation of chemotherapy, and all patients must receive prophylaxis against tumor lysis syndrome before and during their first course of chemotherapy. Prophylaxis includes hydration, alkalinization of the urine, allopurinol, and consideration of rasburicase therapy for rapid lowering of elevated uric acid levels.

Prognosis

A variety of prognostic variables have been identified for NHL, and specific prognostic schemes have been devised for common diseases, including DLBCL, follicular NHL, and mantle cell lymphomas. The predictors for poor survival for most subtypes include advanced stage (III/IV) at onset, involvement of multiple extranodal sites of disease, elevated LDH, B symptoms (e.g., fever, night sweats, weight loss), and poor performance status.

The International Prognostic Index (IPI) stratifies patients based on age, performance status, stage, and number of extranodal sites. The likelihood of cure and long-term, disease-free survival ranges from more than 75% for patients with one or no adverse factors to less than 50% for patients with four or more adverse factors.

Factors associated with shortened survival in follicular NHL include older age, advanced stage, anemia, multiple lymph node sites (more than four), and elevated LDH levels. Patients with three or more of these factors have a median survival of 5 years, roughly one half of that of patients with zero or one risk factor. Cytogenetic and molecular abnormalities that result in increased lymphoma cell proliferation and survival are taking center stage as prognostic variables, with some incremental improvement in outcomes with aggressive upfront treatment strategies and cellular therapies.

Aggressive T-cell lymphomas usually fare more poorly than B-cell NHL, and patients are typically considered candidates for investigational studies and upfront transplantation. Anaplastic large cell lymphoma (ALCL) ALK+, however, has a favorable outcome with chemotherapy alone. The anti-CD30 antibody-drug conjugate brentuximab vedotin has strong activity in ALCL and other types of T-cell lymphomas that express CD30.

细胞免疫治疗中，采集患者的自体T细胞并进行基因改造，使其表达嵌合T细胞受体，该受体能够识别淋巴瘤细胞上的1个或多个表面抗原（如CD19）。对于对挽救性化疗反应不佳的患者，美国食品药品监督管理局（FDA）批准了两款CAR-T产品，即替沙来塞和阿基仑赛。在一组高危的复发淋巴瘤患者中，CAR-T细胞治疗的完全缓解率约为40%。随机对照试验正在比较这些CAR-T细胞治疗和自体SCT。尽管CAR-T细胞治疗的疗效显著，但也可能导致严重的不良反应，包括细胞因子释放综合征、神经毒性、血细胞减少、低丙种球蛋白血症和感染。患者需要由有细胞治疗经验的多学科医生团队进行密切监测。

套细胞淋巴瘤　套细胞淋巴瘤（MCL）占西方国家成人NHL的3%～10%，最常见于老年男性。与其他种族相比，高加索人的发病率更高，发病中位年龄为68岁。MCL是一种成熟B细胞肿瘤，可能起源于淋巴滤泡的外套层，并具有高度特征性的免疫表型，即表达CD5抗原和其他B细胞标志物，但不表达CD23，这可与CLL进行区分。MCL的特征是存在病理性（11;14）染色体易位，该易位使免疫球蛋白重链基因（14q32位点）与 *BCL1* 基因并列，*BCL1* 基因编码生长促进蛋白细胞周期蛋白D1（CCND1）。多数情况下，证明存在该染色体易位或通过免疫组织化学方法证实CCND1蛋白过表达，即可明确诊断。病理分型为母细胞型、多形性亚型或增殖率较高的患者一般肿瘤侵袭性更强，预后更差。*TP53*、*Notch-1* 和 *Notch-2* 突变也与侵袭性临床病程相关。2016年WHO分类体现了两种不同临床表现和分子通路的MCL亚型：①结节型MCL，是最常见的亚型，具有侵袭性临床病程和多种致癌突变；②白血病性非结节型MCL，占10%～20%，患者的临床病程较为惰性，更易出现外周血淋巴细胞增多、脾大和骨髓浸润。

患者通常接受系统性化疗联合利妥昔单抗治疗，但难以实现长期缓解。对于年轻患者，常在首次缓解期间采用大剂量化疗联合自体SCT，可明显延长患者的缓解时间（Ⅱ-1级证据；即数据来自设计合理的非随机对照试验）。存在 *TP53* 突变的患者无法从大剂量化疗中获益，因此首选参加新药临床试验。对于不适合移植和复发的患者，有多种药物和治疗方案可供选择。

Bruton酪氨酸激酶（BTK）抑制剂伊布替尼和阿卡替尼，以及BCL-2抑制剂维奈托克，可与抗CD20单抗联合使用，其在复发的MCL患者中显示出显著疗效。目前有研究尝试将它们与免疫化疗联合作为一线治疗方案，或作为无化疗方案。针对MCL的CAR-T细胞治疗试验正在进行中，为BTK抑制剂治疗后疾病进展的患者带来了希望。alloSCT可使30%的MCL患者获得治愈，因此可考虑用于复发患者和存在 *TP53* 突变的患者。

高级别非霍奇金淋巴瘤　NHL的两种高度侵袭性亚型，即伯基特淋巴瘤（BL）和淋巴母细胞性淋巴瘤，在成人中较为罕见。然而，这些亚型很重要，因为它们通过适当治疗有可能治愈，且由于其高度侵袭性、快速生长及在治疗开始时倾向于发生肿瘤溶解，通常需要在确诊时进行紧急住院治疗。

成人淋巴母细胞性淋巴瘤是一种侵袭性淋巴瘤，被认为是急性T细胞淋巴细胞白血病的淋巴瘤表现形式。B细胞淋巴母细胞性淋巴瘤较少见。淋巴母细胞性淋巴瘤常见于年轻成年男性，可累及纵隔和骨髓，有软脑膜复发倾向。

BL是一种罕见的成人B细胞淋巴瘤，具有高度侵袭性，倾向于累及骨髓和中枢神经系统。BL的细胞遗传学特征为病理性t（8;14）易位，将 *MYC* 癌基因从8号染色体移至14号染色体上的免疫球蛋白重链基因（*IGH* 位点）的增强子附近。在中非国家，BL在儿童中流行，通常与EBV感染相关。然而，在美国，散发性BL很少呈EBV阳性。近期，具有11q异常的伯基特样淋巴瘤已作为暂定亚型被列入WHO分类。11q异常在免疫妥协宿主（如器官移植后患者）中尤其常见。约30%的BL患者存在 *ID3* 基因的复发性突变，*ID3* 被认为是一种肿瘤抑制基因，在BL的发病机制中发挥重要作用。

BL和淋巴母细胞性淋巴瘤需要采用强化多药化疗，包括进行鞘内化疗以预防软脑膜复发。这些淋巴瘤在化疗开始时可能会迅速发生肿瘤溶解，所有患者在化疗前和第一疗程化疗期间必须预防肿瘤溶解综合征。预防措施包括补液、碱化尿液、别嘌醇，并考虑酌情使用拉布立酶快速降低尿酸水平。

预后

目前已确定了多种NHL的预后因素，并为常见亚型（包括DLBCL、滤泡性NHL和MCL）制定了特定的预后方案。大多数亚型的不良预后预测因素包括发病时处于晚期（Ⅲ期/Ⅳ期）、累及多个结外部位、LDH水平升高、B症状（如发热、盗汗、体重减轻）和一般状况差。

国际预后指数（IPI）根据年龄、一般状况、分期和结外受累部位数量对患者进行风险分层。长期无病生存的可能性从＜50%（≥4个不利因素）到＞75%（1个或无不利因素）不等。

与滤泡性NHL患者生存期缩短相关的不利预后因素包括高龄、晚期、贫血、累及多个淋巴结部位（＞4个）和LDH水平升高。具有≥3个不利因素的患者中位生存期为5年，生存期约为仅有1个或无不利因素患者的1/2。导致淋巴瘤细胞增殖和存活增加的细胞遗传学和分子异常正逐渐成为核心预后指标，而一些更加积极的一线治疗策略和细胞治疗也使这些患者的预后得到逐步改善。

侵袭性T细胞淋巴瘤患者的预后通常比B细胞NHL更差，患者通常被推荐参加临床试验或前期进行移植。比较特殊的是，ALK$^+$间变性大细胞淋巴瘤（ALCL）经单纯化疗的预后良好。抗CD30抗体-药物偶联物维布妥昔单抗在ALCL和其他表达CD30的T细胞淋巴瘤患者中具有较好的疗效。

❖ For a deeper discussion of these topics, please see Chapter 176, "Non-Hodgkin's Lymphomas," in *Goldman-Cecil Medicine*, 26th Edition.

Hodgkin Lymphoma

Hodgkin's lymphoma (HL) is a node-based lymphoid malignancy characterized by the neoplastic Reed-Sternberg (RS) cell in an inflammatory background. Hodgkin's lymphoma accounts for 10% of lymphomas, with about 8110 new cases diagnosed in the United States in 2019, and it is the most common lymphoma among young adults. The peak incidence of HL occurs between the ages of 20 and 35. The incidence of HL and death rate have declined in the past decade.

The cause of Hodgkin's lymphoma remains enigmatic. Risk factors include a history of infectious mononucleosis, high socioeconomic status, immunosuppression (e.g., HIV infection, allograft transplantation, immunosuppressive drugs), and autoimmune disorders. Although EBV is frequently detected in patients, a direct causal role has not been established.

Pathology

Hodgkin's lymphoma is diagnosed by identifying the malignant RS cell in involved lymphoid tissue. The classic RS cell is large and binucleate, with each nucleus containing a prominent nucleolus, suggesting the appearance of owl eyes. Although the cellular origin of the RS cell was debated for decades, molecular studies have confirmed that RS cells are B cells with clonal rearrangement of the germline *IG* locus. Unlike NHL, the bulk of the infiltrate in lymph nodes in HL is usually composed of benign reactive inflammatory cells, and the RS cells can be difficult to find. Immunophenotyping of RS cells shows CD30 (Ki-1) and CD15 positivity and negative CD20, CD45, and cytoplasmic or surface immunoglobulin. EBV is identified in the RS cells in about 50% of cases.

The pathologic subtypes of classic HL include four variants—nodular sclerosing (NS), mixed cellularity (MC), lymphocyte depleted (LD), and lymphocyte rich (LR)—plus the non-classic variant, nodular lymphocyte-predominant (NLP). The NS form is the most common variant (60% to 80%) and is characterized by fibrous bands separating the node into nodules and by the lacunar type of RS cells. It is the predominant type encountered in adolescents and young adults and typically involves the mediastinum and supradiaphragmatic nodal sites. In the MC type (15%), band-forming sclerosis is absent, and RS cells are easily identified in a diffuse inflammatory infiltrate that is more heterogeneous than that seen in the NS variant. The LR variant (5%) is characterized by classic RS cells in a background of small lymphocytes. LD is a rare variant (<1%) that is associated with advanced age, HIV infection, and low socioeconomic status. The pathologic hallmarks of LD HL include a notable paucity of inflammatory cells and sheets of RS cells.

The NLP variant is a distinct entity that is more closely related to indolent NHL than to classic HL. The NLP form is characterized by a nodular growth pattern with variants of RS cells that have polylobated nuclei (i.e., popcorn cells); classic RS cells are usually absent. The immunophenotype of these variant cells is distinct from classic RS cells, with expression of B-cell antigens (CD19 and CD20) and CD45 and absence of CD15 and CD30. The existence of CD20 allows the therapeutic use of rituximab, an agent not typically employed in classic Hodgkin's lymphoma. The NLP variant accounts for 5% of Hodgkin's lymphoma cases, has a strong male preponderance, and tends to involve peripheral nodes but spare the mediastinum. The prognosis is excellent, although late relapses are more common than in classic HL.

Clinical Presentation

Hodgkin's lymphoma arises in lymph nodes, most commonly in the mediastinum or neck, and spreads to adjacent contiguous or noncontiguous nodal sites, including retroperitoneal nodes and the spleen. As the disease progresses, it may spread hematogenously to involve extranodal sites, including bone marrow, liver, and lung. Unlike NHL, Hodgkin's lymphoma rarely arises in extranodal sites, although it can involve extranodal sites by contiguous spread from an adjacent lymph node (e.g., vertebrae from retroperitoneal lymph nodes, pulmonary parenchyma from hilar nodes).

Hodgkin's lymphoma usually produces painless enlargement of lymph nodes, most often in the neck. Mediastinal adenopathy may be found incidentally in an asymptomatic patient on routine chest radiography. Massive mediastinal or hilar adenopathy, with or without adjacent pulmonary involvement, may cause cough, shortness of breath, wheezing, or stridor. At clinical presentation, about one third of patients have constitutional symptoms of fever, night sweats, or weight loss (i.e., B symptoms). Generalized pruritus is associated with the NS subtype, and patients may give a history of troubling pruritus for months to years before the diagnosis. Rarely, patients may also complain of prompt marked chest discomfort induced by alcohol, the etiology of which is uncertain, but has been observed in patients with HL and carcinoid syndromes.

If left untreated, the natural history is one of inexorable, albeit often slow, progression to involve multiple nodal sites, followed by hematogenous spread to the bone marrow, liver, and other viscera. As the disease advances, patients experience B symptoms, malaise, cachexia, and infectious complications. Patients with progressive disease ultimately die of complications of bone marrow failure or infection.

Accurate staging of newly diagnosed HL is important for treatment planning, prognosis, and assessing response to therapy. A modification of the Ann Arbor classification is used (see Table 5.4), and the suffix A or B is appended to denote the absence or presence, respectively, of B symptoms. The staging work-up of a newly diagnosed patient is similar to that for patients with NHL (see Table 5.3) and includes a history and physical examination; complete blood work, including erythrocyte sedimentation rate (ESR) and HIV serology; computed tomography (CT) scan of the chest, abdomen, and pelvis; positron emission tomography (PET) scan; and in selected cases, a bone marrow aspirate and biopsy. Additional radiographic tests (e.g., bone films, spinal magnetic resonance imaging [MRI]) should be obtained only if symptoms suggest involvement of these structures. Patients also require evaluation of cardiac and pulmonary function before administration of chemotherapy and testing for hepatitis B due to the risk of reactivation during chemotherapy. The information derived from this noninvasive work-up defines the clinical stage of a patient with HL.

Diagnosis and Differential Diagnosis

The diagnosis requires an adequate biopsy of the involved nodal tissue. Immunophenotyping is routinely performed to confirm the diagnosis made on routine light microscopy and to differentiate HL from morphologically similar NHLs (e.g., T-cell–rich large B-cell lymphoma, anaplastic large cell lymphoma).

Treatment

Hodgkin's lymphoma is highly curable; the cure rate exceeds 80% with the use of current treatment modalities. The optimal treatment, including the duration of chemotherapy and the use and dose of radiation therapy, is determined by the stage (i.e., early stage [I/II] vs. advanced stage [III/IV]) and additional prognostic features. Because most patients are young adults and experience long-term, disease-free survival, the goal of therapy has shifted to minimizing treatment-related morbidity and mortality without sacrificing curative potential. Primary radiation therapy is rarely used because of delayed toxicities, which include a substantial risk of secondary solid tumors within the

❖ 有关此专题的深入讨论，请参阅 *Goldman-Cecil Medicine* 第 26 版第 176 章 "非霍奇金淋巴瘤"。

霍奇金淋巴瘤

霍奇金淋巴瘤（HL）是一种结节性淋巴组织恶性肿瘤，其病理学特征是在炎症背景中出现肿瘤性里-施细胞（RS 细胞）。HL 约占淋巴瘤的 10%，2019 年美国新诊断病例约 8110 例，且 HL 是年轻成人最常见的淋巴瘤类型。HL 的发病高峰年龄为 20～35 岁。在过去十年中，HL 的发病率和死亡率均有所下降。

HL 的病因未明。危险因素包括传染性单核细胞增多症病史、高社会经济地位、免疫抑制（如 HIV 感染、同种异体移植、应用免疫抑制剂）和自身免疫病。尽管在患者中经常可检测到 EBV，但尚未明确其直接致病作用。

病理学

HL 通过受累淋巴组织中的恶性 RS 细胞进行诊断。典型的 RS 细胞体积大且具有双核，每个细胞核中含有 1 个明显的核仁，形似猫头鹰的眼睛。尽管 RS 细胞的起源一直存在争议，但分子研究已证实，RS 细胞是 B 细胞，具有 *IG* 基因位点的克隆性重排。与 NHL 不同，HL 中的淋巴结浸润以良性反应性炎症细胞为主，且 RS 细胞可能难以被发现。RS 细胞的免疫分型呈 CD30（Ki-1）和 CD15 阳性，CD20、CD45 及胞质或表面免疫球蛋白阴性。在约 50% 的病例中，RS 细胞中可检测到 EBV。

经典型 HL 的病理亚型包括 4 种变体：结节硬化（NS）型、混合细胞（MC）型、淋巴细胞消减（LD）型和淋巴细胞为主（LR）型。HL 还包括结节性淋巴细胞为主（NLP）型非经典型 HL。NS 型是最常见的亚型（60%～80%），其特征是纤维带将淋巴结分隔成结节，并存在腔隙型 RS 细胞。NS 型是青少年和年轻成人常见的类型，通常累及纵隔淋巴结。MC 型（15%）中不存在带状硬化，且 RS 细胞在弥漫性炎症浸润背景中易被识别，这种浸润比 NS 型更具有异质性。LR 型（5%）的特征是在小淋巴细胞背景中存在经典 RS 细胞。LD 型是一种罕见亚型（<1%），与高龄、HIV 感染和低社会经济地位相关，其病理学特征包括炎症细胞显著减少和成片的 RS 细胞。

NLP 型是与惰性 NHL 关系更密切的独特亚型。NLP 型以结节性生长模式为特征，其中的 RS 细胞变体具有多叶核（即爆米花细胞），通常无经典 RS 细胞。与经典 RS 细胞不同，这些变体细胞的免疫分型呈 B 细胞抗原（CD19 和 CD20）和 CD45 阳性，CD15 和 CD30 阴性。CD20 阳性使这些患者可以使用利妥昔单抗进行治疗，该药通常不被用于治疗经典型 HL。NLP 型占 HL 病例的 5%，男性明显多于女性，且倾向于累及外周淋巴结，而纵隔则较少受累。NLP 型患者的预后良好，但相比于经典型 HL，其晚期复发更为常见。

临床表现

HL 源于淋巴结，最常见于纵隔或颈部，可扩散至相邻的连续或非连续淋巴结部位，包括腹膜后淋巴结和脾。随着疾病进展，它可能通过血液传播累及结外部位，包括骨髓、肝和肺。与 NHL 不同，HL 很少源于结外部位，但可通过相邻淋巴结的连续扩散（如从腹膜后淋巴结累及椎骨、从肺门淋巴结累及肺实质）累及结外部位。

HL 通常会引起无痛性淋巴结肿大，最常见于颈部。无症状患者可能在常规胸部 X 线检查中偶然发现纵隔肿物。无论是否累及相邻肺组织，巨大的纵隔或肺门肿物可能引起咳嗽、气短、喘息或喘鸣。约 1/3 的患者出现发热、盗汗或体重减轻等全身症状（即 B 症状）。NS 型患者可出现全身瘙痒，且在确诊前数月至数年就可能有瘙痒病史。极少数患者可出现饮酒后明显胸部不适，其病因不明，该表现可见于 HL 和类癌综合征患者。

如果不进行治疗，HL 的自然病程缓慢且持续进展，累及多个淋巴结部位，随后通过血液传播至骨髓、肝和其他内脏器官。随着疾病进展，患者会出现 B 症状、恶病质或感染性并发症。疾病进展的患者最终可能死于骨髓衰竭或感染并发症。

初诊的 HL 患者需进行准确分期，这对于制订治疗方案、预测预后和评估治疗反应非常重要。可采用修订版 Ann Arbor 分类（表 5.4），后缀 A 或 B 分别表示无或有 B 症状。初诊患者的分期检查与 NHL 患者相似（表 5.3），包括病史和体格检查；血液学检查，包括红细胞沉降率（ESR）和 HIV 血清学检查；胸部、腹部和盆腔计算机断层成像（CT）；正电子发射断层成像（PET）；部分患者需进行骨髓穿刺和活检。只有当相关症状提示受累时，才建议进行额外的放射学检查[如骨骼 X 线检查、脊柱磁共振成像（MRI）等]。在开始化疗前，还需要评估患者的心肺功能，并进行乙型肝炎检测，因为化疗期间存在病毒再激活的风险。通过这些无创性检查可确定 HL 患者的临床分期。

诊断和鉴别诊断

确诊需要对受累淋巴结组织进行充分活检。需常规进行免疫分型，以确认普通光学显微镜检查的诊断，并将 HL 与形态学上相似的 NHL（如富于 T 细胞的大 B 细胞淋巴瘤、间变性大细胞淋巴瘤）区分开来。

治疗

HL 具有较高的治愈率；当前治疗方式的治愈率超过 80%。最佳治疗方案（包括化疗的持续时间和放疗的使用及剂量）取决于分期[即早期（Ⅰ期/Ⅱ期）*vs.* 晚期（Ⅲ期/Ⅳ期）]和其他预后特征。由于大多数患者是年轻人且可获得长期无病生存期，因此治疗目标已转变为在不损失治愈率的前提下，尽量降低治疗相关的发病率和死亡率。很少选择单纯放疗，因其可产生远期毒性，包括治疗后 10 年或更长时间内放射区继发性实体瘤的发生率显著升高，如年轻患者罹患乳

radiation field a decade or more after treatment, including a high risk of breast cancer in young patients. Historically noted long-term sequelae of standard doses of chest irradiation include thyroid dysfunction (usually hypothyroidism) and accelerated coronary artery disease.

Most patients with early-stage (I/II) Hodgkin's lymphoma are treated with the ABVD chemotherapy regimen (i.e., doxorubicin [Adriamycin], bleomycin, vinblastine, and dacarbazine) that may be followed by a course of low-dose radiation (<30 Gy) to involved lymph node sites, which has not been associated with an increased risk of secondary solid tumors. The duration of chemotherapy and the dose of radiation depend on whether the patient has favorable or unfavorable early-stage disease. The definition of favorable disease usually incorporates the absence of a large mediastinal mass, a limited number of involved nodal sites, absence of B symptoms, younger age, and a low ESR. Patients with favorable early-stage disease typically receive two to four cycles of ABVD followed by 20 Gy of radiation, whereas four to six cycles of ABVD and 30 Gy of radiation are required for patients with unfavorable disease (level I evidence). The option for limited course chemotherapy without radiotherapy has also been confirmed as feasible in randomized study. The choice of treatment in early-stage disease requires a detailed conversation with the patient regarding the side effects and potential risks of treatment options.

Patients with advanced-stage (III/IV) Hodgkin's lymphoma are treated primarily with chemotherapy. The ABVD regimen is the most widely used initial treatment in the United States. ABVD is more effective and less toxic than the older MOPP regimen (i.e., nitrogen mustard, vincristine, [Oncovin], procarbazine, and prednisone) and does not cause the long-term sequelae of sterility, infertility, or treatment-induced leukemias associated with MOPP (level I evidence). Long-term toxicity concerns with the ABVD regimen include potential for cardiomyopathy (Adriamycin), pulmonary toxicity (bleomycin), and neuropathy (vincristine). Roughly 60% of patients with stage III or IV disease are cured with six cycles of ABVD. A recent randomized trial confirmed the efficacy of ABVD with elimination of bleomycin after two full cycles of treatment in patients with evidence of early response to treatment.

The intensive regimen of BEACOPP (i.e., bleomycin, etoposide, Adriamycin, cyclophosphamide, vincristine, prednisolone, and procarbazine) has been associated with higher rates of complete response and freedom from treatment failure compared with ABVD-based regimens in patients with advanced disease, although overall survival has not been increased in all studies (level I evidence). BEACOPP is used increasingly in selected patients with high-risk features. Gonadal toxicity with permanent infertility may occur after BEACOPP, and an increased risk of secondary leukemia has been reported. Late sequelae and acute toxicities must be considered when choosing this regimen.

Radiation therapy in combination with chemotherapy is typically not used to treat advanced-stage disease. However, in patients with bulky mediastinal disease, consolidative radiation to the mediastinum after completion of chemotherapy has decreased the rate of relapse.

Evaluating the response to therapy involves repetition of the staging evaluation (i.e., physical examination, CT, and PET) during and at the completion of treatment. A mid-treatment PET scan after two full cycles of ABVD for advanced disease is prognostically informative because persistent metabolic activity in tumor sites correlates with resistance or subsequent relapse of disease. Conversely, patients may be cured despite the common finding of a residual abnormality on CT (e.g., enlarged nodes, residual mediastinal mass) when residual disease is not seen on PET imaging. A persistently positive PET scan during or after treatment with residual radiographic abnormalities is associated with a high rate of subsequent relapse, and these patients should be considered for immediate repeat biopsy or salvage therapy. The more intensive BEACOPP regimen may increase the primary cure rate in such cases. Most patients destined to relapse do so within 2 years; relapses after 5 years are rare except for patients with the NLP variant.

Patients who relapse or fail to respond after initial therapy have several options for secondary therapy which may still prove curative. Second-line therapy is often employed with a plan to pursue high-dose chemotherapy and autologous hematopoietic cell transplantation, which may be associated with cure in patients with chemosensitive disease (level I evidence).

Effective novel agents to treat recurrent HL include brentuximab vedotin, an immunotoxin composed of a CD30-directed antibody linked to an antitubulin agent, and the checkpoint inhibitors pembrolizumab and nivolumab. Brentuximab is associated with high response rates, including complete responses in more than 30% of patients with relapsed disease after autologous transplantation (level II-1 evidence). A randomized study of brentuximab versus placebo after transplantation for high-risk HL patients showed a significant prolongation of progression-free survival. The checkpoint inhibitors are also highly active agents in HL patients with recurrent or refractory disease. Roughly two thirds of patients are expected to respond to therapy, although complete responses occur in a minority of patients. Allogeneic transplantation may also be considered for medically fit patients and has curative potential. Novel transplant therapy from haploidentical (half-matched) donors incorporating post-transplant cyclophosphamide has shown encouraging results with lower transplant-related morbidity and is an area of active investigation.

Prognosis

Most patients with Hodgkin's lymphoma are cured. Prognostic factors that influence risk of relapse or survival include MC or LD histology, male sex, large numbers of involved nodal sites, age older than 40 years, B symptoms, high ESR, and bulky disease (i.e., mediastinum widening by more than one third or a mass larger than 10 cm). The International Prognostic Score, based on seven variables at diagnosis, is a validated predictor of outcome in advanced disease.

Lymphoid Leukemias
Acute Lymphocytic Leukemias

The acute lymphocytic leukemias that arise from precursor B or T cells are described in detail in Chapter 2.

Chronic Lymphocytic Leukemia and Small Lymphocytic Lymphoma

Definition and epidemiology. B-cell CLL is a malignant disorder of lymphocytes characterized by expansion and accumulation of small lymphocytes of B-cell origin. CLL is essentially identical to B-cell small lymphocytic lymphoma but represents the leukemic form of the disease. CLL is the most common form of leukemia in the United States and affects twice as many men as women. There were 20,720 estimated new cases in 2019 and 3,930 deaths. Although it can occur at any stage of life, the incidence increases with age, and more than 90% of cases are diagnosed in adults older than 50 years of age.

The cause of CLL is unknown. Familial clustering of CLL suggests a genetic basis in some cases. First-degree relatives of CLL patients have an 8.5-fold increased risk of developing CLL and a 2.6-fold increased risk of developing another indolent lymphoma. The risk of developing CLL is increased by exposure to organic solvents, Agent Orange, and insecticides. Dietary and lifestyle factors have not been associated with an increased risk of CLL.

CLL is preceded by a clinically asymptomatic stage involving a proliferation of clonal B cells. This condition is referred to as a monoclonal B lymphocytosis (MBL). MBL is detectable in more than 5% of people

腺癌的风险增加。标准剂量胸部放疗的远期后遗症包括甲状腺功能障碍（通常为甲状腺功能减退症）和早发冠状动脉疾病。

大多数早期（Ⅰ期/Ⅱ期）HL 患者接受 ABVD 化疗方案（即多柔比星、博来霉素、长春碱和达卡巴嗪）治疗，后续可能对受累淋巴结部位进行低剂量（<30 Gy）放疗，尚未发现该方案与继发性实体瘤风险增加相关。化疗的持续时间和放疗剂量取决于患者的预后和分期。预后良好的定义通常包括无纵隔大肿块、受累淋巴结数量少、无 B 症状、较年轻和 ESR 低。预后良好的早期患者通常接受 2～4 个周期的 ABVD 化疗，随后进行 20 Gy 放疗，而预后不良的患者则需要接受 4～6 个周期的 ABVD 化疗和 30 Gy 放疗（Ⅰ级证据）。随机对照试验也证实了有限疗程化疗且不进行放疗的可行性。早期 HL 的治疗选择需要与患者详细讨论治疗方案的副作用和潜在风险。

晚期（Ⅲ期/Ⅳ期）HL 患者主要以化疗为主。ABVD 方案是美国最常用的初始治疗方案。与既往的 MOPP 方案（即氮芥、长春新碱、丙卡巴肼和泼尼松）相比，ABVD 方案更有效且毒性更低，且不会引起 MOPP 方案相关的远期后遗症，如生育能力受损或治疗相关性白血病（Ⅰ级证据）。ABVD 方案的长期毒性问题包括心肌病（多柔比星）、肺毒性（博来霉素）和神经病变（长春新碱）的潜在风险。约 60% 的Ⅲ期或Ⅳ期患者可通过 6 个周期的 ABVD 化疗获得治愈。近期一项随机试验证实，对于早期对 ABVD 方案有治疗反应的患者，在完成 2 个完整治疗周期后停用博来霉素是有效的。

与基于 ABVD 的方案相比，强化 BEACOPP 方案（即博来霉素、依托泊苷、多柔比星、环磷酰胺、长春新碱、泼尼松龙和丙卡巴肼）在晚期患者中显示出更高的完全缓解率和无治疗失败生存率，但总生存率在所有研究中均未显著提高（Ⅰ级证据）。BEACOPP 方案越来越多地被选择性用于具有高危特征的患者。使用 BEACOPP 方案后可能发生性腺毒性并导致永久性不育，且已有报告继发性白血病风险增加的情况。因此，选择该方案时，必须考虑远期后遗症和急性毒性的相关风险。

化疗联合放疗通常不用于晚期 HL 患者。然而，对于有纵隔大肿块的患者，化疗完成后对纵隔进行巩固性放疗可降低复发率。

评估治疗反应包括在治疗期间和治疗结束时重复进行分期评估（即体格检查、CT 和 PET）。对于晚期患者，完成 2 个完整周期的 ABVD 化疗后进行中期 PET 具有预后意义，因为复查发现肿瘤部位存在持续代谢活性与疾病耐药或后续复发相关。相反，尽管 CT 常可见残留异常（如淋巴结肿大、残留纵隔肿块），但当 PET 未显示残留病变时，患者仍可能处于治愈状态。治疗期间或治疗后 PET 持续阳性且伴有残留影像学异常的患者后续复发率高，应考虑立即重复活检或进行挽救性治疗。在这种情况下，强化 BEACOPP 方案可能提高治愈率。大多数复发的患者发生在 2 年内，5 年后复发的情况很少见，除非患者为 NLP 型 HL。

首次治疗后复发或无反应的患者有多种二线治疗选择，这些治疗仍可能实现治愈。二线治疗通常包括大剂量化疗和自体 SCT，这可能使化疗敏感的患者获得治愈（Ⅰ级证据）。

治疗复发性 HL 的有效新型药物包括维布妥昔单抗（一种由靶向 CD30 的抗体与抗微管蛋白药物偶联而成的免疫毒素），以及免疫检查点抑制剂帕博利珠单抗和纳武利尤单抗。维布妥昔单抗的反应率很高，在自体移植后复发的患者中，超过 30% 的患者可实现完全缓解（Ⅱ-1 级证据）。一项针对高危 HL 患者移植后使用维布妥昔单抗与安慰剂的随机对照试验显示，维布妥昔单抗显著延长了无进展生存期。免疫检查点抑制剂在复发或难治性 HL 患者中也表现出较好的疗效。约 2/3 的患者对治疗有反应，但免疫检查点抑制剂治疗后完全缓解的患者较少。对于身体状况良好的患者，可考虑 alloSCT，有获得治愈的可能。后置环磷酰胺的半相合（半匹配）alloSCT 显示出令人鼓舞的结果，移植相关死亡率更低，是目前热门的研究领域。

预后

大多数 HL 患者可实现治愈。导致复发风险增加或生存期较短的预后因素包括 MC 型或 LD 型组织学亚型、男性、受累淋巴结数量多、年龄 > 40 岁、有 B 症状、ESR 高和伴有巨块病变（即纵隔增宽 > 1/3 或肿块 > 10 cm）。基于诊断时 7 个变量的国际预后评分是晚期患者预后的有效预测指标。

淋巴细胞白血病

急性淋巴细胞白血病

起源于前体 B 细胞或 T 细胞的急性淋巴细胞白血病详见第 2 章。

慢性淋巴细胞白血病和小淋巴细胞淋巴瘤

定义和流行病学 慢性淋巴细胞白血病（CLL）是一种以来源于 B 细胞的小淋巴细胞扩增和积聚为特征的淋巴细胞恶性疾病。CLL 基本等同于小淋巴细胞淋巴瘤，但代表该病的白血病形式。CLL 是美国最常见的白血病类型，男性患者数量是女性的 2 倍。2019 年估计有 20 720 例新发病例，3930 例死亡。尽管 CLL 可发生于任何年龄段，但其发病率随年龄增长而升高，超过 90% 的病例年龄 > 50 岁。

CLL 的病因尚不清楚。CLL 存在明显的家族聚集倾向，表明部分病例具有遗传基础。CLL 患者的一级亲属患 CLL 的风险增加 8.5 倍，患其他惰性淋巴瘤的风险增加 2.6 倍。接触有机溶剂、除草用橙剂和杀虫剂会增加患 CLL 的风险。饮食和生活方式因素与 CLL 风险增加无关。

CLL 发病前有一个临床无症状阶段，伴有克隆性 B 细胞增殖，该阶段被称为单克隆 B 淋巴细胞增多症（MBL）。MBL 在 60 岁以上人群中的发生率 > 5%，其

aged over 60. The risk of transformation into CLL requiring treatment is approximately 1% per year. Such patients are observed.

Pathology. The common form of CLL is a clonal proliferation of mature B cells expressing characteristic mature B-cell markers and low levels of surface immunoglobulin M (IgM) that is light chain restricted, reflecting the clonal origin of this malignancy.

The diagnostic immunophenotype of CLL is unique, with expression of CD5 and CD23 along with the mature B-cell markers CD19, CD20 (dim expression), and CD21. Although a pathognomonic chromosomal abnormality has not been identified, 30% to 50% of patients have cytogenetic abnormalities, more so if sensitive assays such as FISH are employed. The most frequent abnormalities involve chromosomes 12 (often trisomy 12), 13, and 14. Cytogenetic abnormalities of chromosomes 17 and 11 are associated with an adverse prognosis.

Mutations that contribute to the development of CLL may occur at any stage of B-cell development. CLL cells originating from B cells that have not passed through and experienced the lymph node germinal center reaction have unmutated immunoglobulin heavy-chain variable-region (IgVH) genes and are defined as unmutated CLL (U-CLL). CLL cells that have incurred immunoglobulin (Ig) somatic mutation express mutated IgVH genes and are defined as mutated CLL (M-CLL). Unmutated IgVH genes are associated with a more aggressive form of CLL.

The B-cell receptor pathway has been recognized as the most prominent pathway activated in CLL cells. The B-cell receptor in CLL is activated via recognition and binding of autoantigens and antigens that are present in the microenvironment. Multiple kinases including BTK, spleen tyrosine kinase (SYK), and phosphatidylinositol 3-kinase (PI3K) are activated. This triggers a signaling cascade that activates downstream pathways, including *NFκβ* pathway, ultimately promoting malignant B-cell survival and proliferation.

Diagnosis and differential diagnosis. The diagnosis of CLL is often made incidentally on a routine blood cell count that shows a leukocytosis with a predominance of small lymphocytes. Flow cytometric analysis of peripheral blood or bone marrow aspirate reveals the characteristic clonal B-cell population that is CD5 and CD23 positive. There is monoclonal expression of either Ig kappa or lambda and weak or absent expression of CD20, CD79b, FMC7. Smears of the bone marrow or peripheral blood reveal a predominance of small lymphocytes with inconspicuous nucleoli; ruptured cells (i.e., smudge cells) are often observed. Examination of involved lymph nodes reveals a diffuse infiltrate of small lymphocytes effacing the normal architecture.

CLL must be distinguished from reactive causes of lymphocytosis and other forms of lymphoma or leukemia. Mantle cell lymphoma may appear similar morphologically and with a similar immunophenotype, although CD23 is typically absent and cyclin D1 expression is detected. An absolute lymphocytosis of more than 5000 cells/μL is required for the diagnosis of CLL.

Clinical presentation. CLL cells accumulate in bone marrow, peripheral blood, lymph nodes, and spleen, resulting in lymphocytosis, lymphadenopathy, splenomegaly, and ultimately decreased bone marrow function. CLL is also frequently associated with immune dysregulation, exhibited as hypogammaglobulinemia with an increased risk of bacterial infections and autoimmune phenomena such as Coombs-positive hemolytic anemia or immune thrombocytopenia. Some patients exhibit lymphadenopathy, symptoms related to cytopenias, or recurrent infections. As the disease progresses, patients develop generalized lymphadenopathy, hepatosplenomegaly, and bone marrow failure. Death may occur from infectious complications or bone marrow failure after patients have become refractory to treatment. In about 5% of cases, CLL transforms to a highly malignant diffuse large cell lymphoma, which may prove rapidly fatal. This transformation is commonly referred to as Richter syndrome.

Treatment. CLL is a low-grade disease typically characterized by a long natural history with slow progression over years or decades. Median survival is in excess of 6 years. The extent of disease (stage) at onset is the best predictor of survival. Genomic aberrations such as 17p or 11q deletions and unmutated IgVH status predict for significantly shorter median survival in patients with otherwise early stage disease.

Because standard therapy is not curative and CLL may have an asymptomatic phase lasting years, specific treatment is often withheld until signs of disease progression or development of symptoms (e.g., bulky lymphadenopathy, constitutional symptoms such as fevers, cytopenias caused by bone marrow infiltration). The rate of rise of the white blood cell count may also be used to predict development of symptoms and the need for therapy.

When treatment is required, multiple options for therapy are available. The patient's age, medical condition, and cytogenetic abnormalities may influence the choice of therapy. Active chemotherapeutic agents include several alkylating agents (e.g., chlorambucil, cyclophosphamide), the nucleoside analogue fludarabine, or the novel agent bendamustine. The fludarabine/cyclophosphamide (FC) regimen became a standard of care in 2005 combined with rituximab (FCR), achieving high complete remission rates. The FCR regimen was shown to improve overall survival in patients with CLL in a randomized phase 3 trial. This came at the expense of higher infection risks, particularly in older patients who tolerate bendamustine and rituximab (BR) better. There is also a risk of marrow stem cell injury. Patients with del(17p) did not respond to fludarabine-based regimens, however, and had a median survival of only 16 months after first-line treatment. FCR has been shown to provide the greatest benefit to young and fit patients with IgVH mutated CLL. Some of these patients have not relapsed with over 10 years of follow-up and may have been cured. For this subgroup of patients, the potential for cure needs to be balanced against the risks associated with FCR, including secondary malignancies.

The monoclonal anti-CD20 antibody rituximab has activity against CLL, but it is most effectively employed in combination with chemotherapeutic agents.

Most patients respond to therapy with significant reductions in tumor burden. Patients with recurrent or refractory disease may respond to a growing list of monoclonal antibodies. Alemtuzumab, a humanized monoclonal antibody to the CD52 molecule that occurs on most lymphocytes, is efficacious, including in patients with a 17p deletion, though the median response duration for this subset of patients is only 8 months. Additional agents include the anti-CD20 antibodies ofatumumab and obinutuzumab, which were shown to improve remission duration in previously untreated patients when administered in combination with chlorambucil (level I evidence).

Improved understanding of the mechanisms of CLL cell proliferation, mediated through BCR and *NFκβ* signaling, has led to the development of a number of targeted inhibitors with favorable efficacy/toxicity profiles in recent years. In 2013 and 2014, respectively, the BTK inhibitor ibrutinib and the PI3K inhibitor idelalisib were shown to be highly active in patients with refractory and high-risk CLL [del(17p), del(11q) and IgHV unmutated]. At 3 years of follow-up an unprecedented 50% of del(17p) patients taking ibrutinib were alive without progression of disease. In 2016, the BCL-2 inhibitor venetoclax was shown to be active in patients with refractory and high-risk CLL. A randomized phase 3 trial comparing venetoclax-rituximab to bendamustine-rituximab showed a major advantage in 2-year PFS (84.9% vs. 26.3%) in the venetoclax-rituximab group. This was true among patients with del (17p) as well, with 2-year PFS of 81.5% versus 27.8%.

转化为需要治疗的CLL的风险约为每年1%，在此之前仅需随访观察。

病理学 CLL的常见病理学表现为成熟B细胞的克隆性增殖，并表达特征性成熟B细胞标志物和低水平的表面免疫球蛋白M（IgM），且其轻链呈限制性表达，反映出这些B细胞为单克隆肿瘤细胞。

CLL的免疫表型具有诊断意义，其可表达CD5和CD23，以及成熟B细胞标志物CD19、CD20（弱表达）和CD21。尽管尚未发现特异性染色体异常，但30%~50%的患者存在细胞遗传学异常，如果采用FISH等敏感检测方法，这一比例会更高。最常见的异常涉及12号染色体（常为12号染色体三体）、13号染色体和14号染色体。17号染色体和11号染色体的细胞遗传学异常与不良预后相关。

导致CLL的突变可能发生在B细胞发育的任何阶段。起源于未经历淋巴结生发中心反应的B细胞的CLL细胞，其免疫球蛋白重链可变区（IgVH）基因尚未发生突变，被定义为未突变型CLL（U-CLL）。发生免疫球蛋白（Ig）基因体细胞突变的CLL细胞则表达突变的 IgVH 基因，被定义为突变型CLL（M-CLL）。U-CLL的预后更差。

B细胞受体信号通路被认为是CLL细胞中激活最显著的通路。CLL中的B细胞受体通过识别和结合自身抗原或微环境中的抗原而被激活。BTK、脾酪氨酸激酶（SYK）和磷脂酰肌醇3激酶（PI3K）等多种激酶被激活，从而触发信号转导级联反应，激活NF-κB通路等下游通路，最终促进恶性B细胞的存活和增殖。

诊断和鉴别诊断 CLL通常是在常规体检血常规时偶然被发现的，白细胞增多且以小淋巴细胞为主可做出诊断。外周血或骨髓抽吸物流式细胞术分析可发现特征性CD5和CD23阳性克隆性B细胞群。同时存在Igκ或Igλ的单克隆表达，且CD20、CD79b、FMC7的表达较弱或阴性。骨髓或外周血涂片显示以小淋巴细胞为主，核仁不明显；可观察到破裂细胞（即涂抹细胞）。受累淋巴结病理显示小淋巴细胞弥漫性浸润，破坏正常结构。

CLL必须与反应性淋巴细胞增多及其他形式的淋巴瘤或白血病相鉴别。MCL在形态学和免疫表型上可能与CLL类似，但通常CD23表达缺失，且可检测到 CCND1 表达。诊断CLL需要淋巴细胞绝对增多，即>5000/μl。

临床表现 CLL细胞可在骨髓、外周血、淋巴结和脾中聚集，引起淋巴细胞增多、淋巴结肿大、脾大，最终导致骨髓功能下降。CLL通常与免疫功能紊乱相关，表现为低丙种球蛋白血症，伴有细菌感染风险增加和自身免疫现象，如Coombs试验阳性的溶血性贫血或免疫性血小板减少症。一些患者还会出现淋巴结肿大和与血细胞减少相关的症状或反复感染。随着疾病进展，患者可出现全身淋巴结肿大、肝脾大和骨髓衰竭。难治性患者可能因感染并发症或骨髓衰竭而死亡。约5%的CLL会转变为侵袭性更强的弥漫大细胞淋巴瘤，这可能加速致死。这种转化通常被称为 Richter 综合征。

治疗 CLL是一种低度恶性肿瘤，其典型特点是自然病程较长，病情发展缓慢，可持续数年或数十年。中位生存期超过6年。疾病发作时的程度（即疾病分期）是预测生存期的最佳指标。伴有基因组异常（如17p或11q缺失、IgVH未突变状态）预示着患者的中位生存期显著缩短，即使是早期患者。

由于目前应用标准治疗无法治愈CLL，且CLL可能会经历持续数年的无症状阶段，因此通常建议在疾病进展或出现症状［如明显淋巴结肿大、全身症状（如发热）、骨髓浸润导致的血细胞减少］后再进行相关治疗。白细胞计数增多的速度也可用于预测症状的发展和评估治疗的必要性。

CLL患者出现治疗指征时，有多种治疗方案可供选择。年龄、身体状况和细胞遗传学异常可能影响治疗选择。有效的化疗药物包括烷化剂（如苯丁酸氮芥、环磷酰胺）、核苷类似物（如氟达拉滨）或新型化疗药物苯达莫司汀。2005年，氟达拉滨/环磷酰胺（FC）方案联合利妥昔单抗（FCR）成为标准治疗方案，实现了较高的完全缓解率。一项随机Ⅲ期临床试验显示，FCR方案可改善CLL患者的总生存期，但这也增加了感染风险，尤其是老年患者，而这些老年或耐受性差的患者对苯达莫司汀和利妥昔单抗（BR）的耐受性更好。此外，应用FCR方案治疗还存在骨髓干细胞受损的风险。伴有del（17p）的患者对以氟达拉滨为基础的治疗方案的反应较差，一线治疗后的中位生存期仅为16个月。FCR方案可为年轻且身体状况良好的M-CLL患者提供最大获益。在超过10年的随访中，部分患者仍未复发，可能已达到临床治愈。对于这些预后很好的患者，需权衡FCR的潜在治愈效果与继发其他肿瘤等的治疗相关风险。

单克隆抗CD20抗体利妥昔单抗对CLL有效，与化疗药物联合使用时疗效更佳。

大多数患者对治疗有反应，肿瘤负荷显著减小。复发或难治性患者也可能对其他单克隆抗体产生反应。阿仑单抗是一种人源化单克隆抗体，针对大多数淋巴细胞上的CD52分子，对大部分患者有效，也包括伴有17p缺失的患者，但这些患者的中位缓解持续时间仅为8个月。其他药物还包括抗CD20抗体奥法木单抗和奥妥珠单抗，其与苯丁酸氮芥联合治疗可延长初治患者的缓解持续时间（Ⅰ级证据）。

近年来，对BCR和NF-κB信号通路介导的CLL细胞增殖机制的深入了解，促使人们研发出多种疗效良好且副作用少的靶向抑制剂。BTK抑制剂伊布替尼和PI3K抑制剂艾代拉里斯分别于2013年和2014年被证明在难治性和高危CLL患者［即del（17p）、del（11q）和 IgHV 未突变］中具有高度抗肿瘤活性。在3年的随访中，50%伴有del（17p）的患者在服用伊布替尼后存活且未出现疾病进展。2016年，BCL-2抑制剂维奈托克被证明对难治性和高危CLL患者有效。一项随机Ⅲ期临床试验比较了两组患者（维奈托克-利妥昔单抗与苯达莫司汀-利妥昔单抗）的2年无进展生存

Randomized comparisons of ibrutinib with or without rituximab to BR or FCR in untreated patients with CLL also favor ibrutinib-based therapy with improvements in PFS.

With continued use of ibrutinib, resistance mutations may develop and next-generation BTK inhibitors are in development. Combination strategies with BCL-2 inhibitors to circumvent resistance are in phase 3 studies. CAR-T cell therapy has also shown activity in ibrutinib-resistant CLL. While allogeneic transplantation may provide a cure through a graft versus leukemia immune phenomenon, it bears with it potential for significant morbidity and mortality and has been deferred in most CLL treatment algorithms to make room for the promising new targeted therapies.

Patients who develop autoimmune phenomena require treatment with corticosteroids, and intravenous gamma globulin may be used to reduce the frequency of infections in patients who have developed hypogammaglobulinemia. The development of a rapidly enlarging mediastinal mass, constitutional symptoms, and high serum LDH level suggests transformation of the disease to a diffuse large cell lymphoma (i.e., Richter syndrome), which is associated with a poor prognosis.

Plasma Cell Disorders

The plasma cell disorders, or dyscrasias, are a group of clonal B-cell diseases that are related to each other by virtue of their production and secretion of monoclonal immunoglobulin, called the *M protein*. The laboratory hallmark of plasma cell dyscrasias is a homogeneous immunoglobulin molecule (whole or part) that can be detected in the serum or urine by protein electrophoresis. Clinically, these disorders may be characterized by the systemic effects of the M protein and by the direct effects of bone and bone marrow infiltration. Primary amyloidosis, for instance, results in tissue injury through deposition of light chains produced by a clonal population of plasma cells in the absence of an observable proliferation of the plasma cell clone. Waldenström's macroglobulinemia is a disorder with features of NHL and plasma cell disorders. It is discussed in this section because of the distinct clinical effects of the IgM paraprotein produced in this disease.

The most common plasma cell dyscrasia is *monoclonal gammopathy of uncertain significance* (MGUS), followed by multiple myeloma and the closely related plasmacytoma, which is a solitary tumor comprised of clonal plasma cells of bone or extramedullary soft tissue. Less common plasma cell dyscrasias include POEMS (polyneuropathy, organomegaly, endocrinopathy, monoclonal gammopathy and skin abnormalities) syndrome (see later in the chapter), also known as osteosclerotic myeloma, heavy-chain disease, and primary amyloidosis.

When an M protein is found on serum protein electrophoresis from an individual with no apparent associated disease and in the absence of any other laboratory or clinical evidence of a plasma cell disorder, it is designated as MGUS. MGUS is defined by low serum levels of M protein (<3 g/dL), no urinary Bence Jones protein, less than 10% clonal bone marrow plasma cells, and absence of anemia, hypercalcemia, renal failure, and lytic bone lesions. MGUS is more common than myeloma and increases in frequency with aging, occurring in 3% of the population older than 50 years. MGUS is considered a premalignant condition, and patients are at increased risk (7-fold) for overt myeloma or related malignant plasma cell dyscrasias compared with the general population. Nonetheless, progression of MGUS to a frank plasma cell neoplasm occurs only in about 1% of patients per year.

Distinguishing patients with stable, nonprogressive MGUS from patients in whom multiple myeloma will eventually develop is difficult. The risk of progression is greater among patients with IgA or IgM-type M proteins, in patients with initial concentrations of M protein in excess of 1.5 g/dL, and in patients with an abnormal free κ-to-λ light-chain ratio. Although no definitive evidence has been found that monitoring patients with the diagnosis of MGUS improves survival, it is recommended that patients undergo annual evaluation, including serum electrophoresis, to detect progression to multiple myeloma before the onset of overt symptoms or complications.

M proteins can be found in benign and malignant conditions other than the plasma cell dyscrasias (Table 5.6). About 10% of patients with CLL have detectable levels of monoclonal IgG or IgM in their sera. M proteins can also be detected in a variety of autoreactive or infectious disorders.

Multiple Myeloma

Definition and epidemiology. Multiple myeloma is a malignant plasma cell disorder characterized by neoplastic infiltration of the bone marrow and bone and by monoclonal immunoglobulin or light chains in the serum or urine. The cause of myeloma is uncertain.

The disease is more common in men than women and in African Americans than white individuals. Myeloma risk increases with age, with a median age of 69 years at diagnosis (SEER data). There were an estimated 32,110 new cases in the United States in 2019. Myeloma risk is increased for patients with first-degree relatives with a plasma cell dyscrasia. Associations have been described with occupational exposures to organic solvents, pesticides, petroleum products, and ionizing radiation; however, most patients with myeloma have no history of exposure to such agents.

Pathology. The tumor cell exhibits features of a differentiated plasma cell that is adapted to synthesize and secrete immunoglobulin at a high rate. Biopsies of bone marrow or targeted bone biopsies of tumor sites reveal infiltration by plasma cells with light-chain restriction, defining clonality. Cell surface markers useful in identifying and enumerating plasma cells include CD38, CD 138, and immunoglobulin light chains; the B-cell marker CD20 is typically absent and aids in distinguishing other lymphoproliferative disorders from myeloma.

Genetic aberrations are detectable in most patients with myeloma if adequately sensitive tests are applied. Standard karyotyping and FISH are performed routinely on marrow samples to determine abnormalities of prognostic significance, including translocations involving the immunoglobulin heavy-chain locus on chromosome 14, hyperploidy, or abnormalities of chromosomes 1, 13, or 17.

Diagnosis and differential diagnosis. Myeloma must be distinguished from related disorders, including MGUS and plasmacytoma. The diagnosis of multiple myeloma is made by identifying some combination of an increase (>10%) in the number of plasma cells in the bone marrow, a serum M protein other than IgM exceeding 3 g/dL, or a clonal protein in the urine. Asymptomatic myeloma (i.e., stage I myeloma or "smoldering myeloma") is diagnosed when clonal plasma cells are found in 10% to 59% of the bone marrow or monoclonal protein occurs in an amount greater than 3 g/dL in the absence of end organ–related injury, significant elevation in clonal free light chains or evidence of bone disease on advanced imaging (whole body MRI or PET-CT scan).

Patients with disease-related organ dysfunction (e.g., anemia, lytic bone lesions, hypercalcemia, renal dysfunction) are considered to have symptomatic myeloma, for which therapy is indicated. Recurrent infection with hypogammaglobulinemia is also considered a criterion for symptomatic myeloma. Solitary plasmacytoma is diagnosed when a single clonal plasma cell tumor is identified in bone or soft tissue in the absence of bone marrow involvement or other end organ–related injury.

Evaluation of the patient with suspected myeloma includes bone marrow biopsy; measurement of hemoglobin, calcium, renal function, and the serum free κ-to-λ light-chain ratio; serum and urine protein electrophoresis; immunoelectrophoresis; and a skeletal survey. PET

期（PFS），结果显示维奈托克-利妥昔单抗组具有显著优势（84.9% vs. 26.3%），这在伴有 del（17p）患者中也是如此（81.5% vs. 27.8%）。一项随机对照试验比较了伊布替尼单药或联用利妥昔单抗与 BR 或 FCR 治疗在初治 CLL 患者中的疗效，结果显示，以伊布替尼为基础的治疗方案疗效更佳，可延长患者的 PFS。

随着伊布替尼的持续使用，可能会出现耐药突变，目前正在研发下一代 BTK 抑制剂。BTK 抑制剂联用 BCL-2 抑制剂的策略也正处于Ⅲ期临床试验阶段，其可能克服耐药问题。CAR-T 细胞治疗在伊布替尼耐药的 CLL 患者中显示出疗效。虽然 alloSCT 可能通过移植物抗白血病免疫现象提供治愈可能性，但潜在的高并发症发生率和死亡率限制了其应用，因此大多数治疗流程更倾向于选择新型靶向治疗。

出现自身免疫现象的患者需要使用皮质类固醇，静脉注射丙种球蛋白可用于低丙种球蛋白血症患者，以降低感染发生率。若出现纵隔肿块快速增大、全身症状及 LDH 水平升高，常提示已转化为弥漫大细胞淋巴瘤（即 Richter 综合征），患者预后较差。

浆细胞疾病

浆细胞疾病是一组克隆性 B 细胞疾病，可产生和分泌单克隆免疫球蛋白（即 M 蛋白）。浆细胞疾病的实验室检查特征是血清或尿液蛋白电泳可检测到单克隆免疫球蛋白分子（整体或部分）。临床上，这些疾病可能表现为 M 蛋白沉积的系统性改变，或骨和骨髓浸润引发的直接反应。例如，原发性淀粉样变性是由于克隆性浆细胞群产生的轻链沉积于组织而造成组织损伤，但可能无法检测出明显的浆细胞克隆性增殖。瓦尔登斯特伦巨球蛋白血症是一种兼具 NHL 和浆细胞异常特征的疾病，其产生的 IgM 副蛋白具有独特的临床效应（见下文）。

最常见的浆细胞疾病是意义未明单克隆丙种球蛋白血症（MGUS），其次是多发性骨髓瘤和与其密切相关的浆细胞瘤，后者是由骨骼或髓外软组织中的克隆性浆细胞形成的孤立性肿瘤。较少见的浆细胞疾病包括：POEMS（多发性神经病、脏器肿大、内分泌病、M 蛋白血症和皮肤改变）综合征（又称骨硬化性骨髓瘤；见下文）、重链病和原发性淀粉样变性。

当血清蛋白电泳发现 M 蛋白，但患者没有相关症状及任何表明存在其他浆细胞疾病的实验室或临床证据时，应考虑 MGUS。MGUS 的定义为血清 M 蛋白水平低（< 3 g/dl）、无尿本周蛋白、骨髓中克隆性浆细胞< 10%，且无贫血、高钙血症、肾衰竭和溶骨性病变。MGUS 比骨髓瘤更常见，且随年龄增长而增加，50 岁以上人群的发病率为 3%。MGUS 被视为癌前病变，与普通人群相比，MGUS 患者罹患骨髓瘤或其他相关恶性浆细胞疾病的风险增加（7 倍）。然而，MGUS 进展为明显的浆细胞肿瘤的年发生率约为 1%。

病情稳定且无进展的 MGUS 患者与最终将发展为多发性骨髓瘤的 MGUS 患者很难区分。具有 IgA 或 IgM 型 M 蛋白、初始 M 蛋白浓度 > 1.5 g/dl 及游离 κ/λ 轻链比例异常的患者，其病情进展的风险更大。尽管尚未证实持续监测 MGUS 患者能改善生存率，但仍建议患者每年进行 1 次评估，包括血清蛋白电泳，以便在出现明显症状或并发症前检测出病情进展并及时治疗。

M 蛋白还可见于除浆细胞疾病外的其他良性和恶性疾病（表 5.6）。约 10% 的 CLL 患者血清中可检测到单克隆免疫球蛋白 G（IgG）或 IgM。M 蛋白也可在自身免疫病或感染性疾病患者中被检出。

多发性骨髓瘤

定义和流行病学 多发性骨髓瘤是一种恶性浆细胞疾病，其特征是肿瘤浸润骨髓和骨，以及血清或尿液中可检出单克隆免疫球蛋白或轻链。骨髓瘤的病因尚不确定。

多发性骨髓瘤的男性发病率高于女性，非裔美国人的发病率高于白人。骨髓瘤的风险随年龄增长而增加，诊断时的中位年龄为 69 岁（根据 SEER 数据库记录），2019 年美国估计有 32 110 例新发病例。浆细胞疾病患者的一级亲属罹患骨髓瘤的风险增加。研究表明，有机溶剂、农药、石油产品和电离辐射等职业暴露与骨髓瘤的发生相关；然而，大多数骨髓瘤患者并无此类物质暴露史。

病理学 多发性骨髓瘤的肿瘤细胞具有分化的浆细胞特征，这种细胞可快速合成和分泌免疫球蛋白。骨髓活检或肿瘤部位靶向骨活检可见浆细胞浸润并具有轻链限制性，即浆细胞的克隆性。用于识别和计数异常浆细胞的表面标志物包括 CD38、CD138 和免疫球蛋白轻链；B 细胞标志物 CD20 通常缺失，这有助于将其他淋巴增殖性疾病与骨髓瘤区分开来。

如果应用敏感的检测方法，大多数骨髓瘤患者可检测到遗传学异常。常规采用骨髓样本进行核型分析和 FISH 检测，以检出具有预后意义的遗传学异常，包括涉及 14 号染色体上的 IGH 易位、超倍性，以及 1 号、13 号或 17 号染色体异常。

诊断和鉴别诊断 骨髓瘤必须与其他浆细胞疾病进行鉴别，包括 MGUS 和浆细胞瘤。多发性骨髓瘤的诊断依据是骨髓中浆细胞数量增加（> 10%）、除 IgM 外的血清 M 蛋白 > 3 g/dl 或尿液中出现单克隆蛋白。无症状骨髓瘤（即Ⅰ期骨髓瘤或冒烟性骨髓瘤）的诊断依据是骨髓中克隆性血浆细胞占 10%～59%，或单克隆蛋白含量 > 3 g/dl 且无终末器官相关损伤，无克隆性游离轻链显著升高，影像学检查（全身 MRI 或 PET/CT）无骨破坏证据。

对于出现疾病相关器官功能障碍（如贫血、溶骨性病变、高钙血症、肾功能障碍）的患者，应考虑症状性骨髓瘤，需进行系统治疗。反复感染伴低丙种球蛋白血症也被视为症状性骨髓瘤的一种表现形式。孤立性浆细胞瘤的诊断依据是骨骼或软组织中发现单克隆性浆细胞瘤，且无骨髓浸润或其他终末器官相关损伤。

疑似骨髓瘤患者的评估包括骨髓活检；检测血红蛋白、血钙、肾功能和血清游离 κ/λ 轻链比值；血清和尿液蛋白电泳；免疫电泳；骨骼检查。PET 或 MRI 是进一

TABLE 5.6 Classification of Disorders Associated With Monoclonal Immunoglobulin (M Protein) Secretion

Disorder	M Protein Pattern
Plasma Cell Neoplasms	
Multiple myeloma	IgG > IgA > IgD; ± free light chain or light chain alone (κ > λ)
Solitary myeloma of bone	IgG > IgA > IgD; ± free light chain or light chain alone (κ > λ)
Extramedullary plasmacytoma	IgA > IgG > IgD; ± free light chain or light chain alone (κ > λ)
Waldenström's macroglobulinemia	IgM ± free light chain (κ > λ)
Heavy-chain disease	γ, α, μ heavy chain or fragment
Primary amyloidosis	Free light chain (λ > κ)
Monoclonal gammopathy of unknown significance	IgG > IgM > IgA, usually without urinary light-chain secretion
Other B-Cell Neoplasms	
Chronic lymphocytic leukemia	M protein occasionally secreted; IgM > IgG
B-cell non-Hodgkin's lymphomas; Hodgkin's disease	M protein occasionally secreted; IgM > IgG
Nonlymphoid Neoplasms	
Chronic myelogenous leukemia	No consistent patterns
Carcinomas (e.g., colon, breast, prostate)	No consistent patterns
Autoimmune or Autoreactive Disorders	
Cold agglutinin disease	IgM κ most common
Mixed cryoglobulinemia	IgM or IgA
Sjögren's syndrome	IgM
Miscellaneous Inflammatory, Storage, or Infectious Disorders	
Lichen myxedematosus	IgG λ
Gaucher's disease	IgG
Cirrhosis, sarcoid, parasitic diseases, renal acidosis	No consistent pattern

Ig, Immunoglobulin.
Modified from Salmon SE: Plasma cell disorders. In Wyngaarden JB, Smith LH Jr, editors: *Cecil Textbook of Medicine,* ed 18, Philadelphia, 1988, WB Saunders, p 1026.

and MRI are considered to further evaluate bone disease and may be necessary for patients with oligosecretory or nonsecretory disease to define disease and evaluate after therapy. Conventional bone scans are less useful due to the osteolytic nature of myeloma.

About 20% of patients with multiple myeloma do not have detectable serum M protein by standard electrophoresis but have circulating free light chains that may be detectable by serum free light-chain assays. Free light chains may appear in the urine (i.e., Bence Jones protein) and can also be detected in a 24-hour urine collection by urine protein electrophoresis. Free light-chain assays are quite sensitive and may provide measurement of clonal protein in patients thought to have non-secretory disease by other methods. Free light chains have a relatively short half-life (2 to 6 hours) in the circulation compared with a half-life of weeks for intact immunoglobulin molecules and may therefore be used to obtain a more rapid assessment of disease response once therapy is initiated. In rare cases, patients may have true non-secretory myeloma with no detectable serum or urine M protein by any assay.

Clinical presentation. The clinical manifestations of multiple myeloma are the direct effects of bone marrow and bone infiltration by malignant plasma cells, the systemic effects of the M protein, and the effects of the concomitant deficiency in humoral immunity that occurs in this disease. The most common symptom is bone pain. Bone radiographs typically show pure osteolytic punched-out lesions, often in association with generalized osteopenia and pathologic fractures. Bony lesions can show as expansile masses associated with spinal cord compression. Hypercalcemia caused by extensive bony involvement is common in myeloma and may dominate the clinical picture. Anemia occurs in most patients as a result of marrow infiltration and suppression of hematopoiesis and causes fatigue; granulocytopenia and thrombocytopenia are less common.

Patients with myeloma are susceptible to bacterial infections because of impaired production and increased catabolism of normal immunoglobulins. Gram-negative urinary tract infections are common, as are respiratory tract infections caused by *Streptococcus pneumoniae, Staphylococcus aureus, Haemophilus influenzae,* and *Klebsiella pneumoniae.*

Renal insufficiency occurs in about 25% of patients with myeloma. The cause of renal failure is often multifactorial; hypercalcemia, hyperuricemia, infection, and amyloid deposition can contribute. Direct tubular damage from light-chain excretion also occurs. Because of their physicochemical properties, M proteins can cause a host of diverse effects, including cryoglobulinemia, hyperviscosity, amyloidosis, and clotting abnormalities resulting from interaction of the M protein with platelets or clotting factors.

Several staging or classification systems exist for myeloma. The Revised International Staging System (R-ISS) for myeloma identifies three stages with distinct prognoses based on β_2-microglobulin and albumin levels, LDH, and cytogenetic/FISH abnormalities (Table 5.7).

Treatment. Most patients with myeloma exhibit symptomatic, advanced-stage disease and require therapy. Patients with asymptomatic myeloma may have an indolent course and do not always require immediate therapy. Disease progression occurs at a rate of 5% to 10% per year, and patients should be monitored for disease progression

表 5.6　与单克隆免疫球蛋白（M 蛋白）分泌相关的疾病分类	
疾病	M 蛋白类型
浆细胞疾病	
多发性骨髓瘤	IgG ＞ IgA ＞ IgD；± 游离轻链或单独轻链型（κ ＞ λ）
孤立性骨髓瘤	IgG ＞ IgA ＞ IgD；± 游离轻链或单独轻链型（κ ＞ λ）
髓外浆细胞瘤	IgA ＞ IgG ＞ IgD；± 游离轻链或单独轻链型（κ ＞ λ）
瓦尔登斯特伦巨球蛋白血症	IgM± 游离轻链（κ ＞ λ）
重链病	γ、α、μ 重链或片段
原发性淀粉样变性	游离轻链（λ ＞ κ）
意义未明单克隆丙种球蛋白血症	IgG ＞ IgM ＞ IgA，通常无尿轻链分泌
其他 B 细胞肿瘤	
慢性淋巴细胞白血病	偶有 M 蛋白分泌；IgM ＞ IgG
B 细胞非霍奇金淋巴瘤；霍奇金淋巴瘤	偶有 M 蛋白分泌；IgM ＞ IgG
非淋巴系统肿瘤	
慢性粒细胞白血病	无一致模式
实体瘤（如结肠癌、乳腺癌、前列腺癌）	无一致模式
自身免疫病或自身反应性疾病	
冷凝集素病	IgM κ 型最常见
混合性冷球蛋白血症	IgM 或 IgA
干燥综合征	IgM
其他炎症性、沉积性或感染性疾病	
黏液水肿性苔藓	IgG λ
戈谢病	IgG
肝硬化、结节病、寄生虫病、肾性酸中毒	无一致模式

Ig，免疫球蛋白。
改编自 Salmon SE：Plasma cell disorders. In Wyngaarden JB，Smith LH Jr，editors：Cecil Textbook of Medicine, ed 18, Philadelphia, 1988, WB Saunders, p 1026.

步评估骨病变的必要手段，尤其适用于寡分泌型或无分泌型患者，用于确诊和治疗后评估。传统骨扫描对骨髓瘤的诊断价值不大，因为骨髓瘤的溶骨性病变对其不敏感。

约 20% 的多发性骨髓瘤患者通过标准血清蛋白电泳未能检测到血清 M 蛋白，但可能存在循环的游离轻链，可通过血清游离轻链检测来证实。游离轻链可能出现在尿液中（即尿本周蛋白），并能通过尿蛋白电泳在 24 h 尿液中检出。游离轻链检测非常敏感，可在其他检测方法考虑为无分泌型患者中检出克隆性蛋白。游离轻链在循环中的半衰期相对较短（2～6 h），而完整免疫球蛋白分子的半衰期为数周，因此可用于治疗后快速评估治疗反应。罕见情况下，患者为真正的无分泌型骨髓瘤，即任何检测方法均无法测出血清或尿液中的 M 蛋白。

临床表现　多发性骨髓瘤的临床表现由恶性浆细胞浸润骨髓或骨、M 蛋白的系统损害及该病伴随的体液免疫缺陷直接引起。最常见的症状是骨痛。骨 X 线检查通常可见溶骨性、凿孔样病变，常伴有全身性骨质疏松症和病理性骨折。骨病变可表现为膨胀性肿块伴有脊髓压迫。由于广泛的骨浸润，骨髓瘤常引起高钙血症，这可能是患者的主要临床表现。大多数患者可因骨髓浸润和造血抑制而出现贫血，导致疲劳；粒细胞减少和血小板减少较少见。

由于正常免疫球蛋白的生成受限且分解增加，骨髓瘤患者更易出现细菌感染，常见感染包括革兰氏阴性菌尿路感染，以及由肺炎链球菌、金黄色葡萄球菌、流感嗜血杆菌和克雷伯菌引起的呼吸道感染。

约 25% 的骨髓瘤患者伴有肾功能不全。肾衰竭的原因通常是多因素的，如高钙血症、高尿酸血症、感染和淀粉样变性。轻链排泄可直接导致肾小管损伤。由于其物理化学性质，M 蛋白可引起一系列效应，包括冷球蛋白血症、高黏滞综合征、淀粉样变性和凝血异常，这些异常由 M 蛋白与血小板或凝血因子相互作用引起。

目前有多种针对骨髓瘤的分期或分类系统。修订版国际分期系统（R-ISS）根据 β_2- 微球蛋白和白蛋白水平、LDH 及细胞遗传学 /FISH 检测异常将骨髓瘤分为 3 期（表 5.7）。

治疗　大多数骨髓瘤患者表现为有症状的晚期状态，需要启动治疗。无症状骨髓瘤（冒烟性骨髓瘤）患者的病程较缓慢，不需要立即启动治疗。冒烟性骨髓瘤患者每年疾病进展的概率为 5%～10%，应通过定期检测 M 蛋白和血清游离轻链数量，以及评估与疾病

TABLE 5.7 Revised International Staging System for Multiple Myeloma

Stage	Criteria	Survival Rate at 5 Years (Months)
I	B2M <3.5 mg/L Albumin ≥3.5 g/dL LDH ≤ ULN Standard-risk chromosomal abnormalities by FISH	82
II	Not stage I or III	62
III	B2M >5.5 mg/L High-risk chromosomal abnormalities or elevated LDH	40

Palumbo A et al. Revised international staging system for multiple myeloma: a report from International Myeloma Working Group. *J Clin Oncol*, 2015;33:2863.
High-risk chromosomal abnormalities include deletion 17p and/or translocation t(4;14) and/or t(14;16).
B2M, β_2-Microglobulin.

by serial quantification of M protein and serum free light chains and evaluation for disease-related signs or symptoms. For patients with solitary bone or extramedullary plasmacytomas, particularly in the head and neck region, local radiation therapy can induce long-term remissions and is the treatment of choice. Patients with a solitary plasmacytoma of bone are often found on routine MRI of the spine to have asymptomatic bone disease at other sites and should be treated as symptomatic myeloma.

Patients with symptomatic myeloma require systemic therapy and meticulous supportive care. Although myeloma is not a curable malignancy, systemic therapy prolongs survival and dramatically improves quality of life. Options for treatment have expanded in the past two decades to include multiple novel compounds in three broad classes of agents, the immunomodulatory drugs (IMIDs), proteasome inhibitors, and monoclonal antibodies. These agents may be used as single agents or in combinations for more intensive therapy. The novel agents are typically administered in combination with high doses of dexamethasone, which is a potent antimyeloma therapy. The IMIDS include thalidomide, lenalidomide, and pomalidomide. Proteasome inhibitors include bortezomib, carfilzomib, and ixazomib. The anti-CD38 monoclonal antibody daratumumab was approved for use in the United States in 2015. These agents have largely supplanted traditional chemotherapeutic agents as the cornerstone of initial and secondary therapies because they are efficacious and well tolerated. Multiple combination regimens have been devised that also incorporate chemotherapeutic agents in modest doses.

Thalidomide is the first-in-class IMID and was initially used as a sedative in the United Kingdom in the 1960s, but it was found to cause birth defects (phocomelia) when used to combat nausea during pregnancy. The antiangiogenic properties of thalidomide subsequently led to its development as an anticancer agent. The molecular target of the IMID class was recently elucidated as cereblon, an E3 ligase protein crucial to the activity of B cell–specific transcription factors that influence myeloma cell viability. The IMIDs are typically used in combination with dexamethasone, and when used as initial therapy, they have good tolerability and result in high response rates.

Toxicity related to thalidomide includes peripheral neuropathy, constipation, somnolence, and rash. Later-generation IMIDs have a more favorable side effect profile. Myelosuppression is more likely, but neuropathy and constitutional symptoms occur less frequently.

The second-generation IMID lenalidomide is more commonly used in North America due to its favorable tolerability. A troublesome and unique side effect of the IMID-steroid combination programs is development of deep vein thrombosis in up to 25% of patients, and some form of preventative therapy is required.

Bortezomib is the first-in-class proteasome inhibitor and is an important therapy for patients with adverse cytogenetic risk factors. Bortezomib is typically administered subcutaneously and may cause thrombocytopenia, asthenia, and neuropathy.

Most patients respond to initial therapy with a reduction in bone pain, hypercalcemia, and anemia in association with a decline in the M protein level. The selection of initial therapy depends on stage, cytogenetic risk, and candidacy for high-dose chemotherapy and autologous stem cell transplantation. The use of high-dose chemotherapy with alkylating agents followed by autologous peripheral stem cell infusion during first or second remission improves progression-free survival and quality of life compared with conventional therapy. Although this approach is not curative, it does represent an important treatment option for some patients and has an acceptable toxicity profile, even in older patients. Allogenic stem cell or bone marrow transplantation may be associated with durable remission in selected patients, but it carries a high near-term risk of morbidity and mortality. Patients who experience relapse after standard therapy or transplantation may be treated with alternative chemotherapy regimens or with novel combination therapies, including newer agents and chemotherapy drugs. The first-in-class *selective inhibitor of nuclear export,* selinexor was recently added to the antimyeloma armamentarium for patients with relapsed or refractory disease as a fifth-line therapy. CAR-T cell therapy has shown high response rates in clinic trials and is expected to become available as a standard therapy soon.

Supportive care directed toward anticipated complications of myeloma is an important aspect of management. Bone resorption can be reduced with regular injections of the diphosphonates zoledronic acid or pamidronate, reducing pain and pathologic fractures. The monoclonal antibody denosumab targets RANKL, inhibiting osteoclast activity, and may also be used to treat bone disease. Bony lesions, particularly those involving weight-bearing bones, may require palliative irradiation for controlling pain and preventing pathologic fractures. Vertebral bony lesions may lead to spinal cord compression, with increasing back pain and neurologic symptoms. Symptoms suggesting cord compression require prompt evaluation with spinal MRI and, if necessary, local irradiation of involved areas.

Avoidance of nephrotoxins, including intravenous contrast media, is important to prevent renal failure. All patients should receive pneumococcal and *H. influenzae* vaccines, and intravenous gamma globulin may be useful in preventing recurrent infections in patients with profound hypogammaglobulinemia. Use of erythropoietin may alleviate anemia and decrease the need for blood transfusions in patients with treatment-related anemia or concomitant renal insufficiency.

Prognosis. Multiple myeloma is considered incurable, but the overall survival of these patients has improved considerably with the use of newer agents and autologous stem cell transplantation. The five-year survival as reported by the SEER database is 52.2%.

Prognosis depends on stage of disease and cytogenetic profile. Patients with an adverse karyotype, including t(14;16), t(4;14), and 17p deletion, have a less favorable prognosis and are considered for more intensive therapies or clinical investigation. Adverse factors also include advanced stage, impaired renal function, elevated LDH levels, depressed serum albumin levels, and elevated β_2-microglobulin levels.

Waldenström's Macroglobulinemia

Waldenström's macroglobulinemia (WM) is a malignancy of plasmacytoid lymphocytes that secrete large quantities of IgM. It is a chronic

表 5.7	多发性骨髓瘤的修订版国际分期系统（R-ISS）	
分期	分期标准	5 年生存率（%）
Ⅰ期	β_2-微球蛋白 < 3.5 mg/L 白蛋白 ≥ 3.5 g/dl 乳酸脱氢酶 ≤ 正常值上限 FISH 检测为标危型染色体异常	82
Ⅱ期	非Ⅰ期或Ⅲ期	62
Ⅲ期	β_2-微球蛋白 > 5.5 mg/L FISH 检测为高危型染色体异常	40

Palumbo A et al. Revised international staging system for multiple myeloma: a report from International Myeloma Working Group. J Clin Oncol, 2015; 33: 2863.
高危型染色体异常包括 17p 缺失和（或）易位 t（4;14）和（或）t（14;16）。

相关的体征或症状来监测疾病进展状态。对于孤立性骨或髓外浆细胞瘤患者，尤其是发生于头颈部的患者，局部放疗可诱导长期缓解，是首选的治疗方法。孤立性骨浆细胞瘤患者在脊柱 MRI 检查中常会发现其他部位存在无症状骨病，此时应按症状性骨髓瘤进行治疗。

症状性骨髓瘤患者需要全身治疗和支持治疗。尽管骨髓瘤是一种无法治愈的恶性肿瘤，但全身治疗可延长生存期并显著改善生活质量。在过去 20 年中，治疗选择显著增多，目前常用的治疗药物主要分为 3 类：免疫调节药物（IMID）、蛋白酶体抑制剂和单克隆抗体。这些药物可单用或联合使用（强化治疗）。新型药物通常与高剂量地塞米松联用，后者是一种有效的抗骨髓瘤治疗药物。IMID 包括沙利度胺、来那度胺和泊马度胺。蛋白酶体抑制剂包括硼替佐米、卡非佐米和伊沙佐米。抗 CD38 单克隆抗体达雷妥尤单抗于 2015 年在美国获批使用。因其疗效显著且耐受性良好，这些药物目前已在很大程度上取代了传统化疗药物，成为一线治疗和二线治疗的基石。多种联合方案均获得了较好的疗效，其中也包括新药与部分传统化疗药物联用。

沙利度胺是首个 IMID，最初于 20 世纪 60 年代在英国作为镇静剂使用，但后续发现其用于妊娠期止吐会导致胎儿先天性缺陷（短肢畸形）。沙利度胺具有抗血管生成特性，促使其随后被研发为抗癌药物。IMID 的分子靶点为 cereblon，这是一种 E3 连接酶蛋白，对 B 细胞特异性转录因子活性至关重要，而这些转录因子可影响骨髓瘤细胞的存活。IMID 通常与地塞米松联合使用作为患者的初始治疗，具有良好的耐受性且反应率较高。

与沙利度胺相关的毒性包括周围神经病变、便秘、嗜睡和皮疹。新一代 IMID 的骨髓抑制更常见，但神经病变和全身症状的发生率较低。因其良好的耐受性，第二代 IMID 来那度胺在北美较常用。IMID 和类固醇联合治疗方案有一个特殊的副作用，即高达 25% 的患者会出现深静脉血栓，因此需要预防性抗血栓治疗。

硼替佐米是首个蛋白酶体抑制剂类药物，是存在不良细胞遗传学危险因素的患者的重要治疗方法。硼替佐米通常经皮下注射，不良反应包括血小板减少、乏力和神经病变。

大多数患者对初始治疗反应良好，表现为骨痛、高钙血症和贫血相关症状减轻，同时 M 蛋白水平下降。初始治疗的选择取决于疾病分期、细胞遗传学风险及患者是否适合接受大剂量化疗和自体 SCT。与传统治疗相比，在第一次或第二次缓解期使用大剂量烷化剂化疗后进行自体 SCT 可改善患者的无进展生存期和生活质量。尽管这种方法并不能治愈骨髓瘤，但对于适合移植的患者是一个重要的治疗选择，其不良反应在可接受范围内，即使是老年患者。alloSCT 或骨髓移植可使部分患者获得长期缓解，但其近期并发症风险和死亡率较高。接受标准治疗或移植后复发的患者可采用替代化疗方案或新型联合治疗，包括新的靶向药物和化疗药物。近期，首个选择性核输出抑制剂塞利尼索被添加到抗骨髓瘤治疗选择中，作为复发或难治性患者的五线治疗。CAR-T 细胞治疗在临床试验中也显示出较高的反应率，预计很快将成为骨髓瘤的标准治疗。

针对骨髓瘤并发症的支持治疗也是骨髓瘤管理的重要方面。通过定期注射双膦酸盐（如唑来膦酸或帕米膦酸二钠）可减少骨吸收，从而减少骨痛和病理性骨折。靶向 RANKL 的单克隆抗体地舒单抗可抑制破骨细胞活性，从而治疗骨病变。骨病变（尤其是涉及承重骨的病变）可能需要姑息性放疗，以控制疼痛和预防病理性骨折。椎骨病变可能导致脊髓压迫，伴有逐渐加重的背痛和神经症状。出现提示脊髓压迫的症状需尽快进行脊柱 MRI 评估，并在必要时对受累区域进行局部放疗。

避免使用肾毒性物质（包括静脉注射造影剂）对于预防肾衰竭非常重要。所有患者均应接种肺炎球菌和流感嗜血杆菌疫苗，静脉注射免疫球蛋白可能有助于预防低丙种球蛋白血症患者的反复感染。使用促红细胞生成素可能减轻贫血，并减少治疗相关贫血或合并肾功能不全患者的输血需求。

预后 目前认为多发性骨髓瘤不可治愈，但随着新型药物和自体 SCT 的应用，这些患者的总体生存率显著提高。根据 SEER 数据库的报告，患者的 5 年生存率约为 52.2%。

患者的预后取决于疾病分期和细胞遗传学特征。具有不良核型 [包括 t（14;16）、t（4;14）和 17p 缺失] 的患者预后较差，通常需要更大强度的治疗或参加临床试验。不良预后因素还包括分期较晚、肾功能受损、LDH 水平升高、血清白蛋白水平降低和 β_2-微球蛋白水平升高。

瓦尔登斯特伦巨球蛋白血症

瓦尔登斯特伦巨球蛋白血症（WM）是一种浆细胞样淋巴细胞恶性肿瘤，可分泌大量 IgM。它是一种

disorder affecting elderly patients (median age 64 years) that shares features of the low-grade lymphomas and myeloma. Unlike myeloma, Waldenström's macroglobulinemia is associated with lymphadenopathy and hepatosplenomegaly, and although bone marrow involvement invariably occurs, lytic lesions and hypercalcemia are rare. Diagnostic work-up for WM should include polymerase chain reaction analysis for mutation in the MYD88 gene, which is present in most patients and carries diagnostic and therapeutic relevance.

The major clinical manifestations of WM include symptomatic anemia and the hyperviscosity syndrome caused by the physical properties of IgM. In contrast to IgG, IgM remains largely confined to the intravascular space, and as IgM levels rise, plasma viscosity increases. Epistaxis, retinal hemorrhages, dizziness, confusion, and congestive heart failure may occur as a result of the hyperviscosity syndrome. About 10% of IgM proteins have properties of cryoglobulins, and patients show symptoms of cryoglobulinemia or cold agglutinin syndrome demonstrated as acrocyanosis, Raynaud's phenomenon, and vascular symptoms or hemolytic anemia precipitated by exposure to cold. Some patients with WM may develop a peripheral neuropathy that may antedate the appearance of the neoplastic process.

The approach to and treatment of WM is similar to those of other low-grade B-cell lymphomas. The use of fludarabine or an alkylating agent, typically employed in combination with prednisone and rituximab, is effective in decreasing adenopathy and splenomegaly and controlling the M spike but is not curative. Rituximab has activity against WM, as has the proteasome inhibitor bortezomib. The use of rituximab as a single agent may be complicated by initial worsening of hyperviscosity in patients with high IgM burdens. The novel agent ibrutinib, an inhibitor of Bruton tyrosine kinase, is an effective oral therapy for Waldenström's and may be combined with rituximab. Although complete remissions are rare, patients who respond to therapy have median survivals of 4 years, and some patients survive more than a decade.

Rare Plasma Cell Disorders

Heavy-chain disease is a rare lymphoplasmacytoid neoplasm characterized by production of a defective heavy chain of the γ, α, or μ type. The clinical manifestations vary with the type of heavy chain secreted. The γ-type heavy-chain disease is associated with lymphadenopathy, Waldeyer ring involvement with palatal edema, and constitutional symptoms. The α-type heavy-chain disease, also known as Mediterranean lymphoma, is characterized by lymphoid infiltration of the small intestine with associated diarrhea and malabsorption. The μ-type heavy-chain disease is associated with CLL.

Primary amyloidosis. Primary AL amyloidosis is a systemic illness characterized by deposition of immunoglobulin light chains in organs and tissue, resulting in an array of symptoms caused by organ dysfunction. Congestive heart failure, bleeding diathesis, nephrotic syndrome, and peripheral neuropathy are common complications. Patients with primary amyloidosis may respond to selected treatments similar to therapy for myeloma. The combination of bortezomib, cyclophosphamide, and dexamethasone is effective in some patients. Selected patients may respond well to high-dose chemotherapy and autologous stem cell support, but there are increased risks of morbidity and mortality if significant end-organ dysfunction such as cardiomyopathy occurs. It is important to note that not all amyloidosis is AL (light chain), and documentation of the source and type of amyloid protein is vital to appropriate management.

POEMS syndrome. POEMS syndrome is a rare disorder characterized by polyneuropathy, sclerotic bone lesions, endocrinopathy, monoclonal gammopathy, and skin lesions. The cause of POEMS syndrome is unknown, but the disease may be progressive, causing severe disability, third spacing of fluid, and elevated vascular endothelial growth factor (VEGF) levels. Monoclonal λ light chains are typically elevated. Limited bone disease may be treated with radiotherapy. High-dose therapy and autologous stem cell transplantation is effective in patients with extensive disease.

For a deeper discussion of these topics, please see Chapter 178, "Plasma Cell Disorders," and Chapter 179, "Amyloidosis," in *Goldman-Cecil Medicine*, 26th Edition.

CONGENITAL AND ACQUIRED DISORDERS OF LYMPHOCYTE FUNCTION

Several congenital disorders affect lymphocyte maturation or function, resulting in immunodeficiency disorders. Acquired disorders of lymphocyte function are far more common than congenital disorders. HIV infection is the most important infectious cause of acquired immunodeficiency. Patients with HIV infection are at increased risk for NHL. NHLs that occur in the setting of HIV have diffuse, aggressive B-cell histology and include DLBCL and Burkitt lymphoma. They are frequently associated with EBV infection and are often advanced stage (III or IV) at diagnosis, with extranodal sites of involvement.

Patients with HIV-associated NHL are potentially curable with the multidrug chemotherapy regimens used for treating NHL found in the general population. Treatment of the underlying HIV infection with highly active antiretroviral therapy (ART) has improved the outcome and prognosis of patients with HIV-associated NHL.

Patients who have undergone allogeneic organ transplantation require potent immunosuppressive drugs (e.g., cyclosporine, tacrolimus, mycophenolate, corticosteroids, methotrexate) to prevent graft-versus-host disease in the case of bone marrow transplantation or allograft rejection in the case of solid organ transplantation. These medications cause defects in T-cell function with an associated immunodeficiency state, which increases risk for a post-transplant lymphoproliferative disorder (PTLD). PTLD is an EBV-associated lymphoproliferative disorder characterized by a polymorphous or monomorphous population of B cells that can be monoclonal or polyclonal. Patients are treated by reducing doses of immunosuppressive drugs whenever possible. Patients with polymorphous disease early after organ transplantation may respond well to this approach. Patients who are not candidates for withdrawal of immunosuppression because of allograft rejection or who develop late monophorphic disease may respond better to treatment with rituximab alone or in combination with chemotherapy.

SUGGESTED READINGS

Canellos GP, Anderson JR, Propert KJ, et al: Chemotherapy of advanced Hodgkin's disease with MOPP, ABVD, or MOPP alternating with ABVD, N Engl J Med 327:1478–1484, 1992.

Cheson B, Fisher R, Barrington S, et al: Recommendations for initial evaluation, staging, and response assessment of Hodgkin and non-Hodgkin lymphoma: the Lugano classification, J Clin Oncol 32:3059–3068, 2014.

Coiffier B, Lepage E, Briere J, et al: CHOP chemotherapy plus rituximab compared with CHOP alone in elderly patients with diffuse large-B-cell lymphoma, N Engl J Med 346:235–242, 2002.

Dispenzieri A: POEMS Syndrome: 2019 Update on diagnosis, risk-stratification, and management, Am J Hematol 94(7):812–827, 2019.

Engert A, Plütschow A, Eich HT, et al: Reduced treatment intensity in patients with early-stage Hodgkin's lymphoma, N Engl J Med 363:640–652, 2010.

Fisher RI, Gaynor ER, Dahlberg S, et al: Comparison of a standard regimen (CHOP) with three intensive chemotherapy regimens for advanced non-Hodgkin's lymphoma, N Engl J Med 328:1002–1006, 1993.

主要见于老年人（中位年龄为64岁）的慢性疾病，兼具低级别淋巴瘤和骨髓瘤的特征。与骨髓瘤不同，WM可能导致淋巴结肿大和肝脾大，尽管骨髓受累非常常见，但溶骨性病变和高钙血症较罕见。WM的诊断性检查包括聚合酶链反应（PCR）检测MYD88基因突变，该突变可见于大多数患者，并可指导诊断和治疗选择。

WM的主要临床表现包括症状性贫血和IgM引起的高黏滞综合征。与IgG不同，IgM主要局限于血管内，随着IgM水平升高，血浆黏度增加。高黏滞综合征可导致鼻出血、视网膜出血、头晕、意识模糊和充血性心力衰竭等。约10%的IgM蛋白具有冷球蛋白的特性，患者可表现为冷球蛋白血症或冷凝集素综合征的症状，如肢端发绀、雷诺现象、与寒冷相关的血管症状或溶血性贫血。部分WM患者可出现周围神经病，其症状可能在诊断肿瘤之前就已表现出来。

接诊和治疗WM的方法与其他低级别B细胞淋巴瘤相似。氟达拉滨或烷化剂治疗（通常与泼尼松和利妥昔单抗联合使用）可有效缓解淋巴结肿大和脾大，并降低M蛋白水平，但不能治愈疾病。利妥昔单抗和蛋白酶体抑制剂硼替佐米对WM均有效。对于IgM负荷高的患者，单用利妥昔单抗可能一过性加重高黏滞综合征。新型靶向药物伊布替尼是一种BTK抑制剂，可有效治疗WM，并可与利妥昔单抗联合使用。尽管WM的治疗较少能达到完全缓解，但有治疗反应的患者中位生存期为4年，部分患者生存期可超过10年。

罕见的浆细胞疾病

重链病是一种罕见的淋巴浆细胞样肿瘤，其特征是产生有缺陷的γ、α或μ重链。临床表现根据分泌的重链类型而异。γ重链病易出现淋巴结肿大、累及Waldeyer环引起的腭部水肿和全身症状。α重链病（又称地中海淋巴瘤）的特征是淋巴细胞累及小肠并伴有腹泻和吸收不良。μ重链病与CLL相关。

原发性淀粉样变性
原发性轻链（AL）型淀粉样变性是一种全身性疾病，其特征是免疫球蛋白轻链在器官和组织中沉积，导致器官功能障碍而引起的一系列症状。充血性心力衰竭、出血倾向、肾病综合征和周围神经病是常见的并发症。原发性淀粉样变性患者可能对治疗骨髓瘤的药物有反应。硼替佐米、环磷酰胺和地塞米松的联合方案对部分患者有效。部分患者可能对大剂量化疗和自体SCT反应较好，但如果发生严重终末器官功能障碍（如心肌病），则并发症发生率和死亡率均升高。值得注意的是，并非所有淀粉样变性都是AL型，确定淀粉样蛋白的来源和类型对于疾病管理至关重要。

POEMS综合征
POEMS综合征是一种罕见疾病，其特征为多发性神经病、骨硬化性病变、内分泌病、单克隆丙种球蛋白病和皮肤病变。POEMS综合征的病因尚不清楚，但该病可能呈进行性发展，导致严重残疾、浆膜腔积液和血管内皮生长因子（VEGF）水平升高。单克隆λ轻链水平通常升高。局限性骨病可采用放疗。大剂量化疗和自体SCT对广泛病变的患者有效。

有关此专题的深入讨论，请参阅 *Goldman-Cecil Medicine* 第26版第178章"浆细胞疾病"和第179章"淀粉样变性"。 ❖

先天性和获得性淋巴细胞功能障碍

多种先天性疾病可影响淋巴细胞的成熟或功能，导致免疫缺陷性疾病。获得性淋巴细胞功能障碍比先天性疾病更为常见。HIV感染是获得性免疫缺陷最重要的感染性原因。HIV感染者患NHL的风险增加。HIV相关NHL具有弥漫性、侵袭性B细胞的组织学特征，包括DLBCL和伯基特淋巴瘤。它们通常与EBV感染有关，且诊断时通常处于晚期（Ⅲ或Ⅳ期），并伴有结外部位受累。

HIV相关NHL患者一般采用NHL的多药化疗方案，有潜在治愈可能。高效抗逆转录病毒治疗（ART）可改善HIV感染相关NHL患者的预后。

接受过同种异体移植的患者需使用强效免疫抑制剂（如环孢素、他克莫司、霉酚酸酯、皮质类固醇、甲氨蝶呤）来预防骨髓移植后的移植物抗宿主病或实体器官移植后的同种异体移植排斥。这些药物会导致T细胞功能障碍，并伴随免疫缺陷状态，从而增加移植后淋巴增殖性疾病（PTLD）的风险。PTLD是一种与EBV感染相关的淋巴增殖性疾病，其特征是可检出多形性或单形性B细胞群，可为单克隆或多克隆。患者可通过尽可能减小免疫抑制剂的剂量来进行治疗。器官移植后早期出现多形性疾病的患者可能对此种方法反应良好。因同种异体移植排斥而无法停用免疫抑制剂或晚期出现单形性疾病的患者，使用利妥昔单抗单药治疗或与化疗联合治疗的效果可能更好。

推荐阅读

Canellos GP, Anderson JR, Propert KJ, et al: Chemotherapy of advanced Hodgkin's disease with MOPP, ABVD, or MOPP alternating with ABVD, N Engl J Med 327:1478–1484, 1992.

Cheson B, Fisher R, Barrington S, et al: Recommendations for initial evaluation, staging, and response assessment of Hodgkin and non-Hodgkin lymphoma: the Lugano classification, J Clin Oncol 32:3059–3068, 2014.

Coiffier B, Lepage E, Briere J, et al: CHOP chemotherapy plus rituximab compared with CHOP alone in elderly patients with diffuse large-B-cell lymphoma, N Engl J Med 346:235–242, 2002.

Dispenzieri A: POEMS Syndrome: 2019 Update on diagnosis, risk-stratification, and management, Am J Hematol 94(7):812–827, 2019.

Engert A, Plütschow A, Eich HT, et al: Reduced treatment intensity in patients with early-stage Hodgkin's lymphoma, N Engl J Med 363:640–652, 2010.

Fisher RI, Gaynor ER, Dahlberg S, et al: Comparison of a standard regimen (CHOP) with three intensive chemotherapy regimens for advanced non-Hodgkin's lymphoma, N Engl J Med 328:1002–1006, 1993.

Geisler CH, Kolstad A, Laurell A, et al: Long-term progression-free survival of mantle cell lymphoma after intensive front-line immunochemotherapy with in vivo purged stem cell rescue: a nonrandomized phase 2 multicenter study by the Nordic Lymphoma Group, Blood 112:2687–2693, 2008.

Hasenclever D, Diehl V: A prognostic score for advanced Hodgkin's disease. International prognostic factors project on advanced Hodgkin's disease, N Engl J Med 339:1506–1514, 1998.

Howlader N, Noone AM, Krapcho M, et al (eds): SEER Cancer Statistics Review, Bethesda, MD, 1975-2016, National Cancer Institute, based on November 2018 SEER data submission, posted to the SEER web site. https://seer.cancer.gov/csr/1975_2016/. Accessed April 2019.

Kyle RA, Therneau TM, Rajkumar SV, et al: A long-term study of prognosis in monoclonal gammopathy of undetermined significance, N Engl J Med 346:564–569, 2002.

Maloney DG, Grillo-Lopez AJ, White CA, et al: IDEC-C2B8 (rituximab) anti-CD20 monoclonal antibody therapy in patients with relapsed low-grade non-Hodgkin's lymphoma, Blood 90:2188–2195, 1997.

McSweeney PA, Niederwieser D, Shizuru JA, et al: Hematopoietic cell transplantation in older patients with hematologic malignancies: replacing high-dose cytotoxic therapy with graft-versus-tumor effects, Blood 97:3390–3400, 2001.

Philip T, Guglielmi C, Hagenbeek A, et al: Autologous bone marrow transplantation as compared with salvage chemotherapy in relapses of chemotherapy-sensitive non-Hodgkin's lymphoma, N Engl J Med 33:1540–1545, 1995.

Rummel MJ, Niederle N, Maschmeyer G, et al: Bendamustine plus rituximab versus CHOP plus rituximab as first-line treatment for patients with indolent and mantle-cell lymphomas: an open-label, multicentre, randomised, phase 3 non-inferiority trial, Lancet 381:1203–1210, 2013.

Singhal S, Mehta J, Desikan R, et al: Antitumor activity of thalidomide in refractory multiple myeloma, N Engl J Med 341:1565–1571, 1999.

Swerdlow SH, Harris NL, Jaffe ES, et al: World Health Organization classification of tumours of hematopoietic and lymphoid tissues, revised ed 4, Lyon, 2017, IARC Press.

Wang ML, Rule S, Martin P: Targeting BTK with ibrutinib in relapsed or refractory mantle-cell lymphoma, N Engl J Med 369:507–516, 2013.

Geisler CH, Kolstad A, Laurell A, et al: Long-term progression-free survival of mantle cell lymphoma after intensive front-line immunochemotherapy with in vivo purged stem cell rescue: a nonrandomized phase 2 multicenter study by the Nordic Lymphoma Group, Blood 112:2687–2693, 2008.

Hasenclever D, Diehl V: A prognostic score for advanced Hodgkin's disease. International prognostic factors project on advanced Hodgkin's disease, N Engl J Med 339:1506–1514, 1998.

Howlader N, Noone AM, Krapcho M, et al (eds): SEER Cancer Statistics Review, Bethesda, MD, 1975-2016, National Cancer Institute, based on November 2018 SEER data submission, posted to the SEER web site. https://seer.cancer.gov/csr/1975_2016/. Accessed April 2019.

Kyle RA, Therneau TM, Rajkumar SV, et al: A long-term study of prognosis in monoclonal gammopathy of undetermined significance, N Engl J Med 346:564–569, 2002.

Maloney DG, Grillo-Lopez AJ, White CA, et al: IDEC-C2B8 (rituximab) anti-CD20 monoclonal antibody therapy in patients with relapsed low-grade non-Hodgkin's lymphoma, Blood 90:2188–2195, 1997.

McSweeney PA, Niederwieser D, Shizuru JA, et al: Hematopoietic cell transplantation in older patients with hematologic malignancies: replacing high-dose cytotoxic therapy with graft-versus-tumor effects, Blood 97:3390–3400, 2001.

Philip T, Guglielmi C, Hagenbeek A, et al: Autologous bone marrow transplantation as compared with salvage chemotherapy in relapses of chemotherapy-sensitive non-Hodgkin's lymphoma, N Engl J Med 33:1540–1545, 1995.

Rummel MJ, Niederle N, Maschmeyer G, et al: Bendamustine plus rituximab versus CHOP plus rituximab as first-line treatment for patients with indolent and mantle-cell lymphomas: an open-label, multicentre, randomised, phase 3 non-inferiority trial, Lancet 381:1203–1210, 2013.

Singhal S, Mehta J, Desikan R, et al: Antitumor activity of thalidomide in refractory multiple myeloma, N Engl J Med 341:1565–1571, 1999.

Swerdlow SH, Harris NL, Jaffe ES, et al: World Health Organization classification of tumours of hematopoietic and lymphoid tissues, revised ed 4, Lyon, 2017, IARC Press.

Wang ML, Rule S, Martin P: Targeting BTK with ibrutinib in relapsed or refractory mantle-cell lymphoma, N Engl J Med 369:507–516, 2013.

6

Normal Hemostasis

Lauren Shevell, Alfred I. Lee

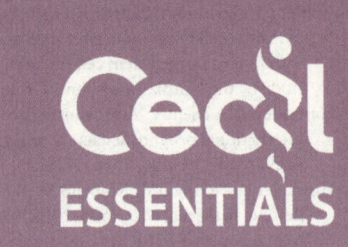

INTRODUCTION

Hemostasis is the physiologic balance of procoagulant and anticoagulant forces that provide structural integrity of vasculature while maintaining circulating blood flow. Vascular damage initiates clotting, which results in a localized platelet-fibrin plug at the site of injury to prevent blood loss. This is followed by clot containment, wound healing, eventual clot dissolution, and tissue regeneration. In healthy individuals, procoagulant and anticoagulant reactions occur continuously and in a balanced fashion so that bleeding is contained while blood vessels simultaneously remain patent to deliver adequate organ blood flow. If any of these processes is disrupted, either from inherited defects or acquired abnormalities, disordered hemostasis may result in either bleeding diatheses or thromboembolic disease.

Traditionally, hemostasis has been conceptualized in two parts: *primary hemostasis*, resulting in adhesion and activation of platelets, and *secondary hemostasis*, resulting in activation and regulation of the coagulation cascade. More recent studies, however, demonstrate a considerable amount of interplay between primary and secondary hemostatic components.

This chapter briefly details the physiologic and interdependent mechanisms of vascular hemostasis, including the normal balance of procoagulant and anticoagulant functions of the blood vessel wall and platelets, receptor-ligand interactions that are critical for hemostasis, as well as the highly complex, interwoven pathways that represent the coagulation cascade.

VASCULATURE PHYSIOLOGY

Blood flow in the arterial system differs from that in the venous system and imposes different coagulation requirements. In the pressurized arteries, relatively minor vascular damage can rapidly result in massive exsanguination; therefore, the procoagulant response in the arteries must rapidly arrest bleeding. Platelets are critical to the arterial response; they initially contain the blood loss and then provide an active surface for soluble coagulation factors to both localize and accelerate formation of fibrin for a strong fibrin clot. In contrast, the slower flow rates in the venous circulation produce slower bleeding, a feature that makes platelets less critical; instead, the balance of venous hemostasis is most dependent on the rate of thrombin generation. These differences are underscored clinically by the antithrombotic agents used in these distinct clinical settings: antiplatelet agents such as aspirin and clopidogrel are used to prevent coronary and cerebral artery thrombosis, whereas anticoagulants such as heparins, warfarin, and direct oral anticoagulants (e.g., direct thrombin inhibitors like dabigatran, or Xa inhibitors like rivaroxaban or apixaban) are used for the treatment and prophylaxis of venous disease.

Vascular endothelial cells (ECs) that line the luminal surfaces of blood vessels contribute both procoagulant and anticoagulant forces depending on circumstances. When the vasculature is intact, healthy ECs exert anticoagulant activity to maintain blood fluidity. This is done through several mechanisms. First, ECs act as a barrier, separating blood from subendothelial procoagulants such as tissue factor (TF) and collagen (Fig. 6.1 A). ECs also contribute to hemostatic balance by secreting several products including prostacyclin, nitric oxide, adenosine diphosphatase, and tissue factor pathway inhibitor (TFPI). Prostacyclin and nitric oxide release by ECs leads to vascular smooth muscle relaxation, reducing shear injury. These chemicals also promote the generation of cyclic adenosine monophosphate (cAMP), thus inhibiting platelet activation and aggregation. Adenosine diphosphatase degrades extracellular platelet-released ADP, inhibiting platelet recruitment into the growing platelet clot. TFPI acts by blunting the initiation of the coagulation cascade (described in more detail in the "Termination of Clotting" section).

When ECs are physically damaged or activated, their balance of coagulant properties is shifted to favor a procoagulant state. This is mediated by both the ECs themselves and subendothelial matrix that is exposed when the vascular wall is disrupted. Activated ECs express ligands on their surfaces allowing for platelet adhesion and increased inflammatory responses. These include E-selectin and P-selectin, β_1 and β_2 integrins, platelet EC adhesion molecule-1 (PECAM-1), and von Willebrand factor (VWF) multimers (Table 6.1). On the activated EC surface, VWF multimers localize and promote platelet adhesion, whereas integrins mediate adhesion and subsequent transendothelial migration of leukocytes into the tissues. After EC damage, the exposed subendothelial matrix also binds VWF multimers to further enhance platelet adhesion. Subendothelial procoagulant proteins such as thrombospondin, fibronectin, and especially collagen function both as ligands to capture platelets and as activators of adherent platelets. Collagen, in particular, is both a platelet ligand and a strong platelet agonist and causes platelets to undergo alpha and dense granule release and to express conformationally active ligands such as glycoprotein IIb/IIIa (GPIIb/IIIa, also known as integrin $\alpha_{IIb}\beta_3$) (described in detail later). Another critical procoagulant mediator exposed by EC damage is TF, which is constitutively expressed by subendothelial smooth muscle cells and fibroblasts. As outlined further later, TF is the major initiator of the soluble coagulation system that, along with activated platelets, results in the formation of a definitive platelet-fibrin clot.

VON WILLEBRAND FACTOR

VWF is an essential component of coagulation. Produced by ECs and megakaryocytes, the VWF protein is stored within platelets in alpha granules and within ECs in rodlike granules known as Weibel-Palade

正常止血

代新岳 译 薛峰 杨仁池 审校 王建祥 通审

引言

止血过程是促凝和抗凝反应之间的生理平衡，在维持循环血流的同时，保持血管结构的完整性。血管损伤会启动凝血过程，从而在损伤部位形成局部血小板-纤维蛋白血栓，防止血液流失。随后，血凝块形成被抑制、伤口愈合，最终血凝块溶解和组织再生。在健康人体内，促凝和抗凝反应是一个持续平衡的过程，从而在控制出血的同时保持血管通畅，以提供足够的器官血流。如果其中任何一个过程因遗传缺陷或获得性异常而受到干扰，失调的止血机制可能导致出血倾向或血栓栓塞性疾病。

止血在概念上分为两个部分：①初级止血，导致血小板黏附和活化；②次级止血，导致凝血级联反应的激活和调节。然而，近期研究表明，初级和次级止血之间存在相当多的相互作用。

本章简要介绍血管止血中相互依赖的生理学机制，包括血管壁和血小板促凝和抗凝功能的平衡、对止血至关重要的受体-配体相互作用，以及代表凝血级联的高度复杂且相互交织的途径。

血管生理学

动脉系统中的血流与静脉系统不同，对凝血的要求也不同。在血管内压力较大的动脉中，相对较小的血管损伤即可迅速导致大量失血；因此，动脉中的促凝反应必须能够迅速止血。血小板是动脉促凝反应的关键；它们在起始时控制失血，然后为可溶性凝血因子提供活性表面，使其定位并加速形成纤维蛋白，从而形成坚固的纤维蛋白凝块。相比之下，静脉循环中由于血流速度较慢，出血也较慢，这一特点使得血小板变得不那么重要；相反，静脉止血的平衡主要依赖于凝血酶的生成速度。在不同临床情况下使用的抗血栓药物凸显了这些差异：阿司匹林和氯吡格雷等抗血小板药物用于预防冠状动脉和脑动脉血栓形成，而肝素、华法林和直接口服抗凝剂［直接凝血酶抑制剂（如达比加群等）或Xa抑制剂（如利伐沙班、阿哌沙班）］等抗凝药物则用于治疗和预防静脉血栓性疾病。

血管内皮细胞（EC）排列于血管腔内表面，可根据不同情况发挥促凝和抗凝作用。当血管壁完整时，健康的EC会通过多种机制发挥抗凝作用，以保持血液的流动性。EC先发挥屏障作用，将血液与内皮下促凝物质［如组织因子（TF）和胶原蛋白］隔开（图6.1A）。EC还可通过分泌前列环素、一氧化氮、腺苷二磷酸酶和组织因子途径抑制物（TFPI）等多种物质来促进止血平衡。EC释放的前列环素和一氧化氮可使血管平滑肌松弛，减少剪切损伤。这些化学物质还能促进环磷酸腺苷（cAMP）的生成，从而抑制血小板的活化和聚集。腺苷二磷酸酶能降解细胞外血小板释放的ADP，抑制血小板被募集到不断增大的血小板凝块中。TFPI通过抑制凝血级联反应的启动来发挥作用（详见下文"凝血终止"）。

当EC受到物理损伤或被激活时，其凝血平衡会发生变化，转为倾向于促凝状态，这是由EC本身和血管壁被破坏时暴露的内皮下基质介导的。活化的EC在其表面表达配体，使血小板得以黏附并增加炎症反应。这些配体包括E选择素和P选择素、β_1和β_2整合素、血小板内皮细胞黏附分子1（PECAM-1）和血管性血友病因子（vWF）多聚体（表6.1）。vWF多聚体定位于活化的EC表面，并促进血小板黏附，而整合素则介导白细胞黏附并随后跨内皮迁移到组织中。EC损伤后，暴露的内皮下基质会结合vWF多聚体，进一步增强血小板黏附。内皮下促凝蛋白［如血小板应答蛋白（TSP）、纤维连接蛋白、胶原蛋白］既可作为捕获血小板的配体，又可作为黏附血小板的激活剂。尤其是胶原蛋白，其既是血小板配体，又是一种强效血小板激动剂，可使血小板释放α颗粒和致密颗粒，并表达构象活性配体，如糖蛋白Ⅱb/Ⅲa（GPⅡb/Ⅲa，又称整合素$\alpha_{IIb}\beta_3$）（见下文）。EC损伤暴露的另一种重要促凝介质是TF，它由内皮下平滑肌细胞和成纤维细胞表达。TF是可溶性凝血系统的主要启动因子，它与活化的血小板共同导致血小板-纤维蛋白凝块的形成。

血管性血友病因子

vWF是凝血系统的重要组成部分。vWF蛋白由EC和巨核细胞产生，储存在血小板内的α颗粒和EC内的棒状颗粒（即Weibel-Palade小体）中。在血小板

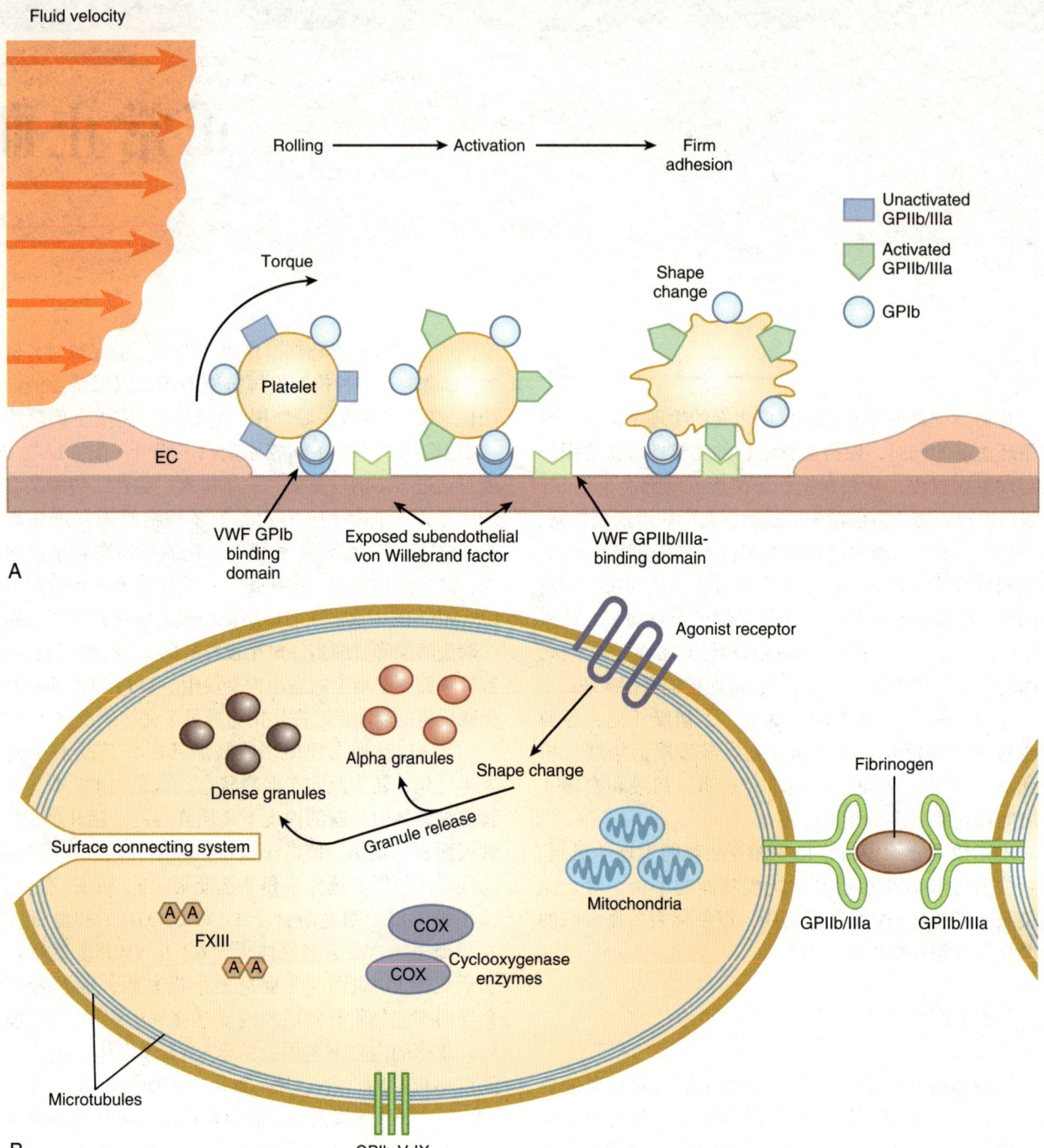

Fig. 6.1 (A) The adhesive interactions that produce stable platelet attachment to subendothelial von Willebrand factor (VWF). The initial attachment between platelet glycoprotein Ib (GPIb) and its binding domain on VWF is rapid but has a short half-life, and the result is a rolling movement caused by torque generated by flowing blood. The VWF-GPIb interaction produces transmembrane signaling that activates the platelet to change shape and simultaneously transforms GPIIb/IIIa into an activated conformation capable of binding to a distinct arginine-glycine-aspartate domain on VWF. This secondary adhesion causes the platelet to firmly adhere to the exposed subendothelial VWF. (B) The internal and external anatomy of a platelet. The platelet consists of several important external, transmembrane, and internal components that help to promote platelet activation, adhesion, aggregation/agglutination, and general coagulation factor–based hemostasis. The most important and most clinically relevant aspects of platelet anatomy are shown. Details regarding the steps leading to platelet activation and release of granules and cytosolic contents are discussed in the text. *A*, A subunits of factor XIII; *COX*, cyclooxygenase; *EC*, endothelial cell; *FXIII*, factor XIII; *GP*, glycoprotein complex.

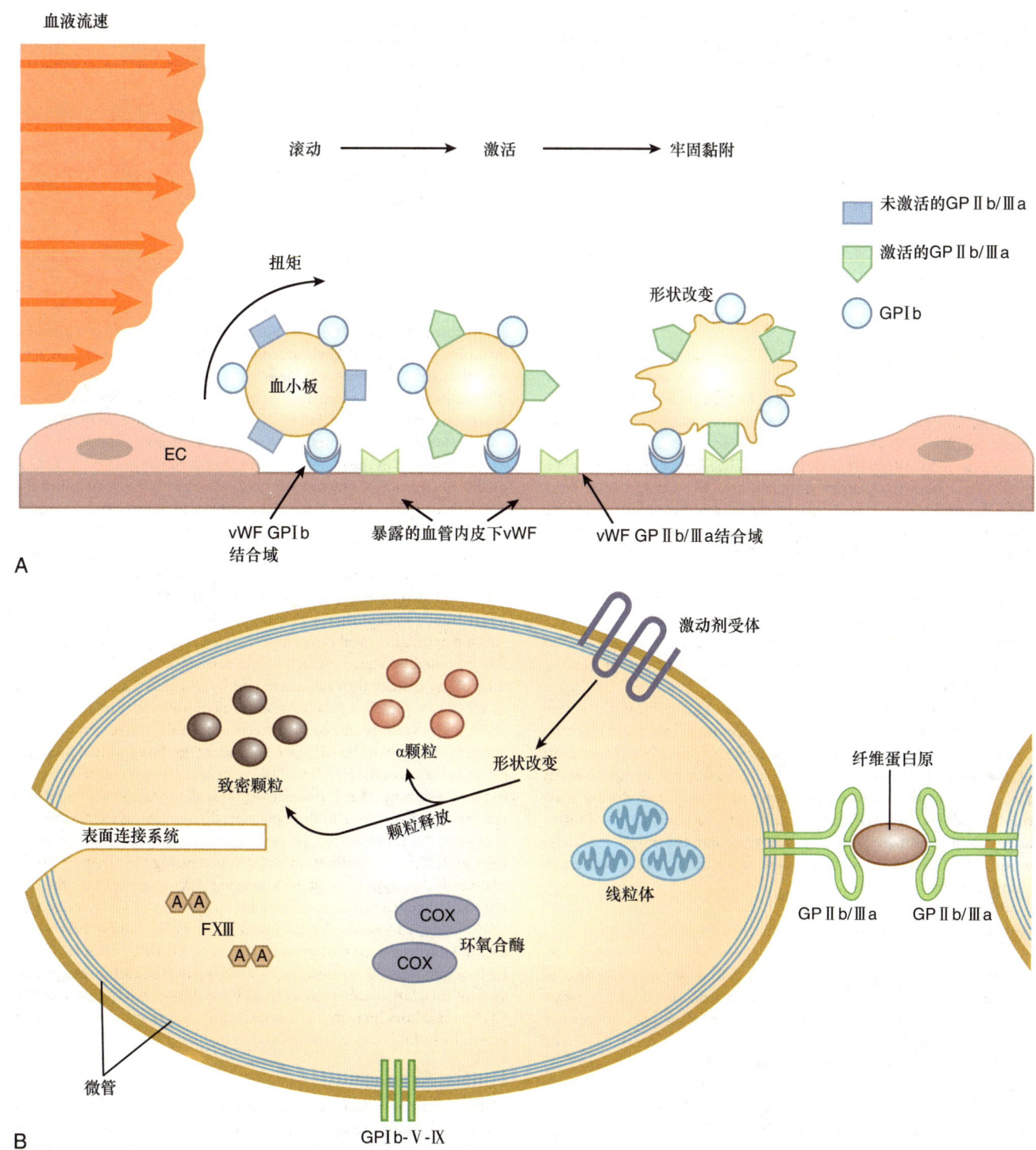

图 6.1 **A**. 黏附相互作用使血小板稳定附着于内皮下血管性血友病因子（vWF）。血小板糖蛋白Ⅰb（GPⅠb）与其在vWF上的结合域的初始附着是快速的，但半衰期很短，其结果是由血液流动产生的扭矩引起的滚动运动。vWF-GPⅠb相互作用会产生跨膜信号，激活血小板，从而改变其形状，同时将GPⅡb/Ⅲa转变为活化构象，能够与vWF上独特的精氨酸-甘氨酸-天冬氨酸结构域结合。这种二次黏附使血小板牢固地附着于暴露的内皮下vWF。**B**. 血小板的内部和外部解剖结构。血小板由多种重要的外部、跨膜和内部成分组成，它们有助于促进血小板活化、黏附、聚集/凝集和基于凝血因子的一般止血反应。图中展示了血小板解剖学中最重要、最具临床意义的方面。有关导致血小板活化和释放颗粒及细胞膜内容物的详细步骤见正文。A，凝血因子ⅩⅢ的A亚基；COX，环氧合酶；EC，内皮细胞；FⅩⅢ，凝血因子ⅩⅢ；GP，糖蛋白复合物

TABLE 6.1 Properties of Endothelial Cell Coagulants

Procoagulant	Anticoagulant
Collagen	Vasodilation
Factor VIII	Adenosine diphosphatase
Fibronectin	Heparan sulfates
Integrins	Nitric oxide
Platelet-endothelial cell adhesion molecule-1 (PECAM-1)	Prostacyclin
Selectins (E and P)	Thrombomodulin
Vasoconstriction	Tissue factor pathway inhibitor
von Willebrand factor	Tissue plasminogen activator

bodies. In both platelets and ECs, VWF proteins multimerize in the Golgi apparatus; about 95% of VWF multimers are constitutively released into the plasma and can be detected on electrophoretic gels as high-, intermediate-, and low-molecular-weight VWF forms. The remaining 5% of VWF multimers are stored either in platelet alpha granules or in EC Weibel-Palade bodies in the form of ultra-large VWF multimers. Following platelet stimulation or EC damage, ultra-large VWF multimers are released into the plasma and have high affinity for platelets and subendothelial collagen, forming string-like structures that must then be cleaved into smaller VWF proteins for proper function. Cleavage of ultra-large VWF multimers is performed by a metalloproteinase, ADAMTS13 (a disintegrin and metalloproteinase with a thrombospondin type 1 motif, member 13). In addition to platelet and subendothelial collagen binding, VWF in the plasma serves as a second role in binding and stabilizing coagulation factor VIII and preventing its degradation.

The importance of VWF is underscored clinically by von Willebrand disease (VWD), the most common inherited bleeding condition in the world, characterized by defects in either the amount or the activity of VWF protein; and alternatively by thrombotic thrombocytopenic purpura, an inherited or acquired disease arising from defects in ADAMTS13 that lead to accumulation of ultra-large VWF multimers, causing microvascular thrombosis, platelet consumption, shearing of red blood cells and multiple end-organ complications.

PLATELET PHYSIOLOGY

Platelets are anucleated cells measuring 2 to 4 μm in diameter and are derived from megakaryocyte cytoplasm (Fig. 6.1B). Each megakaryocyte contributes 1000 to 3000 platelets in its lifetime. After platelets are released into the circulation, they survive 7 to 10 days. The normal platelet count ranges between 150,000 to 450,000/μL; only approximately 7100 platelets/μL are required for hemostasis per day if vascular structures are intact (i.e., in the absence of any recent surgeries or trauma) and if there is no increase in normal platelet consumption (e.g., as might occur in sepsis or disseminated intravascular coagulation).

The bleeding time, an in vivo measure of hemostasis, is usually less than 8 minutes if the platelet count is within the normal limit. It is used as a screening test for platelet function defects, VWD, and sometimes other bleeding disorders. The bleeding time is dependent on the platelet count and will naturally be prolonged if the platelet count falls to less than 100,000/μL. Therefore, in the setting of thrombocytopenia, a prolonged bleeding time cannot be used to determine whether bleeding is caused by abnormal platelet function, VWD, another bleeding problem, or thrombocytopenia. Because the bleeding time is an operator-dependent, highly variable in vivo assay that causes trauma to patients, most laboratories now use the Platelet Function Analyzer-100 (PFA-100) (Fig. 7.2.), which uses anticoagulated blood to examine the amount of time required for platelets to form a plug in response to either collagen and ADP or collagen and epinephrine (i.e., the "closure time"). The PFA-100 is similar to the bleeding time test in that both may be used to assess platelet function and to screen for VWD but are unable to distinguish between thrombocytopenia and abnormal platelet function when the platelet count is lower than 100,000/μL.

Platelet Activation

In the setting of vascular injury, platelets are recruited to the area by exposure to local agonists (collagen, epinephrine and thrombin) and by release of agonists within platelets into the local microenvironment (ADP, thromboxane). The most potent platelet activators, collagen and thrombin, interact with their specific platelet receptors to strongly activate platelets. Epinephrine alone is not a powerful platelet agonist, but stimulation of the α-adrenergic receptor on platelets primes them for synergistic activation by relatively weak agonists such as ADP. Platelets also release activating compounds, including thromboxane A2 (TXA_2), which is formed in the platelet cytosol after cyclooxygenase 1 (COX1)-mediated cleavage of arachidonic acid, which is then released into the clot milieu. TXA_2 is both a platelet agonist and vasoconstrictor and is rapidly degraded to its inert by-product, thromboxane B2. Notably, the exact roles of different platelet agonists depend on a spatial hierarchy within the platelet plug. Thrombin activates platelets within the core of the hemostatic plug, whereas ADP and TXA_2 activate platelets in the loosely packed shell surrounding the core.

Of particular clinical importance, platelet COX1 activity is irreversibly inhibited by aspirin, which blocks formation of TXA_2 for the lifetime of the platelet through a covalent bond causing steric hindrance of the active site. In contrast, nonsteroidal anti-inflammatory drugs (NSAIDs) reversibly and competitively bind at the active site; thus, the antiplatelet effects of NSAIDs are dependent on the continual presence of plasma levels of the NSAID. COX2 is an induced isoform of the cyclo-oxygenase enzyme that is present within leukocytes and that mediates inflammation and pain. Mature platelets do not possess COX2 activity, providing the rationale for the development of selective COX2 inhibitors to decrease inflammation without increasing the bleeding risk of platelet dysfunction (as well as decreasing risk for gastrointestinal side effects, which will not be addressed here). However, ECs are reliant on COX2 activity to synthesize the antithrombogenic compound prostacyclin. Downregulation of prostacyclin, coupled with preserved platelet function, tips the hemostatic balance in favor of clot formation. In view of this, large-scale clinical trials have shown that highly selective COX2 inhibitors increase the likelihood of hypertension and vascular events including myocardial infarction and stroke.

Platelet Adhesion

Platelet activation leads to a functional shape change of the platelet from a disk to an irregular sphere with pseudopod extensions, as well as exposure of platelet binding domains. This enhances platelet adhesion capabilities and maximizes the interaction of coagulation factors with the platelet surface. Initial platelet adhesion is primarily mediated by the glycoprotein 1b-IX-V (GP1b-IX-V) complex on the platelet surface binding to multimeric VWF, which is immobilized by adherence to exposed subendothelial collagen. The weak binding of GP1b-IX-V to VWF contributes to transmembrane signaling with downstream effects that include a change in platelet shape (see Fig. 6.1A) and a change in GPIIb/IIIa (integrin $\alpha_{IIb}\beta_3$) from a low-affinity to a high-affinity state, facilitating binding of the latter to fibrinogen and VWF (see Fig. 6.1B). A deficiency of the GP1b-IX-V complex leads to

表6.1　内皮细胞凝血的特性	
促凝剂	抗凝剂
胶原蛋白	血管扩张
因子Ⅷ	腺苷二磷酸酶
纤维连接蛋白	硫酸肝素
整合素	一氧化氮
血小板内皮细胞黏附分子1（PECAM-1）	前列环素
选择素（E选择素和P选择素）	凝血酶调节蛋白
血管收缩	组织因子途径抑制物
血管性血友病因子	组织纤溶酶原激活物

和EC中，vWF蛋白在高尔基体内发生多聚体化；约95%的vWF多聚体会持续释放到血浆中，可在电泳凝胶上检测到高分子量、中分子量和低分子量vWF。其余5%的vWF多聚体以超大型vWF多聚体的形式储存在血小板α颗粒或EC Weibel-Palade小体中。当血小板受到刺激或EC受损后，超大型vWF多聚体会释放到血浆中，与血小板和内皮下胶原蛋白高度亲和，形成串状结构，然后必须被裂解为较小的vWF蛋白才能发挥正常功能。超大型vWF多聚体的裂解是由金属蛋白酶ADAMTS13（一种具有血小板应答蛋白1型基序的去整合素和金属蛋白酶）来完成的。除了与血小板和内皮下胶原蛋白结合外，血浆中的vWF还能发挥第二种作用，即结合和稳定凝血因子Ⅷ并防止其降解。

在临床上，血管性血友病（vWD）和血栓性血小板减少性紫癜（TTP）都凸显了vWF的重要性，前者是最常见的遗传性出血性疾病，其特征是vWF蛋白数量或功能缺陷；后者是一种遗传性或获得性疾病，由ADAMTS13缺陷导致超大vWF多聚体积聚所致，引起微血管血栓形成、血小板消耗、红细胞剪切和多种终末器官并发症。

血小板的生理功能

血小板是无核细胞，直径为2～4μm，来源于巨核细胞胞质（图6.1B）。每个巨核细胞可释放1000～3000个血小板。血小板进入血液循环后，可存活7～10天。正常血小板数量为（150 000～450 000）/μl；如果血管结构完好无损（如近期没有任何手术或外伤）且没有大量的血小板消耗（如感染中毒症或弥散性血管内凝血），每天仅需约7100/μl的血小板即可满足生理性止血需求。

出血时间（BT）是反映体内生理性止血的指标，如果血小板计数在正常范围内，通常BT＜8 min。它可用于筛查血小板功能缺陷、vWD或其他出血性疾病。BT取决于血小板计数，如果血小板计数降至100 000/μl以下，BT自然会延长。因此，血小板减少时BT延长无法鉴别出血原因（如血小板功能异常、vWD、其他出血问题或血小板减少症）。由于BT试验依赖于操作者，体内检测的变异性大，且会对患者造成创伤，目前大多数实验室使用血小板功能分析仪-100（PFA-100）（图7.2），该仪器使用抗凝血检测血小板在胶原蛋白和ADP或胶原和肾上腺素作用下形成血栓所需的时间（即"闭合时间"）。与BT试验类似，PFA-100可用于评估血小板功能和筛查vWD，但当血小板计数＜100 000/μl时，则无法区分血小板减少症和血小板功能异常。

血小板活化

在血管损伤后，通过暴露的局部激动剂（胶原蛋白、肾上腺素和凝血酶）及释放到局部微环境中的血小板内激动剂（ADP、血栓素）募集血小板。胶原蛋白和凝血酶是最强效的血小板激动剂，通过与其特定的血小板受体相互作用，强效激活血小板。肾上腺素本身并不是强效的血小板激动剂，但刺激血小板上的α肾上腺素受体可使血小板在ADP等相对较弱的激动剂的影响下发生协同激活。血小板还会释放激活化合物，包括血栓素A_2（TXA_2），它由环氧合酶1（COX1）催化介导花生四烯酸裂解后在血小板胞质溶胶中形成，然后释放到血凝块环境中。TXA_2既是血小板激动剂，也是血管收缩剂，会迅速代谢为无活性的副产物血栓素B_2。需要注意的是，不同血小板激动剂的确切作用取决于血小板栓子内的空间层次结构。凝血酶激活止血栓子核心内的血小板，而ADP和TXA_2则激活核心周围松散包裹着的外壳内的血小板。

尤为重要的是，阿司匹林会不可逆地抑制血小板COX1的活性，通过共价键导致活性位点的空间位阻，在血小板的整个寿命周期内阻止TXA_2的形成，这具有独特的临床意义。相反，非甾体抗炎药（NSAID）可逆且竞争性地与活性位点结合；因此，NSAID的抗血小板作用取决于血浆中NSAID的持续存在。COX2是环氧合酶的一种诱导型异构体，存在于白细胞中，可介导炎症和疼痛。成熟的血小板不具有COX2活性，这一特性为研发选择性COX2抑制剂提供了理论依据，可在不增加血小板功能障碍出血风险（以及降低胃肠道副作用的风险）的情况下减轻炎症。然而，EC依赖COX2的活性来合成抗血栓形成的化合物前列环素。前列环素下调和血小板功能的保持使止血平衡倾向于形成血栓。鉴于此，大规模临床试验表明，高选择性COX2抑制剂会升高高血压和血管事件（包括心肌梗死和卒中）的发生率。

血小板黏附

血小板活化会导致血小板发生功能性形状改变，从圆盘状变为具有伪足延伸的不规则球状，并暴露血小板结合域。这增强了血小板的黏附能力，并使凝血因子与血小板表面的相互作用最大化。最初的血小板黏附主要由血小板表面的糖蛋白Ib-Ⅸ-V（GPⅠb-Ⅸ-V）复合物与vWF多聚体结合来介导，后者通过黏附于暴露的内皮下胶原蛋白而被固定。GPIb-Ⅲ与vWF的弱结合有助于跨膜信号转导，其下游效应包括血小板形状改变（图6.1A）和GPⅡb/Ⅲa（整合素$α_{Ⅱb}β_3$）从低亲和力状态转变为高亲和力状态，从而促进后者与纤维蛋白原和vWF的结合（图6.1B）。GP1b-Ⅸ-V复合物缺乏会导致巨血小

Bernard-Soulier syndrome, a congenital bleeding disorder characterized by giant platelets that are dysfunctional.

GPIIb/IIIa (integrin $\alpha_{IIb}\beta_3$) is a member of the integrin superfamily and the most abundant receptor on the platelet surface. Prior to platelet activation, the GPIIb/IIIa ($\alpha_{IIb}\beta_3$) receptor sits on the platelet surface and has low affinity for binding. However, upon platelet activation and its consequent conformational changes, the GPIIb/IIIa receptor adopts a high-affinity conformation that facilitates binding both to VWF, securing platelets strongly on the subendothelial surface, and to fibrinogen, linking platelets together and reinforcing the platelet plug. Further, after binding to VWF, the cytosolic side of the GPIIb/IIIa ($\alpha_{IIb}\beta_3$) receptor binds to the cytoskeleton of the platelet, fostering further changes to platelet shape change and spreading via cytoskeletal reorganization. These roles of GPIIb/IIIa ($\alpha_{IIb}\beta_3$) in platelet adhesion and platelet plug formation provide the rationale for use of GPIIb/IIIa ($\alpha_{IIb}\beta_3$) antagonists in treatment of coronary artery disease. Of note, mutations in the gene encoding GPIIb/IIIa ($\alpha_{IIb}\beta_3$) lead to Glanzmann thrombocythemia, another congenital bleeding disorder leading to platelet dysfunction.

Platelet Secretion

After activation, dense granules and alpha granules within platelets fuse with the canalicular membrane and liberate their procoagulant contents into the extracellular fluid. Dense granules contain serotonin, ADP, ATP, ionized calcium, and histamine. Serotonin and ADP both activate and recruit platelets to sites of vascular injury. Additionally, serotonin, similarly to TXA_2, acts as a vasoconstrictor. ADP acts purely as a platelet agonist through the G protein–linked P2RY12 receptor and has no vasoactive properties. The importance of dense-granule release is illustrated by the severe bleeding seen in patients with congenital dense-granule deficiencies such as Hermansky-Pudlak syndrome or Chediak-Higashi syndrome.

Alpha granules contain numerous proteins including many adhesive molecules (fibrinogen, VWF, thrombospondin), cellular mitogens (platelet-derived growth factor, transforming growth factor beta), coagulation factors (factor V), and physiologically important receptors (P-selectin, $\alpha_{IIb}\beta_3$). The importance of platelet alpha granules is illustrated in patients with gray platelet syndrome, an inherited deficiency of alpha granules leading to bleeding. Other components within platelets, including factor XIII, are also released upon platelet activation and act as clot stabilizers (see Fig. 6.1B).

COAGULATION

Coagulation Cascade Model

The classical coagulation cascade (Fig. 6.2A), first described over 50 years ago, features two starting points, the intrinsic and extrinsic pathways, that flow in a step-wise waterfall of proteolytic reactions and converge in a common pathway. The common pathway culminates with the generation of thrombin, which converts fibrinogen to fibrin. Fibrin then cross-links platelets and strengthens the platelet plug.

In the classical model, coagulation begins with the extrinsic pathway, which is initiated by the exposure of TF and activated factor VIIa, leading to activation of factor X in the common pathway.

The intrinsic pathway is initiated by the activation of proteins circulating in plasma—namely, factor XII (Hageman factor), high-molecular-weight kininogen (HMWK, also known as Fitzgerald factor), and prekallikrein (PK, also known as Fletcher factor). This pathway is also referred to as the contact activation pathway because these proteins are activated by contact with negatively charged surfaces. Factor XIIa and HMWK activate factor XI, leading to the activation of factor IX, which in conjunction with factor VIII activates factor X to initiate the common pathway (see Fig. 6.2AB). The importance of the intrinsic coagulation cascade is demonstrated in patients with hemophilias, which are congenital bleeding disorders due to deficiencies in factor VIII (hemophilia A), factor IX (hemophilia B), or factor XI (hemophilia C).

Notably, all procoagulants are produced almost exclusively in the liver aside from factor VIII, which is produced in both liver sinusoidal cells and ECs, and VWF, which is produced in ECs and megakaryocytes. The procoagulant factors II, VII, IX, and X, and the anticoagulant proteins C and S, all undergo post-translational modification in the form of vitamin K–dependent g-carboxylation of the amino terminal domains, which is critical for calcium binding and determining the three-dimensional structure of proteins. The importance of vitamin K–dependent g-carboxylation is demonstrated by the anticoagulant warfarin, which acts by blocking vitamin K epoxide reductase, thereby reducing the generation of these specific proteins.

In the classical coagulation model, the prothrombin time (PT) serves as a measure of extrinsic pathway activity while the activated partial thrombin time (aPTT) measures activity of the intrinsic pathway. Therapeutically, the PT and aPTT are used to guide warfarin and heparin dosing, respectively. Although the classical model of coagulation is workable for some clinical scenarios, more recent models have made strides to more accurately elucidate and depict the physiology and complex interplay of different components of coagulation.

Cell-Based Model of Coagulation

The cell-based coagulation model (see Fig. 6.2B) has largely been established as the most physiologically accurate in vivo model of coagulation. This model proposes that coagulation takes place on the surfaces of different cells in a three-step fashion: initiation, amplification, and propagation.

The *initiation phase* begins as exposed TF on the EC surface binds to picomolar amounts of factor VIIa, present in the circulation at all times. The VIIa-TF complex (termed the extrinsic Xase) activates factors IX and X. The conversion of a small amount of X to Xa produces a tiny amount of thrombin. The nearly trivial amount of thrombin sparks feedback to activate factor XI, leading to *amplification* of thrombin generation. Factor VIII, conveniently brought to the bleeding site by its carrier VWF, is also activated by thrombin, a step that causes release of VWF. Factor VIIIa then complexes with the picomolar amounts of factor IXa generated by the TF-VIIa complex during the initiation phase to create the VIIIa-IXa complex, known as the intrinsic Xase complex. Notably, IXa generation by the TF-VIIa complex is limited by TFPI, so factor IX is secondarily activated by platelet-bound factor XIa (catalyzed by factor XIIa in conjunction with high molecular weight kininogen), providing sufficient amounts of factor IXa in the intrinsic Xase complex. The formation of this complex on the platelet surface heralds the *propagation phase*, and the switch of the primary path of Xa generation from the TF-VIIa complex, the extrinsic Xase complex, to the intrinsic Xase. This switch is of significant kinetic advantage, with the intrinsic Xase complex exhibiting a 50-fold higher efficiency than the extrinsic Xase. More than 96% of the total thrombin that is generated during clotting occurs during the propagation phase. The bleeding diathesis associated with hemophilia is a testament to the physiologic importance of the exuberant thrombin generation engendered by the switch from extrinsic to intrinsic Xase. The aPTT, which measures the initiation phase of clotting begun by an artificial in vitro stimulant, is prolonged by severe deficiencies of either VIII or IX, but it is thrombin generation during the propagation phase, a function not evaluated by the aPTT, that is more impaired in hemophilia.

Thrombin generated during the initiation phase is a potent platelet activator. The activated platelet expresses receptors for VIIIa and IXa, and binding of these active proteases in complex with membrane phosphatidylserine enhances the binding of the enzyme's substrate,

板综合征（Bernard-Soulier 综合征），其是一种以伴有功能障碍的巨大血小板为特征的先天性出血性疾病。

GPⅡb/Ⅲa 是整合素超家族成员，也是血小板表面最丰富的受体。在血小板活化前，GPⅡb/Ⅲa 受体位于血小板表面，其结合亲和力较低。然而，当血小板活化并随之发生构象变化时，GPⅡb/Ⅲa 受体会采用一种高亲和力构象，这种构象既有利于与 vWF 结合，使血小板牢固地固定在内皮下表面，也有利于与纤维蛋白原结合，将血小板连接在一起并加固血小板栓子。此外，在与 vWF 结合后，GPⅡb/Ⅲa 受体的胞质侧与血小板的细胞骨架结合，促进血小板形状的进一步改变，并通过细胞骨架重组而扩散。GPⅡb/Ⅲa 在血小板黏附和血小板栓子形成中的这些作用为使用 GPⅡb/Ⅲa 拮抗剂治疗冠心病提供了理论依据。编码 GPⅡb/Ⅲa 的基因突变会导致血小板无力症（格兰茨曼血小板功能不全），这是另一种导致血小板功能障碍的先天性出血性疾病。

血小板分泌

血小板活化后，其内的致密颗粒和 α 颗粒与管状膜融合，并将其促凝物质释放到细胞外液中。致密颗粒含有血清素、ADP、ATP、钙离子和组胺。血清素和 ADP 能激活血小板并将其募集到血管损伤部位。此外，与 TXA_2 类似，血清素也是一种血管收缩剂。ADP 仅通过与 G 蛋白相连的 P2RY12 受体发挥血小板激动剂的作用，无血管活性特性。先天性致密颗粒缺乏症（如 Hermansky-Pudlak 综合征或 Chediak-Higashi 综合征）患者的严重出血说明了致密颗粒释放的重要性。

α 颗粒含有多种蛋白质，包括许多黏附分子（纤维蛋白原、vWF、血小板应答蛋白），细胞促有丝分裂原（血小板源性生长因子、转化生长因子 β），凝血因子（因子 V）和具有重要生理学意义的受体（P 选择素、$α_{Ⅱb}β_3$）。灰色血小板综合征患者说明了血小板 α 颗粒的重要性，该综合征是一种会导致出血的遗传性 α 颗粒缺乏症。血小板内的其他成分（包括因子 XⅢ）也会在血小板活化时释放，并起到血凝块稳定剂的作用（图 6.1B）。

凝血

凝血级联模型

经典的凝血级联模型（图 6.2A）于 50 多年前被首次描述，它有两个起点，即内源性凝血途径和外源性凝血途径，这两个途径呈现逐级引发的瀑布式蛋白质水解反应，最后汇聚到共同途径。共同途径最终产生凝血酶，凝血酶将纤维蛋白原转化为纤维蛋白。随后，纤维蛋白与血小板交联，形成强化血小板栓子。

在经典模型中，凝血始于外源性凝血途径，由暴露的 TF 和活化因子 Ⅶa 启动，导致共同途径中因子 X 的活化。

内源性凝血途径通过激活血浆中循环的蛋白质来启动，这些蛋白质包括因子 Ⅻ（Hageman 因子）、高分子量激肽原（HMWK；又称 Fitzgerald 因子）和前激肽释放酶（PK；又称 Fletcher 因子）。该途径也被称为接触激活途径，因为这些蛋白质是通过与带负电荷的表面接触而被激活的。因子 Ⅻa 和 HMWK 激活因子 Ⅺ，从而激活因子 Ⅸ，因子 Ⅸ 与因子 Ⅷ 共同激活因子 X，从而启动共同途径（图 6.2）。内源性凝血级联反应的重要性在血友病患者中得到证实，血友病是由缺乏因子 Ⅷ（血友病 A）、因子 Ⅸ（血友病 B）或因子 Ⅺ（血友病 C）而导致的先天性出血性疾病。

需注意，所有促凝因子几乎均在肝内产生，除了因子 Ⅷ（在肝窦细胞和 EC 中产生）和 vWF（在 EC 和巨核细胞中产生）。促凝因子 Ⅱ、Ⅶ、Ⅸ 和 X，以及抗凝蛋白质 C 和 S 的氨基末端结构域均会发生依赖维生素 K 的 γ-羧化形式的翻译后修饰，这对于钙结合和确定蛋白质的三维结构至关重要。抗凝剂华法林通过阻断维生素 K 环氧化物还原酶而减少这些特定蛋白质的生成，证明了维生素 K 依赖性 γ-羧化的重要性。

在经典的凝血模型中，凝血酶原时间（PT）是衡量外源性凝血途径活性的指标，而活化部分凝血活酶时间（APTT）是衡量内源性凝血途径活性的指标。在治疗上，PT 和 APTT 分别用于指导华法林和肝素的治疗剂量。虽然经典凝血模型在某些临床情况下是可行的，但新模型在更准确地阐明和描述凝血不同成分的生理学和复杂相互作用方面取得了长足进步。

基于细胞的凝血模型

目前公认基于细胞的凝血模型（图 6.2B）是最符合生理学原理的体内凝血模型。该模型提出，凝血通过以下 3 个步骤发生在不同细胞的表面：启动、放大和扩增。

当 EC 表面暴露的 TF 与循环中始终存在的皮摩尔（pmol）量级的因子 Ⅶa 结合时，即进入启动阶段。Ⅶa-TF 复合物（即外源性 X 酶复合物）可激活因子 Ⅸ 和 X。少量因子 X 转化为因子 Xa 会产生微量的凝血酶。凝血酶引发反馈来激活因子 Ⅺ，导致凝血酶生成的放大效应。因子 Ⅷ 易被其载体 vWF 带到出血部位，也能被凝血酶激活，从而导致 vWF 释放。随后，因子 Ⅷa 与 TF-Ⅶa 复合物在启动阶段产生的皮摩尔量级的因子 Ⅸa 结合，形成 Ⅷa-Ⅸa 复合物（即内源性 X 酶复合物）。值得注意的是，由 TF-Ⅶa 复合物生成的因子 Ⅸa 受到 TFPI 的限制，因此因子 Ⅸ 会被血小板结合因子 Ⅺa（由因子 Ⅻa 和 HMWK 共同催化）二次激活，从而为内源性 X 酶复合物的形成提供足量的因子 Ⅸa。该复合物在血小板表面的形成预示着凝血扩增阶段的开始，也预示着因子 Xa 生成的主要途径从 Ⅶa-TF 复合物（即外源性 X 酶复合物）转变为内源性 X 酶复合物。这种转换具有显著的动力学优势，内源性 X 酶复合物的效率比外源性 X 酶复合物高 50 倍。凝血过程中产生的凝血酶总量的 96% 以上发生在扩增阶段。与血友病相关的出血倾向证明了从外源性 X 酶复合物到内源性 X 酶复合物的转换所产生的大量凝血酶的生理学重要性。APTT 可评估人工体外刺激物引发的凝血启动阶段，当因子 Ⅷ 或 Ⅸ 严重缺乏时，APTT 会延长，但血友病患者在扩增阶段凝血酶生成受损更严重，而 APTT 无法评估这一过程。

启动阶段产生的凝血酶是一种强效的血小板激活

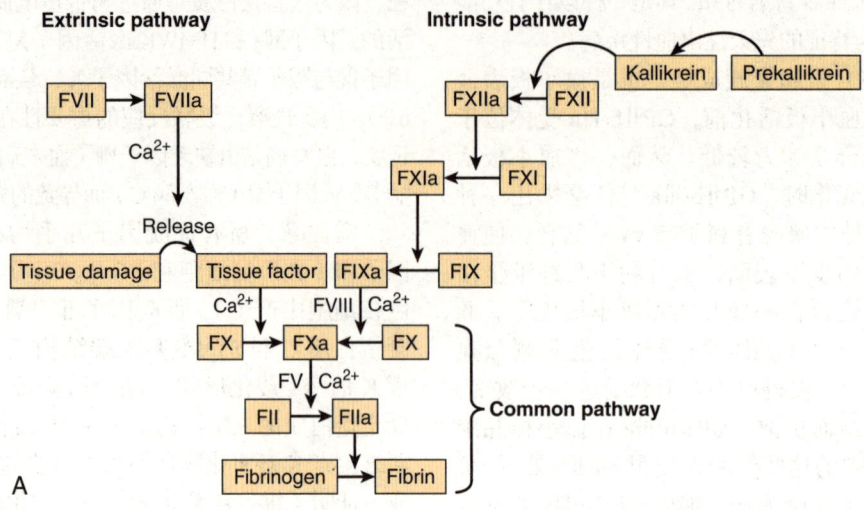

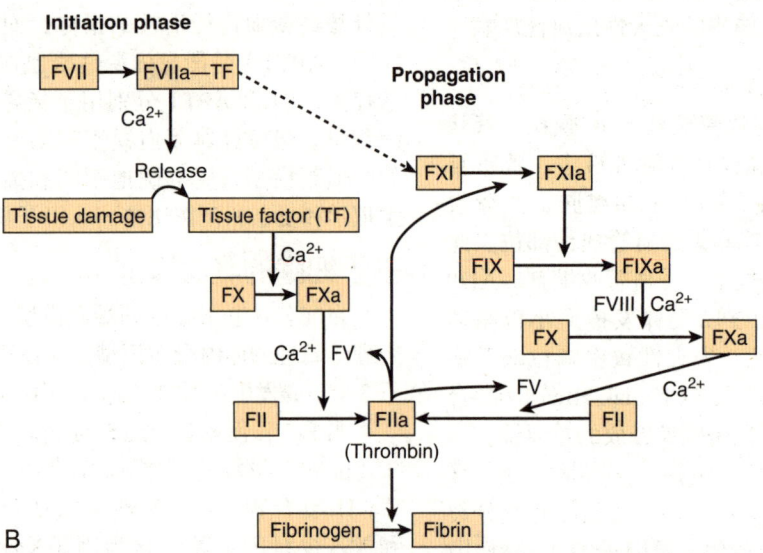

Fig. 6.2 (A) The classic view of the coagulation cascade. The laboratory-defined *extrinsic* and *intrinsic* pathways allow monitoring of anticoagulation by serial measurements of the prothrombin time (PT) and partial thromboplastin time (PTT), respectively. The PT primarily monitors factor VII activity, whereas the PTT is the best measure of XI and the hemophilic factors IX and VIII; both assays will detect deficiency of the common pathway factors (X, V, and II). (B) In the more modern view of the coagulation cascade, initiation of clotting begins with exposure to tissue factor (TF), which combines with small amounts of circulating factor (F) VIIa to form the extrinsic tenase (Xase) complex and generate FXa. FXa forms the prothrombinase complex with FVa and FII, generating small amounts of thrombin (FIIa), which begins to cleave fibrinogen into weak fibrin monomers in the initiation phase of coagulation. Thrombin's ability to activate factors, especially on the activated platelet surface, is responsible for propagation of the coagulant response. Thrombin generates FXIa, which in turn activates FIX; the TF-VIIa complex (before it is shut down by TFPI) also generates FIXa. Thrombin-activated FVIIIa then combines with IXa to form the intrinsic Xase complex, generating large amounts of FXa and prothrombinase complex on the platelet surface to further amplify thrombin generation. The large amounts of thrombin now generate enough fibrin monomers to form stable polymers and fibrin clot. *HMWK,* High-molecular-weight kininogen; *PK,* prekallikrein; *TFPI,* tissue factor pathway inhibitor.

factor X, increasing the kinetic efficiency of the intrinsic Xase complex. The activated platelet (Table 6.2) also enhances coagulation by supplying the developing clot with an activated platelet surface membrane (i.e., anionic lipids, primarily phosphatidylserine) and abundant factor V, stored in platelet granules. Factor V is then promptly activated to Va by the trace amount of thrombin produced by TF-VIIa complex. In combination with membrane phospholipids and calcium, activated Xa and its cofactor Va form the prothrombinase complex, which cleaves prothrombin to thrombin. The prothrombinase complex is several hundred thousand times more efficient at converting prothrombin to thrombin than free factor Xa acting on prothrombin alone. The role of the procoagulant effects of activated platelets on thrombosis is

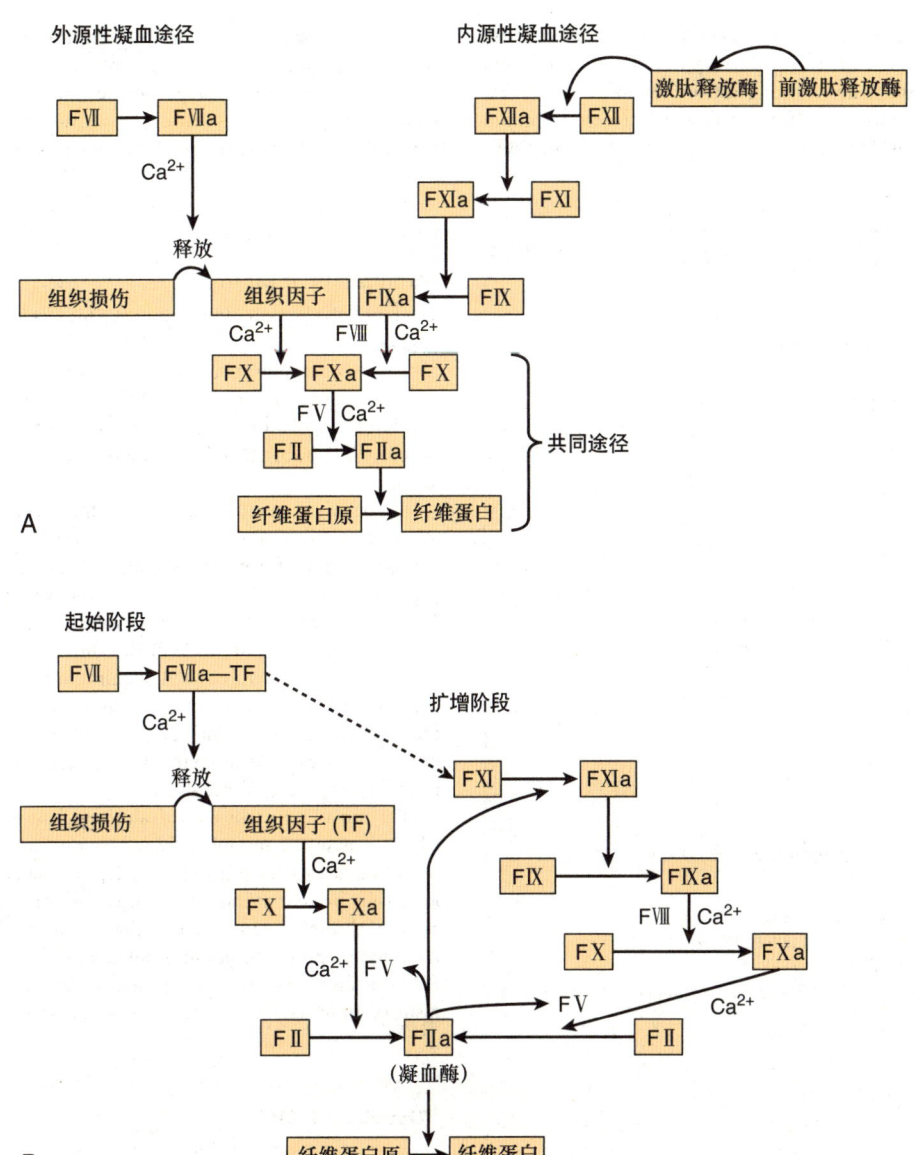

图6.2 **A**. 经典凝血级联模型。可通过分别连续检测实验室指标凝血酶原时间（PT）和活化部分凝血活酶时间（APTT）来监测外源性和内源性凝血途径。PT主要监测因子Ⅶ活性，而APTT是因子Ⅺ和血友病因子Ⅸ和Ⅷ的最佳监测指标；两种检测方法均可检出共同途径因子（Ⅹ、Ⅴ和Ⅱ）缺乏。**B**. 在新凝血级联模型中，凝血的启动阶段始于暴露于组织因子（TF），TF与少量循环因子（F）Ⅶa结合形成外源性Ⅹ酶复合物并生成FⅩa。FⅩa与FⅤa和FⅡ形成凝血酶原酶复合物，生成少量凝血酶（FⅡa），在凝血的起始阶段开始将纤维蛋白原裂解为弱纤维蛋白单体。凝血酶能够激活因子，尤其是激活血小板表面的因子，从而引起凝血反应的扩增。凝血酶可生成FⅪa，进而激活FⅨ；TF-Ⅶa复合物（在受TFPI限制前）也可生成FⅨa。凝血酶激活的FⅧa与Ⅸa结合形成内源性Ⅹ酶复合物，在血小板表面生成大量FⅩa和凝血酶原酶复合物，进一步增强凝血酶生成。大量的凝血酶生成足够的纤维蛋白单体，从而形成稳定的聚合物和纤维蛋白凝块。TFPI，组织因子途径抑制物

剂。活化的血小板表达因子Ⅷa和Ⅸa的受体，这些活性蛋白酶与膜磷脂酰丝氨酸的结合增强了酶底物与因子Ⅹ的结合，从而提高内源性Ⅹ酶复合物的动力学效率。活化的血小板（表6.2）还能为正在形成的血凝块提供活化的血小板表面膜（即阴离子脂质，主要是磷脂酰丝氨酸）和储存在血小板颗粒中丰富的因子Ⅴ，从而增强凝血功能。因子Ⅴ随后被TF-Ⅶa复合物产生的微量凝血酶迅速活化为因子Ⅴa。活化的因子Ⅹa及其辅因子Ⅴa与磷脂膜和钙结合，形成凝血酶原酶复合物，其可将凝血酶原裂解为凝血酶。凝血酶原酶复合物将凝血酶原转化为凝血酶的效率比游离因子Ⅹa单独作用于凝血酶原高出数10万倍。斯科特综合征（Scott

highlighted by Scott syndrome, a condition in which the platelet phospholipid membrane does not change in response to activation, and thus phosphatidylserine is not rearranged from the inner membrane surface to the outer membrane surface, leading to decreased thrombin generation and prolonged bleeding as a result of platelet dysfunction.

TABLE 6.2 Procoagulant Properties of Platelets

Receptor-Ligand Interactions Promoting Adhesion
[a]GPIb-IX-V-VWF
[b]GPIIb/IIIa-fibrinogen and GPIIb/IIIa-VWF
[c]GPIa/IIa-collagen
[d]P-selectin–P-selectin glycoprotein ligand-1

Receptor-Ligand Interactions Mediating Activation
GPV-thrombin
GPVI-collagen

Secreted Alpha-Granule Proteins
Ligands (fibrinogen, fibronectin, thrombospondin, vitronectin, von Willebrand factor)
Enzymes (α_2-antiplasmin; factors V, VIII, and XI)
Antiheparin (platelet factor 4)

Secreted Dense-Granule Agonists
Adenosine diphosphate, serotonin

Components and Functions of Platelets That Promote Coagulation
Thromboxane A_2 formation, phosphatidylserine expression

GP, Glycoprotein.
[a]GPIb-IX-V complex is also known as CD42.
[b]GPIIb/IIIa (integrin $\alpha_{IIb}\beta_3$) complex is also known as CD41.
[c]GPIIa is also known as CD29.
[d]P-selectin is also known as CD62P and P-selectin glycoprotein ligand-1 as CD162.

Of note, polyphosphate has been shown to have a critical role in coagulation and acts as a procoagulant, initiating clotting through several mechanisms. First, polyphosphate contains numerous negatively anionic charged surfaces leading to activation of plasma factor XII, HMWK, and PK that set off the intrinsic pathway. Polyphosphate also mitigates the inhibitory effects of TFPI, enhances the activation of factor V and factor IX, and leads to thickened fibrin fibrils by increasing fibrin polymerization.

Termination of Clotting

The rapid production of thrombin at a localized site of vascular injury could quickly lead to extensive clotting if left unchecked; thus, there are several mechanisms in place to ensure proper modulation. This includes endogenous inhibitors of the coagulation pathway (Fig. 6.3) that limit coagulation initiation, dilution of procoagulants at the site of injury by flowing blood, and removal and inactivation of activated factors.

Endogenous anticoagulants can either prevent thrombin generation or inactivate formed thrombin. Among endogenous anticoagulants that target thrombin generation, the earliest in the coagulation process is TFPI. TFPI acts by both inactivating factor Xa and the TF-VIIa complex. TFPI is constitutively released by ECs into the microvasculature. Nascent TFPI has direct activity only against Xa, but after exposure to Xa, TFPI acquires activity against the TF-VIIa complex. Notably, C1 esterase inhibitor also inhibits factors early in the coagulation cascade, including factor XIIa and PK, although a deficiency of C1 esterase inhibitor, which causes angioedema, does not result in a hypercoagulable state.

The most important natural anticoagulant is antithrombin (AT), which inactivates several activated factors in the clotting cascade including factors IIa (thrombin), IXa, Xa, XIa and XIIa. AT is physiologically present at more than twice the concentration of the highest local thrombin concentration that can be reached during clotting. AT activity against thrombin is potentiated 1000-fold by endogenous EC-associated heparin sulfate proteoglycans. This is also the mechanism of anticoagulation employed by the anticoagulant medications

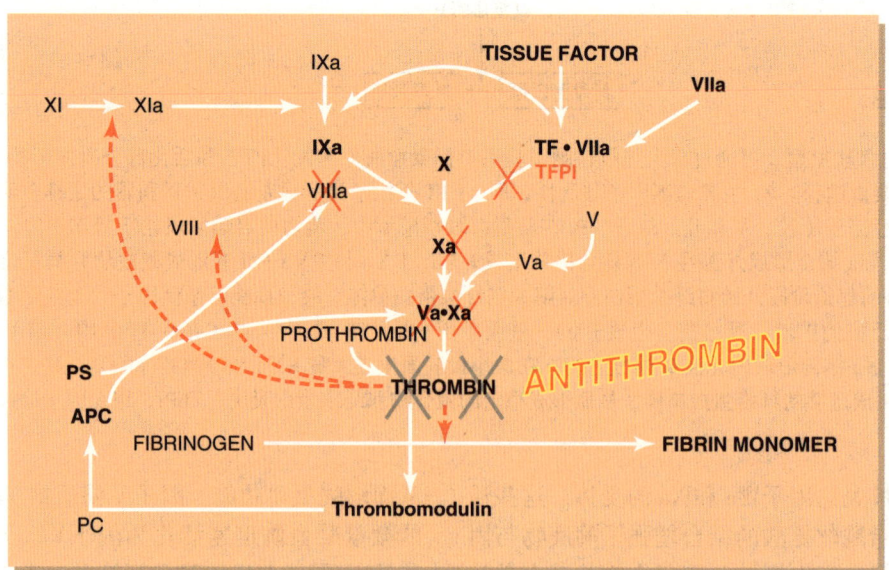

Fig. 6.3 Endogenous anticoagulant pathways. Tissue factor pathway inhibitor (TFPI) shuts off tissue factor (TF) stimulation and blocks the TF-VIIa-X complex; in addition, the clotting cascade is further downregulated by the natural anticoagulants. This inhibition is partly generated by thrombin, which activates thrombomodulin. Circulating antithrombin inhibits thrombin activity and Xa generation of thrombin. The complex of thrombin and thrombomodulin activates protein C (PC) to become activated protein C (APC), which combines with protein S (PS) to cleave and inactivate VIIIa and Va, further blocking thrombin generation.

综合征）凸显了活化血小板的促凝作用在血栓形成中的重要性，该综合征患者的血小板磷脂膜在活化后不会发生变化，使磷脂酰丝氨酸不能从内膜表面重新排列到外膜表面，引起血小板功能障碍，从而导致凝血酶生成减少和出血时间延长。

多磷酸盐已被证明是一种在凝血过程中发挥关键作用的促凝剂，可通过多种机制启动凝血过程。多磷酸盐含有大量带负电荷的表面，可激活血浆中的因子XII、HMWK 和 PK，从而启动内源性凝血途径。多磷酸盐还能减弱 TFPI 的抑制作用，增强因子 V 和因子 IX 的活化，并通过增加纤维蛋白的聚合作用使纤维蛋白的纤维增厚。

凝血终止

血管损伤局部可快速产生凝血酶，如果不加以控制，很快会导致大面积凝血；因此，多种机制可确保适当调节，包括凝血途径中限制凝血启动的内源性抗凝剂（图 6.3）、损伤部位的血液流动稀释促凝剂，以及清除和灭活活化因子。

内源性抗凝剂既可阻止凝血酶生成，也可使形成的凝血酶失活。在针对凝血酶生成的内源性抗凝剂中，TFPI 在凝血过程中最早起作用。TFPI 通过灭活因子 Xa 和 TF-VIIa 复合物而发挥作用。TFPI 由 EC 持续释放到微血管中。新生成的 TFPI 仅直接作用于因子 Xa，但暴露于因子 Xa 后，TFPI 即可获得对抗 TF-VIIa 复合物的能力。值得注意的是，C1 酯酶抑制剂也能抑制凝血级联早期的因子，包括因子 XIIa 和 PK，虽然 C1 酯酶抑制剂缺乏会导致血管性水肿，但不会导致高凝状态。

最重要的天然抗凝剂是抗凝血酶（AT），它可灭活凝血级联中的多种活化因子，包括因子 IIa（凝血酶）、IXa、Xa、XIa 和 XIIa。在凝血过程中，AT 的生理浓度可达到局部凝血酶最高浓度的 2 倍以上。内源性 EC 相关硫酸乙酰肝素蛋白聚糖可使 AT 对抗凝血酶的活性增强 1000 倍，这也是抗凝药物肝素、低分子量肝素、磺达肝素的抗凝机制。血小板表面膜和血小板因子 4 可保护凝血酶免于在血凝块处失活。然而，任何逃逸到

表 6.2 血小板的促凝特性

受体-配体相互作用促进黏附
[a]GP Ib-IX-V-vWF
[b]GP IIb/IIIa- 纤维蛋白原和 GP IIb/IIIa-vWF
[c]GP Ia/IIa- 胶原蛋白
[d]P 选择素 -P 选择素糖蛋白配体 1

受体-配体相互作用介导激活
GPV- 凝血酶
GPVI- 胶原蛋白

α 颗粒分泌的蛋白质
配体（纤维蛋白原、纤维连接蛋白、血小板应答蛋白、玻连蛋白、vWF）
酶（α_2-纤溶酶抑制物；因子 V、VIII 和 XI）
抗肝素（血小板因子 4）

致密颗粒分泌的激动剂
二磷酸腺苷、血清素

血小板的促凝成分和功能
血栓素 A_2 形成、磷脂酰丝氨酸表达

GP，糖蛋白。
[a] GP Ib-IX-V 复合物又称 CD42。
[b] GP IIb/IIIa（整合素 $\alpha_{IIb}\beta_3$）又称 CD41。
[c] GP IIa 又称 CD29。
[d] P 选择素又称 CD62P，P 选择素糖蛋白配体 1 又称 CD162。

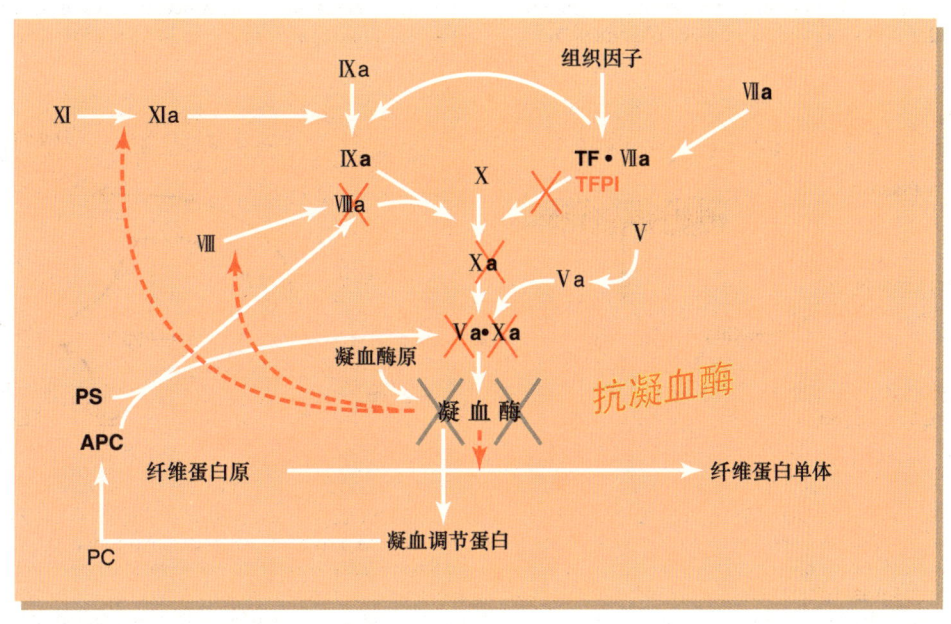

图 6.3 内源性抗凝途径。组织因子途径抑制物（TFPI）可关闭组织因子（TF）刺激并阻断 TF-VIIa-X 复合物；此外，天然抗凝剂可进一步下调凝血级联。这种抑制作用部分由激活凝血调节蛋白的凝血酶产生。循环抗凝血酶可抑制凝血酶活性和凝血酶生成因子 Xa。凝血酶和凝血调节蛋白的复合物可激活蛋白 C（PC）成为活化蛋白 C（APC），后者与蛋白 S（PS）结合，裂解并灭活因子 VIIIa 和 Va，进一步阻断凝血酶生成

heparin, low-molecular-weight heparin, and fondaparinux. Platelet surface membranes and platelet factor 4 protect thrombin from inactivation at the clot. However, any thrombin that escapes into the circulation is immediately inhibited by AT, and free thrombin is neutralized instantaneously. Therefore, early thrombin generation is critically dependent on protection by the activated platelet membrane to allow sufficient time to make the transition from initiation to propagation phase. Notably, during the initiation phase, platelet-bound factor Xa is protected from inactivation by both TFPI and AT.

Activated protein C (APC) has anticoagulant, anti-inflammatory, and profibrinolytic properties that make it an important regulator of both thrombosis and inflammation. Like TFPI, protein C becomes activated only after coagulation is underway. Formed thrombin binds to thrombomodulin, a proteoglycan associated with endothelial and monocyte cell surfaces. Thrombomodulin-bound thrombin loses its procoagulant abilities such as activating platelets and fibrin clot formation and instead activates protein C. On the EC surface, nascent protein C binds to EC protein C receptor (EPCR), which positions it for activation by the adjacent thrombomodulin-bound thrombin. In a reaction that is enhanced by EPCR and protein S, APC inactivates factors VIIIa and Va (components of the Xase and prothrombinase complexes, respectively), thereby limiting procoagulant self-amplification. Notably, a common mutation in factor V known as factor V Leiden results in the arginine at position 506 being replaced by glutamine, rendering the mutated factor V resistant to cleavage by APC and resulting in a hypercoagulable state. As with other coagulation factors, the activated platelet membrane protects VIIIa and Va from APC inactivation. In addition to its effects on thrombin generation, APC neutralizes plasminogen activator inhibitor-1 (PAI-1, described further in the fibrinolysis section) to enhance clot remodeling. APC has anti-inflammatory properties as well; recombinant APC reduces production of tumor necrosis factor-α after endotoxin challenge, and protein C–deficient mice exhibit higher levels of proinflammatory cytokines.

Several other molecules have been identified as contributing to antithrombotic effects. As discussed previously, prostacyclin and nitric oxide, both released from ECs, exert antithrombotic properties through vasodilation and inhibition of platelet aggregation and adhesion. Poly(adenosine 5′-diphosphate [ADP]-ribose) polymerase (PARP) protein regulates TF mRNA levels. Activated macrophages and monocytes express TF on their surfaces, and modulating TF mRNA may prevent some degree of thrombosis in the setting of inflammation. Thrombospondin 5 (also known as cartilage oligomeric matrix protein), an extracellular matrix protein, has been shown to inhibit thrombin and thrombin-dependent platelet aggregation in mouse models.

Fibrin Clot Architecture

The architecture of the fibrin clot is surprisingly variable. Although genetic factors unquestionably play a role in determining clot structure, two dominant factors are the local concentrations of thrombin and fibrinogen, whose reactions yield the fibrin strands. A thrombin-rich microenvironment typically results in thinner, more tightly cross-linked fibers, making the overall fibrin clot virtually impermeable to lytic enzymes. In thrombin-poor locations, the fibrin strands are thicker and the structure more porous, making the clot vulnerable to thrombolysis. Similarly, high fibrinogen concentrations are associated with larger thrombi whose tight, rigid meshwork makes them less deformable and more resistant to lysis. Low fibrinogen concentrations produce a less compact clot that is highly lysis prone. As mentioned previously, one of the major roles of polyphosphate on thrombosis is contributing to thicker fibrin fibrils.

Factor XIII plays a critical role in stabilization of the forming clot. Factor XIII circulates in the plasma and is also stored within platelets (see Fig. 6.1B). Notably, 50% of the total fibrin-stabilizing activity in blood resides in the platelet and is released by activation. Thrombin-activated factor XIIIa binds to fibrin and cross-links the fibrin units, thereby rendering them less permeable and more resistant to lysis. Furthermore, factor XIIIa cross-links the major plasmin inhibitor, α_2-antiplasmin, directly to fibrin, positioning it for neutralization of any invading plasmin.

Fibrinolysis

The fibrinolytic system (Fig. 6.4) operates to restore patency and prevent fibrin from occluding healthy vessels. During clot formation, factor Xa and thrombin stimulate healthy ECs to release tissue-type plasminogen activator (t-PA) and urokinase-type plasminogen activator (u-PA), both of which activate plasminogen to plasmin. Plasmin then cleaves the fibrin strands of the platelet plug, producing fibrin degradation products, including D-dimer. Additionally, factor XIIIa is also cleaved by plasmin, further destabilizes the platelet plug by reducing fibrin cross-linking.

The vast excess of plasminogen in the plasma dictates that under normal circumstances, the concentrations of t-PA and u-PA comprise the rate-limiting step for plasmin formation. The kinetic efficiency of

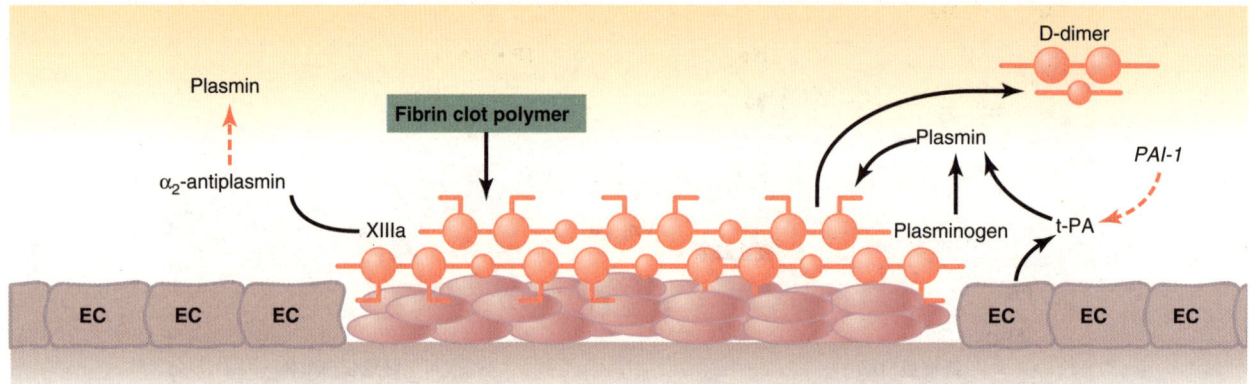

Fig. 6.4 Balanced fibrinolysis limits the platelet-fibrin clot. The platelet plug and fibrin matrices are strengthened by incorporation of factor XIIIa into the fibrin clot. Factor XIIIa also binds α_2-antiplasmin to the clot to protect it from plasmin-mediated fibrinolysis. At the same time, nearby intact endothelial cells (ECs) secrete tissue plasminogen activator (t-PA). t-PA that evades plasminogen activator inhibitor-1 (PAI-1) converts clot-bound plasminogen to plasmin and leads to fibrin clot degradation and release of soluble fibrin peptides and D-dimer. Therefore, detection of circulating D-dimer usually indicates active fibrinolysis.

循环中的凝血酶都会立即被 AT 抑制，而游离凝血酶则会立即被中和。因此，早期凝血酶生成主要依赖于活化血小板膜的保护，以便有足够的时间从启动阶段过渡到扩增阶段。在启动阶段，血小板结合因子 Xa 可以保护其免于 TFPI 和 AT 导致的失活。

活化蛋白 C（APC）具有抗凝、抗炎和促纤维蛋白溶解特性，是血栓形成和炎症的重要调节因子。与 TFPI 相同，蛋白 C 仅在凝血过程开始后才会被激活。形成的凝血酶与凝血调节蛋白结合，后者是一种与 EC 和单核细胞表面相关的蛋白聚糖，结合后的凝血酶失去其促凝能力，如激活血小板和纤维蛋白凝块形成，转而激活蛋白 C。在 EC 表面，新生成的蛋白 C 与 EC 蛋白 C 受体（EPCR）结合，使其被周围与凝血调节蛋白结合的凝血酶激活。在 EPCR 和蛋白 S 的帮助下，APC 可灭活因子 VIIIa 和 Va（分别是 X 因子酶复合物和凝血酶原酶复合物的成分），从而限制了促凝成分的自我扩增。需要注意的是，一种常见的因子 V 突变（即因子 V 莱登突变）可导致 506 位点的精氨酸被谷氨酰胺取代，使突变的因子 V 无法被 APC 裂解，从而导致高凝状态。与其他凝血因子一样，活化的血小板膜可保护 VIIIa 和 Va 免受 APC 的破坏。除了对凝血酶生成的影响外，APC 还可中和纤溶酶原激活物抑制物 -1（PAI-1；见下文"纤维蛋白溶解"）以增强血凝块重塑。APC 还具有抗炎特性，重组 APC 可减少内毒素刺激后肿瘤坏死因子 α 的产生，而缺乏蛋白 C 的小鼠表现出更高水平的促炎细胞因子。

其他几种分子也被认为具有抗血栓作用。如前所述，前列环素和一氧化氮均由 EC 释放，通过血管扩张、抑制血小板聚集和黏附来发挥抗血栓特性。多腺苷二磷酸核糖聚合酶（PARP）蛋白可调节 TF mRNA 的水平。活化的巨噬细胞和单核细胞在其表面表达 TF，在炎症情况下，调节 TF mRNA 可在一定程度上预防血栓形成。血小板应答蛋白 5（又称软骨寡聚基质蛋白）是一种细胞外基质蛋白，其在小鼠模型中已被证明可抑制凝血酶和凝血酶依赖的血小板聚集。

纤维蛋白凝块结构

纤维蛋白凝块的结构高度可变。虽然遗传因素在决定凝块结构方面明确发挥作用，但凝血酶和纤维蛋白原的局部浓度也是主要因素，它们发生反应而产生纤维蛋白链。在富含凝血酶的微环境中，通常会产生薄而紧密的交联纤维，使整个纤维蛋白凝块几乎无法被水解酶渗透。在凝血酶缺乏的部位，纤维蛋白链更厚，具有多孔结构，使血凝块更易被溶解。同样，高浓度纤维蛋白原与较大的血栓有关，血栓致密的网状结构使其不易变形，更耐溶解。低浓度纤维蛋白原产生的血凝块较疏松，极易被水解酶溶解。如前所述，多磷酸盐在血栓形成中的主要作用之一是增加纤维蛋白纤维的厚度。

因子 XIII 在稳定已形成的血凝块方面发挥关键作用。因子 XIII 在血浆中循环，也有部分储存在血小板中（图 6.1B）。需注意，血液中 50% 具有稳定活性的纤维蛋白存在于血小板中，并在激活后释放出来。凝血酶激活的因子 XIIIa 与纤维蛋白结合形成交联单位，使其渗透性降低，抗裂解能力增强。此外，因子 XIIIa 还能与主要的纤溶酶抑制剂 α2- 纤溶酶抑制物交联，直接作用并定位于纤维蛋白，使所有入侵的纤溶酶失活。

纤维蛋白溶解

纤维蛋白溶解系统（图 6.4）的作用是恢复血管通畅，防止纤维蛋白堵塞健康血管。在血栓形成过程中，因子 Xa 和凝血酶可刺激健康 EC 释放组织型纤溶酶原激活物（t-PA）和尿激酶型纤溶酶原激活物（u-PA），这两种物质都能将纤溶酶原激活为纤溶酶。纤溶酶随后裂解血小板栓子的纤维蛋白链，产生纤维蛋白降解产物，包括 D- 二聚体。此外，纤溶酶还可裂解因子 XIIIa，通过减少纤维蛋白交联进一步破坏血小板栓子的稳定性。

血浆中大量的纤溶酶原决定了在正常情况下 t-PA 和 u-PA 的浓度是纤溶酶形成的限速步骤。在纤维蛋白存在的

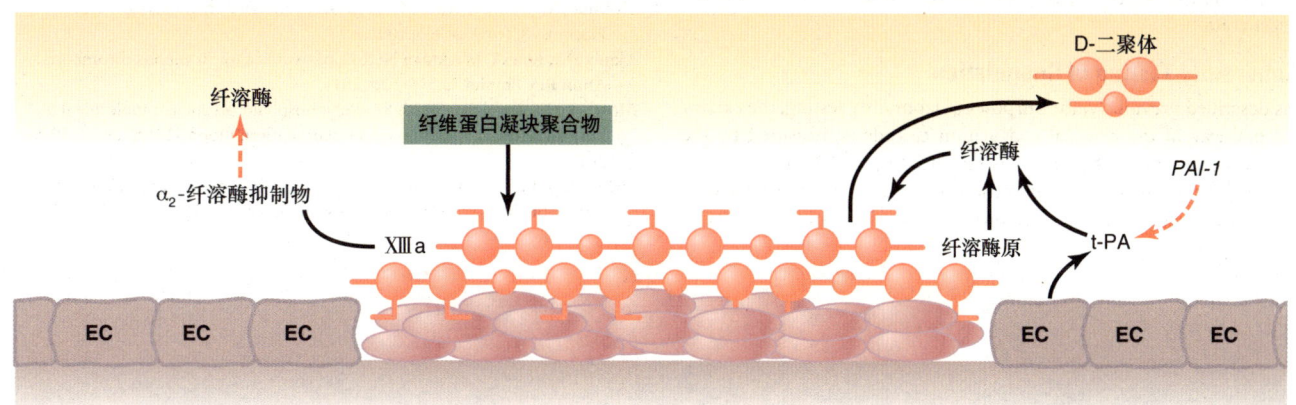

图 6.4 平衡的纤维蛋白溶解限制血小板-纤维蛋白凝块。血小板栓子和纤维蛋白基质通过因子 XIIIa 与纤维蛋白凝块的结合而得到加强。因子 XIIIa 使 α2- 纤溶酶抑制物与血凝块结合，以保护其不受纤溶酶介导的纤维蛋白溶解。同时，附近完整的内皮细胞（EC）分泌组织型溶酶原激活物（t-PA）。t-PA 可避开纤溶酶原激活物抑制物 -1（PAI-1），将凝块结合的纤溶酶原转化为纤溶酶，导致纤维蛋白凝块降解，并释放可溶性纤维蛋白肽和 D- 二聚体。因此，检测到循环中的 D- 二聚体通常表明纤维蛋白溶解活跃

t-PA is improved by at least an order of magnitude in the presence of fibrin. This helps to keep t-PA most active in the microenvironment of the clot. By contrast, u-PA appears to require binding to activated platelets for its ability to liberate plasmin.

Acting to contain fibrinolysis are plasma mediators that either inactivate formed plasmin (e.g., α_2-antiplasmin and possibly α_2-macroglobulin) or block plasmin formation (e.g., PAI-1). α_2-Antiplasmin rapidly inactivates plasmin in plasma but is present in lower concentrations than plasminogen and thus can become depleted while plasmin continues to be formed. Additionally, the α_2-antiplasmin protein cross-links to the fibrin clot providing resistance to cleavage by plasmin. PAI-1 is present in several-fold molar excess in the plasma and is also released by both ECs and activated platelets, thereby protecting clots from premature lysis. Plasma levels of PAI-1 are highly variable due to a circadian pattern of secretion; polymorphisms of the *PAI-1* gene leading to higher PAI-1 levels are associated with a higher risk for thromboembolic disease, whereas rare congenital deficiencies in PAI-1 protein are associated with increased bleeding tendencies.

Another mediator that limits fibrinolysis in the vicinity of the clot is thrombin activator fibrinolysis inhibitor (TAFI). TAFI is synthesized in an inactive form by the liver and circulates in the plasma, possibly in a complex with plasminogen. TAFI cleaves specific fibrin lysine residues that would otherwise promote binding of fibrinolytic enzymes (e.g., plasmin). TAFI requires either plasmin or thrombin for activation; however, thrombin activation of TAFI requires extraordinarily large amounts of free thrombin. By contrast, EC-associated thrombomodulin increases thrombin-induced TAFI activation 1250-fold, making this an essential cofactor and one that is predominantly available only at the interface between the blood and the vessel wall.

In addition to the EC surface, macrophages are also critical to fibrinolysis. Macrophages degrade the fibrin clot through lysosomal proteolysis by a plasmin-independent mechanism. The macrophage binds to fibrin and fibrinogen through its surface integrin receptor, CD11b/18; this binding is followed by internalization of the complex into the lysosome, where fibrin and fibrinogen are degraded.

Tissue repair and regeneration are the physiologic end points of clotting, and they eventually lead to dissolution of the fibrin-based clot. Besides t-PA and u-PA, the intrinsic pathway activators kallikrein, factor XIIa, and factor XIa also generate active plasmin from plasminogen. Plasminogen binding to cell surface receptors promotes its own activation to plasmin by placing it in proximity to t-PA and the fibrin clot and protects plasmin from inactivation by circulating α_2-antiplasmin. Plasmin eventually dissolves the fibrin matrix to produce soluble fibrin peptides and D-dimer and also activates metalloproteinases that further degrade damaged tissue. Fibroblasts and leukocytes migrate into the wound, the latter mediated by selectin binding, and these inflammatory cells act in concert with growth factors secreted by leukocytes and activated platelets to enhance vascular repair and tissue regeneration.

Laboratory Testing of Coagulation

As described previously, for purposes of laboratory testing, the extrinsic pathway of the classical coagulation cascade is measured by the PT, while the intrinsic pathway is measured by the aPTT. The PT is assessed by measuring the interaction of circulating factor VIIa with exogenously added TF (also known as thromboplastin). The PT is highly sensitive to deficiencies in factors II, V, VII, and X, all of which may be associated with bleeding, but is unaffected by deficiencies in intrinsic pathway factors (i.e., factors XII, XI, IX, or VIII).

Because factors II, VII, and X are also vitamin K–dependent factors, with factor VII having the shortest half-life, the PT is also the main lab test used for monitoring warfarin therapy. The degree of prolongation of the PT by warfarin depends on the strength of the particular thromboplastin agent and the specific coagulation instrument used for the assay. A blood test known as the international normalized ratio (INR), calculated by dividing the patient's PT by a mean control PT, takes these factors into account in order to standardize variations among laboratories in PT measurements and is the preferred test for warfarin monitoring.

The aPTT measurement is based on in vitro contact activation (e.g., plasma stimulation with a negatively charged compound such as kaolin). The aPTT is sensitive to deficiencies of factors in the contact (i.e., PK, HMWK, and factor XII), intrinsic (factors XI, IX, and X), and common (factors II, V, and X) pathways but not in the extrinsic pathway (factor VII). As detailed previously, deficiencies of factors VIII, IX, or XI comprise the basis of the congenital hemophilias A, B, and C, respectively, all of which are characterized by bleeding. By contrast, deficiencies of PK, HMWK, and factor XII, while all prolonging the aPTT, do not result in significant bleeding.

The aPTT is also highly sensitive to unfractionated heparin and is used to monitor heparin activity although the therapeutic index of the aPTT in patients on heparin is rather wide owing to natural fluctuations in aPTT measurements. Alternatively, heparin, low-molecular-weight heparin, and fondaparinux activity may be measured via an anti-Xa activity, which assesses the level of inhibition of factor Xa.

In surgical settings, trauma units, and intensive care units, there may be a need for immediate turnaround in coagulation testing. One specific point-of-care test used for real-time coagulation testing is thromboelastography (TEG), a global test of hemostasis. TEG uses whole blood to monitor all components of hemostasis, including the initiation and termination phases of the coagulation cascade, fibrinolysis, and platelet function. TEG has been demonstrated to improve outcomes in trauma by guiding transfusion therapy and may have roles in surgery and in assessing coagulation status in patients with advanced liver disease, although its utility outside of these indications is uncertain.

SUGGESTED READINGS

Büller HR, Bethune C, Bhanot S, et al: Factor XI antisense oligonucleotide for prevention of venous thrombosis, N Engl J Med 372(3):232–240, 2015.

Esmon CT: The protein c pathway, Chest 124(26s), 2003.

Ho K, Pavey W: Applying the cell-based coagulation model in the management of critical bleeding, Anaesth Intensive Care 45(2):166–176, 2017.

Hoffman M, Monroe 3rd DM: A cell-based model of hemostasis, Thromb Haemost 85(6):958–965, 2001.

Manly DA, Boles J, Mackman N: Role of tissue factor in venous thrombosis, Annu Rev Physiol 73:515–525, 2011.

Morrissey JH, Choi SH, Smith SA: Polyphosphate: an ancient molecule that links platelets, coagulation, and inflammation, Blood 119(25):5972–5979, 2012.

Shen J, Sampietro S, Wu J, et al: Coordination of platelet agonist signaling during the hemostatic response in vivo, Blood Adv 1(27):2767–2775, 2017.

情况下，t-PA 的动力学效率至少会提高一个数量级。这有助于使 t-PA 在血凝块的微环境中保持最活跃的状态。相比之下，u-PA 似乎需要与活化的血小板结合才能释放纤溶酶。

血浆调节物质可通过使已形成的纤溶酶（如 α_2-纤溶酶抑制物，可能还有 α_2-巨球蛋白）失活或阻止纤溶酶的形成（如 PAI-1）来抑制纤维蛋白溶解。α_2-纤溶酶抑制物能迅速使血浆中的纤溶酶失活，但其浓度低于纤溶酶原，因此在纤溶酶连续形成的同时，α_2-纤溶酶抑制物也会被耗尽。此外，α_2-纤溶酶抑制物蛋白可与纤维蛋白凝块交联，从而抵抗纤溶酶的裂解。PAI-1 在血浆中以数倍于 t-PA 的摩尔浓度存在，且同样由 EC 和活化的血小板释放，从而防止凝块过早溶解。由于 PAI-1 的分泌具有昼夜节律，因此其血浆水平变化很大；*PAI-1* 基因多态性可导致 PAI-1 水平较高，与血栓栓塞性疾病风险升高相关，而罕见的先天性 PAI-1 蛋白缺乏症与出血倾向增加有关。

另一种限制血凝块附近纤维蛋白溶解的调节物质是凝血酶活化纤维蛋白溶解抑制物（TAFI）。TAFI 在肝内合成其未激活形式，并在血浆中循环，可能与纤溶酶原形成复合体。TAFI 可裂解特定的纤维蛋白赖氨酸残基，否则这些残基会促进纤维蛋白与纤维蛋白溶解酶（如纤溶酶）的结合。TAFI 需要纤溶酶或凝血酶来激活；然而，通过凝血酶直接激活 TAFI 需要大量的游离凝血酶。相比之下，EC 相关的凝血调节蛋白可使凝血酶介导的 TAFI 活化增强 1250 倍，这使得凝血调节蛋白成为一种重要的辅因子，且其主要存在于血管壁与血流的交界处。

除了 EC 表面，巨噬细胞在纤维蛋白溶解中也具有重要作用。巨噬细胞通过非纤溶酶依赖的机制经由溶酶体蛋白水解酶来降解纤维蛋白凝块。巨噬细胞通过其表面的整合素受体 CD11b/CD18 与纤维蛋白和纤维蛋白原结合，随后复合体内化进入溶酶体中，将纤维蛋白或纤维蛋白原降解。

组织修复和再生是凝血的生理终点，最终导致纤维蛋白凝块溶解。除了 t-PA 和 u-PA，内源性凝血途径激活因子（激肽释放酶、因子XIIa 和XIa）也能将纤溶酶原激活为纤溶酶。纤溶酶原与细胞表面受体结合后，可通过接近 t-PA 和纤维蛋白凝块来促进自身活化为纤溶酶，并保护纤溶酶不被循环中的 α_2-纤溶酶抑制物灭活。纤溶酶最终溶解纤维蛋白多聚体，产生可溶性纤维蛋白多肽和 D-二聚体；纤溶酶还可激活金属蛋白酶，进一步降解受损组织。成纤维细胞和白细胞可迁移到伤口处，后者由选择素结合诱导，这些炎症细胞与白细胞和活化血小板分泌的生长因子协同作用，加强血管修复和组织再生。

凝血的实验室检查

在实验室检查中，经典凝血级联的外源性凝血途径可通过 PT 来检测，而内源性凝血途径可通过 APTT 来检测。

PT 通过检测循环因子VIIa 与外源添加的 TF（又称凝血活酶）的相互作用来评估。PT 对缺乏因子 II、V、VII 和 X 高度敏感，这些因子均可能与出血有关，但不受内源性凝血途径因子（即因子XII、XI、IX 或VIII）缺乏的影响。

由于因子 II、VII 和 X 依赖于维生素 K，且因子 VII 的半衰期最短，因此 PT 也是用于监测华法林治疗的主要实验室检测指标。华法林延长 PT 的程度取决于特定凝血活酶试剂的性能和用于检测的专用凝血仪器。国际标准化比值（INR）由患者的 PT 值除以平均对照 PT 值计算得出，它将以上因素考虑在内，从而统一各实验室 PT 值的检测差异，是华法林治疗的首选监测方法。

APTT 的检测基于体外接触活化（如用高岭土等带负电荷的化合物刺激血浆）。APTT 对缺乏接触途径因子（即 PK、HMWK 和因子XII）、内源性凝血途径因子（因子XI、IX 和 X）和共同途径因子（因子 II、V 和 X）敏感，但对缺乏外源性凝血途径因子（因子VII）则不敏感。如前所述，因子VIII 或IX 的缺乏分别导致先天性血友病 A 或 B，这些疾病均以出血为特征。相比之下，PK、HMWK 和因子XII缺乏虽然也会延长 APTT，但不会导致严重出血。

APTT 对普通肝素高度敏感，可用于监测肝素活性，但由于 APTT 检测值的自然波动，使用肝素治疗的患者的 APTT 治疗指数相当宽泛。此外，可通过抗因子 Xa 活性来检测肝素、低分子量肝素和磺达肝素的活性，其活性可评估因子 Xa 的抑制水平。

在外科、创伤科和重症监护病房，可能需要立即进行凝血检测，以快速纠正凝血异常。血栓弹力图（TEG）是用于实时凝血检测的特异性即时诊断检测，是一种全面的止血检测方法。TEG 需使用全血监测止血的所有组成部分，包括凝血级联反应的启动和终止阶段、纤维蛋白溶解和血小板功能。研究表明，TEG 可通过指导输血治疗来改善创伤患者的预后，并可用于外科手术和评估晚期肝病患者的凝血状态，但其在这些适应证之外的用途尚不确定。

推荐阅读

Büller HR, Bethune C, Bhanot S, et al: Factor XI antisense oligonucleotide for prevention of venous thrombosis, N Engl J Med 372(3):232–240, 2015.

Esmon CT: The protein c pathway, Chest 124(26s), 2003.

Ho K, Pavey W: Applying the cell-based coagulation model in the management of critical bleeding, Anaesth Intensive Care 45(2):166–176, 2017.

Hoffman M, Monroe 3rd DM: A cell-based model of hemostasis, Thromb Haemost 85(6):958–965, 2001.

Manly DA, Boles J, Mackman N: Role of tissue factor in venous thrombosis, Annu Rev Physiol 73:515–525, 2011.

Morrissey JH, Choi SH, Smith SA: Polyphosphate: an ancient molecule that links platelets, coagulation, and inflammation, Blood 119(25):5972–5979, 2012.

Shen J, Sampietro S, Wu J, et al: Coordination of platelet agonist signaling during the hemostatic response in vivo, Blood Adv 1(27):2767–2775, 2017.

7

Disorders of Hemostasis: Bleeding

Aric Parnes

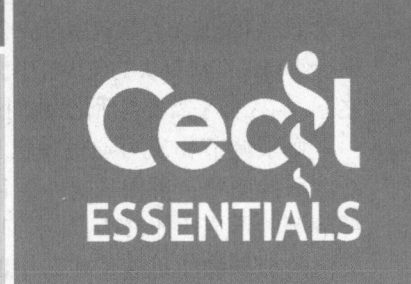

INTRODUCTION

The complex network maintaining a balance between bleeding and clotting functions in fine equilibrium. However, each component of this network can falter. This chapter describes the imbalances that result in bleeding. It covers platelet disorders, vascular abnormalities, and clotting factor deficiencies. In addition to reviewing the pathophysiology and clinical manifestations of these disorders, it covers a general approach to the evaluation of a bleeding patient and how to treat each disease. How the equilibrium shifts to favor coagulation is covered in a separate chapter.

HEMOSTASIS

Hemostasis, the ability to stop bleeding, can be simplified into two phases called primary and secondary hemostasis. However, the reality is more complex than this because primary and secondary hemostasis frequently interact and blend together. Primary hemostasis reflects an initial phase of platelet activation, adhesion, and aggregation with help from von Willebrand factor. Secondary hemostasis involves the coagulation factors activating in a cascade to augment and stabilize clotting. The clotting cascade is explained in more detail in Chapter 6. To initiate bleeding, the integrity of the endothelium is disrupted most commonly by trauma or surgery but sometimes through a vascular defect. Regardless of the inciting event, collagen and other platelet activators are released from endothelial tissue triggering primary hemostasis, whereas the release of tissue factor activates the clotting cascade.

CLINICAL EVALUATION OF BLEEDING

The evaluation of bleeding requires a careful history and physical examination. The history includes the details of the current bleeding event as well as past bleeding events. Spontaneous bleeding without a traumatic event points to a severe defect in hemostasis. Lifelong recurring bleeding events and a family history of such suggest congenital disease whereas new bleeding despite previous "hemostatic stress tests" such as surgery or dental extraction without bleeding favor an acquired disorder or a medication effect. Disorders of primary hemostasis including causes of thrombocytopenia or platelet dysfunction or diseases of von Willebrand factor lead to mucocutaneous superficial bleeding, but disorders of secondary hemostasis with missing coagulation factors cause deeper bleeding, for example muscle hematomas, hemarthroses, and intracranial hemorrhages. Superficial bleeding can be easy bruising, gum bleeding when brushing teeth, frequent epistaxis, and heavy menstrual bleeding. When uncovering family history, distinguishing between X-linked genetic disease (e.g., hemophilia A and B) and autosomal disease, such as most von Willebrand disease cases, can be vital. The X-linked inheritance pattern for hemophilia A and B means that more severe disease manifests in males than in females and subsequently may appear to skip generations.

Similar distinctions appear in the physical examination. Hemarthroses result in joint swelling, tenderness, and moderate warmth, and multiple joint hemorrhages cause arthritis and deformity. Without imaging or laboratory tests, hemarthrosis can be indistinguishable from septic arthritis or other causes of joint pain. Platelet disorders classically result in petechiae, small subcutaneous hemorrhages that typically appear on the legs, a result of gravity dependence. Sometimes vascular anomalies can be seen on physical examination. For example, small ectatic vessels, prone to bleeding, can be seen on oral mucosa in hereditary hemorrhagic telangiectasia.

Liver disease can cause bleeding through a decline in production of coagulation factors and a decline in platelet count, due to hypersplenism and decreased thrombopoietin production by the liver. Hallmark features of liver disease can be obvious on examination, such as jaundice and abdominal distension from ascites, but can be overlooked if not searched for. This includes spider angioma, gynecomastia, Dupuytren contracture, and asterixis.

Rare causes of aplastic anemia can be determined by physical examination. Fanconi anemia patients have short stature, café au lait spots, hypoplastic thenar eminences, and absent radii. Dyskeratosis congenita, a disease of short telomeres, leads to leukoplakia, nail dystrophy, and hyperpigmented macules.

Importantly, the timing of a thorough examination and subsequent laboratory testing must be tempered in order to control rapid bleeding and hemodynamic instability. Airway, breathing, and circulation, the A-B-C's, take precedence in emergency situations, and recognizing that bleeding can evolve quickly is critical. Life-threatening hemorrhage requires immediate treatment while simultaneously pursuing diagnostic testing. Life-threatening blood loss is not limited to trauma or gastrointestinal sites but also includes small bleeds near the airway or neck and hemorrhages around other vital organs. Heart rate and blood pressure are first steps in assessing volume of blood loss.

LABORATORY EVALUATION OF BLEEDING

The initial laboratory assessment of the bleeding patient (Table 7.1) should include complete blood cell counts (CBC), prothrombin time (PT), activated partial thromboplastin time (aPTT), and fibrinogen (Fig. 7.1). The CBC marks a critical first step in this evaluation because it includes the platelet count as well as hemoglobin and hematocrit, which are essential for monitoring the rate of blood loss (as are vital signs). The CBC also contains the mean corpuscular volume (MCV), measuring the size of the red blood cell. A low MCV can suggest a slower chronic blood loss resulting in iron deficiency. A peripheral blood smear should be examined to confirm thrombocytopenia. Pseudothrombocytopenia occurs when platelets clump from EDTA

止血障碍：出血

孙婷 译 张磊 杨仁池 审校 王建祥 通审

引言

出血和凝血之间存在着复杂的调控网络并维持着精细的平衡。然而，该复杂网络中的任何一个组成部分都有可能出现异常。本章将探讨导致出血的各种失衡，包括血小板疾病、血管异常和凝血因子缺陷。除了对这些出血性疾病的病理生理学和临床表现进行回顾之外，本章还涵盖了评估出血患者的一般方法及治疗。出凝血平衡如何向凝血方向转化将在第 8 章中阐述。

止血

止血过程可简化为两个阶段，即初级止血和次级止血。然而，实际情况更加复杂，因为初级止血和次级止血经常相互作用并相互融合。初级止血反映了血小板在血管性血友病因子（vWF）的帮助下活化、黏附和聚集的初始阶段。次级止血涉及凝血级联反应（见第 6 章）或凝血"瀑布"中的多种凝血因子，以加强和稳定已形成的血凝块。出血时，血管内皮的完整性被破坏，最常见的原因是创伤或手术，也可能是由于血管本身的缺陷。无论引发出血的原因是什么，胶原蛋白和其他血小板激活物质均可从内皮组织释放，触发初级止血，而组织因子（TF）的释放则激活凝血级联反应。

出血的临床评估

出血的评估需要详细的病史询问和体格检查。患者病史应包括对当前出血事件及既往出血事件的详细描述。无创伤事件的自发性出血常提示严重的止血缺陷。长期反复发作的出血事件并有相关家族史提示先天性疾病，而既往"止血压力试验"（如手术或拔牙）无出血的新发出血则提示获得性疾病或药物作用。初级止血障碍（包括血小板减少或功能障碍及 vWF 相关疾病所致的止血障碍）可导致皮肤黏膜浅表出血，表现为容易瘀伤、刷牙时牙龈出血、频繁鼻出血和月经量大等；凝血因子缺陷所致的次级止血障碍则可引起更深部位的出血，如肌肉血肿、关节出血和颅内出血。询问家族史对于鉴别 X 连锁遗传病（如血友病 A、血友病 B）和常染色体病（如大多数血管性血友病）至关重要。血友病 A 和血友病 B 的 X 连锁遗传特征导致男性比女性表现更严重，并可能出现隔代遗传的现象。

体格检查也有类似的鉴别意义。关节出血可导致关节肿胀、压痛和一定程度的发热，多个关节出血可导致关节炎症和畸形。但是，如果不进行影像学或实验室检查，则无法区分关节出血与化脓性关节炎或其他原因引起的关节疼痛。血小板疾病通常表现为瘀点，即皮下小出血点，由于重力原因常见于腿部。体格检查中有时可观察到血管异常，如在遗传性出血性毛细血管扩张症患者的口腔黏膜上可见易出血的扩张小血管。

肝病可引起脾功能亢进及肝合成的血小板生成素（TPO）减少，导致血小板计数下降和凝血因子合成减少，从而引起出血。肝病的特征性表现在体格检查时可能很明显，如黄疸和腹腔积液引起的腹部膨隆。有些表现可能被忽视，包括蜘蛛痣、男性乳房发育、掌腱膜挛缩和扑翼样震颤。

再生障碍性贫血的罕见病因可通过体格检查得以确定。范科尼贫血患者有身材矮小、咖啡牛奶色素斑、大鱼际发育不全和桡骨发育不全等表现。先天性角化不良是一种端粒过短的疾病，可导致白斑、指甲营养不良和色素斑等。

需要注意的是，在有活动性出血和血流动力学不稳定的情况下，必须权衡全面体格检查和后续实验室检查的时机。在紧急情况下，需要优先开通气道、进行呼吸支持和循环支持（A-B-C），意识到出血可能迅速发展至关重要。危及生命的出血需要立即治疗，同时进行诊断性检查。危及生命的出血不仅限于创伤或胃肠道出血，还包括气道或颈部附近小血管出血及其他重要器官出血。心率和血压是评估失血量的第一步。

出血的实验室评估

对出血患者的初始实验室评估（表 7.1）应包括全血细胞计数（CBC）、凝血酶原时间（PT）、活化部分凝血活酶时间（APTT）和纤维蛋白原检测（图 7.1）。CBC 是出血评估中关键的第一步，包括血小板计数、血红蛋白和血细胞比容，这些指标对于监测失血速度和生命体征至关重要。CBC 还包含平均红细胞体积（MCV；反映红细胞大小的指标），MCV 降低提示慢性失血并导致铁

TABLE 7.1 Screening Assays for Hemostasis

Laboratory Test	Aspect of Hemostasis Tested	Causes of Abnormalities
Blood counts (CBC) and peripheral blood smear	Platelet count and morphologic features	Thrombocytopenia, thrombocytosis, gray platelet and giant platelet syndromes
Prothrombin time (PT)	Factor VII–dependent pathways	Vitamin K deficiency and warfarin, liver disease, DIC, factor deficiency (VII, V, X, II), factor inhibitor
Partial thromboplastin time (aPTT)	Factor XI–, IX–, and VIII–dependent pathways	Heparin, DIC, lupus anticoagulant[a], VWD, factor deficiency (XII[a], XI, IX, VIII, V, X, II), factor inhibitor
Thrombin time	Fibrinogen	Heparin, hypofibrinogenemia, dysfibrinogenemia, DIC
Platelet aggregation and platelet function analysis	Platelet and VWF function	Aspirin, VWD, storage pool disease
Mixing study	Factor inhibitors or deficiencies	Abnormal clotting time corrects for a factor deficiency; does not correct for an inhibitor

DIC, Disseminated intravascular coagulation; *VWD,* von Willebrand disease; *VWF,* von Willebrand factor.
[a]Lupus anticoagulant and factor XII deficiency are not associated with bleeding.

antibodies and are then read as white blood cells instead of platelets by automated counters. Other helpful findings on a peripheral blood smear include schistocytes, suggesting microangiopathic hemolytic anemia. Teardrop cells with immature white and red blood cells characterize the myelophthisic blood smear, indicative of marrow replacement by solid tumor, lymphoma, granuloma, or fibrosis.

PT and aPTT are two commonly used broad measures of the coagulation cascade. PT assesses the extrinsic and common pathways, that is clotting factors, in order of activation: VII, X, V, II, and fibrinogen. aPTT covers the intrinsic and common pathways: Clotting factors XII, XI, IX, VIII, X, V, II, and fibrinogen. Both PT and aPTT become abnormal with deficiencies of the common pathway (X, V, II, and fibrinogen) or multiple clotting factor deficiencies involving both the intrinsic and extrinsic pathways. The International Normalized Ratio (INR) represents a standardized correlate of PT so that measurements of vitamin K–dependent anticoagulation can be compared despite interlaboratory variation. Abnormal PT and aPTT should be repeated to verify the elevation was not in error. Specific factor deficiencies may be suspected based on elevations in PT or aPTT and these factor activities can be tested to confirm the diagnosis and monitor effects of treatment.

Factor deficiencies can be congenital (e.g., hemophilia A) or acquired (e.g., acquired hemophilia, liver disease, disseminated intravascular coagulopathy [DIC]). A mixing study can distinguish a factor deficiency resulting from a decline in production from a decline due to inhibition from an autoantibody. Mixing studies combine patient plasma with control plasma so that missing factors are replaced and the abnormal clotting times correct (i.e., prolonged PT or PTT becomes normal). A positive mixing study does not correct because of the presence of an inhibitor, blocking the factor from the normal control plasma. Mixing studies can also be useful in finding a lupus anticoagulant, which is important for the diagnosis of antiphospholipid syndrome (see Chapter 8), but a lupus anticoagulant does not affect bleeding and should not be in the differential diagnosis of the bleeding patient.

Fibrinogen can be decreased through a decline in production or consumption, as in DIC. The assay is an easy, rapid, and cheap test to run and should be run early in the evaluation of the bleeding patient. Many fibrinogen assays incorporate function into the quantitative measurement, but since this information may not be readily available, thrombin time is able to measure the function of fibrinogen by adding thrombin to plasma and then measuring the conversion of fibrinogen to fibrin.

Similarly, platelet function may be helpful if a defect in primary hemostasis is suspected, but platelet count and von Willebrand factor testing are normal. Platelet dysfunction disorders can be induced by many different medications, although they are often not clinically significant and rarely are congenital. Platelet function can be assessed by platelet aggregation studies or Platelet Function Analyzer-100 (PFA-100; Fig. 7.2), which both use platelet activators to trigger platelet activation and aggregation. Different platelet activators such as adenosine diphosphate (ADP), collagen, epinephrine, and ristocetin may detect subtle differences in platelet function. These tests, not surprisingly, fail to work when platelets are absent or low. Bleeding time, a test measuring the time it takes to stop bleeding after making a small incision in the forearm as a gauge of platelet function, should no longer be performed because numerous studies have shown poor sensitivity, specificity, and reproducibility with significant technician variability.

Testing for von Willebrand disease (VWD) is as complicated as the disease, which has multiple subtypes, each with different means of diagnosing. A typical von Willebrand factor (VWF) panel includes VWF activity (a functional test measured by ristocetin-mediated binding of VWF to platelets, VWF antigen (the quantitative level), and clotting factor VIII, which declines without the presence of its stabilizer, VWF. Other tests that may be required to determine the subtype of VWD include VWF multimer analysis, VWF-factor VIII binding assay, and a measure of platelet aggregation as induced by ristocetin (RIPA). As with any congenital disorder, gene sequencing may be the only way to confirm the diagnosis, but it adds time and expense and is frequently normal in mild cases of VWD.

Additional laboratory tests useful in evaluating bleeding include factor Xa activity for measurement of low-molecular-weight heparin effect, heparin neutralization (with heparinase, hexadimethrine bromide [Polybrene], or protamine), and euglobulin clot lysis time as a measure of fibrinolysis, the time to dissolve a fibrin clot. Currently, the new class of anticoagulants, direct oral anticoagulants (DOACs), do not have readily available methods for measurement of plasma concentrations or activity. Because vitamin C deficiency (scurvy) can cause bleeding, measuring ascorbic acid can be helpful when nutrient deficiency is suspected. Thromboelastography (TEG) and rotational thromboelastometry (ROTEM) use torque to measure clotting of whole blood. These methods have many proponents but remain investigational. A rapid approach to identifying possible causes of bleeding (Fig. 7.3) considers several major disease categories: (1) VWD, thrombocytopenia, or abnormal platelet function; (2) low levels of multiple coagulation factors resulting from vitamin K deficiency, liver disease, or DIC; (3) single-factor deficiency (usually inherited); and, more rarely, (4) an acquired inhibitor to a coagulation factor such as factor VIII. The laboratory evaluation is most efficient when it is performed in this context.

表7.1 止血相关筛查检测		
实验室检查	止血检查项目	异常的原因
全血细胞计数（CBC）和外周血涂片	血小板计数及其形态学特征	血小板减少症、血小板增多症、灰色血小板综合征和巨血小板综合征
凝血酶原时间（PT）	因子Ⅶ依赖性途径	维生素K缺乏、华法林、肝病、DIC、因子缺乏（Ⅶ、Ⅴ、Ⅹ、Ⅱ）、因子抑制物
活化部分凝血活酶时间（APTT）	因子Ⅹ、Ⅸ和Ⅷ依赖性途径	肝素、DIC、狼疮抗凝物ª、vWD、因子缺乏（Ⅻª、Ⅺ、Ⅸ、Ⅷ、Ⅴ、Ⅹ、Ⅱ）、因子抑制物
凝血酶时间（TT）	纤维蛋白原	肝素、低纤维蛋白原血症、异常纤维蛋白原血症、DIC
血小板聚集和血小板功能分析	血小板和vWF功能	阿司匹林、vWD、贮存池病
混合试验	因子抑制物或因子缺陷	异常凝血时间被纠正，提示因子缺陷；若不能被纠正，则存在因子抑制物

DIC，弥散性血管内凝血；vWD，血管性血友病；vWF，血管性血友病因子。
ª 狼疮抗凝物和因子Ⅻ缺陷与出血无关。

缺乏。血小板减少应进行外周血涂片检查以明确诊断。当乙二胺四乙酸（EDTA）抗凝剂引起血小板聚集时，自动计数器会误将血小板计作白细胞，从而出现假性血小板减少症。外周血涂片中发现破碎红细胞提示微血管病性溶血性贫血。泪滴状细胞伴有未成熟的白细胞和红细胞是骨髓疾病血涂片的特征性表现，提示骨髓可能被实体瘤、淋巴瘤、肉芽肿侵犯或发生骨髓纤维化。

PT和APTT是评估凝血级联反应的两个常用指标。PT测定可评估外源性凝血途径和共同途径，包括凝血因子（按激活顺序排列）Ⅶ、Ⅹ、Ⅴ、Ⅱ和纤维蛋白原。APTT测定可评估内源性凝血途径和共同途径，包括凝血因子Ⅻ、Ⅺ、Ⅸ、Ⅷ、Ⅹ、Ⅴ、Ⅱ和纤维蛋白原。当共同途径（Ⅹ、Ⅴ、Ⅱ和纤维蛋白原）缺陷或涉及内外源性凝血途径的多种凝血因子缺陷时，PT和APTT均异常。国际标准化比值（INR）对PT测定值进行了标准化，校正了各实验室之间的差异，使得对维生素K依赖性抗凝效应的测定结果具有可比性。如果检测结果显示PT或APTT异常，应重复检测以确认结果。PT或APTT延长提示特定凝血因子缺乏，可通过检测这些凝血因子的活性来进一步确诊并监测治疗效果。

凝血因子缺乏可以是先天性（如血友病A）或获得性［如获得性血友病、肝病、弥散性血管内凝血（DIC）］。混合试验可鉴别合成减少所致的凝血因子缺乏和自身抗体所致的凝血因子缺陷。混合试验是将患者血浆与对照血浆混合，使缺失的凝血因子得到补充，以纠正异常的凝血时间（如延长的PT或APTT恢复到正常范围）。混合试验阳性（即未被纠正）提示存在凝血因子抑制物，抑制了正常对照血浆中的凝血因子。混合试验还有助于发现狼疮抗凝物，这对诊断抗磷脂综合征非常重要（见第8章），但狼疮抗凝物不会影响出血，故无须被列入出血患者的鉴别诊断中。

纤维蛋白原可因生成减少或消耗增多而减少，如在DIC中。纤维蛋白原的检测方法简单、快速且便宜，应在出血患者的早期评估中进行。许多纤维蛋白原检测方法纳入了定量测定，但这一信息不易获得，凝血酶时间（TT）可通过将凝血酶添加到血浆中，然后测定纤维蛋白原向纤维蛋白的转化来反映功能性纤维蛋白原的水平。

如果血小板计数和vWF相关检查结果正常，但仍怀疑初级止血异常，可进行血小板功能检测。血小板功能障碍可由多种药物诱发，但通常没有临床意义，也很少是先天性的。血小板功能可通过血小板聚集功能检测或血小板功能分析仪-100（PFA-100；图7.2）进行评估，两者均使用血小板激活剂来触发血小板活化和聚集。不同的血小板激活剂［如腺苷二磷酸（ADP）、胶原蛋白、肾上腺素和瑞斯托霉素］可检测出血小板功能的细微差异。但是，当血小板缺乏或显著减少时，这些检测将失效。出血时间（BT）是在患者前臂做小切口后通过测量止血所需的时间来衡量血小板功能的方法，由于其敏感性、特异性和可重复性较差及显著的技术差异，目前已不再采用。

血管性血友病（vWD）的检查和疾病本身一样复杂，该病有多种亚型，每种亚型有不同的诊断方法。经典的vWF检测组合包括血浆vWF活性测定（检测瑞斯托霉素诱导的vWF与血小板的结合能力）、血浆vWF抗原测定（定量）及血浆凝血因子Ⅷ活性测定（在缺少vWF作为其稳定剂的情况下活性会下降）。确定vWD的亚型需要其他检测，包血浆vWF多聚体分析、血浆vWF与因子Ⅷ结合试验及瑞斯托霉素诱导的血小板聚集（RIPA）。与其他先天性疾病一样，基因检测可能是确诊的唯一方法，但这会增加诊断所需的时间和费用，且轻度vWD患者的基因检测结果通常是正常的。

可用于评估出血的其他实验室检查包括：血浆因子Xa活性测定（用于评估低分子量肝素效应）、肝素中和测定［使用肝素酶、溴化己二甲胺（聚凝胺）或鱼精蛋白］，以及优球蛋白溶解时间（作为衡量纤维蛋白溶解的指标）。直接口服抗凝剂（DOAC）是新型抗凝药，目前尚无方法测量其血浆浓度或活性。由于维生素C缺乏症（坏血病）会导致出血，因此当怀疑患者营养缺乏时，检测抗坏血酸可能有所帮助。血栓弹力图（TEG）和旋转式血栓弹力图（ROTEM）使用扭矩来评估全血的凝固情况，这些方法虽然有许多证据支持，但目前仍处于研究阶段。为了快速识别可能的出血原因（图7.3），应考虑以下几类主要疾病：①vWD、血小板减少症或血小板功能异常；②由维生素K缺乏、肝病或DIC引起的多种凝血因子水平降低；③单一凝血因子缺乏（通常为遗传性）；④获得性凝血因子（如因子Ⅷ）抑制物（较罕见）。在这些情况下进行实验室评估最为有效。

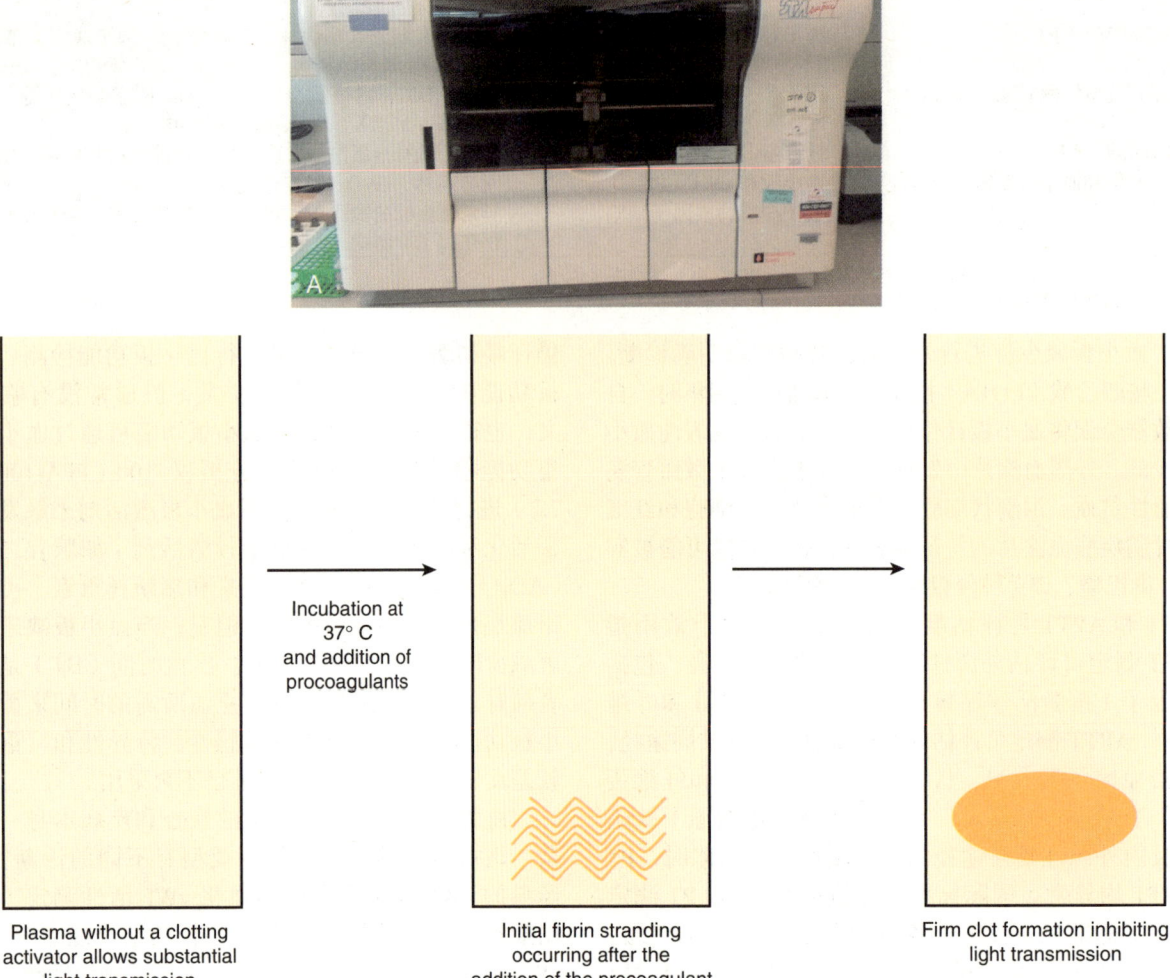

Fig. 7.1 Basic methodology underlying measurement of prothrombin (PT) and activated partial thromboplastin time (aPTT). (A) Typical laboratory instrument used to perform basic and complex coagulation assays. (B) Plasma specimens are incubated at 37° C and then mixed with tissue factor and phospholipid (PT) or a surface activator and phospholipid (aPTT). The time it takes for clot formation to block light passage through the specimen is measured and compared with a reference range. Prolongation of the PT or aPTT clotting time can be associated with many congenital or acquired coagulation factor defects. Abnormal PT or aPTT values are typically followed by more specific coagulation factor assays, depending on the type of prolongation and the suspected underlying clinical disease.

BLEEDING CAUSED BY VASCULAR DISORDERS

Vascular purpura (i.e., bruising) is defined as bleeding caused by intrinsic structural abnormalities of blood vessels or by inflammatory infiltration of blood vessels (i.e., vasculitis). Although vascular purpura usually causes bleeding in the setting of normal platelet counts and normal coagulation tests, vasculitis and vessel damage may be severe enough to cause secondary consumption of platelets and coagulation factors.

Collagen breakdown and thinning of the subcutaneous tissue that overlies blood vessels is often observed in older patients (i.e., senile purpura), and similar atrophic skin changes are a common effect of steroid therapy. Another acquired cause of vascular purpura is scurvy (i.e., deficiency of vitamin C [ascorbic acid]). Patients with scurvy have bleeding around individual hair fibers (i.e., perifollicular hemorrhage) and corkscrew-shaped hair. Bruising occurs in a classic saddle pattern over the upper thighs. The bleeding gums are caused by gingivitis and not by the subcutaneous tissue defect. Edentulous patients with scurvy do not have bleeding gums, and scurvy should not be excluded on this basis.

Congenital defects of the vessel wall can cause bruising. These rare syndromes include pseudoxanthoma elasticum, a defect of the elastic fibers of the vasculature associated with severe gastrointestinal (GI) and genitourinary bleeding, and Ehlers-Danlos syndrome, which is characterized by abnormal collagen in blood vessels and subcutaneous tissue. Both syndromes cause bruising in the skin, but only patients with pseudoxanthoma elasticum develop significant GI bleeding.

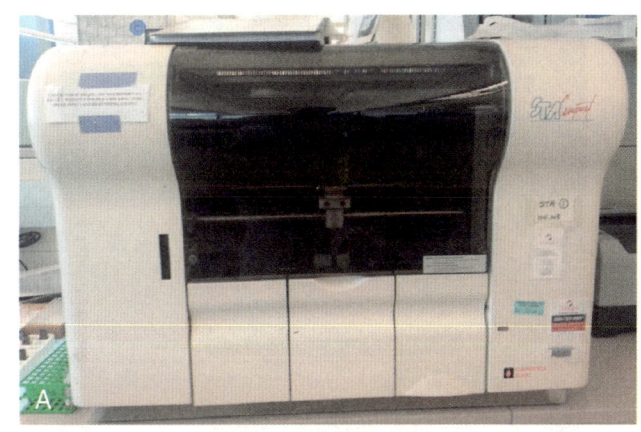
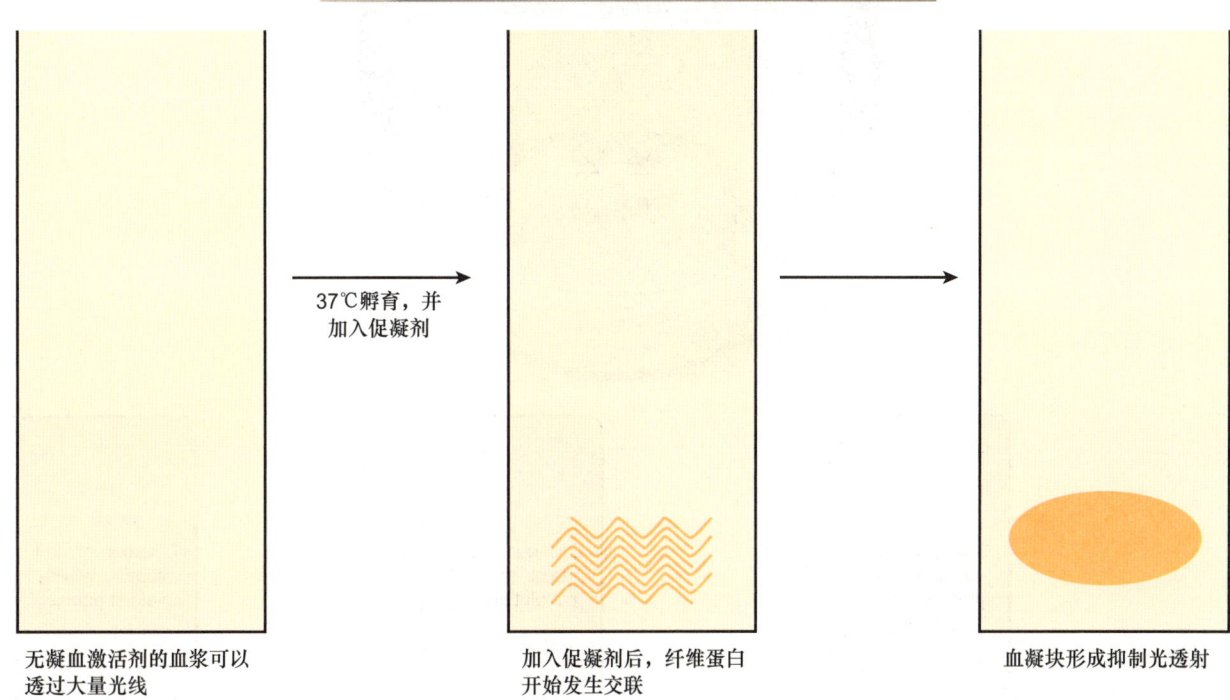

图 7.1 测定凝血酶原时间（PT）和活化部分凝血活酶时间（APTT）的基本方法。A.用于进行基础和复杂凝血试验的典型实验室仪器。B.将血浆样品置于37℃下孵育，然后与组织因子和磷脂混合（测定 PT 时），或与表面激活剂和磷脂混合（测定 APTT 时）。血凝块形成可阻断光通过样品，测量光通过所用的时间并与参考范围进行比较。PT 或 APTT 延长可与多种先天性或获得性凝血因子缺陷有关。根据延长的类型和疑诊的潜在疾病，出现 PT 或 APTT 异常值后通常可进行更具特异性的凝血因子检测

由血管疾病引起的出血

血管性紫癜（即瘀斑）的定义是由血管内在结构异常或血管炎症浸润（即血管炎）引起的出血。虽然血管性紫癜通常在患者血小板计数和凝血检查结果正常的情况下引起出血，但血管炎和血管损伤可能严重到足以引起继发性血小板和凝血因子消耗。

老年患者通常存在覆盖血管的皮下组织菲薄和胶原蛋白分解，从而引起老年性紫癜，类固醇治疗也常导致类似的萎缩性皮肤变化。血管性紫癜的另一种获得性病因是坏血病［即维生素 C（抗坏血酸）缺乏症］。坏血病患者可出现毛发周围出血（即毛囊周围出血）和毛发卷曲。瘀斑常在大腿上部形成经典的鞍形图案。牙龈出血由牙龈炎引起，而不是由皮下组织缺损引起。缺齿的坏血病患者可以没有牙龈出血症状，据此不能排除坏血病。

先天性血管壁缺陷可引起瘀斑。这些罕见的综合征包括：①弹性纤维假黄瘤，一种脉管系统弹性纤维缺陷病，可伴有严重胃肠道和泌尿生殖道出血；②埃勒斯-当洛综合征，其特征是血管和皮下组织中存在异常胶原蛋白。这两种综合征均可引起皮肤瘀斑，但只有弹性纤维假黄瘤患者会发生严重的胃肠道出血。

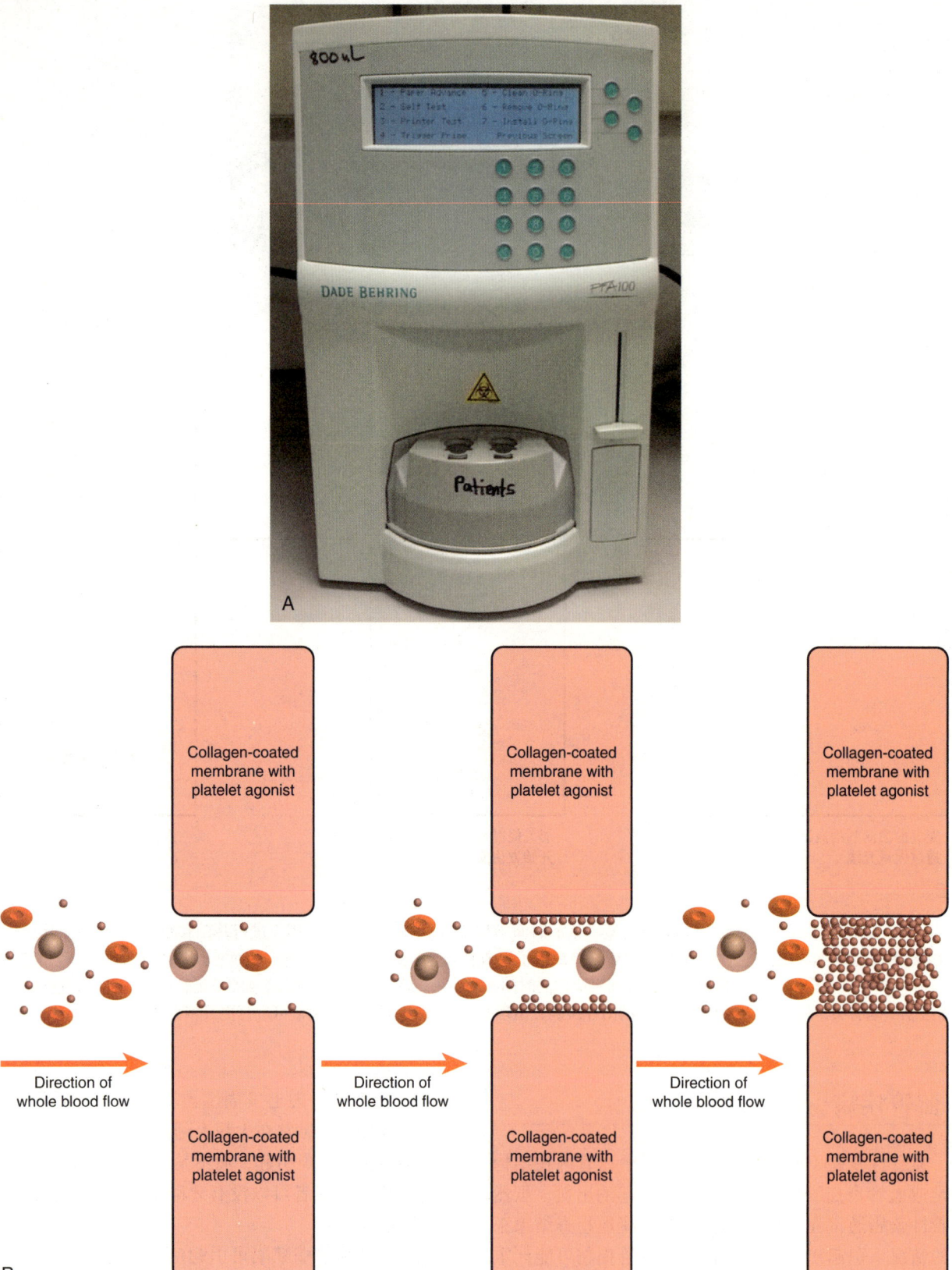

Fig. 7.2 Methodology underlying the Platelet Function Analyzer-100 (PFA-100). (A) Whole blood platelets are streamed toward a collagen-based aperture. The membrane is infused with a potent platelet agonist (i.e., adenosine diphosphate or epinephrine). (B) Streaming the platelets through the instrument channels induces shear-based activation, which in conjunction with the agonists should yield an initial wave of platelet adhesion and aggregation. Over time, activated platelets continue to aggregate, closing off the aperture to whole blood flow. The time it takes for aperture closing is measured in seconds and compared with a reference range. Abnormally prolonged closure times can be associated with von Willebrand disease due to the reliance on adhesion in this assay or with a platelet functional defect due to the reliance on aggregation for complete aperture closure.

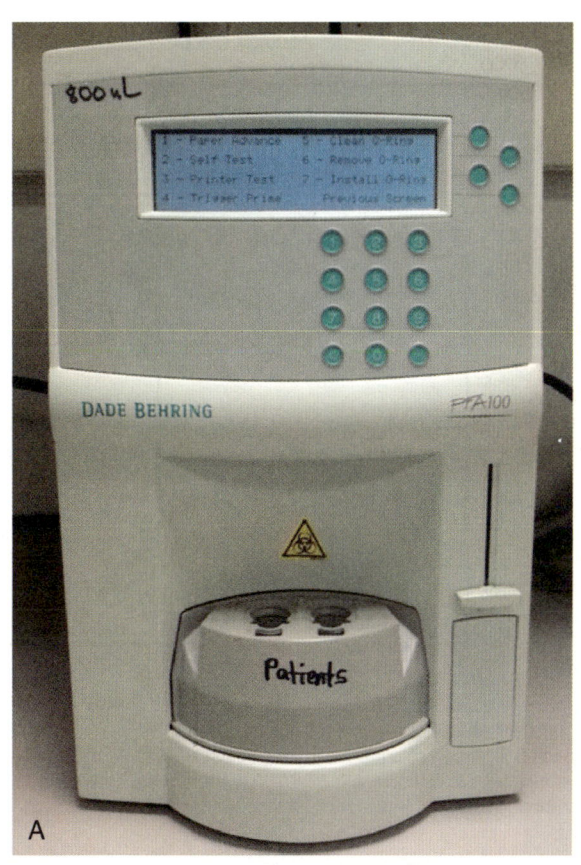

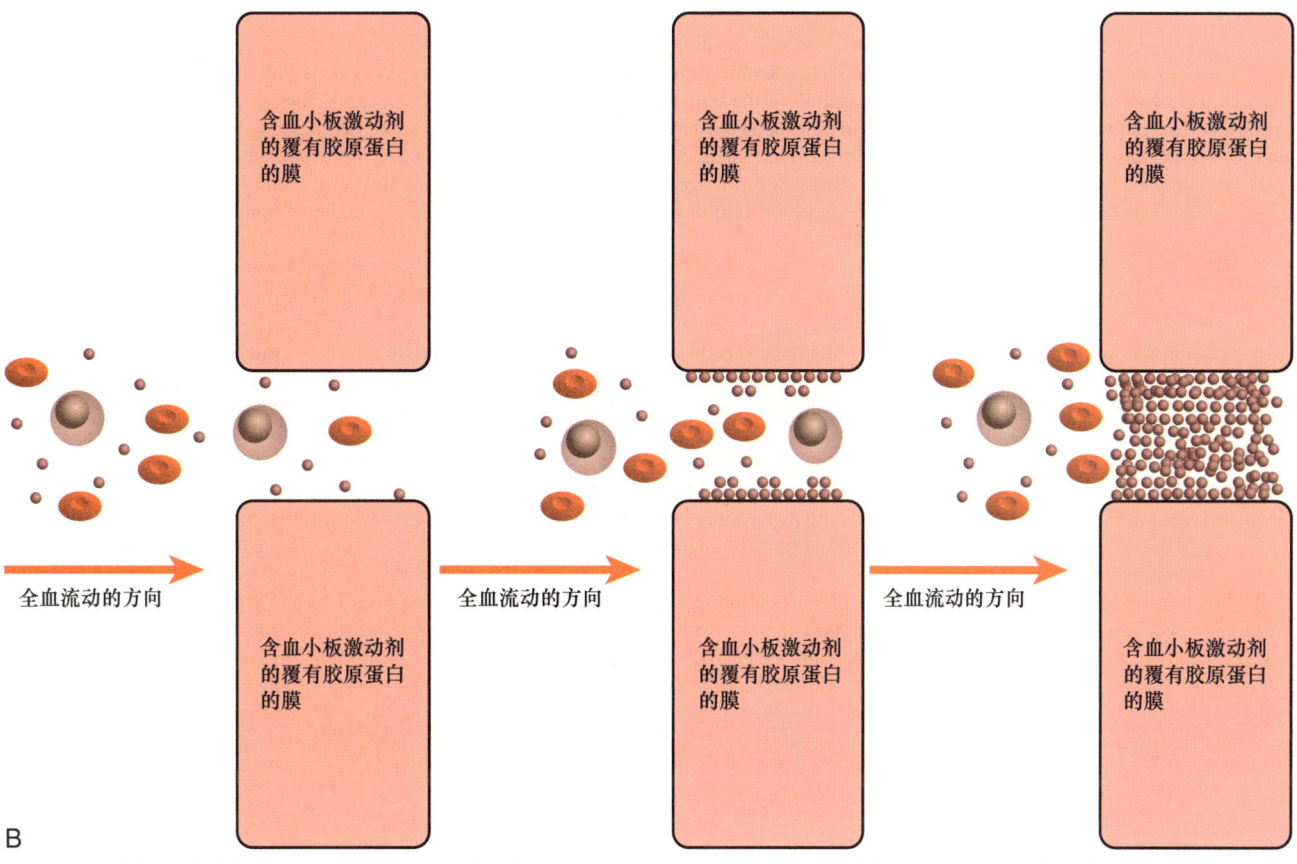

图 7.2 血小板功能分析仪-100（PFA-100）的基本原理。**A**. 全血中的血小板流向覆有胶原蛋白的孔道。将强效血小板激动剂（即腺苷二磷酸或肾上腺素）注入膜。**B**. 在仪器通道的流动中，血小板被高剪切力激活，同时在激动剂作用下产生血小板黏附和聚集的初始波。随着时间的推移，活化的血小板继续聚集，关闭孔道阻断全血血流。孔道关闭所需的时间以秒为单位进行测量，并与参考范围进行比较。闭合时间延长可能与 vWD 相关，因为该试验依赖于血小板黏附，也可能与血小板功能缺陷有关，因为完全闭合有赖于血小板聚集

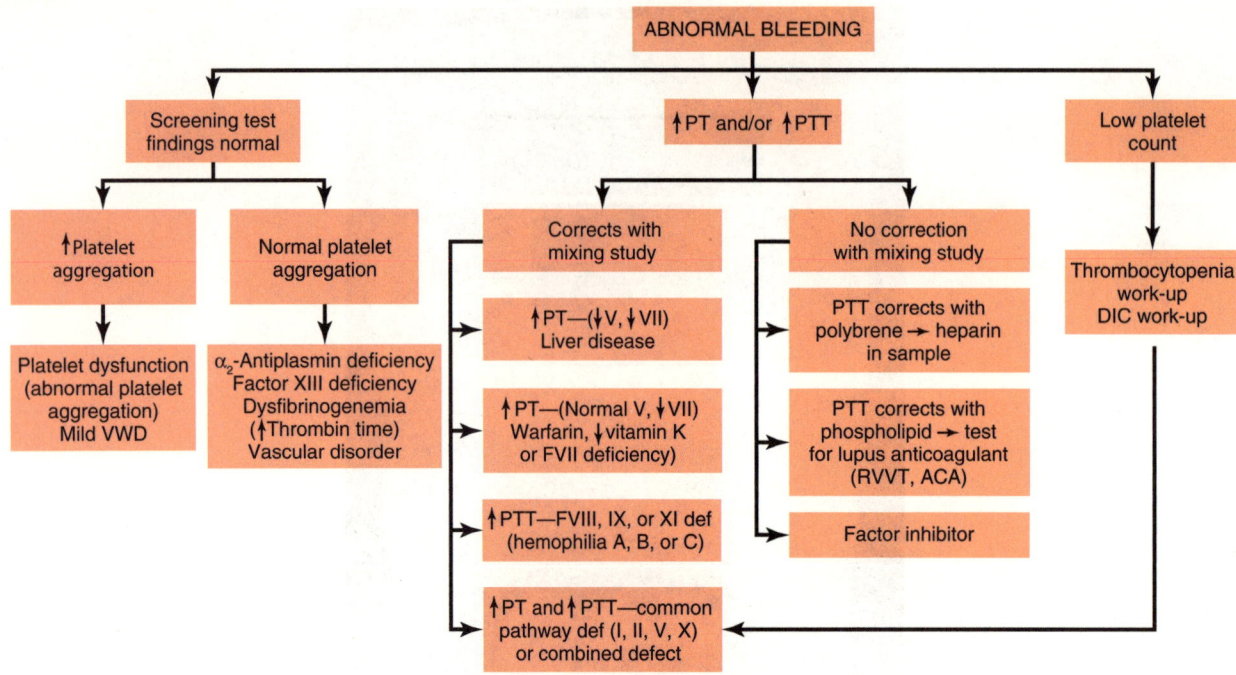

Fig. 7.3 Algorithm for the evaluation of bleeding. Screening laboratory tests for platelet and factor deficiencies are used to narrow the work-up for bleeding, followed by specific factor and other coagulation studies (e.g., mixing studies, D-dimer) to confirm the diagnosis. *ACA,* Anticardiolipin antibody; *DIC,* disseminated intravascular coagulation; *FVIII,* factor VIII; *PFA-100,* Platelet Function Analyzer-100; *PT,* prothrombin time; *PTT,* partial thromboplastin time; *RVVT,* Russell viper venom time; *VWD,* von Willebrand disease; ↑, increased; ↓, decreased.

Another inherited vessel wall defect associated with GI bleeding is hereditary hemorrhagic telangiectasia (Osler-Weber-Rendu syndrome). This disorder is characterized by degeneration of the blood vessel wall that results in angiomatous lesions resembling blood blisters on mucous membranes, including the lips and GI tract. The frequency of bleeding caused by breakdown of these lesions increases with age, and GI lesions commonly cause significant chronic bleeding, resulting in iron deficiency anemia.

The sudden onset of palpable purpura (i.e., localized, raised hemorrhages in the skin) associated with rash and fever may be caused by aseptic or septic vasculitis. Septic vasculitis can be caused by meningococcemia and other bacterial infections and is often accompanied by thrombocytopenia and prolongation of clotting times. One cause of aseptic vasculitis in young children and adolescents is Henoch-Schönlein purpura, a vasculitis of the skin, GI tract, and kidneys that is usually accompanied by abdominal pain from bleeding into the bowel wall. This syndrome may occur after a viral prodrome and appears to be caused by an immunoglobulin A (IgA) hypersensitivity reaction, as evidenced by serum IgA immune complexes and renal histopathologic features resembling IgA nephropathy.

The therapy for bleeding from vascular disorders depends upon the diagnosis. Senile purpura and steroid-induced purpura do not usually require treatment. Scurvy is corrected by vitamin C supplementation. In congenital disorders, including Ehlers-Danlos syndrome, hereditary hemorrhagic telangiectasia, and pseudoxanthoma elasticum, patients should avoid medications (e.g., aspirin) that may aggravate their bleeding tendencies, and they should receive supportive therapy (e.g., iron supplementation, red blood cell transfusion). Systemic administration of estrogen to patients with hereditary hemorrhagic telangiectasia may help to decrease epistaxis by inducing squamous metaplasia of the nasal mucosa, which protects lesions from trauma.

Treatment of septic vasculitis focuses on appropriate antibiotic therapy. In the case of aseptic vasculitis, steroids and immunosuppressive agents are most effective. When vasculitis is severe enough to cause consumption of platelets and coagulation factors (see section on disseminated intravascular coagulation), transfusions of platelets, cryoprecipitate, and fresh-frozen plasma (FFP) may be indicated.

BLEEDING CAUSED BY THROMBOCYTOPENIA

With thrombocytopenia, bleeding does not occur until platelets are less than 20,000/μL unless platelet dysfunction accompanies the thrombocytopenia as it frequently does in myelodysplastic syndromes or when aspirin or nonsteroidal anti-inflammatory drugs have been used (Fig. 7.4). Platelets less than 100,000/μL can be problematic after trauma or during surgery. Since most patients do not bleed from mild thrombocytopenia (50,000 to 150,000/μL), treatment is often not required, but thrombocytopenia should be investigated to determine the cause, expected trajectory, and a plan for when treatment is needed. Broadly, thrombocytopenia results from a decline in platelet production, hypersplenism/sequestration, or destruction/consumption. However, determining which category to focus attention on can be challenging. Bone marrow biopsy can help because megakaryocyte hyperplasia implies increased production, a means of compensating for peripheral platelet destruction, whereas megakaryocyte hypoplasia suggests decreased platelet production. Still, bone marrow biopsy is often unnecessary in the evaluation. Hypersplenism is usually associated with an enlarged spleen, but splenic overactivity can be seen when the spleen is normal

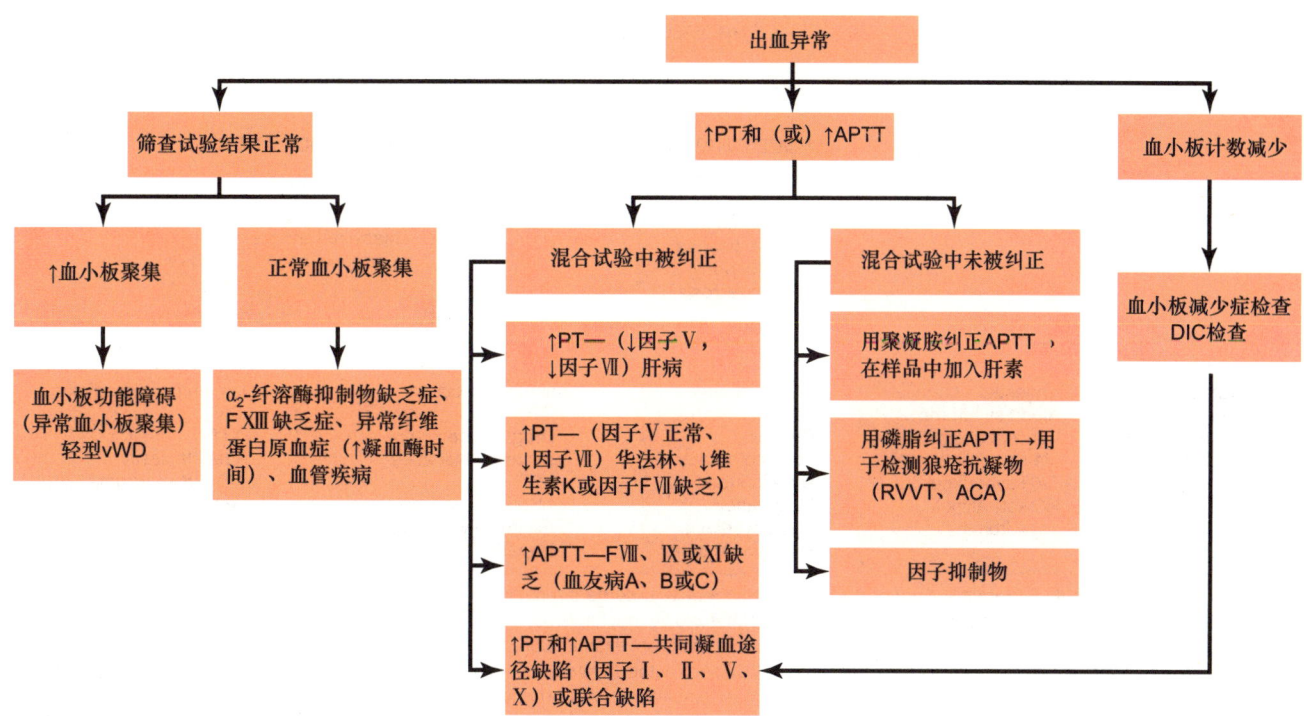

图7.3 评估出血的流程图。对血小板和因子缺乏进行实验室筛查可锁定检查的方向，随后根据特异性因子和其他凝血试验（如混合试验、D-二聚体）以明确诊断。ACA，抗心磷脂抗体；DIC，弥散性血管内凝血；FⅧ，因子Ⅷ；PFA-100，血小板功能分析仪-100；PT，凝血酶原时间；APTT，活化部分凝血活酶时间；RVVT，蝰蛇毒时间；vWD，血管性血友病；↑，增加或延长；↓，减少

与消化道出血相关的另一种先天性血管壁缺陷是遗传性出血性毛细血管扩张症（即Osler-Weber-Rendu综合征）。这种疾病的特征为血管壁变性，引起血管瘤样病变，与黏膜表面（包括唇和胃肠道）的血疱类似。随着年龄增长，由这些病灶破裂引起的出血也随之增加，胃肠道病变通常引起明显的慢性出血，导致铁缺乏。

突然发生的可触性紫癜（即皮肤局部出血，突出皮面）伴皮疹和发热可能由无菌性或感染中毒性血管炎引起。感染中毒性血管炎可由脑膜炎球菌败血症和其他细菌感染引起，且通常伴有血小板减少和凝血时间延长。幼儿和青少年无菌性血管炎的原因之一是过敏性紫癜（HSP），其为一种可发生于皮肤、胃肠道和肾的血管炎，常伴有因肠道出血而引起的腹痛。该综合征可发生在病毒性前驱症状后，可能由免疫球蛋白A（IgA）超敏反应引起，血清IgA免疫复合物和类似IgA肾病的肾组织病理学特征证实了这一点。

由血管疾病引起的出血的治疗取决于诊断。老年性紫癜和类固醇引起的紫癜通常不需要治疗。坏血病可通过补充维生素C来纠正。先天性疾病（包括埃勒斯-当洛综合征、遗传性出血性毛细血管扩张症和弹性纤维假黄瘤）患者应避免使用可能加重出血倾向的药物（如阿司匹林），且应接受支持治疗（如补铁、红细胞输注）。对于遗传性出血性毛细血管扩张症患者，全身使用雌激素可诱导鼻黏膜的鳞状上皮化生，从而减少外伤所致的鼻出血。

感染中毒性血管炎处理的重点是应用恰当的抗生素治疗。对于无菌性血管炎，类固醇激素和免疫抑制剂是最有效的治疗。当血管炎严重到足以引起血小板和凝血因子消耗（见下文"弥散性血管内凝血"）时，可以考虑输注血小板、冷沉淀或新鲜冰冻血浆（FFP）。

由血小板减少症引起的出血

在血小板减少症患者中，一般血小板计数 < 20 000/µl时才会发生出血症状，除非血小板减少合并血小板功能障碍，如骨髓增生异常综合征（MDS）或使用阿司匹林或非甾体抗炎药时（图7.4）。创伤后或手术期间血小板 < 10 000/µl可能引发出血。大多数患者不会因轻度血小板减少（即血小板计数为50 000～150 000/µl）而出血，因此轻度血小板减少通常不需要治疗，但应明确血小板减少的病因、预估进展及确定治疗时机。总体上，血小板减少主要是由血小板生成减少、脾功能亢进/血小板滞留及破坏/消耗引起。但是，确定寻找病因的方向具有一定挑战性。骨髓活检有助于诊断，因为巨核细胞增殖活跃意味着血小板生成增加，这是代偿外周血小板破坏的一种方式，而巨核细胞发育不良则表明血小板生成减少。骨髓活检在评估过程中不是必须的。脾功能亢进通常伴有脾大，

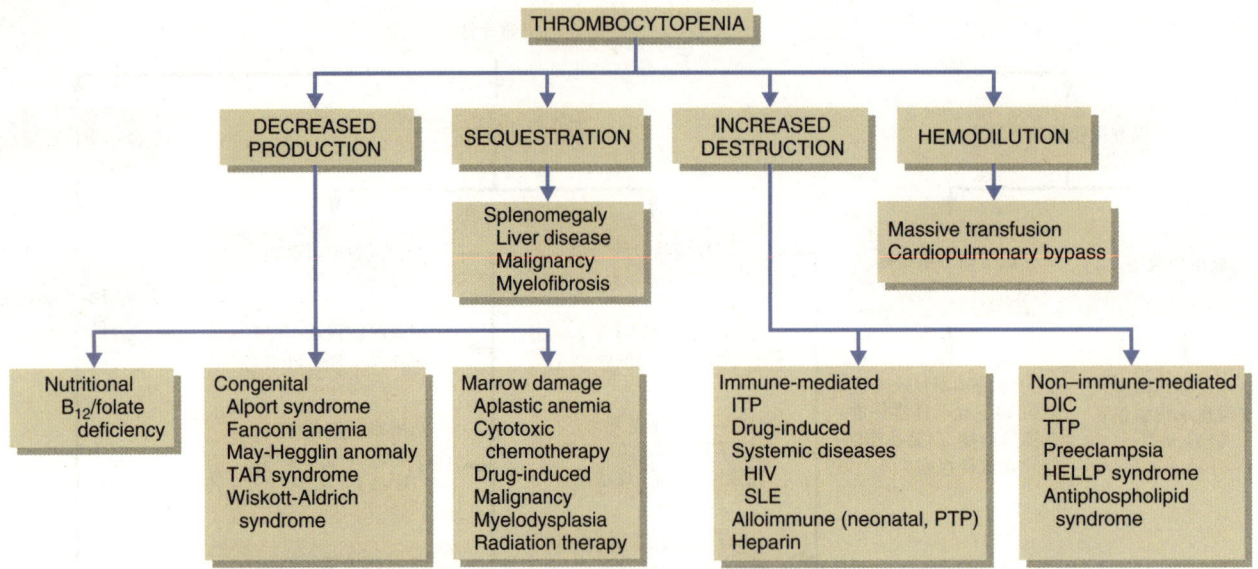

Fig. 7.4 Differential diagnosis of thrombocytopenia. Disorders resulting in a decreased circulating platelet number can be classified by four main pathophysiologic mechanisms: hypoproduction, sequestration, peripheral destruction, and hemodilution. The history, physical examination, and bone marrow evaluation usually narrow the range of possible causes. *DIC*, Disseminated intravascular coagulation; *HELLP*, hemolysis, elevated liver enzymes, and low-platelet count in association with pregnancy; *HIV*, human immunodeficiency virus; *ITP*, immune thrombocytopenic purpura; *PTP*, post-transfusion purpura; *SLE*, systemic lupus erythematosus; *TAR*, thrombocytopenia-absent radius syndrome; *TTP*, thrombotic thrombocytopenic purpura.

in size, as it is in immune thrombocytopenic purpura. Conversely, not all enlarged spleens are associated with hypersplenism (see Fig. 7.4).

Decreased Marrow Production of Platelets

Decreased production of platelets in the bone marrow is characterized by decreased or absent megakaryocytes on the bone marrow aspirate and biopsy. Suppression of normal megakaryopoiesis occurs after marrow damage and destruction of stem cells (such as occurs with cytotoxic chemotherapy); destruction of the normal marrow micro-environment and replacement of normal stem cells by invasive malignant disease, aplasia, infection (e.g., miliary tuberculosis), or myelofibrosis; specific but rare intrinsic defects of the megakaryocytic stem cells; and metabolic abnormalities affecting megakaryocyte maturation.

Drug-Associated Thrombocytopenia

Many drugs cause immune-mediated thrombocytopenia. However, some can have a direct cytotoxic effect on stem cells and megakaryocytes, causing a decline in platelet production. The classic example of this is cytotoxic chemotherapy used to treat malignancies. These medications are used to stop malignant cells from dividing, but they have the same effect on nonmalignant proliferating cells such as in the bone marrow. This myelosuppression frequently results in thrombocytopenia as well as neutropenia and anemia. Other drugs including thiazide diuretics and alcohol can have similar effects. Diagnostic confirmation comes from recovery of platelets after withdrawal of the medication. Recovery usually occurs within 7 days but can take several weeks. After repeated injury, stem cells may not recover, resulting in chronic thrombocytopenia.

Nutrition-Associated Thrombocytopenia

Deficiencies in copper, folate, and vitamin B_{12} can cause thrombocytopenia. However, they typically will cause other cytopenias prior to affecting platelet production. Megaloblastic anemia refers to the effects of impaired DNA synthesis on bone marrow causing dyssynchrony between slowed maturation of the nucleus and continued maturation of cytoplasm with unimpaired protein synthesis. This process results in large erythroid precursors called megaloblasts and mature large red blood cells (macrocytes). Certain medications can have this effect: azathioprine, 5-fluorouracil, methotrexate, and others. Folate and vitamin B_{12} deficiencies are classic causes of megaloblastic anemia and when severe can cause pancytopenia. These deficiencies are most commonly caused by poor absorption either from autoimmune interference of intrinsic factor (pernicious anemia), other causes of atrophic gastritis, celiac disease, or previous gastrointestinal surgery. Less commonly, folate and vitamin B_{12} deficiency arise from a poor diet (e.g., strict vegans and alcoholics), an inherited defect in transcobalamin, or competition for vitamin B_{12} absorption from *Diphyllobothrium latum* parasitic infection.

Copper deficiency causes leukopenia and anemia before affecting platelet production. It occurs in two settings, first through malabsorption from celiac disease and past bowel surgeries, and second, through copper transport blockage from zinc excess. Zinc levels should be tested when copper is found to be low. Zinc excess occurs from zinc-containing denture cream and improper use of zinc supplements.

Bone Marrow Invasion

When the bone marrow is replaced by non-marrow elements, space for hematopoiesis becomes limited. In addition, the microenvironment necessary to supply proper nutrients, growth factors, and neuroendocrine stimulation is damaged. The prototypic disease of marrow invasion is myelofibrosis, either primary (a chronic myeloproliferative disease) or secondary, from other myeloproliferative

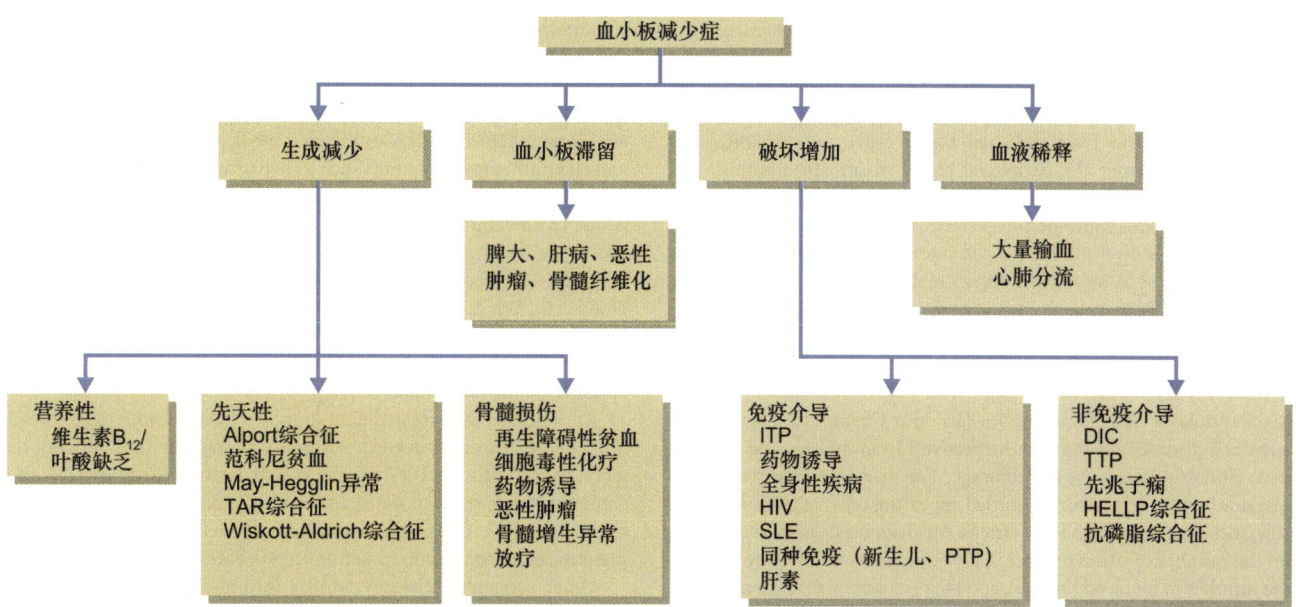

图 7.4 血小板减少症的鉴别诊断。导致循环血小板数量减少的疾病可通过 4 种主要病理生理学机制进行分类：生成减少、滞留、外周破坏增加和血液稀释。病史、体格检查和骨髓评估可缩小鉴别范围。DIC，弥散性血管内凝血；HELLP，与妊娠相关的溶血、肝酶水平升高和血小板计数减少；HIV，人类免疫缺陷病毒；ITP，免疫性血小板减少性紫癜；PTP，输血后紫癜；SLE，系统性红斑狼疮；TAR，血小板减少伴桡骨缺失；TTP，血栓性血小板减少性紫癜

但即使脾大小正常，也可能出现脾功能亢进，如免疫性血小板减少性紫癜。同样，不是所有脾大均与脾功能亢进有关（图 7.4）。

骨髓血小板生成减少

骨髓血小板生成减少的特征是骨髓穿刺和活检标本显示巨核细胞减少或缺失。正常巨核细胞生成抑制可见于骨髓损伤和干细胞破坏（如使用细胞毒性化疗药物）；侵袭性恶性疾病、再生障碍性疾病、感染（如粟粒性结核）或骨髓纤维化破坏正常骨髓微环境并替代正常干细胞；特异但罕见的先天性巨核干细胞缺陷；影响巨核细胞成熟的代谢异常。

药物相关的血小板减少症

许多药物可引起免疫介导的血小板减少症。但是，部分药物会对干细胞和巨核细胞产生直接的细胞毒性作用，导致血小板生成减少。典型的例子是用于治疗恶性肿瘤的细胞毒性化疗药物可阻止恶性细胞分裂，但对骨髓中的非恶性增殖细胞也具有同样的作用。这种骨髓抑制常导致血小板减少症、中性粒细胞减少症和贫血。其他有类似作用的药物包括噻嗪类利尿剂和酒精。如果停药后血小板计数恢复，则有利于确诊。血小板计数通常在 7 天内恢复，但也可能需要数周。反复损伤后，干细胞可能无法恢复，导致慢性血小板减少症。

营养相关的血小板减少症

铜、叶酸和维生素 B_{12} 缺乏会导致血小板减少症。但是，它们通常会在影响血小板生成之前引起其他血细胞减少。巨幼细胞贫血是由于骨髓 DNA 合成障碍，导致细胞核成熟减慢与蛋白质合成未受损的细胞质持续成熟之间的不同步。这一过程会产生大的红系前体细胞，包括巨幼红细胞和大红细胞（即成熟的大的红细胞）。某些药物可产生这种作用，如硫唑嘌呤、5-氟尿嘧啶和甲氨蝶呤等。叶酸和维生素 B_{12} 缺乏是巨幼细胞贫血的常见病因，严重时可导致全血细胞减少。导致叶酸和维生素 B_{12} 缺乏最常见的原因是吸收不良，如由于自身免疫因素对内因子的影响（恶性贫血）、各种原因所致的萎缩性胃炎、乳糜泻或既往接受胃肠道手术。较少见的引起叶酸和维生素 B_{12} 缺乏的情况包括：不良饮食（如严格素食和酗酒）、先天性钴胺素转运蛋白缺陷或由于阔节裂头绦虫感染而竞争性吸收维生素 B_{12}。

铜缺乏会导致白细胞减少和贫血，继而影响血小板生成。它可见于两种情况，第一种是由乳糜泻或既往肠道手术导致的吸收不良，第二种是由锌过量导致的铜转运受阻。当发现铜含量低时，应检测锌的含量。含锌义齿乳膏和锌补充剂使用不当可导致锌过量。

骨髓侵犯

当骨髓被非骨髓成分取代时，造血空间变得有限，提供营养物质、生长因子和神经内分泌刺激所必需的骨髓微环境也遭到破坏。骨髓侵犯的典型疾病是骨髓纤维化，包括原发性骨髓纤维化（如慢性骨髓增生性疾病），以及继发性于其他骨髓增生性疾病（如真性红细胞增多症和原发性血小板增多症）、血液系统恶性肿瘤、自身免

disease (polycythemia vera, essential thrombocythemia), hematologic malignancy, autoimmune disease, or infection. Rarely, myelofibrosis is associated with systemic mastocytosis and osteogenesis imperfecta. In myelofibrosis, the marrow is replaced by fibrotic strands causing immature erythroid (nucleated red blood cells) and myeloid cells ("left-shift") to enter the peripheral blood stream. In addition, red blood cells become deformed (teardrop cells) as they squeeze between narrow spaces. This combination of teardrop cells and immature blood cells is called the myelophthisic blood smear. It can be seen when bone marrow is replaced by fibrotic tissue, malignant cells, or granuloma from sarcoidosis or tuberculosis. Confirmation of marrow invasion requires a bone marrow biopsy.

Myelodysplastic Syndrome

Myelodysplastic syndrome (MDS) (see also Chapter 2) is a clonal stem cell disorder resulting in ineffective hematopoiesis and cytopenias, either unilineage or multilineage. The diagnosis requires a bone marrow biopsy. Dysplasia (abnormal appearing cells) in the bone marrow and cytopenias fulfill the criteria for diagnosis. Subtypes depend on the number of blasts present in the bone marrow (must be <20%), the number of involved lineages, and the presence or absence of ringed sideroblasts, a nucleated erythroid cell with iron-laden mitochondria surrounding the nucleus (requires iron stain to see). The cytopenias tend to progress slowly, over months to years. MDS causes infection through neutropenia, symptoms of anemia, and easy bleeding/bruising from thrombocytopenia. It is also a precursor to acute myelogenous leukemia (AML).

Prior to the advent of next-generation sequencing (NGS), proving clonality in MDS was challenging because about one third of cases have normal cytogenetics. Now, NGS has become a routine part of the diagnostic evaluation and provides prognostic information as well as occasionally targetable mutations for treatment. RUNX1 is a transcription factor that leads to upregulation of the thrombopoietin receptor. When RUNX1 has a pathologic mutation as part of MDS or leukemia, patients become thrombocytopenic.

Recent studies have found MDS-associated mutations in people with normal blood counts. These mutations, for example DNMT3A, TET2, and ASXL1 among others, confer an increased risk for MDS/AML (and cardiac disease). The state of having MDS-associated mutations but normal blood counts is called clonal hematopoiesis of indeterminate potential (CHIP). Gene sequencing data are rapidly being incorporated into the pathogenesis, diagnosis, and treatment of MDS and other hematologic malignancies.

Other Hematologic Malignancies

Any hematologic malignancy can cause thrombocytopenia through marrow invasion, particularly common in acute leukemias and aggressive lymphomas. Chronic lymphocytic leukemia (CLL) progresses slowly, eventually causing thrombocytopenia from marrow invasion (defined as Rai stage IV). Additionally, CLL at any stage can cause thrombocytopenia through immune-mediated platelet destruction.

Aplastic Anemia

Aplastic anemia can cause severe pancytopenia and occurs when the bone marrow hematopoietic elements are replaced by adipose cells. The diagnosis requires a bone marrow biopsy to show decreased cellularity (hypoplasia). Once the diagnosis is established, the cause for marrow failure must be explored. Aplastic anemia can be caused by congenital or acquired diseases. Congenital causes include Fanconi anemia (mutations in the *FANC* gene leading to chromosomal instability), dyskeratosis congenital (mutations in the telomerase complex leading to short telomeres), Shwachman-Diamond syndrome (mutation on the *SBDS* gene leading to ribosomal dysfunction), and amegakaryocytic thrombocytopenia (mutations in the thrombopoietin or thrombopoietin receptor c-mpl genes).

Acquired causes of aplastic anemia include medication effects such as chloramphenicol, sulfa, antithyroid medications, gold, allopurinol, and chemotherapy; infections such as hepatitis, HIV, and Epstein-Barr virus (EBV); and paroxysmal nocturnal hemoglobinuria (PNH). PNH is due to an acquired mutation in the gene *PIG-A*, which provides a protective coating around red blood cells (CD55 and CD59). CD55 and CD59 prevent complement from binding and hemolyzing red blood cells. When they are absent as in PNH, patients develop chronic hemolysis, causing the dark urine that accumulates overnight, thus the name nocturnal hemoglobinuria. PNH patients frequently develop aplastic anemia (see Chapter 1).

Aplastic anemia is treated with supportive transfusions of red blood cells and platelets as needed, immunosuppression (anti thymocyte globulin and cyclosporine), platelet growth factors (eltrombopag), and sometimes stem cell transplant. Interestingly, the platelet growth factor eltrombopag increases white blood cells and red blood cells as well as platelets, because thrombopoietin receptors are also on stem cells.

Other congenital diseases causing thrombocytopenia will be discussed in the later sections on platelet dysfunction.

Platelet Sequestration

Up to 30% of circulating platelets are normally sequestered within the spleen at any time. Thrombocytopenia due to sequestration is common when the spleen is enlarged as in advanced liver disease. Platelets continue to decline the larger the spleen becomes. Rarely are platelets less than 50,000/μL. Besides chronic liver disease, splenic lymphomas, chronic myelogenous leukemia and other myeloproliferative diseases, hemoglobinopathies, and Gaucher's disease, an inherited glycolipid storage disease, can cause splenomegaly with cytopenias.

The diagnosis of platelet sequestration may be suspected by physical examination findings or imaging studies demonstrating splenomegaly. Bone marrow studies typically reveal normal megakaryocyte numbers and morphology. Given the lack of specific tests for platelet sequestration, the diagnosis often is one of exclusion of other causes of thrombocytopenia.

Treatment of thrombocytopenia due to splenomegaly frequently depends on the underlying cause of increased spleen size. Splenectomy immediately resolves the thrombocytopenia when the thrombocytopenia is caused by hypersplenism. However, this must be weighed against the potential complications of surgery, an increased risk of thrombosis, and a lifelong increased risk of infection.

Platelet Destruction

Platelets can be removed from circulation by various means. One common process is through an immune mechanism, where antibodies target platelets, either from autoimmune disease (e.g., immune thrombocytopenic purpura [ITP]) or a drug effect. Another manner of platelet destruction is by consumption, for instance the rapid dissipation of platelets in DIC or hemophagocytic lymphohistiocytosis (HLH).

Immune-Mediated Platelet Destruction

Immune platelet destruction typically refers to antibody-mediated clearance. Platelet destruction can be further divided into autoimmune forms (i.e., antibody against self-antigens) and alloimmune forms (i.e., antibody against nonself-antigens). Autoimmune thrombocytopenia is the most commonly encountered form of immune-mediated platelet destruction. It may be a primary disorder directed only at platelets or a secondary complication of another autoimmune disease, such as systemic lupus erythematosus (SLE). Alloimmune-mediated platelet

疫病或感染的骨髓纤维化。罕见情况下，骨髓纤维化与系统性肥大细胞增多症和成骨不全有关。在骨髓纤维化中，骨髓被纤维条索取代，导致未成熟的红系细胞（有核红细胞）和髓系细胞（"核左移"）进入外周血中。此外，红细胞在狭窄的空间受到挤压时会变形，形成泪滴状红细胞。当外周血涂片中出现泪滴状红细胞和不成熟的血细胞时被称为"骨髓病性"血涂片，可出现于骨髓组织被纤维化组织、恶性肿瘤细胞及结节病或结核的肉芽肿组织取代时。进一步确诊骨髓侵犯需要进行骨髓活检。

骨髓增生异常综合征

MDS（见第 2 章）是一种克隆性干细胞疾病，可导致单系或多系无效造血和血细胞减少。明确诊断需要进行骨髓活检。诊断标准包括骨髓病态造血（出现形态异常的细胞）和血细胞减少。MDS 的亚型取决于骨髓中的原始细胞数量（必须 < 20%）、受累谱系的数量及是否有环状铁粒幼细胞[一种细胞核周围有含铁线粒体的有核红细胞（需要进行铁染色才能观察到）]。MDS 的血细胞减少往往进展缓慢，持续数月至数年。MDS 的临床表现与外周血中性粒细胞减少、贫血和血小板减少有关，可分别导致感染、贫血症状和易出血/瘀伤。MDS 也可能进展为急性髓系白血病（AML）。

由于约 1/3 的 MDS 患者没有明显的细胞遗传学异常，因此在二代测序（NGS）出现之前，确定 MDS 的克隆性极具挑战性。现在，NGS 已成为 MDS 诊断性评估的常规手段，并能提供预后信息，有时也能发现可用于治疗的靶基因突变。RUNX1 是一种导致血小板生成素受体上调的转录因子，当 MDS 或白血病患者发生 *RUNX1* 致病性突变时，会出现血小板减少。

近期研究发现，在血细胞计数正常的人群中也可能存在与 MDS 相关的基因突变。这些突变（如 *DNMT3A*、*TET2* 和 *ASXL1*）会增加患 MDS、AML 及心脏病的风险。具有 MDS 相关基因突变但血细胞计数正常的状态被定义为潜能未定克隆性造血（CHIP）。基因测序数据正在被迅速运用于 MDS 和其他血液系统恶性肿瘤的发病机制研究、诊断和治疗中。

其他血液系统恶性肿瘤

任何血液系统恶性肿瘤均可通过侵犯骨髓而引起血小板减少，尤其常见于急性白血病和侵袭性淋巴瘤。慢性淋巴细胞白血病（CLL）进展缓慢，最终可导致骨髓浸润而出现血小板减少（定义为 Rai Ⅳ 期）。此外，任何阶段的 CLL 都可能通过免疫介导的血小板破坏而引起血小板减少。

再生障碍性贫血

在再生障碍性贫血中，当骨髓造血细胞被脂肪细胞取代时，即可引发严重的全血细胞减少。诊断需要符合骨髓活检显示细胞增生减低。一旦确诊，必须探究骨髓衰竭的原因。再生障碍性贫血可由先天性或获得性疾病引起。先天性疾病包括范科尼贫血（*FANC* 基因突变导致染色体不稳定性）、先天性角化不良（端粒酶复合体突变导致端粒缩短）、施-戴综合征（*SBDS* 基因突变导致核糖体功能障碍）和无巨核细胞血小板减少症（血小板生成素或血小板生成素受体 *c-mpl* 基因突变）。

再生障碍性贫血的获得性因素包括药物作用，如氯霉素、磺胺类药物、抗甲状腺药物、金、别嘌醇和化疗药物等；感染，如肝炎病毒、HIV 和 EB 病毒（EBV）等；阵发性睡眠性血红蛋白尿症（PNH）。PNH 由 *PIG-A* 基因获得性突变所致，该基因为红细胞提供了一层保护层（CD55 和 CD59）。CD55 和 CD59 可阻止补体与红细胞结合，以避免溶血。当 CD55 和 CD59 缺失时，PNH 患者会出现慢性溶血，导致夜间深色尿液累积，即夜间血红蛋白尿。PNH 患者常发生再生障碍性贫血（见第 1 章）。

再生障碍性贫血的治疗包括按需输注红细胞和血小板进行支持治疗、使用免疫抑制剂（抗胸腺细胞球蛋白和环孢素）、血小板生长因子（艾曲泊帕）或干细胞移植。由于干细胞上也有血小板生成素受体，血小板生长因子艾曲泊帕在增加血小板的同时也可以增加白细胞和红细胞。

其他引起血小板减少的先天性疾病详见下文"血小板功能障碍"。

血小板滞留

正常情况下，多达 30% 的循环血小板会被滞留在脾中。滞留引起的血小板减少在脾大时（如肝病晚期）很常见。脾越大，血小板越少。血小板很少低于 50 000/μl。除了慢性肝病外，脾淋巴瘤、慢性髓细胞性白血病和其他骨髓增生性疾病、血红蛋白病和戈谢病（一种遗传性糖脂贮积症）也可引起脾大伴血细胞减少。

血小板滞留的诊断需通过体格检查或影像学检查发现脾大。骨髓检查通常显示巨核细胞数量和形态正常。由于缺乏血小板滞留的特异性检查，通常是在排除血小板减少的其他原因后做出诊断。

由脾大引起的血小板减少症的治疗通常取决于导致脾大的原发疾病。当血小板减少由脾功能亢进引起时，脾切除术可立即改善血小板减少。但是，必须权衡手术潜在的并发症，如血栓形成风险增加和感染的终身风险增加。

血小板破坏

血小板在循环中可通过多种方式被清除，其中一种常见的方式是通过免疫机制，即自身免疫病[如免疫性血小板减少性紫癜（ITP）]或药物作用产生的抗血小板抗体所介导的血小板清除。另一种破坏血小板的方式是消耗增加，如在 DIC 或噬血细胞性淋巴组织细胞增生症（HLH）中血小板被快速消耗。

免疫介导的血小板破坏

免疫介导的血小板破坏通常指抗体介导的血小板清除。血小板破坏可进一步分为自身免疫型（即抗自身抗原的抗体）和同种免疫型（即针对非自身抗原的抗体）。自身免疫性血小板减少症是最常见的免疫介导的血小板破坏形式。它可以是仅针对血小板的原发性疾病，或是继发于另一种自身免疫病（如系统性红斑狼疮）的并发症。同种免疫介

destruction is rare and encountered in neonates as a result of maternal antibodies formed against fetal platelet antigens or in chronically transfused individuals, who form alloantibodies against foreign platelet antigens.

In autoimmune and alloimmune thrombocytopenia, immune platelet destruction is caused by increased levels of polyclonal antiplatelet antibodies directed against platelet membrane glycoprotein receptors, most often cryptic neoepitopes of glycoprotein IIb/IIIa (GPIIb/IIIa) and less commonly glycoprotein Ib (GPIb) or human leukocyte antigens (HLAs). Coating of the platelet with these antibodies leads to opsonization of platelets by Fc receptors on macrophages in the reticuloendothelial system (RES). Antibody-coated platelets are cleared by the spleen and, to a lesser extent, by the liver.

These disorders involve a dramatic increase in marrow platelet production reflected by increased numbers of marrow megakaryocytes. The younger platelets produced have relatively high granule contents, providing increased hemostatic function. Bone marrow examination for increased or normal megakaryocyte numbers can help distinguish platelet destruction from decreased production.

Thrombocytopenia resulting from immune clearance may be severe, and platelet survival is often reduced from the normal 7 to 10 days to less than 1 day. Despite severe thrombocytopenia, serious bleeding or hemorrhagic death is uncommon, partly because the function of young platelets is increased and partly because the number of circulating platelets required to maintain vascular integrity is relatively low, estimated at 7100/μL per day.

Immune thrombocytopenic purpura. Autoimmune destruction of platelets is referred to as ITP. This can be primary or secondary to other autoimmune diseases (e.g., SLE), hematologic malignancy (especially CLL), or infections, mostly viral. ITP in children is self-limiting in more than 80% of cases and they often recover without treatment. In adults, however, it frequently remains a chronic relapsing and remitting disease. Presentations in children and adults are the same with petechiae on examination and mucocutaneous bleeding. Platelet count is varied but can be extremely low, frequently less than 10,000/μL and occasionally below the limit of detection. Blood blisters in the mouth (wet purpura) may carry a higher risk for life-threatening hemorrhage such as in the central nervous system and warrant rapid intervention. Hemorrhagic deaths are rare in children (<2%), but mortality is higher if the ITP is chronic. Fatal hemorrhage in adults is approximately 5%.

A characteristic feature of ITP is that the other cell lines are intact, so that only the platelets are affected. There are two caveats to this rule. First, bleeding patients can become anemic, and second, ITP can overlap with warm autoimmune hemolytic anemia (AIHA). When ITP occurs in conjunction with AIHA, the disease is called Evans syndrome and tends to be more resistant to treatment. The confirmatory test for the warm autoimmune hemolytic component is a direct antiglobulin Coombs test, which adds anti-IgG and anti-C3 sera to the patient's serum. The added antibodies bind to the autoantibodies, which are bound to the red blood cells, causing the red blood cells to agglutinate. The agglutination, the mark of a positive test, can be visualized in a test tube.

Besides the Coombs test for Evans syndrome, there is no confirmatory test for ITP, making it a diagnosis of exclusion. Antiplatelet antibody testing has poor sensitivity and specificity and should not factor into treatment decision making, so its diagnostic role is doubtful. Similarly, mean platelet volume (MPV) tends to be increased in ITP because younger platelets are larger, but MPV lacks sensitivity and specificity and cannot be relied upon. Revealing increased megakaryocytes as the bone marrow tries to compensate for the peripheral platelet destruction, bone marrow biopsy can be helpful, particularly in unclear cases, but is not usually necessary. More often, confirmation of the diagnosis of ITP stands in its response to treatment.

ITP can be associated with HIV and hepatitis. It can also be the presenting manifestation of SLE. Patients should be screened for these diseases and treated if any are present because treating the underlying disease will also help control the ITP.

Therapy for ITP starts with corticosteroids, although treatment is not necessary if platelets are stable above 20 to 50,000/μL. A recent randomized control trial found faster time to response and more complete responses when using pulse dexamethasone 40 mg daily for 4 days repeated in monthly cycles compared to a prolonged taper of prednisone. An added benefit was decreasing the total long-term exposure to steroids, which comes with many complications including weight gain, infection, and osteoporosis. Response rates were high, but so were relapses. In patients who relapse, repeating cycles of dexamethasone may help, but additional therapeutic options are often necessary. Intravenous immunoglobulins (IVIG) 1 g/kg daily for 1 to 2 days or 400 mg/kg daily for 5 days are two common regimens used as first-line therapy with or without corticosteroids. Its response rates are similar to corticosteroids and it works by mopping up the autoantibody as well as blocking the Fc receptors on splenic macrophages. The order of second-line therapy for ITP is unclear and controversial. Splenectomy, with response rates of approximately 50%, offers a potential cure, but patients frequently opt for noninvasive approaches. Relapses after splenectomy warrant a search for an accessory spleen missed during surgery.

Rituximab is a chimeric monoclonal antibody that targets CD20, a B-cell antigen, thus working by decreasing the autoantibody production. It is given by intravenous infusion, weekly for 4 weeks. Response rates are around 60% but can take weeks to work and relapses often occur after 1 year. Hypersensitivity infusion reactions are common with rituximab. Infection, though rare, is also a concern. Thrombomimetics are a newer class with high efficacy. They work as thrombopoietin agonists and come as a subcutaneous injectable called romiplostim, given in weekly doses, or an oral agent called eltrombopag, mentioned previously as a treatment for aplastic anemia. The newest therapeutic option in ITP is fostamatinib, a small molecule Syk inhibitor, preventing macrophage binding to opsonized platelets, thus decreasing platelet consumption without affecting autoantibody production, similar to one of the mechanisms of IVIG. All of these newer targeted therapies are expensive, so patients need to be intolerant to or have failed steroids before using them.

There are many other treatment options that have been used with moderate success. Anti-Rh(D) immunoglobulin can be used to saturate Fc receptors on splenic macrophages, preventing these cells from consuming platelets. There is probably competitive inhibition and blockade of the mononuclear phagocytic system/RES by sensitized red blood cells in the spleen. However, this only works if patients are blood type Rh(D)+, still have their spleen, and do not have concomitant hemolytic anemia. Danazol, azathioprine, mycophenolate, cyclosporine, and cyclophosphamide can regulate autoimmunity. Platelet transfusions are necessary in bleeding patients even though the transfused platelets will be destroyed along with the endogenous platelets. Platelet transfusions should be continued until bleeding stops.

Drug-induced platelet destruction. Immune-mediated platelet destruction associated with specific drugs is an often overlooked cause of thrombocytopenia. Unlike some of the drugs mentioned earlier (e.g., chemotherapeutic agents) that act by directly suppressing megakaryocyte production, drugs in this category of thrombocytopenia induce an immune response against platelet antigens.

Drugs may induce an autoimmune response by several mechanisms. One is the development of an antibody response against soluble

导的血小板破坏比较罕见，通常仅在新生儿或长期输血的个体中发生，前者是由于母体形成抗胎儿血小板抗原的抗体，后者是由于形成针对外源血小板抗原的同种抗体。

在自身免疫和同种免疫介导的血小板减少症中，免疫性血小板破坏是由直接针对血小板膜糖蛋白受体的多克隆抗血小板抗体增加引起的，最常见的是针对糖蛋白Ⅱb/Ⅲa（GPⅡb/Ⅲa）隐性新表位的抗体，而抗糖蛋白Ⅰb（GPⅠb）或人类白细胞抗原（HLA）的抗体较少见。抗体包被的血小板可诱发网状内皮系统中的巨噬细胞通过Fc受体吞噬破坏血小板。抗体包被的血小板被脾清除，小部分被肝清除。

这些疾病导致骨髓血小板生成急剧增加，表现为骨髓巨核细胞数目增加。新生成的血小板具有相对较高的颗粒含量，从而增强止血功能。骨髓检查中巨核细胞数目增加或正常有助于区分血小板破坏与生成减少。

免疫清除引起的血小板减少可能很严重，血小板存活时间通常从正常的7～10天减少至<1天。虽然该类血小板减少很严重，但严重出血或出血性死亡并不常见，部分原因是新生成的血小板功能增加，另一部分原因是维持血管完整性所需的循环血小板数量相对较少，估计每日为7100/μl。

免疫性血小板减少性紫癜 自身免疫性血小板破坏被称为ITP。ITP可为原发性，也可继发于其他自身免疫病（如SLE）、血液系统恶性肿瘤（尤其是CLL）或感染（主要是病毒感染）。80%以上的儿童ITP具有自限性，通常无须治疗即可康复。但在成人中，ITP通常是一种慢性复发性疾病。儿童和成人的临床表现相同，均可表现为瘀点和皮肤黏膜出血。血小板计数差异较大，但可能极低，通常<10 000/μl，有时甚至低于检测下限。口腔血疱（湿性紫癜）导致危及生命的出血（如中枢神经系统出血）的风险可能更高，需要快速干预。儿童患者中出血性死亡很少见（<2%），但慢性ITP的死亡率升高。成人患者致死性出血的发生率约为5%。

ITP的一个特征是其他细胞系不受影响，只有血小板减少。但需注意两点：①出血患者可能会贫血；②ITP可能合并温抗体型自身免疫性溶血性贫血（AIHA）。ITP与AIHA同时发生被称为伊文思综合征（Evans综合征），其治疗通常更加困难。温抗体型自身免疫性溶血的特异性检查是直接抗球蛋白试验（直接Coombs试验）。该试验将抗IgG和抗C3血清添加到患者血清中。添加的抗体与自身抗体结合，自身抗体又与红细胞结合，导致红细胞凝集。试管中观察到凝集反应是Coombs试验阳性的标志。

除了诊断Evans综合征的Coombs试验外，尚无用于ITP的确诊试验，因此ITP的诊断是排除性诊断。抗血小板抗体检测的敏感性和特异性较差，其诊断价值存疑，不应将其作为影响治疗决策的因素。同样，由于新生成的血小板体积较大，因此ITP患者的平均血小板体积（MPV）通常增大，但MPV检测缺乏敏感性和特异性，不能依赖MPV诊断ITP。骨髓活检有助于发现巨核细胞增多（代偿外周血小板破坏），尤其是在原因不明的病例中，但通常并非必须。多数情况下，ITP的确诊取决于其对治疗的应答。

ITP可能与HIV感染和肝炎有关，也可能是系统性红斑狼疮的表现。患者应完善相关疾病的筛查，如果存在这些疾病则应进行治疗，治疗基础病也有助于控制ITP。

ITP的一线治疗是皮质类固醇，但如果患者血小板计数稳定在20 000～50 000/μl以上，一般无须治疗。近期一项随机对照试验显示，与延长泼尼松减量时间相比，地塞米松冲击治疗（40 mg/d，共4天，每月1次）的起效时间更快，完全缓解率更高。这种治疗方法的另一个好处是减少了类固醇的长期总暴露量，长期使用类固醇可导致许多并发症，包括体重增加、感染和骨质疏松症。虽然治疗缓解率高，但复发率也高。对于复发的患者，重复应用地塞米松治疗可能有帮助，但通常需要联合其他药物。常用的一线治疗方案是静脉注射免疫球蛋白（IVIG）[1.0 g/（kg·d）×（1～2）天；或0.4 g/（kg·d）×5天]，可单独给药或与皮质类固醇联用。免疫球蛋白通过清除自身抗体和阻断脾巨噬细胞上的Fc受体来发挥作用，其缓解率与类固醇激素相似。ITP二线治疗的顺序尚存争议。脾切除术的缓解率约为50%，是一种潜在的治愈方法，但患者常选择无创性方法。脾切除术后复发的患者需要明确是否存在副脾。

利妥昔单抗是一种靶向B细胞抗原CD20的嵌合单克隆抗体，通过减少自身抗体的产生来发挥作用。利妥昔单抗经静脉输注给药，每周1次，共4次，缓解率约为60%。但可能需要数周才能起效，且通常在1年后复发。利妥昔单抗治疗中常见过敏性输液反应。虽然感染较罕见，但也需要考虑。促血小板生成药以血小板生成素激动剂的形式发挥作用，是一类疗效较好的新型药物，包括：①罗米司亭，皮下注射，每周1次；②艾曲泊帕，口服，也可用于治疗再生障碍性贫血。目前ITP最新的治疗选择为福他替尼[一种小分子脾酪氨酸激酶（Syk）抑制剂]，可阻止巨噬细胞与血小板结合，从而在不影响自身抗体产生的情况下减少血小板消耗，类似于IVIG的作用机制之一。但是，所有较新的靶向治疗都很昂贵，因此在患者对类固醇治疗无效、不耐受或复发时才考虑这些治疗。

还有许多其他的治疗方案也取得了一定成功。抗Rh（D）免疫球蛋白可使脾巨噬细胞上的Fc受体饱和，从而阻止这些细胞破坏血小板。脾中的致敏红细胞可能竞争性抑制和阻断单核吞噬细胞系统/网状内皮系统（RES）。但是这种治疗仅适用于Rh（D）⁺血型、仍有脾和不伴有溶血性贫血的患者。达那唑、硫唑嘌呤、麦考酚酯、环孢素和环磷酰胺可调节自身免疫。虽然输注的血小板会与内源性血小板一起被破坏，但对于出血患者，血小板输注是必要的，应持续输注血小板直至出血停止。

药物诱导的血小板破坏 与特定药物相关的免疫介导的血小板破坏是血小板减少症常被忽视的病因。与上文所述的通过直接抑制巨核细胞生成发挥作用的药物（如化疗药物）不同，该类药物可诱导针对血小板抗原的免疫应答。

药物可通过多种机制诱导自身免疫应答。一种是针对可溶性药物分子产生抗体应答。当可溶性药物与

drug molecules. When soluble drugs bind to the platelet membrane, drug-induced antibodies act to destroy circulating platelets through the RES. Other mechanisms of drug-induced thrombocytopenia include formation of an immunogenic neoantigen through drug-platelet interactions (hapten response) with autoantibodies against drugs cross-reacting with platelet antigens. Occasionally, immune complexes that include the drug and circulating platelets are formed.

Historically, quinidine or quinine-based formulations were among the first class of drugs to be associated with platelet antibodies. The antibodies can be detected by tests using a drug coupled to a carrier protein. As awareness of drug-induced thrombocytopenia has grown, scores of drugs, including antibiotics, anticonvulsants, psychotropic drugs, and antiplatelet agents, have been reported to mediate platelet destruction (Table 7.2).

Heparin also induces thrombocytopenia, but unlike other drugs, this reaction paradoxically leads to a prothrombotic state referred to as heparin-induced thrombocytopenia (HIT) syndrome. The mechanism of heparin-induced thrombocytopenia and its prothrombotic effects are discussed in greater detail in Chapter 8.

When eliciting the medical history from patients with acute-onset thrombocytopenia, a careful review of all medications, particularly those initiated just before the development of low platelet counts, may help to deduce the cause and reverse the platelet count decline. Regardless of the mechanism of induction, development of thrombocytopenia is temporally related to exposure to the drug and is usually rapid. Discontinuation of the offending drug results in an increase in platelet count over days to weeks. For some patients with prolonged thrombocytopenia after drug removal, immunosuppression with steroids or IVIG (2 g/kg in two to three divided doses) may restore baseline platelet counts.

Although confirmation of drug-induced thrombocytopenia can often be made by testing for antibodies with drug specificities, these tests are not routinely available, are performed only by specialty reference laboratories, and take weeks to complete, by which time the offending drug has already been identified by stopping it and recovering the platelet count. When drug-induced thrombocytopenia is suspected, clinicians should not wait for results of drug-specific antibody tests before discontinuing potential offending agents.

Platelet alloimmunization. Patients who receive multiple platelet transfusions such as those with MDS may develop alloantibodies to platelets rendering future platelet transfusions less beneficial. Some do not respond to platelet transfusion at all. Alloimmunization can be assessed by measuring serial platelet counts after receiving a platelet transfusion to confirm the expected rise. Panel reactive antibody testing can also help. This test provides a percentage of HLA antigens that react with the patient's antibodies, giving the likelihood that the patient will consume a random platelet transfusion. In order to overcome this platelet destruction for those who are alloimmunized, HLA-matched platelets can be transfused, but this can take the blood bank days to find the right matched units (see "Platelet Transfusion Failure and Platelet Refractoriness" section).

Fetal and neonatal alloimmune thrombocytopenia. Fetal and neonatal alloimmune thrombocytopenia (FNAIT) occurs when a mother is homozygous for an uncommon platelet alloantigen, most often human platelet antigen 1b (HPA-1b) on the platelet GPIIIa receptor, and a fetus expresses the HPA-1a haplotype inherited from the father. The pathogenesis of alloimmune thrombocytopenia is analogous to the mechanism by which Rh(D) sensitization induces hemolytic disease of the newborn. The mother is exposed to the HPA-1a antigen during a first pregnancy, and during that or subsequent pregnancies, she produces high-titer IgG antibody against HPA-1a.

TABLE 7.2 Commonly Used Drugs Associated With Immune Thrombocytopenia

Drug Class	Examples
Antibiotics	Penicillins
	Cephalosporins (cephalothin, ceftazidime)
	Vancomycin
	Sulfonamides (sulfisoxazole)
Antiepileptics, antipsychotics, and sedative-hypnotics	Rifampin
	Linezolid
	Quinine
	Benzodiazepines (diazepam)
	Haloperidol
	Carbamazepine
	Lithium
	Phenytoin
Antihypertensives	Diuretics (chlorothiazide)
	Angiotensin-converting enzyme inhibitors (ramipril)
	Methyldopa
Analgesics and anti-inflammatories	Acetaminophen
	Ibuprofen
	Naproxen
Antiplatelet agents	Abciximab
	Tirofiban
Anticoagulants	Heparin
	Low-molecular-weight heparin

These antibodies cross the placenta, react with HPA-1a–positive fetal platelets, and cause peripheral platelet destruction through the RES.

A diagnosis of FNAIT is frequently suspected when in utero fetal bleeding is observed by imaging studies or when an otherwise healthy newborn has unexpected bleeding or bruising associated with thrombocytopenia (typically with platelet counts of 50,000 to 75,000/μL or lower). A maternal history of FNAIT is a strong predictor of its occurrence during future pregnancies.

After a diagnosis of FNAIT is suspected, it may be confirmed by examining maternal sera for anti-HPA alloantibodies and through platelet typing of the mother and father. Although bleeding may be severe in cases of FNAIT, the antibody does not necessarily predict whether bleeding will occur in utero, at delivery, or in the first days of life, and it is used primarily for confirmatory purposes.

Transfusion of washed maternal platelets (washed to remove the mother's anti-HPA-1a antibodies) or random platelets lacking the HPA-1a antigen and IVIG are useful for treating bleeding and restoring the platelet count. For newborns who recover from bleeding, there are few long-lasting deficits from FNAIT after circulating maternal antibodies are cleared from the circulation. For future pregnancies, IVIG with or without corticosteroids is given weekly throughout the second and third trimesters to prevent FNAIT.

Post-transfusion purpura. Alloimmune thrombocytopenia can occur in adults after transfusion, known as post-transfusion purpura (PTP). As in neonates, this condition is based on exposure to a common platelet alloantigen that is not present on the patient's native platelets. For instance, PTP can occur after transfusion of a blood product in an individual who lacks HPA-1a and who has been previously alloimmunized to this antigen during a prior pregnancy or transfusion. Because more than 95% of blood donors express HPA-1a and the antigen is shed by platelets, any blood product

血小板膜结合时，药物诱导的抗体通过 RES 破坏循环血小板。药物诱导的血小板减少症的其他机制包括通过药物-血小板相互作用（半抗原反应）形成免疫源性新抗原，药物依赖性自身抗体可与血小板抗原发生交叉反应。有时也会形成药物-循环血小板免疫复合物。

奎尼丁或奎宁类制剂是与血小板抗体相关的第一类药物。通过偶联至载体蛋白上的药物试验可检测到抗体。随着对药物诱导的血小板减少症的认识不断加深，已报道了数十种可介导血小板破坏的药物，包括抗生素、抗惊厥药、精神药物和抗血小板药（表 7.2）。

肝素也可以诱导血小板减少症，但与其他药物不同，这种相互作用会导致看似矛盾的血栓形成，即肝素诱导的血小板减少症（HIT）。HIT 的机制及其促血栓形成作用详见第 8 章。

询问急性血小板减少症患者的病史时，应仔细回顾所有用药情况，特别是血小板计数降低之前应用的药物，可能有助于推断病因并纠正血小板计数降低。无论诱导的机制如何，血小板减少症通常迅速发生，且在时间上与服用的药物相关。停用可疑药物后血小板计数通常在数天至数周内上升。对于停用药物后仍存在长期血小板减少的患者，使用 IVIG（2 g/kg，分 2～3 次应用）或类固醇可使血小板计数恢复至基线水平。

尽管可通过检测具有药物特异性的抗体来确诊药物诱导的血小板减少症，但这些并不是常规检查，且只能在专业实验室进行，并需要数周才能完成，当检测结果回报时，致病药物往往已通过停药和血小板计数恢复而被确定。因此，如果疑诊药物引起的血小板减少症，临床医生应停用潜在的可疑药物，不必等待特异性抗体检测结果。

同种免疫性血小板减少症　频繁输注血小板的患者（如 MDS 患者）可能会产生血小板的同种抗体，导致血小板输注效果欠佳，甚至无效。可通过在血小板输注后连续测定血小板计数来判断血小板是否升高至预期水平，从而评估是否发生了同种免疫。群体反应性抗体的检测对诊断也有一定帮助，该检测可提供与患者抗体发生反应的 HLA 百分比，为患者接受随机血小板输注提供了可能。为了避免同种免疫所致的血小板破坏，可输注 HLA 相合的血小板，但血库可能需要几天时间才能找到匹配的血小板（见下文"血小板输注失败和血小板无效输注"）。

胎儿和新生儿同种免疫性血小板减少症（FNAIT）　FNAIT 发生在母亲为罕见的血小板同种异体抗原纯合子时，最常见的是血小板 GPⅢa 受体上的人血小板抗原 1b（HPA-1b），而胎儿表达遗传自父亲的 HPA-1a 单倍体基因型。同种免疫性血小板减少的发病机制类似于 Rh（D）致敏诱导的新生儿溶血性疾病。母亲第一次妊娠时暴露于 HPA-1a 抗原，在这期间或随后的妊娠

表 7.2	与免疫性血小板减少症相关的常用药物
药物类别	举例
抗生素	青霉素
	头孢菌素（头孢噻吩、头孢他啶）
	万古霉素
	磺胺类药物（磺胺异噁唑）
	利福平
	利奈唑胺
	奎宁
抗癫痫药、抗精神病药和镇静催眠药	苯二氮䓬类（地西泮）
	氟哌啶醇
	卡马西平
	锂剂
	苯妥英
抗高血压药	利尿剂（氯噻嗪）
	血管紧张素转换酶抑制剂（雷米普利）
	甲基多巴
镇痛药和抗炎药	对乙酰氨基酚
	布洛芬
	萘普生
抗血小板药	阿昔单抗
	替罗非班
抗凝剂	肝素
	低分子量肝素

过程中产生抗 HPA-1a 的高滴度 IgG 抗体。这些抗体穿过胎盘，与 HPA-1a 阳性胎儿血小板发生反应，并通过 RES 引起外周血小板破坏。

当影像学检查发现宫内胎儿出血，或健康新生儿出现意外出血或瘀伤并伴有血小板减少时（通常血小板计数为 50 000～75 000/μl 或更低），应考虑 FNAIT 的诊断。孕产妇 FNAIT 病史可提示其未来妊娠期间再次发生 FNAIT 的可能性较大。

疑诊 FNAIT 后，可通过检查母体血清中抗 HPA 同种抗体和父母血小板抗体分型来确诊。虽然 FNAIT 患者的出血可能很严重，但抗体不一定能预测子宫内、分娩时或出生后最初几天是否会发生出血，抗体检测主要用于确诊。

洗涤母体血小板（洗涤以去除母体的抗 HPA-1a 抗体）或无 HPA-1a 抗原的随机血小板和 IVIG 的输注可用于治疗出血和恢复血小板计数。对于已纠正出血的新生儿，从循环中清除母体抗体后，FNAIT 几乎不会造成长期伤害。对于未来妊娠，可在妊娠中期和晚期每周给予 IVIG（联用或不联用皮质类固醇）以预防 FNAIT。

输血后紫癜　成人输血后可出现同种免疫性血小板减少症［即输血后紫癜（PTP）］。如同在新生儿中，这种情况是由于患者暴露于其自身血小板不表达的常见血小板同种抗原。例如，缺乏 HPA-1a 及既往在妊娠或输血时已经对该抗原形成同种免疫的个体，在输血后均可发生 PTP。由于超过 95% 的献血者表达 HPA-1a，且抗原随血小板而分散，故任何血液制品都可能含有 HPA-1a。

TABLE 7.3 Molecular Basis for Alloimmune Thrombocytopenia

Glycoprotein	Alleles (Alloantigens)	Phenotype/Frequency	Amino Acid and Location
IIIa	HPA-1a/1b	0.98/0.25	Leucine/proline; 33
Ib	HPA-2a/2b	0.99/0.14	Threonine/methionine; 145
IIb	HPA-3a/3b	0.91/0.70	Isoleucine/serine; 843
IIIa	HPA-4a/4b	0.99/0.01	Arginine/glutamine; 143
Ia	HPA-5a/5b	0.99/0.21	Glutamic acid/lysine; 505
IIIa	HPA-6a/6b	NA	Proline/glutamic acid; 407
IIIa	HPA-7a/7b	NA	Proline/glutamic acid; 407
IIIa	HPA-8a/8b	NA	Arginine/cystine; 636

HPA, Human platelet antigen; *NA*, data not available.

TABLE 7.4 Causes of Disseminated Intravascular Coagulation

Sepsis or Endotoxin
Gram-negative bacteremia

Tissue Damage
Trauma
Closed-head injury
Burns
Hypoperfusion or hypotension

Malignant Disease
Adenocarcinoma
Acute promyelocytic leukemia

Primary Vascular Disorders
Vasculitis
Giant hemangioma (Kasabach-Merritt syndrome)
Aortic aneurysm
Cardiac mural thrombus

Exogenous Causes
Snake venom
Activated-factor infusions (prothrombin-complex concentrate)

---

can contain HPA-1a. Although not clearly understood, some investigators have speculated that soluble HPA antigens are deposited onto endogenous platelets, resulting in their rapid clearance by anti-HPA alloantibodies.

The diagnosis of PTP can be confirmed by demonstrating anti-HPA antibodies in the serum of an affected individual. Patients are typically treated with IVIG, and additional transfusions must be derived from donors lacking the implicated HPA. Although HPA-1a is the most common cause of alloimmune thrombocytopenia, other platelet alloantigens can cause this clinical syndrome (Table 7.3).

Non–Immune-Mediated Platelet Destruction

Disseminated intravascular coagulation. One of the most common and potentially life-threatening causes of nonimmune platelet destruction is DIC, which is associated with sepsis, malignancy, advanced liver disease, and other disorders that trigger endotoxin release or cause severe tissue damage (Table 7.4). In DIC caused by bacterial sepsis, circulating endotoxin induces expression of tissue factor on circulating monocytes and endothelial cells, a process leading to overwhelming thrombin and fibrin generation. Deposition of fibrin occurs throughout the vasculature, with relatively inadequate concurrent fibrinolysis, leading to a thrombotic microangiopathic vasculopathy and subsequent organ damage. Thrombin activation of platelets and circulating factors eventually overwhelms the bone marrow and liver synthetic capability, respectively, resulting in thrombocytopenia and prolongation of the PT and aPTT.

Although the primary lesion of DIC is thrombin and clot generation, the clinical end point is usually a consumptive coagulopathy with depletion of platelets and coagulation factors. Mucosal bleeding, especially in the GI tract and oozing from intravenous puncture sites are signs of DIC.

Fibrinogen levels decrease in DIC but may be normal in earlier compensated stages and from the acute phase reaction to the underlying disorder, which increases fibrinogen production and secretion. DIC should not be ruled out because fibrinogen is in the normal range. Fibrinolysis in DIC is triggered by fibrin clot formation and the action of tissue-type plasminogen activator. Laboratory testing shows increased levels of fibrin split products (i.e. cleavage of fibrin monomers) and D-dimer (i.e., cleavage of fibrin-fibrin bonds), although these findings are nonspecific. The peripheral blood smear often contains schistocytes. Schistocytes are seen in other microangiopathic hemolytic anemias such as thrombotic thrombocytopenic purpura and hemolytic uremic syndrome (TTP/HUS), but these lead to excessive clotting, not bleeding (see Chapter 8).

Chronic DIC may be triggered by consumption of platelets and factors in large blood clots associated with aneurysms, hemangiomas, and mural thrombi. Another cause of chronic DIC is malignant disease, often adenocarcinoma or acute promyelocytic leukemia. Malignant cells in these disorders promote thrombin formation through secretion of tissue factor, cysteine proteases that activate factor X, induction of platelet-ligand binding, and upregulation of endothelial cell plasminogen activator inhibitor-1 (PAI-1) or cyclooxygenase 2 (COX2). Chronic DIC associated with malignancy usually causes enough factor consumption that the PT and aPTT are prolonged. Clinically, patients exhibit migratory thrombophlebitis (i.e., Trousseau syndrome) or nonbacterial thrombotic (marantic) endocarditis.

Therapy for DIC should be aimed at (1) treatment of the underlying disorder, such as antibiotics for sepsis or chemotherapy for malignant disease; (2) supportive hemostatic therapy, including platelets, cryoprecipitate (for fibrinogen), and FFP (for clotting factors); and (3) disruption of the activation of coagulation factors and platelets. For the last approach, anticoagulation is usually not indicated unless the balance of procoagulant and anticoagulant activity actively favors clotting, such as arterial thromboemboli with mural thrombus or migratory thrombophlebitis. These thrombotic complications of chronic DIC are often resistant to warfarin therapy and usually require more intensive anti-Xa therapy with unfractionated or low-molecular-weight heparin.

表 7.3　同种免疫性血小板减少症的分子基础

糖蛋白	等位基因（同种抗原）	表型/频率	氨基酸和位置
Ⅲa	HPA-1a/1b	0.98/0.25	亮氨酸/脯氨酸；33
Ⅰb	HPA-2a/2b	0.99/0.14	苏氨酸/甲硫氨酸；145
Ⅱb	HPA-3a/3b	0.91/0.70	异亮氨酸/丝氨酸；843
Ⅲa	HPA-4a/4b	0.99/0.01	精氨酸/谷氨酰胺；143
Ⅰa	HPA-5a/5b	0.99/0.21	谷氨酸/赖氨酸；505
Ⅲa	HPA-6a/6b	NA	脯氨酸/谷氨酸；407
Ⅲa	HPA-7a/7b	NA	脯氨酸/谷氨酸；407
Ⅲa	HPA-8a/8b	NA	精氨酸/胱氨酸；636

HPA，人血小板抗原；NA，数据不可用。

表 7.4　弥散性血管内凝血的病因

感染中毒症或内毒素
革兰氏阴性菌血症

组织损伤
创伤
闭合性头部损伤
烧伤
低灌注或低血压

恶性疾病
腺癌
急性早幼粒细胞白血病

原发性血管疾病
血管炎
巨大血管瘤（Kasabach-Merritt 综合征）
主动脉瘤
心脏附壁血栓

外源性病因
蛇毒
输注活化因子（凝血酶原复合体浓缩物）

虽然尚未完全明确，一些研究者推测可溶性 HPA 抗原可沉积在内源性血小板上，导致它们被抗 HPA 同种抗体快速清除。

PTP 可通过检测患者的血清中存在抗 HPA 抗体来确诊。患者通常使用 IVIG 治疗，且后续输血必须来源于无相关 HPA 的供者。虽然 HPA-1a 是同种免疫性血小板减少症的最常见原因，但其他血小板同种抗原也可引起该临床综合征（表 7.3）。

非免疫介导的血小板破坏

弥散性血管内凝血（DIC）　非免疫性血小板破坏中最常见和潜在危及生命的原因之一是 DIC，其与感染中毒症、恶性肿瘤、晚期肝病，以及引发内毒素释放或引起严重组织损伤的其他疾病相关（表 7.4）。在由细菌性感染中毒症引起的 DIC 中，循环内毒素诱导循环单核细胞和内皮细胞表达组织因子，导致生成大量的凝血酶和纤维蛋白。纤维蛋白沉积可发生在整个血管系统中，同时纤维蛋白溶解相对不足，导致血栓性微血管病性血管病变及随后的器官损伤。血小板和循环因子的凝血酶活化最终分别远远超过骨髓和肝的合成能力，导致血小板减少及 PT 和 APTT 延长。

虽然 DIC 的原发性损害是凝血酶和凝块产生的，但临床终点通常是消耗性凝血病，表现为血小板和凝血因子的耗竭。黏膜出血，特别是胃肠道出血及静脉穿刺部位渗血，是 DIC 的早期征兆。

DIC 患者的纤维蛋白原水平降低，但由于潜在疾病的急性期反应可增加纤维蛋白原的生成和分泌，早期代偿阶段纤维蛋白原水平可正常。因此，不能因为纤维蛋白原在正常范围内而排除 DIC。纤维蛋白凝块形成和组织型纤溶酶原激活物可触发 DIC 中的纤维蛋白溶解。实验室检查显示 DIC 患者纤维蛋白裂解产物（即纤维蛋白单体的裂解片段）和 D-二聚体（即纤维蛋白-纤维蛋白二聚体的裂解片段）水平增加，但这并不特异。患者外周血涂片通常含有破碎红细胞。但破碎红细胞也可见于其他微血管病性溶血性贫血，如血栓性血小板减少性紫癜/溶血性尿毒综合征（TTP/HUS），但这些疾病会导致过度凝血，而不是出血（见第 8 章）。

与动脉瘤、血管瘤和附壁血栓等相关的大血块可导致血小板和凝血因子消耗，从而诱导慢性 DIC。慢性 DIC 的另一原因是恶性疾病，通常是腺癌或急性早幼粒细胞白血病。这些疾病中的恶性细胞通过以下几个方面促进凝血酶形成：①分泌组织因子；②合成可激活因子 X 的半胱氨酸蛋白酶；③诱导血小板-配体结合；④上调内皮细胞纤溶酶原激活物抑制剂-1（PAI-1）或环氧合酶 2（COX-2）的表达。与恶性肿瘤相关的慢性 DIC 通常会引起大量凝血因子消耗，使 PT 和 APTT 延长。患者表现为迁移性血栓性静脉炎（即 Trousseau 综合征）或非细菌性血栓性（消耗性）心内膜炎。

DIC 的治疗应针对以下方面：①治疗潜在疾病，如感染中毒症给予抗生素或恶性疾病给予化疗；②支持性止血治疗，包括输注血小板、冷沉淀（含纤维蛋白原）和 FFP（含凝血因子）；③阻断凝血因子和血小板的活化。对于最后一点，通常不建议抗凝治疗，除非抗凝和促凝的平衡明显倾向于凝血，如伴随附壁血栓的动脉血栓栓塞或迁移性血栓性静脉炎。慢性 DIC 的这些血栓性并发症一般对华法林治疗耐药，通常需要使用普通肝素或低分子量肝素等高强度抗因子 Xa 治疗。

TABLE 7.5 Disorders Causing Abnormal Platelet Aggregation

Disorder	Epinephrine	Adp	Collagen	Arachidonic Acid	Ristocetin
Aspirin and NSAIDs	PW	PW	NL, ↓[a]	↓	NL
Glanzmann disease	Absent	Absent	Absent	Absent	PW
Bernard-Soulier syndrome	NL	NL	NL	NL	Absent
Storage pool disease	↓	PW	↓	NL, ↓	PW
Hermansky-Pudlak syndrome	↓	PW	↓	NL	PW
Gray platelet syndrome	↓	↓	↓	NL	NL
von Willebrand disease	NL	NL	NL	NL	↓, NL[b]

ADP, Adenosine diphosphate; *NL*, normal; *NSAIDs*, nonsteroidal anti-inflammatory drugs; *PW*, primary wave aggregation only; *↓*, decreased.
[a]Aspirin results in decreased aggregation with most collagen doses.
[b]In von Willebrand disease type 2B, patients have increased aggregation with low-dose ristocetin and decreased or normal aggregation with standard doses of ristocetin.

Thrombocytopenia with pregnancy-induced hypertension. Mild thrombocytopenia in pregnant women called gestational thrombocytopenia represents an effect of hemodilution as plasma volume increases through pregnancy, a normal physiologic response that can bring platelet counts into the range of 100,000 to 150,000/μL; these counts are not associated with maternal or fetal bleeding. However, pregnancy-induced hypertension can result in platelet counts of less than 100,000/μL, and these conditions can be associated with complications.

The spectrum of pregnancy-induced hypertension includes hypertension progressing to proteinuria and renal dysfunction (i.e., preeclampsia) and then to cerebral edema and seizures (i.e., eclampsia). Thrombocytopenia may appear as a late finding accompanying pregnancy-induced hypertension, often occurring at the time of delivery or late in the third trimester. HELLP syndrome in pregnancy (characterized by *h*emolysis, *e*levated *l*iver enzymes, and *l*ow *p*latelet counts) is occasionally associated with hypertension. The thrombocytopenia associated with pregnancy-induced hypertension or HELLP may result from abnormal vascular prostaglandin metabolism or placental dysfunction that leads to platelet consumption, vasculopathy, and microvascular occlusions. Both disorders are usually reversed by delivery of the fetus and placenta. Occasionally, IVIG or plasmapheresis is required when the disorder does not resolve after delivery.

Hemophagocytic lymphohistiocytosis. HLH is a deadly disease of T-cell and NK-cell dysregulation causing macrophage activation and extreme cytokine inflammatory responses. Histiocytes ingest blood in bone marrow and other organs. Cytopenias, fever, splenomegaly, liver function abnormalities, coagulopathy, and high levels of ferritin (typically >1000) ensue. In children, congenital causes can be found in perforin or granule fusion defects. In adults, an underlying malignancy (usually lymphoma) catalyzes the syndrome and is fatal without a stem cell transplant. Treatment otherwise entails chemotherapy with etoposide, steroids, and other immunosuppression. When associated with a rheumatologic disease, the name macrophage activation syndrome is used.

Consumption and dilutional thrombocytopenia. In addition to sequestration, hypoproductive, and destructive causes of thrombocytopenia, low platelet counts occasionally result from consumption and hemodilution. The pathophysiology of thrombocytopenia in these cases is directly attributable to the underlying cause of the bleeding, frequently large-scale trauma.

Overwhelming hemorrhage causes the consumption of endogenous platelets in an attempt to curb bleeding, and platelets are consumed faster than they can be released by the spleen or generated in the bone marrow. Resuscitative efforts after trauma, including infusion of massive volumes of intravenous fluids, red blood cells, and FFP, result in the dilution of circulating platelet numbers. The combination of platelet consumption and dilution during trauma can have catastrophic consequences and historically has been a leading cause of death in this setting. In addition to identifying the source of a large bleed, aggressive platelet transfusions in the setting of trauma may provide the greatest benefit in overcoming the effects of consumption and dilution (discussed in the "Standard Platelet Therapy" section).

BLEEDING CAUSED BY PLATELET FUNCTION DEFECTS

The ability of platelets to adhere to damaged vasculature and to recruit additional platelets into the clot is essential for primary hemostasis, especially when patients are challenged by trauma or surgery. Unlike bleeding caused by thrombocytopenia, individuals with platelet function defects bleed because their platelets cannot adhere or aggregate appropriately in response to in vivo stimuli.

These qualitative platelet disorders are most frequently encountered in individuals with normal or near-normal platelet counts. Evaluation often relies on tests that assess the function (rather than the number) of circulating platelets. From an epidemiologic standpoint, acquired qualitative platelet defects are much more frequently encountered than their congenital counterparts.

Acquired Causes of Platelet Dysfunction
Antiplatelet Therapy

The patient's history and preoperative screening should assess whether patients are taking medications that interfere with platelet function, such as aspirin and nonsteroidal anti-inflammatory drugs (NSAIDs). Aspirin irreversibly blocks arachidonic acid metabolism, and all exposed platelets are irreversibly affected so that affected platelets do not respond to stimulation even after aspirin is discontinued. The characteristic aspirin-induced platelet aggregation pattern is shown in Table 7.5 and Fig. 7.5.

Nonsteroidal anti-inflammatory drugs (NSAIDs) (e.g., indomethacin) reversibly inhibit cyclooxygenase (COX), and platelet function is restored within 48 hours after discontinuing the drug. Bleeding after most surgical procedures that is associated with aspirin or NSAIDs is

表 7.5 引起血小板聚集异常的疾病

疾病	对激动剂的反应				
	肾上腺素	ADP	胶原蛋白	花生四烯酸	瑞斯托霉素
阿司匹林和 NSAID	PW	PW	NL、↓[a]	↓	NL
格兰茨曼血小板功能不全（血小板无力症）	缺失	缺失	缺失	缺失	PW
巨血小板综合征	NL	NL	NL	NL	缺失
贮存池病	↓	PW	↓	NL、↓	PW
赫尔曼斯基-普德拉克综合征	↓	PW	↓	NL	PW
灰色血小板综合征	↓	↓	↓	↓	NL
血管性血友病	NL	NL	NL	NL	↓、NL[b]

ADP，腺苷二磷酸；NL，正常；NSAID，非甾体抗炎药；PW，仅有主要波聚集；↓，下降。
[a] 在大多数胶原蛋白剂量下，阿司匹林会导致血小板聚集减少。
[b] 在 2B 型血管性血友病患者中，低剂量瑞斯托霉素可使血小板聚集增加，而标准剂量的瑞斯托霉素使血小板聚集减少或保持正常。

妊娠高血压综合征伴血小板减少症 妊娠期女性出现的轻度血小板减少症被称为妊娠期血小板减少症，这是妊娠期间血浆容量增加导致血液稀释的结果，是一种正常的生理学反应，其可使血小板计数降至 100 000～150 000/μl，但不会导致母亲或胎儿出血。然而，妊娠高血压综合征可导致血小板计数＜100 000/μl，可能引发并发症。

妊娠高血压综合征的范围可从高血压进展为蛋白尿和肾功能障碍（即先兆子痫），到进展为脑水肿和癫痫发作（即子痫）。血小板减少症是妊娠高血压综合征的晚期表现，通常发生在分娩时或妊娠晚期。妊娠期 HELLP 综合征（以溶血、肝酶水平升高和血小板计数降低为特征）偶尔伴有高血压。与妊娠高血压综合征或 HELLP 综合征相关的血小板减少症可能是由血管前列腺素代谢异常或胎盘功能失调引起血小板消耗、血管病变和微血管闭塞所致。这两种疾病通常随胎儿和胎盘的娩出而好转。少数情况下，分娩后血小板减少症未缓解，应给予 IVIG 或血浆置换治疗。

噬血细胞性淋巴组织细胞增生症（HLH） HLH 是一种由 T 细胞和 NK 细胞失调引起巨噬细胞活化和过度细胞因子炎症反应的致死性疾病。组织细胞在骨髓和其他器官中吞噬血细胞，继而出现血细胞减少、发热、脾大、肝功能异常、凝血功能障碍和铁蛋白水平升高（通常＞1000 μg/L）。在儿童中，遗传性病因包括穿孔素或颗粒融合缺陷。在成人中，HLH 常继发于潜在的恶性肿瘤（通常是淋巴瘤），患者如不进行干细胞移植可能有生命危险。其他治疗包括使用依托泊苷、类固醇和其他免疫抑制药物进行化疗。若 HLH 与风湿病相关，则被称为巨噬细胞活化综合征。

消耗和稀释性血小板减少症 除血小板滞留、生成减少和破坏等原因导致血小板减少外，低血小板计数偶尔由消耗和血液稀释引起。在这些患者中，出血的潜在原因通常是大规模创伤，这是直接造成血小板减少的病理生理学原因。

严重出血时，血小板试图止血，导致内源性消耗，并且其消耗速度远快于脾释放或骨髓生成血小板的速度。创伤后的复苏措施（包括大量静脉补液、输注红细胞和 FFP）可导致循环血小板被稀释。创伤期间血小板消耗和血液稀释的联合作用可能造成严重后果，这也是既往创伤后死亡的主要原因。除了确定大出血的来源外，创伤后积极输注血小板可以最有效地克服血小板消耗和稀释的影响（见下文"标准血小板治疗"）。

由血小板功能缺陷引起的出血

血小板黏附至损伤血管并将额外的血小板募集到血块中的能力对于初级止血，特别是当患者面临创伤或手术时是必要的。与血小板减少症引起的出血不同，血小板功能缺陷个体的出血是因为血小板不能对体内刺激产生合适的黏附或聚集等应答。

这些血小板质量缺陷疾病最常见于血小板计数正常或接近正常的个体。评估通常依赖于检测循环血小板功能（而不是数量）。从流行病学角度看，获得性血小板质量缺陷比先天性血小板缺陷更常见。

血小板功能障碍的获得性病因
抗血小板治疗

应通过病史和术前筛查评估患者是否正在服用干扰血小板功能的药物，如阿司匹林等非甾体抗炎药（NSAID）。阿司匹林不可逆地阻断花生四烯酸的正常代谢，且所有暴露的血小板均受到不可逆的影响，因此即使停用阿司匹林，血小板也不能对刺激做出反应。阿司匹林诱导的血小板聚集模式见表 7.5 和图 7.5。

NSAID（如吲哚美辛）可逆地抑制 COX，在停药 24～48 h 后血小板功能可以恢复。与阿司匹林等 NSAID 相关的大多数术后出血通常为轻度，因此术前

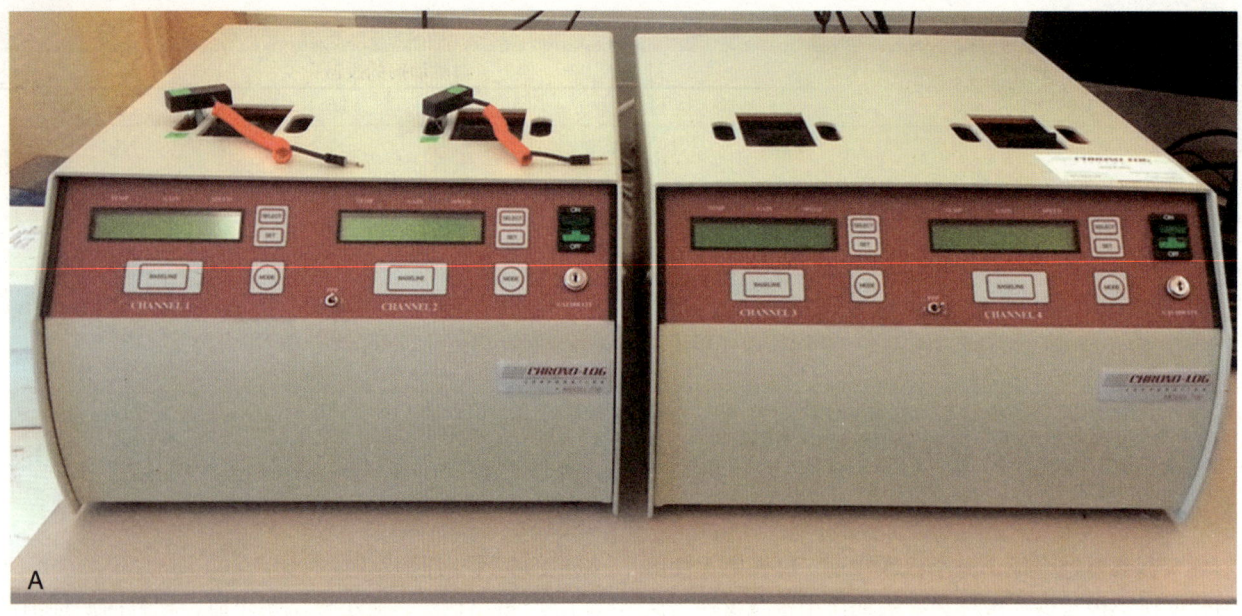

Fig. 7.5 Methodology underlying light transmission aggregometry. (A) Typical laboratory light transmission aggregometer. (B) Platelet function is directly proportional to light transmission in this assay. Platelet-rich plasma, which prevents light transmission, is exposed to various agonists (i.e., adenosine diphosphate, epinephrine, collagen, arachidonic acid, and ristocetin). As platelets begin to aggregate or agglutinate, light transmission increases over time and is typically reflected as a primary or secondary wave of aggregation for most agonists. Low or no increase in light transmission typically correlates with diminished platelet function.

usually mild, so aspirin may not need to be discontinued before surgery, especially considering aspirin-induced platelet dysfunction is desirable in patients at risk for stroke or myocardial infarction.

The aspirin effect is restricted to COX1, and various NSAIDs have different relative affinities for COX1 and COX2. COX2 is an inducible enzyme that is synthesized in endothelial cells in response to inflammatory cytokines. Suppression of COX2 reduces synthesis of endothelial cell prostaglandin I_2 (i.e., prostacyclin), a molecule that exhibits antithrombotic effects through inhibition of platelet aggregation. The net effect of nonselective NSAIDs on the prothrombotic or antithrombotic balance favors bleeding because NSAID-induced COX1 inhibition means that thromboxane A_2 production in platelets is blocked. In contrast, the increased cardiovascular risk with administration of more selective COX2 inhibitors is probably attributable to the COX2-induced lack of endothelial cell prostacyclin production, coupled with intact platelet function (i.e., no inhibition of thromboxane A_2 by COX2 blockade).

Another category of antiplatelet agents acts independently of the COX1/2 pathways. These drugs are P2Y12 receptor antagonists (e.g., clopidogrel, prasugrel). They disrupt function by irreversibly binding

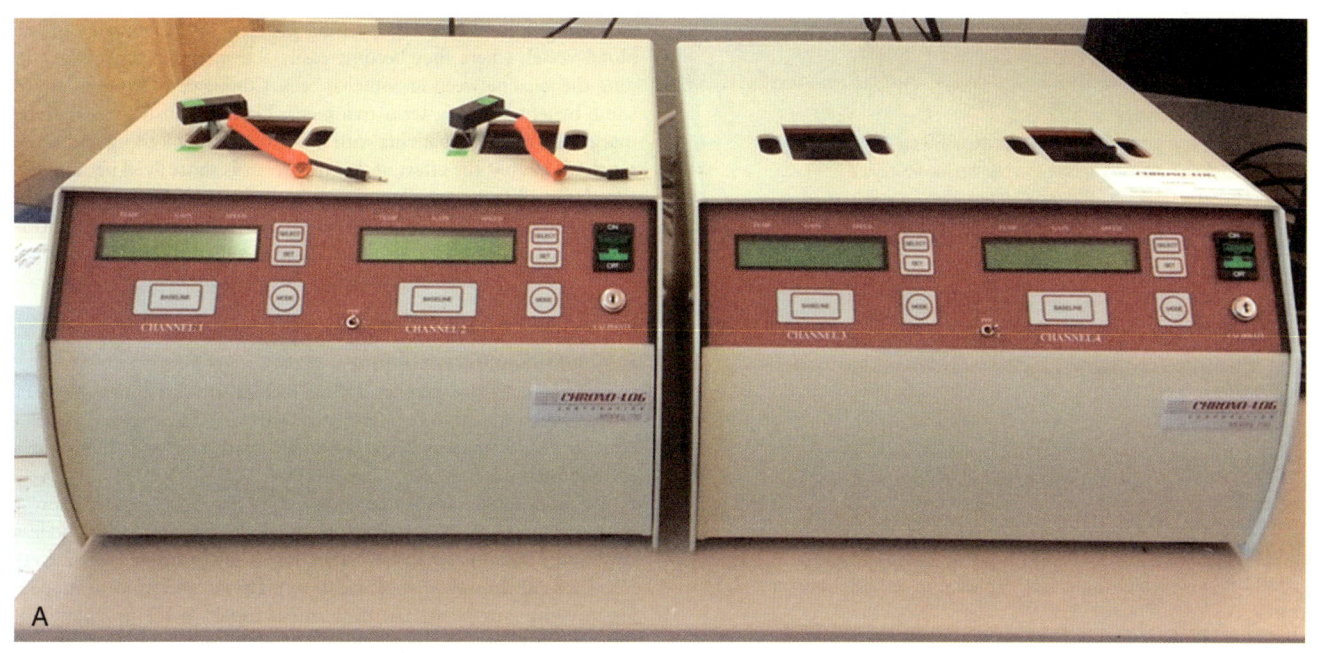

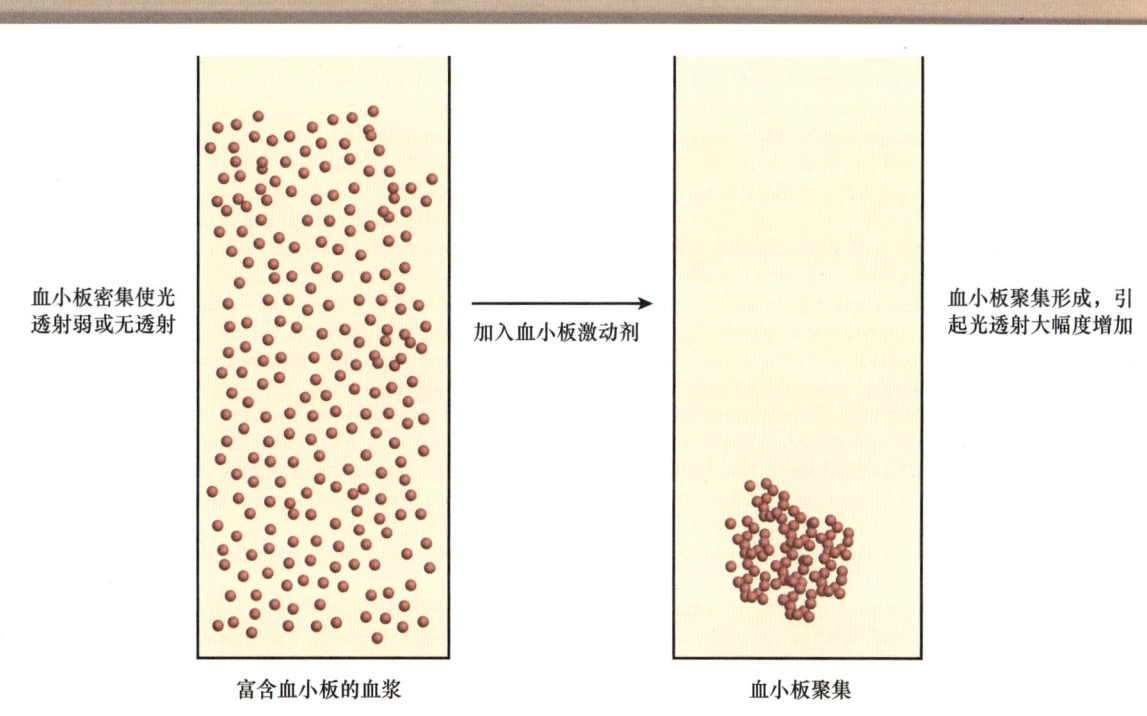

图 7.5 光电比浊法检测血小板聚集的方法。A. 典型的实验室光电比浊法血小板聚集仪。B. 在该检测中，血小板功能与光的透射率成正比。富含血小板的血浆可阻止光透过，将其暴露于各种血小板激动剂（即腺苷二磷酸、肾上腺素、胶原蛋白、花生四烯酸和瑞斯托霉素）后，随着血小板开始聚集或凝集，光透射量逐渐增加，大多数激动剂可导致主要或次要聚集波。光透射较低或无增加通常与血小板功能减弱有关

可能不需要停用阿司匹林，尤其是对于有卒中或心肌梗死风险的患者，阿司匹林诱导的血小板功能障碍是有利的。

阿司匹林的效应仅限于 COX-1，各种 NSAID 对 COX-1 和 COX-2 的相对亲和力不尽相同。COX-2 是在炎症细胞因子作用下在内皮细胞中合成的诱导酶。抑制 COX-2 可减少内皮细胞前列腺素 I_2（即前列环素）的合成，该物质可通过抑制血小板聚集而表现出抗血栓形成作用。非选择性 NSAID 在促血栓或抗血栓平衡中的净效应是倾向于出血，因为 NSAID 诱导的 COX-1 抑制意味着血小板中血栓素 A_2 的生成被阻断。相反，应用选择性更强的 COX-2 抑制剂会出现心血管风险增加，这可能归因于 COX-2 诱导的内皮细胞前列环素生成不足，以及血小板功能未受影响（即阻断 COX-2 没有抑制血栓素 A_2）。

另一类抗血小板药物不通过 COX-1/2 通路发挥作用。这些药物是 P2Y12 受体拮抗剂（如氯吡格雷、普拉格雷）。它们通过不可逆地结合血小板激动剂 ADP

TABLE 7.6	Drugs Affecting Platelet Function
Strong Inhibitors	
Abciximab (and other anti-GPIIb/IIIa or anti-RGD compounds)	
Aspirin (often contained in over-the-counter medications)	
Clopidogrel, ticlopidine (ADP-receptor blockers)	
Nonsteroidal anti-inflammatory drugs	
Moderate Inhibitors	
Antibiotics (penicillins, cephalosporins, nitrofurantoin)	
Dextran	
Fibrinolytics	
Heparin	
Hetastarch	
Weak Inhibitors	
Alcohol	
Nitroglycerin	
Nitroprusside	

ADP, Adenosine diphosphate; *GP*, glycoprotein; *RGD*, arginine-glycine-aspartate.

to the surface receptor for the platelet agonist, ADP. P2Y12 receptor antagonists are primarily used as adjunctive anticoagulant therapy for individuals at risk for thrombosis associated with coronary artery disease and stroke. These drugs can inhibit platelet activation at the site of injury, not unlike the effect in an individual taking aspirin, and further potentiate bleeding.

Regardless of the type of agent used, discontinuing an antiplatelet drug is a reasonable first step for a patient who has moderate to severe bleeding while on the therapy. Discontinuation of aspirin will not help the affected platelets because its inhibition is irreversible, but this will allow newly produced platelets to be free of drug effect and function appropriately at the site of an injury.

Beyond stopping the offending drug, bleeding caused by aspirin or other antiplatelet agents may be addressed by infusion of 1-deamino-(8-D-arginine)-vasopressin (DDAVP, desmopressin), although the results of small clinical trials have been mixed regarding its benefit to platelet function and bleeding cessation. Occasionally, platelet transfusion is necessary. In most cases, a single platelet transfusion of 4 to 6 random donor units (or one apheresis unit) contributes enough normal platelets (>10% of total circulating number) to restore primary hemostasis. Platelet dysfunction and bleeding caused by other drugs is similarly treated by discontinuing the drug and providing platelet transfusions when needed (Table 7.6).

Uremic Platelet Dysfunction

Renal insufficiency can be associated with the accumulation of toxic proteins, which induce high levels of nitric oxide formation by vascular endothelial cells and inhibit platelet function. The uremic state can also suppress platelet secretory pathways and platelet adhesion to exposed endothelium through mechanisms that are not well understood. Nonetheless, the uremic state does put an individual at risk for platelet dysfunction–related bleeding. Because no formal tests are available, the diagnosis should be suspected in individuals with acute or chronic renal failure who demonstrate bleeding.

Short-term treatment of uremic platelet dysfunction includes administration of DDAVP. This increases circulating von Willebrand factor, which can help to overcome some of the uremia-associated platelet deficits. Transfusion of red blood cells also seems to help by increasing volume, thereby pushing platelets to the margins of the blood vessel, where they become easily activated and more likely to plug the gaps between endothelial cells. Conjugated estrogens are of some benefit for long-term treatment. Platelet transfusions may be marginally useful in patients with life-threatening bleeding and acute renal failure, but the effect of this treatment is short lived because the transfused platelets rapidly acquire the uremic defect. Platelet transfusion should not be considered as a first-line therapy for most forms of uremic bleeding. Ultimately, renal replacement therapy, including dialysis or renal transplantation, may be necessary.

Congenital Causes of Platelet Dysfunction
Platelet Glycoprotein Defects

Inherited qualitative platelet defects include abnormalities of platelet receptors and granules. Two rare but well-characterized platelet receptor disorders are Bernard-Soulier syndrome and Glanzmann thrombasthenia.

Bernard-Soulier syndrome is caused by decreased surface expression of platelet GPIb, a key receptor for von Willebrand factor and less commonly by diminished GPIb function. The syndrome is characterized by mild thrombocytopenia, large platelets, and mild to moderate bleeding symptoms. The diagnosis is usually made in childhood, but some patients may be discovered in adulthood. Laboratory testing for Bernard-Soulier syndrome shows an absent platelet aggregation response to ristocetin (see Table 7.5 and Fig. 7.5) despite adequate VWF activity.

Glanzmann thrombasthenia is characterized by an increased bleeding time and abnormally low levels of expression of platelet GPIIb/IIIa (receptor for VWF and fibrinogen) or, less commonly, normal expression but absent GPIIb/IIIa function, while platelet count remains normal. Patients usually exhibit bleeding in childhood. Whereas patients with Bernard-Soulier syndrome have an elevated mean platelet volume (MPV), MPV is normal in Glanzmann thrombasthenia. In cases of Glanzmann thrombasthenia, platelet aggregation testing confirms an absent or diminished response to all agonists except ristocetin (see Table 7.5 and Fig. 7.5).

Platelet transfusions correct the bleeding in Bernard-Soulier syndrome and Glanzmann thrombasthenia. However, because of the high risk for alloimmunization with frequent platelet transfusions (particularly because patients lack GPIb or GPIIb/IIIa), this therapy should be used sparingly. Instead, factor VIIa can be used with high efficacy for both diseases. DDAVP has some benefit in Bernard-Soulier syndrome.

Platelet Granule or Secretory Defects

Inherited platelet granule disorders are defined by the type of granule that is absent or defective. Storage pool disease is characterized by a relative decrease or absence of dense granules and correspondingly moderate to severe mucosal bleeding. Release of dense granule contents that recruit and activate platelets is impaired. Storage pool disease has a diminished or absent secondary wave of aggregation in response to most agonists (see Table 7.5 and Fig. 7.5).

Hermansky-Pudlak syndrome is a dense granule deficiency associated with oculocutaneous albinism, nystagmus, and pulmonary fibrosis. Multiple gene defects have been attributed to Hermansky-Pudlak syndrome and cause lysosome dysfunction. Patients may have spontaneous bleeding, but bleeding more often occurs with surgical procedures or trauma. This can be particularly problematic for the patients who undergo lung transplant for pulmonary fibrosis.

Chédiak-Higashi syndrome is a rare dense granule disorder characterized by mild bleeding, partial albinism, and recurrent pyogenic infections. It is caused by a mutation in the *LYST* gene leading to lysosome dysregulation. Large, irregular, gray-blue inclusions (granules)

表 7.6　影响血小板功能的药物
强效抑制剂 阿昔单抗（及其他抗 GPⅡb/Ⅲa 或抗 RGD 化合物） 阿司匹林（通常包含在非处方药物中） 氯吡格雷、噻氯吡定（ADP 受体阻滞剂） 非甾体抗炎药
中效抑制剂 抗生素（青霉素类、头孢菌素类、呋喃妥因） 右旋糖酐 纤溶剂 肝素 羟乙基淀粉
弱效抑制剂 酒精 硝酸甘油 硝普钠

ADP，腺苷二磷酸；GP，糖蛋白；RGD，精氨酸-甘氨酸-天冬氨酸。

的表面受体来破坏血小板功能。P2Y12 受体拮抗剂主要用于具有冠状动脉疾病和脑卒中相关血栓形成风险个体的辅助抗凝治疗。这些药物可抑制损伤部位的血小板活化，与服用阿司匹林的效果类似，并进一步促进出血。

无论使用何种药物，中重度出血最合理的第一步治疗是停用抗血小板药物。停用阿司匹林对受累血小板没有影响，因为其抑制作用是不可逆的，但新生成的血小板不受药物影响并能在损伤部位发挥作用。

除了停用药物外，由阿司匹林或其他抗血小板药物诱发的出血也可通过输注 1-去氨基-(8-D-精氨酸) 血管升压素（DDAVP；去氨加压素）来处理，但关于其对血小板功能和止血益处的小型临床试验结果不一致。患者有时需要输注血小板。在大多数情况下，单纯输注 4~6 U 随机供者血小板（或 1 U 单采血小板）可提供足够的正常血小板（> 10% 的总循环数）以恢复初始止血。由其他药物引起的血小板功能障碍和出血也可通过停药并在需要时输注血小板进行治疗（表 7.6）。

尿毒症性血小板功能障碍

肾功能不全可与毒性蛋白的累积相关，其可诱导血管内皮细胞形成高水平的一氧化氮，以抑制血小板功能。尿毒症状态也可抑制血小板分泌途径，并抑制血小板黏附到暴露的内皮，其机制尚不明确。然而，尿毒症状态会使个体处于血小板功能障碍相关的出血风险中。由于没有正式的检测手段，对于表现为出血的急性或慢性肾衰竭患者，应疑诊尿毒症性血小板功能障碍。

尿毒症性血小板功能障碍的短期治疗包括给予 DDAVP，以增加循环中的 vWF，这有助于纠正尿毒症相关的血小板缺陷。输注红细胞也可能有帮助，其可通过增加血容量将血小板推到血管边缘，使其更易被激活，更有可能堵塞内皮细胞之间的间隙。联用雌激素对长期治疗有一定益处。输注血小板对危及生命的出血和急性肾衰竭患者可能略有帮助，但治疗效果短暂，因为输注的血小板会快速获得尿毒症缺陷，血小板输注不应作为大多数尿毒症性出血的一线治疗方法。患者最终可能需要进行肾脏替代治疗，包括透析或肾移植。

血小板功能障碍的先天性病因

血小板糖蛋白缺陷

遗传性血小板质量缺陷包括血小板受体和颗粒的异常。两种罕见但特征明显的血小板受体疾病是巨血小板综合征（Bernard-Soulier 综合征）和格兰茨曼血小板功能不全（血小板无力症）。

巨血小板综合征由血小板表面 GPⅠb（vWF 的关键受体）表达下降引起，少数情况由 GPⅠb 功能减弱引起。该综合征的特点是轻度血小板减少、大血小板和轻中度出血症状。该病通常在儿童期被诊断，但部分患者可能在成年时才确诊。尽管 vWF 活性正常，但实验室检查可见患者的血小板对瑞斯托霉素的诱导无聚集反应（表 7.5 和图 7.5）。

格兰茨曼血小板功能不全的特点是出血时间延长、血小板 GPⅡb/Ⅲa（即 vWF 和纤维蛋白原的受体）异常低水平表达，少数也可表现为 GPⅡb/Ⅲa 表达正常但功能缺失，但血小板计数保持正常。患者通常在儿童期出现出血。巨血小板综合征患者的平均血小板体积（MPV）增大，而格兰茨曼血小板功能不全患者的 MPV 正常。在格兰茨曼血小板功能不全患者中，血小板聚集试验可见患者对所有血小板激动剂（除瑞斯托霉素外）均无反应或反应减弱（表 7.5 和图 7.5）。

血小板输注可纠正巨血小板综合征和格兰茨曼血小板功能不全引起的出血。但是，由于频繁输注血小板引起的同种免疫的风险很高（尤其是因为患者缺乏 GPⅠb 或 GPⅡb/Ⅲa），应谨慎使用该治疗。因子Ⅶa 对这两种疾病均有很好的疗效。DDAVP 对巨血小板综合征有一定疗效。

血小板颗粒或分泌缺陷

遗传性血小板颗粒疾病由缺失或缺陷的颗粒类型来定义。贮存池病的特点是血小板的致密颗粒相对减少或缺失，以及相应的中重度黏膜出血。招募和激活血小板的致密颗粒内容物的释放受损。贮存池病对大多数血小板激动剂的继发聚集效应减弱或消失（表 7.5 和图 7.5）。

赫尔曼斯基-普德拉克综合征（Hermansky-Pudlak 综合征）是一种伴有眼皮肤白化病、眼球震颤和肺纤维化的致密颗粒缺陷疾病。其归因于多种基因缺陷导致的溶酶体功能障碍。患者可出现自发性出血，但出血更多见于外科手术或创伤中。严重患者可能因为肺纤维化而需要接受肺移植手术。

白细胞异常色素减退综合征（Chédiak-Higashi 综合征）是一种罕见的致密颗粒疾病，以轻度出血、局部皮肤白化病和反复发作的化脓性感染为特征。它由 *LYST* 基因突变导致溶酶体失调引起，在中性粒细胞和其他白

are seen in neutrophils and other white blood cells. Many patients with Chédiak-Higashi syndrome develop an accelerated phase with HLH.

Gray platelet syndrome is characterized by colorless or gray platelets that lack normal staining on the peripheral smear. Electron microscopy confirms the loss of α-granules or their contents. A mutation in the gene *NBEAL* disrupts vesicle trafficking, leading to a deficiency of the α-granules. Patients with gray platelet syndrome have a history of mild bleeding, and aggregation testing detects diminished responses to epinephrine, ADP, and collagen.

Thrombocytopenia with small platelets is characteristic of Wiskott-Aldrich syndrome, an X-linked recessive disorder with eczema and immunodeficiency that can be diagnosed by the lack of CD43 expression on T lymphocytes. A *WAS* gene mutation results in a defect in the actin cytoskeleton followed by a deficiency in platelet dense granules. Most patients with Wiskott-Aldrich syndrome will not survive without a stem cell transplant.

May-Hegglin anomaly and related myosin heavy-chain 9 gene (*MYH9*) diseases are characterized by giant platelets and Döhle bodies (i.e., basophilic inclusions in leukocytes). Platelet count is low and a family history of bleeding is common because the inheritance pattern is autosomal dominant. Unlike the other diseases in this section, *MYH9* diseases have normal granules and normal platelet aggregation, but the *MYH9* mutation impairs the platelet cytoskeleton, which affects clot retraction. With thrombopoietin agonists, the additional platelets produced are also dysfunctional, but the quantitative increase in platelets may be enough to stop bleeding.

All the platelet dysfunction disorders are treated by avoiding antiplatelet drugs, using hormonal control of menses in women, and transfusing platelets when bleeding occurs.

Platelet Transfusion Therapy
Standard Platelet Therapy

Platelet transfusions derived from the whole blood of healthy donors can be used to stop or prevent bleeding. The two broad categories of platelet transfusion support are based on the conditions previously discussed: prophylactic platelet transfusions for thrombocytopenia in nonbleeding patients and platelet transfusion for acute bleeding.

For the nonbleeding thrombocytopenic patient, several triggers can prompt platelet transfusion in the absence of frank hemorrhage. Patients receiving chemotherapy may be severely thrombocytopenic and should be transfused when their platelet counts are less than 10,000/μL to prevent spontaneous bleeding. This is a safe and appropriate threshold for patients with relatively uncomplicated clinical pictures without fever, sepsis, or bleeding. The threshold of 10,000/μL, which was rigorously established through several prospective, randomized, controlled trials, significantly decreases the frequency of platelet transfusion and thereby reduces risks associated with multiple blood product exposures. If the patient has complicating circumstances, prophylactic transfusions may be given when platelet counts are lower than 20,000/μL, although this threshold is not rigorously based on clinical trial evidence.

For patients undergoing invasive procedures or who suffer trauma, it is reasonable to transfuse platelets when counts are lower than 50,000/μL. Higher platelet counts (>100,000/μL) are recommended for patients undergoing neurologic surgery. The thresholds of 50,000/μL and 100,000/μL are based primarily on experience and published guidelines. Clinical trials are lacking in these settings.

For the acutely bleeding patient, the decision to transfuse platelets depends on several factors, of which thrombocytopenia is the most straightforward and useful criterion. Platelet counts higher than 50,000/μL are a reasonable goal for most cases of acute bleeding, whereas counts higher than 100,000/μL may be necessary for neurologic bleeding.

Congenital or acquired platelet dysfunction must be considered for acutely bleeding patients. Those with significant bleeding who have taken an antiplatelet drug such as aspirin may benefit from platelet transfusion regardless of baseline counts. Another consideration is the volume of blood products and fluids received. Trauma patients may receive more than 10 units of transfused red blood cells in addition to plasma, volume expanders, and saline solutions. Resuscitation with large fluid volumes (≥10 units transfused) reduces the platelet count to less than 50% of baseline, resulting in a significant dilutional coagulopathy. In these scenarios, repeated platelet counts must be obtained and platelets liberally transfused to maintain adequate hemostasis. Similarly, clotting factors need repletion during massive transfusion (see "Dilutional Coagulopathy" section).

Blood banks provide random-donor pooled platelets and apheresis platelets. Random-donor pooled platelets consist of platelet concentrates from four to six donors combined (pooled) into one large dose. For the adult patient with uncomplicated thrombocytopenia, a single random-donor platelet concentrate unit typically raises the platelet count by about 8000 to 10,000/μL. Between 4 and 6 units pooled together can be expected to raise counts by 30,000 to 60,000 platelets/μL. Apheresis platelets are collected from one donor using automated apheresis instruments. The dose of these *single-donor platelets* is almost equivalent to that of a 6-unit platelet pool and is estimated to increase platelet count by up to 50,000/μL in an uncomplicated patient.

Based on the expected increments and typical transfusion goals outlined previously, one random-donor platelet pool (6 units pooled together) or one apheresis platelet product should sufficiently raise platelet counts to improve thrombocytopenia and prevent spontaneous bleeding. These doses should also be sufficient to stop or prevent bleeding associated with thrombocytopenia in the setting of invasive procedures, mild to moderate trauma, or bleeding associated with platelet dysfunction. For the complicated patient (e.g., thrombocytopenia with intracranial hemorrhage, massive trauma), additional platelet doses may be necessary to achieve adequate hemostasis.

Platelet Transfusion Failure and Platelet Refractoriness

Platelet transfusions in thrombocytopenic patients are not successful in all cases. Uremia causes an acquired dysfunction of transfused platelets, limiting their hemostatic capabilities in vivo. Patients who are thrombocytopenic due to conditions such as ITP usually do not show increased platelet counts after transfusion because circulating autoantibodies cause rapid destruction of both endogenous and infused (exogenous) platelets. This phenomenon, known as platelet transfusion refractoriness, can be caused by many other recipient problems, including fever, sepsis, splenomegaly, and DIC. Although the pathophysiology of refractoriness is well understood for conditions such as ITP or DIC (in which platelets are cleared from the circulation), few data are available to suggest why individuals with conditions such as fever or infection have an inappropriate response to platelet transfusion.

When approaching a patient with platelet transfusion refractoriness, the physician should consider whether it is mediated by nonimmune or immune factors. Immune refractoriness indicates antibody-mediated clearance. For nonimmune-mediated refractoriness, as in fever or DIC, the underlying conditions usually decrease transfused platelet survival over time but do not affect immediate platelet recovery.

A standard diagnostic approach to platelet refractoriness involves measuring the platelet count 10 minutes to 1 hour after completion of the platelet transfusion. The patient with non–immune-mediated

细胞中可见大的、不规则的、灰蓝色包涵体（颗粒）。许多白细胞异常色素减退综合征患者可进展为 HLH。

灰色血小板综合征的特征是外周血涂片可见缺乏正常染色的无色或灰色血小板。电子显微镜可证实 α 颗粒或其内容物的缺失。NBEAL 基因突变可破坏囊泡运输，导致 α 颗粒缺失。灰色血小板综合征患者可有轻度出血病史，聚集试验显示其对肾上腺素、ADP 和胶原蛋白的反应减弱。

血小板减少伴血小板变小是威-奥综合征（Wiskott-Aldrich 综合征）的特征，这是一种伴有湿疹和免疫缺陷的 X 连锁隐性遗传病，可通过检测到 T 淋巴细胞上缺乏 CD43 表达来诊断。WAS 基因突变可导致肌动蛋白细胞骨架缺陷，进而出现血小板致密颗粒缺陷。如果不进行干细胞移植，大多数威-奥综合征患者无法存活。

梅-黑异常［May-Hegglin 异常（MHA）］及其相关的肌球蛋白重链 9 基因（MYH9）疾病的特征是巨大血小板和 Döhle 小体（即白细胞内的嗜碱性包涵体）。由于该病呈常染色体显性遗传，故血小板计数减低、出血家族史很常见。与本章中的其他疾病不同，MYH9 疾病患者的血小板颗粒和血小板聚集功能正常，但 MYH9 突变会破坏血小板细胞骨架，从而影响血凝块收缩。使用血小板生成素激动剂时，新产生的血小板也会发生功能障碍，但血小板数量的增加可能足以发挥止血功能。

所有血小板颗粒疾病的治疗均包括避免应用抗血小板药物、激素控制女性月经、出血时给予血小板输注。

血小板输注治疗

标准血小板治疗

输注来自健康献血者全血中的血小板可用于止血或预防出血。基于上文讨论的情况，血小板输注支持治疗可分为两大类：未出血的血小板减少症患者的预防性血小板输注和急性出血时的血小板输注。

对于未出血的血小板减少症患者，多个触发因素可在未出血的情况下提示需要进行血小板输注。接受化疗的患者可能出现严重血小板减少症，当其血小板计数 < 10 000/μl 时应输注血小板，以防止自发性出血。对于没有发热、感染中毒症或出血等临床病情相对简单的患者，10 000/μl 是安全、合适的阈值，并已经过多项前瞻性随机对照试验的严格验证，可显著降低血小板输注的频率，从而降低与多种血液制品暴露相关的风险。如果患者的情况复杂，当血小板计数 < 20 000/μl 时，可进行预防性输注，但这一阈值并非基于严格的临床试验证据。

对于接受有创性操作或创伤患者，当血小板计数 < 50 000/μl 时，输注血小板是合理的。对于接受神经系统手术的患者，建议使用更高的血小板计数阈值（> 100 000/μl）。采用 50 000/μl 或 100 000/μl 作为阈值主要是基于临床经验和已发布的指南，但缺乏相应的临床试验证据。

对于急性出血患者，是否输注血小板取决于多个因素，其中血小板减少是最直接、最有效的标准。对于大多数急性出血，合理的目标是血小板计数 > 50 000/μl，而神经系统出血则可能需要血小板计数 > 100 000/μl。

急性出血患者必须考虑先天性或获得性血小板功能障碍。服用抗血小板药物（如阿司匹林）的患者出现严重出血时，无论基线血小板计数如何，都可能从血小板输注中获益。另一个考虑因素是血液制品的输注量和补液量。创伤患者除输注血浆、扩容剂和生理盐水外，还可以接受 > 10 U 的红细胞输注。大量液体复苏（输血量 ≥ 10 U）可将血小板计数降至基线的 50% 以下，导致显著的稀释性凝血功能障碍。在这些情况下，必须反复监测血小板计数，并输注足量的血小板以维持充分的止血功能。同样，大量输血时也需要补充凝血因子（见下文"稀释性凝血功能障碍"）。

血库能够提供随机供者富集血小板和单采血小板。随机供者富集血小板由 4～6 名供者的血小板浓缩物组成（合并）一个大剂量。对于无并发症的成人血小板减少症患者，1 个单位随机供者血小板浓缩物通常可将血小板计数提高 8000～10 000/μl。4～6 个单位合并在一起预计可将血小板增加 30 000～60 000/μl。单采血小板是使用自动化单采仪采集 1 名供者的血小板。这些单供者血小板的剂量几乎相当于 6 个单位浓缩血小板的剂量，预计可使无合并症患者的血小板计数增加 50 000/μl。

基于上文所述的预期增量和特定输血目标，1 份随机供者富集血小板（6 个单位合并）或 1 份单采血小板制品应足以提高血小板计数至改善血小板减少症，并防止自发性出血。在血小板减少症患者进行有创性操作、发生轻中度创伤时，以及血小板功能障碍患者发生出血时，这些剂量足以止血或预防出血。对于病情复杂的患者（如血小板减少症伴颅内出血、严重创伤），可能需要更大的血小板剂量以达到有效止血。

血小板输注失败和血小板无效输注

输注血小板并非对所有血小板减少症患者都有效。尿毒症会导致输注的血小板出现获得性功能障碍，限制其在体内的止血能力。由于循环中的自身抗体会快速破坏内源性和输注（外源性）的血小板，因此输血后 ITP 等疾病所致的血小板减少通常不会改善。这种现象被称为血小板无效输注，可由多种受血者问题所致，包括发热、感染中毒症、脾大和 DIC。尽管 ITP 或 DIC 等情况引起血小板无效输注的病理生理学机制已被阐明（血小板从循环中被清除），但有关发热或感染等疾病患者血小板输注疗效欠佳的机制，目前仍所知甚少。

当接诊血小板无效输注的患者时，医生应考虑其是由非免疫因素还是免疫因素介导的。免疫介导的无效输注是指抗体介导的清除。对于非免疫介导的无效输注，如发热或 DIC 时，基础疾病通常会随着时间推移而降低输注血小板的存活率，但不影响血小板的即刻恢复。

血小板无效输注的标准诊断方法包括在血小板输

refractoriness typically shows an initial increase at 10 minutes but then a blunted increase in the platelet count 1 hour after transfusion, with a subsequent decline at a steeper rate than expected because of the underlying disorder. For patients with this type of platelet refractoriness, addressing the underlying illness often increases the effectiveness of platelet transfusions.

For patients with immune-mediated platelet refractoriness, there is virtually no increase in the platelet count, even minutes after completion of a transfusion. The antiplatelet antibodies are most frequently encountered in individuals who have been recurrently transfused. Repeated exposures to transfused products can induce alloantibodies, most commonly to HLA antigens. Over time and with multiple transfusion exposures, the titer of alloantibodies can increase sharply and cause rapid clearance of incompatible platelets after infusion.

For the alloimmunized patient, immunosuppression fails to decrease platelet alloantibodies, and efforts to improve platelet recovery after transfusion are focused on finding compatible platelet units. The first step in managing transfusion of the alloimmunized patient is to provide ABO antigen–matched platelets to minimize clearance caused by naturally occurring ABO antibodies; this is often helpful because platelets express A and B antigens on their surface. If this step fails to yield increases in platelet counts, donor platelets that lack target antigens for the detected alloantibodies should be pursued. One strategy is to use the patient's serum to crossmatch platelet donor units, with selection of those units demonstrating compatibility for subsequent transfusion.

If crossmatch-compatible platelets fail to induce adequate platelet recovery, blood banks should provide platelets that are matched to the recipient's HLA system in the hope of evading HLA-based antibodies. HLA-matched platelets are collected from compatible donors using apheresis at frequent intervals until the patient's platelet count recovers and they are no longer transfusion dependent. Many blood banks and transfusion services have attempted to address the problem of platelet HLA alloimmunization through prevention. They provide blood products that have undergone filtration to reduce their white blood cell content, a process called *leukoreduction*. Because contaminating leukocytes are the primary sources of exposure to HLAs, their removal can be quite effective in preventing subsequent alloimmunization, even in chronically transfused patients.

BLEEDING CAUSED BY VON WILLEBRAND DISEASE

Von Willebrand disease is caused by either a deficiency or dysfunction of von Willebrand factor. Because VWF is a key component to primary hemostasis, its deficiency results in easy bleeding, typically superficial (bruising, mucosal). However, VWF is a stabilizer of factor VIII and when VWF is low, factor VIII is rapidly cleared, resulting in declining factor VIII levels and an elevated aPTT. If factor VIII levels are low enough, patients can have deeper bleeding as in hemophilia A and B with muscle hematomas, hemarthroses, and bleeding into the central nervous system. VWF is synthesized in endothelial cells and megakaryocytes and functions in plasma to mediate platelet adhesion to the damaged site. VWF is a large, multimeric protein; the largest multimers contain the greatest number of adhesive sites and confer greater hemostatic ability than smaller VWF molecules. In patients with low VWF levels, platelet adhesion to damaged vessels is delayed.

VWD is grouped into three main subtypes. Type 1 VWD results from a decline in VWF antigen. Decline in VWF antigen parallels a decline in VWF activity. Type 2 VWD represents a dysfunctional VWF, leading to a more significant decline in VWF activity than VWF antigen. Type 3 VWD is the most severe type. Patients with type 3 VWD do not make any VWF.

Type 1 von Willebrand Disease

Type 1 VWD is the most common type. Although severity can vary significantly, it tends to be mild. The cause is not always clear because many cases of type 1 VWD have a normal VWF gene sequence. Therefore, other factors must be in play such as the rate of VWF secretion, storage, and clearance. Blood type O is associated with a 25% decline in VWF levels. However, this decline does not affect bleeding rates, possibly due to enhanced secretion and decreased clearance of VWF with age. Inheritance of type 1 VWD tends to be autosomal dominant. VWF antigen levels decline in parallel with VWF activity, reported as VWF:ristocetin (RCo), and increasing severity. VWF:RCo measures the ability of the patient's VWF (plasma) to agglutinate normal platelets in the presence of ristocetin. VWF:RCo 30% to 49% is referred to as "low VWF" but not true VWD. Diagnostic criterion for VWD is VWF:RCo less than 30%. Repeating VWF testing is wise because significant variability occurs within individuals and between labs.

VWF levels also increase with age, inflammation, liver disease, and estrogen such as while on oral contraception or during pregnancy. Patients with mild and moderate VWD rarely have bleeding during pregnancy as the baseline VWF levels increase. However, days to weeks after delivery, bleeding becomes more common as levels fall back to the original baseline. Pregnant women should be alerted to this possibility so they contact a provider if postpartum bleeding occurs. Postpartum bleeding should be carefully assessed so it is not dismissed as expected lochia.

Treatment for VWD focuses on modalities to increase VWF. DDAVP increases production of VWF and its release from stores in the Weibel-Palade bodies in endothelial cells. It also increases factor VIII levels. Increased VWF levels can be detected within minutes of DDAVP administration, either intravenous or intranasal. Prior to relying on DDAVP for prevention of bleeding with surgeries or treatment of acute bleeds, a DDAVP challenge should be undertaken, where VWF and factor VIII levels are measured at baseline and then at specified timed intervals (e.g., 1 hour, 2 hours, and 6 hours) after administration of DDAVP to confirm an adequate response. Once this is done, intravenous DDAVP 0.3 μg/kg (capped at 20 μg max dose) can be given 30 to 60 minutes prior to surgeries, and intranasal DDAVP can be prescribed so patients can self-treat at home for bleeds or heavy menstrual periods.

The drawbacks to DDAVP include common side effects such as flushing, headache, malaise, and nausea, but also importantly hyponatremia, which becomes more severe with every dose. This can be circumvented by instructing patients to incorporate a 1-week drug holiday after every three doses and to limit free water intake during DDAVP days. A drug holiday is also important because tachyphylaxis develops, meaning that subsequent doses have diminishing returns on their ability to raise VWF levels (i.e., the third dose does not work as well as the first dose) as VWF stores become depleted. When DDAVP responses are inadequate or when patients do not tolerate DDAVP, VWF concentrates must be used. VWF concentrates come as plasma-derived or recombinant. Recombinant VWF contains no factor VIII, while plasma-derived VWF has factor VIII attached. This is important for treatment decisions because many patients with VWD also have low factor VIII levels. In that situation, both VWF and factor VIII need to be replaced to effectively treat acute bleeding. Thus, if recombinant VWF is used, a separate infusion of factor VIII concentrate also needs to be infused if factor VIII is low. For severely affected patients who need prophylaxis (regularly infused VWF to prevent spontaneous bleeding), either type of product is adequate because factor VIII levels become normal several hours after VWF is infused since the VWF stabilizes endogenous factor VIII. If baseline VWF levels of zero are assumed, VWF concentrates of 50 U/kg intravenous will bring

注完成后 10 min 至 1 h 检测血小板计数。非免疫介导的无效输注患者通常在输血后 10 min 血小板计数开始增加，但在 1 h 后增加减慢，由于潜在疾病的存在，随后血小板计数下降的速度比预期快。对于这种血小板无效输注的患者，解决潜在疾病通常能提高血小板输注的有效性。

对于免疫介导的血小板无效输注患者，即使在输血后数分钟，血小板计数也没有增加。抗血小板抗体最常见于反复输血的患者。反复暴露于输血制品可诱导同种抗体的产生，最常见的是针对 HLA 抗原的抗体。随着时间推移和多次输血暴露，同种抗体的滴度会急剧增加，并导致输注后不相容的血小板被快速清除。

对于同种免疫的患者，免疫抑制不能减少血小板的同种抗体，因此努力寻找相容的血小板是目前改善输血后血小板恢复的关键。管理同种免疫患者输血的第一步是提供 ABO 抗原匹配的血小板，以减少天然产生的 ABO 抗体引起的血小板清除；这通常是有效的，因为血小板表面表达 A 和 B 抗原。如果这一步骤不能使血小板计数增加，则应寻找缺乏检测到的同种抗体靶抗原的供者血小板。一种方法是使用患者的血清来交叉匹配供者血小板，选择相容的血小板后进行输注。

如果交叉匹配相容的血小板不能使血小板计数提升到目标水平，血库应提供与受者 HLA 相匹配的血小板，以避免 HLA 相关抗体的产生。可使用血小板单采术从相容的供者中反复采集 HLA 匹配的血小板，直到患者的血小板计数恢复且不再需要输注。许多血库和输血服务机构试图通过预防来解决血小板 HLA 同种免疫的问题。他们提供的血液制品经过过滤以减少白细胞含量，这一过程被称为"白细胞去除"。由于污染的白细胞是暴露于 HLA 的主要来源，因此去除白细胞可以非常有效地防止随后的同种免疫，甚至在长期输血的患者中也是如此。

由血管性血友病引起的出血

vWD 是由 vWF 缺乏或功能障碍引起。由于 vWF 是初级止血的关键组成部分，其缺乏会导致易出血，通常是浅表出血（瘀伤、黏膜出血）。然而，vWF 是因子Ⅷ的稳定剂，当 vWF 水平较低时，因子Ⅷ会迅速被清除，导致因子Ⅷ水平下降和 APTT 延长。如果因子Ⅷ水平足够低，患者会像血友病 A 和血友病 B 一样出现较严重的出血，如肌肉血肿、关节血肿和中枢神经系统出血。vWF 在内皮细胞和巨核细胞中合成，在血浆中发挥作用，介导血小板黏附到损伤部位。vWF 是一种大的多聚体蛋白，最大的多聚体包含的黏附位点最多，较小的 vWF 分子具有更强的止血能力。在 vWF 水平较低的患者中，血小板黏附到受损血管的时间延长。

vWD 主要分为 3 个亚型。1 型 vWD 由 vWF 抗原水平下降引起，其与 vWF 活性下降平行。2 型 vWD 为 vWF 功能障碍，vWF 活性下降比 vWF 抗原水平下降更显著。3 型 vWD 是最严重的类型，患者不产生任何 vWF。

1 型血管性血友病

1 型 vWD 是最常见的类型，虽然严重程度可有很大差异，但出血往往为轻度。许多 1 型 vWD 患者的 vWF 基因序列正常，因此其病因有时难以明确，因此，其他因素也会参与发病，如 vWF 的分泌、储存和清除。O 型血的个体 vWF 水平下降 25%。但是，这种下降并不影响出血发生率，可能是由于 vWF 随年龄增长而分泌增加且清除减少。1 型 vWD 通常呈常染色体显性遗传。1 型 vWD 中 vWF 抗原水平和 vWF 活性同步下降，以 vWF：瑞斯托霉素（RCo）表示，下降越多，疾病越严重。vWF：RCo 检测了患者血浆中的 vWF 在瑞斯托霉素作用下黏附聚集正常血小板的功能。vWF：RCo 为 30%～49% 被称为"低 vWF 水平"，但此时并不诊断 vWD。vWD 的诊断标准为 vWF：RCo < 30%。由于个体和实验室之间存在很大差异，建议重复检测 vWF。

vWF 水平会随年龄增加、炎症、肝病和雌激素水平升高（如口服避孕药或妊娠期间）而升高。由于 vWF 基线水平升高，轻中度 vWD 患者在妊娠期间很少发生出血。但在分娩后的数天至数周内，随着 vWF 水平回落到基线水平，患者常会发生出血。孕妇应警惕这种可能性，以便在产后出血时及时联系医务人员。应仔细评估产后出血，以避免将其视为常见的恶露而漏诊或误诊。

vWD 的治疗重点是提高 vWF 水平。DDAVP 能增加内皮细胞中 vWF 的产生及其从 Weibel-Palade 小体（W-P 小体）中的释放，同时还能提高因子Ⅷ的水平。给予（静脉或鼻内）DDAVP 后数分钟内即可检测到 vWF 水平升高。在使用 DDAVP 预防手术出血或治疗急性出血之前，应进行 DDAVP 预试验，即先检测 vWF 和因子Ⅷ的基线水平，然后在给予 DDAVP 后的指定时间（如 1 h、2 h 和 6 h）检测 vWF 和因子Ⅷ，以确认是否充分应答。完成上述试验后，可在手术前 30～60 min 静脉注射 0.3 μg/kg（最大剂量 20 μg）DDAVP，鼻内使用 DDAVP 便于患者在家中自行治疗出血或月经过多。

DDAVP 常见的副作用包括潮红、头痛、乏力和恶心，但最需注意低钠血症，随着给药次数的增加，低钠血症会越来越严重，可通过指导患者每 3 次给药后停药 1 周及使用 DDAVP 期间限制水摄入量来避免。暂停用药也很重要，因连续服用同一种药物可能会发生快速耐受，即随着给药次数增多，vWF 储备逐渐耗尽，后续剂量提高 vWF 水平的能力逐渐下降（即第 3 次给药效果不如第 1 次）。当患者对 DDAVP 反应不佳或不能耐受时，必须使用 vWF 浓缩物，包括血浆源性 vWF 浓缩物和重组 vWF 浓缩物。重组 vWF 不含因子Ⅷ，而血浆源性 vWF 含因子Ⅷ。这对于治疗决策很重要，因为许多 vWD 患者的因子Ⅷ水平降低，需同时补充 vWF 和因子Ⅷ才能有效治疗急性出血。因此，在因子Ⅷ水平低的情况下，若使用重组 vWF，还需单独输注因子Ⅷ浓缩物。对于需要预防性治疗（定期输注 vWF 以预防自发性出血）的重症患者，两种制品都可选用，因为 vWF 可稳定内源性的因子Ⅷ，在输注 vWF 数小时后，因子Ⅷ水平也会恢复正常。假设 vWF 基线水平为零，那么静脉注射 50 U/kg

VWF to 100%. The half-life of these products is about 12 hours, so doses need to be repeated every 12 to 24 hours.

Type 2 von Willebrand Disease

Type 2 VWD is characterized by heterozygous mutations that produce a qualitative defect in the VWF molecule. Because the defect causes a dysfunction in VWF, DDAVP, which will increase the dysfunctional endogenous VWF levels, may not work as well as it does for type 1 VWD.

A variety of VWF mutations can cause VWD type 2A, which result in decreased VWF secretion or increased clearance through ADAMTS-13 (a disintegrin and metalloprotease with thrombospondin-1-like-domains-13). These patients show disproportionately low VWF:RCo activity compared with the VWF antigen level (VWF RCo:Ag < 0.6) and large or high-molecular-weight VWF multimers are absent. Platelet aggregation is decreased in response to ristocetin. Patients with type 2A VWD respond to VWF concentrate and less commonly to DDAVP.

Type 2B VWD represents a gain-of-function mutation in exon 28 of VWF that augments VWF binding to the platelet GP1b receptor. This leads to mild thrombocytopenia that worsens with exposure to DDAVP. Therefore, DDAVP is contraindicated in type 2B VWD. High-molecular-weight multimers are absent and platelet aggregation is increased by ristocetin. Patients are treated with VWF concentrate.

The same scenario can be found with platelet-type VWD (previously called pseudo-VWD), where the mutation is not on VWF but instead on the GP1b receptor, and this also augments the interaction of VWF with GP1b. GP1b can be sequenced to verify the diagnosis. These patients are treated with platelet transfusions, not VWF, because the VWF is normal.

Type 2M VWD has a VWF mutation causing decreased binding to GP1b, the opposite of type 2B VWD. These patients have normal platelet counts and normal VWF multimers. Gastrointestinal bleeding is more common in type 2M VWD than in other types. Some patients with type 2M VWD respond to DDAVP, but most require VWF concentrate. The platelet version of type 2M VWD is called Bernard-Soulier syndrome, which is caused by a mutation in GP1b leading to decreased VWF binding (see "Congenital Causes of Platelet Dysfunction").

In type 2N VWD, the abnormal VWF molecule has decreased binding affinity for factor VIII, which decreases factor VIII survival and produces a bleeding phenotype similar to hemophilia A (e.g., hemarthroses) except that it affects males and females equally because it has an autosomal recessive inheritance pattern, unlike the X-linked hemophilia A and B. The diagnosis of type 2N VWD should be considered in females who have hemophilia A. VWF levels are normal because the mutated region is isolated to the factor VIII binding site and not affecting the other functions of VWF. To confirm the diagnosis, tests for VWF binding to factor VIII are available in reference laboratories. The low factor VIII levels respond poorly to factor VIII infusions because the infused factor is rapidly cleared without functioning VWF to stabilize it. Instead, type 2N VWD is treated with VWF concentrates with or without factor VIII concentrates.

Type 3 von Willebrand Disease

Patients with type 3 VWD have a complete deficiency of VWF, often as a result of the inheritance of two abnormal VWF alleles (i.e., compound heterozygous). This VWD type is the most severe and can mimic hemophilia because factor VIII levels are also severely decreased without VWF protection. It does not respond to DDAVP and requires VWF with factor VIII concentrates to treat bleeding. Many patients with type 3 VWD require regular prophylaxis of VWF concentrates infused every 2 to 3 days to prevent spontaneous bleeding.

Acquired von Willebrand Disease

The acquired form of VWD usually appears as a severe, type 2A–like defect without larger VWF multimers in a patient with no history of bleeding. Acquired VWD is caused by abnormal clearance of the larger VWF multimers and is associated with essential thrombocythemia, monoclonal gammopathies, multiple myeloma, lymphoproliferative disorders, and other malignancies. For some patients, no etiology is apparent. Unlike ITP, acquired VWD is not associated with pregnancy. Acquired VWD has been successfully treated with IVIG and treatment for the underlying disorder. Another cause of abnormal VWF multimer clearance resulting in acquired VWD is critical aortic stenosis (Heyde syndrome). It is corrected with successful surgical repair.

BLEEDING CAUSED BY COAGULATION FACTOR DISORDERS

Unlike disorders of platelets and von Willebrand factor, which favor mucocutaneous bleeding, coagulation factor defects generally cause deeper hemorrhages, such as bleeding into muscle and joints. Because the initial platelet plug is not solidified by secondary hemostasis, the effects are clot breakdown and at times delayed bleeding.

Most patients with significant factor deficiencies have abnormal screening laboratory test results, although patients with mild deficiencies can have bleeding and only borderline-abnormal coagulation factor values. Like other hemostasis abnormalities previously discussed, coagulation factor problems can be classified as congenital deficiencies or acquired.

Congenital Factor Deficiencies

Hemophilia A and B

After VWD, hemophilia A and B are the two most common factor deficiencies, corresponding to factor VIII and factor IX deficiency, respectively. Hemophilia A, with an incidence of 1:10,000 live male births, is approximately four times more common than hemophilia B. They are both X-linked and clinically indistinguishable from each other. Although more prominent in males, females can also have hemophilia as symptomatic carriers and by skewing of X chromosomal inactivation (i.e., favoring one chromosome over the other).

More than 2000 different mutations have been reported to cause hemophilia A and more than 1000 to cause hemophilia B. About 50% of severe hemophilia A patients have an inversion of a major portion of the gene at intron 22 (inversion 22) that results in complete loss of activity. Smaller missense mutations tend to result in mild or moderate disease. One third of cases are de novo, therefore there is no family history.

Hemophilia A and B are stratified by severity: Severe hemophilia is defined as a factor activity of less than 1%, moderate hemophilia as a factor activity of 1% to 5%, and mild hemophilia as a factor activity of 6% to 40%. These distinctions appear small, but are not. Severely affected patients bleed often and spontaneously. Moderately affected patients occasionally bleed spontaneously, whereas mildly affected patients typically bleed only after trauma or surgery. The most common locations for hemorrhages are joints and muscles, but bleeding can occur anywhere. They can be life-threatening, particularly when intracranial. Hemarthroses cause intra-articular inflammation and synovial hyperplasia. Subsequent cartilage and bone damage worsens with repeated hemorrhages. Hemophilic arthropathy results in chronic pain and limitations in joint function. Prior to the advent of prophylaxis, patients often needed joint replacement surgery early in life.

Currently, patients who bleed frequently take factor prophylaxis by self-infusing factor intravenously every few days to maintain detectable baseline factor levels so that spontaneous bleeding does

的vWF浓缩物可使vWF达到100%。这些制品的半衰期约为12 h，因此需要每12～24 h重复给药1次。

2型血管性血友病

2型vWD的特点是杂合突变导致vWF分子的质量缺陷，进而导致vWF功能障碍，由于DDAVP增加的是功能缺陷的内源性vWF水平，因此其对2型vWD的疗效可能不及1型vWD。

多种vWF突变可引起2A型vWD，导致vWF分泌减少或通过ADAMTS13（具有血小板应答蛋白-1样结构域的去整合素和金属蛋白酶）使vWF清除增加。患者表现出与vWF抗原水平不成比例的低vWF：RCo活性（vWF RCo：Ag＜0.6），且缺乏大分子量或高分子量vWF多聚体。瑞斯托霉素诱导的血小板聚集反应降低。2A型vWD患者对vWF浓缩物有反应，而对DDAVP的反应较差。

2B型vWD中vWF的第28号外显子发生功能获得突变，增强vWF与血小板GPIb受体的结合，导致轻度血小板减少症，且DDAVP会加重血小板减少。因此，2B型vWD患者禁用DDAVP。患者缺乏高分子量多聚体，且瑞斯托霉素可增加血小板聚集。患者可使用vWF浓缩物进行治疗。

血小板型vWD（既往称假性vWD）也会出现同样的情况，其突变在GPIb受体上（而不是vWF），这会增强vWF与GPIb的相互作用。对GPIb进行测序可明确诊断。由于vWF正常，故需要输注血小板，而不是vWF。

2M型vWD存在vWF突变，导致其与GPIb结合减少，与2B型相反。这些患者的血小板计数和vWF多聚体均正常。胃肠道出血多见于2M型vWD。一些2M型vWD患者对DDAVP有反应，但大多数需输注vWF浓缩物。2M型vWD中的血小板可导致巨血小板综合征，由GPIb突变导致vWF结合减少引起（见上文"血小板功能障碍的先天性病因"）。

在2N型vWD中，异常vWF分子对因子Ⅷ的亲和力降低，从而降低了因子Ⅷ的稳定性，产生类似于血友病A（如关节血肿）的出血表现，但与X连锁血友病A和血友病B不同的是，2N型vWD呈常染色体隐性遗传模式，对男性和女性的影响相同。考虑为血友病A的女性患者应鉴别2N型vWD。2N型vWD中，由于突变区域仅限于因子Ⅷ结合位点，而不影响vWF的其他功能，因此vWF水平正常。为明确诊断，可进行vWF与因子Ⅷ的结合试验。当因子Ⅷ水平低时，对输入的因子Ⅷ的反应较差，因为没有正常的vWF来稳定因子Ⅷ，输入的凝血因子会被迅速清除。2N型vWD的治疗需使用含或不含因子Ⅷ浓缩物的vWF浓缩物。

3型血管性血友病

3型vWD患者的vWF完全缺陷，通常是由于遗传了两个异常vWF等位基因（即复合杂合子）。这种vWD类型最为严重，可能类似血友病，因为在没有vWF保护的情况下，因子Ⅷ水平也会严重下降。3型vWD对DDAVP无反应，需使用含有因子Ⅷ浓缩物的vWF来治疗出血。许多此型患者需常规预防，每2～3天输注1次vWF浓缩物，以预防自发性出血。

获得性血管性血友病

获得性vWD常表现为严重的2A型vWD，患者没有较大的vWF多聚体，既往没有出血史。获得性vWD由较大的vWF多聚体被异常清除引起，与原发性血小板增多症、单克隆丙种球蛋白病、多发性骨髓瘤、淋巴增殖性疾病及其他恶性肿瘤有关。部分患者病因不明。与ITP不同，获得性vWD与妊娠无关。应用IVIG和治疗基础疾病可成功治疗获得性vWD。导致获得性vWD的vWF多聚体清除异常的另一个原因是严重的主动脉狭窄（Heyde综合征），可通过修复手术成功纠正。

由凝血因子障碍引起的出血

血小板和vWF相关疾病易引起皮肤、黏膜出血，而凝血因子缺陷通常导致更深层（如肌肉和关节）的出血。由于凝血因子异常，初始形成的血小板栓子未被次级止血固化，血凝块易分解和破裂，有时会导致延迟出血。

大多数凝血因子显著缺乏的患者会出现实验室筛查结果异常，但轻度缺乏的患者可能会出血，且凝血因子仅为临界异常值。与上文提及的其他止血异常一样，凝血因子问题可分为先天性缺陷或获得性缺陷。

先天性凝血因子缺陷

血友病A和血友病B

血友病A和血友病B是两种最常见的凝血因子缺乏症，仅次于vWD，其分别对应于因子Ⅷ和因子Ⅸ缺乏。血友病A在男性新生儿中的发病率为1/10 000，约为血友病B的4倍。两者均为X连锁遗传，在临床上难以区分。虽然男性更易患病，但女性也可作为有症状的携带者或通过X染色体失活偏倚（即倾向于两条X染色体中的一条失去活性）而患血友病。

据报道，超过2000种突变可导致血友病A，超过1000种突变可导致血友病B。约50%的重度血友病A的发生是由于基因22号内含子的主要部分发生倒位（倒位22），导致活性完全丧失。较小的错义突变通常导致轻中度血友病。1/3的病例为新发病例且没有家族史。

根据严重程度，血友病A和血友病B可分为：①重度血友病，定义为凝血因子活性＜1%；②中度血友病，定义为凝血因子活性为1%～5%；③轻度血友病，定义为凝血因子活性为6%～40%。这些差别看起来很小，其实不然。重度患者常出现自发性出血，中度患者偶尔出现自发性出血，而轻度患者通常只在创伤或手术后出血。最常见的出血部位是关节和肌肉，但可发生于任何部位。出血可能会危及生命，尤其是颅内出血。关节血肿可引起关节内炎症和滑膜增生，反复出血会加重后续的软骨和骨质损伤。血友病性关节病可导致慢性疼痛和关节功能受限。在预防性治疗出现之前，患者通常需要在早期进行关节置换手术。

目前，频繁出血的患者可通过每隔几天自行注射凝血因子来进行预防性治疗，以维持一定的基线凝血因子水平，避免自发性出血。当急性出血时，应指导

not occur. When acute hemorrhages occur, patients are instructed to infuse factor as early as possible. Most severely affected patients know how to self-infuse intravenously at home. DDAVP, given intravenously or intranasally, can rapidly raise factor VIII levels in mild hemophilia A patients but not in patients who are severely affected. It does not raise factor IX levels in hemophilia B patients either.

A newly approved therapy for prophylaxis is emicizumab, a bispecific antibody that mimics the function of factor VIII by binding to factors IXa and X. This has several advantages over traditional factor products. First, administration is subcutaneous, not intravenous like all other previous factor products. Second, the half-life is substantially longer. Traditional factor's half-life was roughly 12 hours, some extended to nearly 24 hours by the addition of extra moieties such as polyethylene glycol, albumin, or the Fc receptor domain of immunoglobulin, all slowing the metabolism of factor VIII. Emicizumab's half-life is 30 days. The third advantage of emicizumab is that it is not a clotting factor and, therefore, factor VIII inhibitors do not interfere with its efficacy. The disadvantages of emicizumab are that clotting assays (PTT, factor VIII, and others) no longer provide accurate results and that emicizumab is only used for prophylaxis, so acute bleeds are still treated by infusing factor VIII, although acute bleeds are significantly less common with emicizumab versus traditional factor VIII prophylaxis. Emicizumab works only for factor VIII deficiency, not in hemophilia B.

Inhibitors remain the largest problem for hemophilia patients. In up to one third of hemophilia A patients (much less common in hemophilia B), an alloantibody against factor VIII or IX forms, blocking the utility of factor infusions. In this situation, a bypass to work around the inhibitor in the clotting cascade is required to treat hemorrhage. There are two types of bypass agents: activated factor VII and activated 4-factor prothrombin complex concentrates (aPCC), which contain activated factors II, VII, IX, and X. Inhibitor titers can be measured in Bethesda units (BU); 1 BU is defined as the amount of inhibitor that neutralizes 50% of factor activity. High-titer inhibitors (>5 BU) completely neutralize the activity of infused factor concentrates, while low-titer inhibitors can be out-competed by using higher doses of factor, but at the risk of subsequently increasing the titer level. Inhibitors are sometimes transient, sometimes permanent, and sometimes able to be eradicated by immune tolerance induction, by giving frequent high doses of factor infusions to desensitize patients to the factor. Patients with inhibitors have more severe disease and poorly respond to available treatments. Inhibitors make an already costly disease much more expensive.

Not just a footnote in history, many hemophilia patients continue to struggle with the sequelae of human immunodeficiency virus (HIV) and viral hepatitis after contracting them from contaminated blood and factor products in the 1980s and 1990s. In fact, a large percentage of hemophilia patients died from complications of these infections. Recombinant factor was developed in the 1990s and most patients switched even though plasma-derived factor products became safe again through viral testing and inactivation procedures. In addition, a large randomized control trial has shown that plasma-derived factor leads to fewer inhibitors than recombinant, yet most patients remain on recombinant products.

The future has taken a rapid upward swing for hemophilia patients, with curative therapies for hepatitis C, emicizumab, other novel agents coming soon from development and the imminent arrival of gene therapy through coagulation factor DNA deployed into the liver by a viral vector. Multiple studies for gene therapy have shown early success and are already in phase III trials with approval for wider use expected in the coming years.

Hemophilia C

Hemophilia C refers to factor XI deficiency. Although one step prior to factor IX in the clotting cascade, factor XI deficiency is very different than hemophilia A and B. First of all, bleeding tends to be mucocutaneous, similar to platelet and VWF disorders. Second, bleeding risk does not parallel factor activity level and tends to be mild. For example, some patients with zero factor XI activity rarely bleed. Bleeding risk is best determined by a patient's bleeding history; therefore, the need for presurgical factor replacement depends on whether or not a patient tends to bleed. Factor XI replacement is done with fresh-frozen plasma (FFP) in the United States. Some countries have an available factor XI concentrate. Hemophilia C is inherited autosomal recessively and is common in Ashkenazi Jewish people.

Other Congenital Factor Deficiencies

Factor deficiencies can occur in any clotting factor. Patients with factor V deficiency usually lack plasma factor V and platelet factor V and have joint and muscle bleeding similar to patients with hemophilia. Some patients who are plasma factor V deficient are asymptomatic until they are challenged with the stress of surgery or trauma, and these patients are thought to have normal platelet factor V levels. Rarely, patients inherit combinations of factor deficiencies, such as combined factors V and VIII deficiencies. Some factor deficiencies have specific factor concentrations available for treatment such as factor VIIa, factor X, and factor XIII. However, others do not have specific concentrates available; those would be treated with FFP.

In neonates, factor XIII deficiency manifests with late umbilical stump bleeding or intracranial hemorrhage. Bleeding is delayed, but severe. Factor XIII deficiency does not affect PT or aPTT. It is diagnosed by screening for increased clot solubility in urea; if the clot dissolves abnormally quickly, an enzyme-linked immunosorbent assay for the precise factor XIII level should be performed. Factor XIII deficiency is treated with factor XIII concentrate or cryoprecipitate. Because of the long half-life of factor XIII, prophylactic therapy for severe deficiency is provided only in single doses on a 3- to 4-week recurring schedule.

Fibrinogen (factor I) functions as a bridging ligand for the platelet receptor GPIIb/IIIa in the platelet-platelet matrix at sites of vascular damage. It also functions in the final steps of the coagulation cascade to form the fibrin clot after activation from thrombin (factor IIa). This dual role leads to a varied phenotype of bleeding with superficial and deeper bleeding when defects in fibrinogen exist. Congenital abnormalities of fibrinogen include low levels (hypofibrinogenemia), absent fibrinogen (afibrinogenemia), and abnormally functioning fibrinogen (dysfibrinogenemia). The diagnosis can be established by screening assays, laboratory assays to measure fibrinogen levels, and tests such as thrombin time that are designed to measure fibrinogen function. Reptilase time can also confirm dysfibrinogenemia; heparin does not interfere with this assay like it does with thrombin time. PT and aPTT are prolonged in disorders of fibrinogen. Fibrinogen concentrates can be used for replacement, but if not available, cryoprecipitate offers high concentrations of fibrinogen compared to FFP.

Acquired Factor Inhibitors

Acquired inhibitors can occur in congenital hemophilia as described above (see "Hemophilia A and B" section), but they can also occur in those born with a normal coagulation system. Acquired factor VIII inhibitors are the most common and are associated with pregnancy, autoimmune disease, and malignancy, especially lymphoproliferative disorders. Some are idiopathic. The mechanisms underlying acquired factor inhibitors remain poorly understood.

患者尽早输注凝血因子。大多数重度血友病患者可在家中自行输注。DDAVP（静脉或鼻腔给药）可迅速提高轻度血友病A患者的因子Ⅷ水平，但对重度血友病A患者无效，也不会提高血友病B患者的因子Ⅸ水平。

艾美赛珠单抗是一种被批准用于预防性治疗的新药，它是一种双特异性抗体，通过与因子Ⅸa和X结合来模拟因子Ⅷ的功能，与传统凝血因子制品相比，艾美赛珠单抗具有多种优势。第一，可通过皮下注射给药，而既往所有凝血因子制品均需静脉给药。第二，半衰期大大延长。传统凝血因子的半衰期约为12h，部分制品通过添加额外成分（如聚乙二醇、白蛋白或免疫球蛋白的Fc受体结构域，以减缓因子Ⅷ的代谢）将半衰期延长至近24h，而艾美赛珠单抗的半衰期为30天。第三，艾美赛珠单抗不是凝血因子，故因子Ⅷ抑制物不会干扰其疗效。艾美赛珠单抗的缺点是会影响凝血检测（APTT、因子Ⅷ检测等）结果的准确性。与传统的凝血因子Ⅷ预防性治疗相比，艾美赛珠单抗预防性治疗可显著降低急性出血发生率，但艾美赛珠单抗仅用于预防性治疗，急性出血仍需通过输注因子Ⅷ进行治疗。艾美赛珠单抗仅对因子Ⅷ缺乏有效，对血友病B无效。

凝血因子抑制物仍然是血友病患者面临的最大问题。多达1/3的血友病A患者（血友病B患者中较少见）存在针对因子Ⅷ或Ⅸ的同种抗体，影响凝血因子输注的效用。此情况下，需绕过凝血级联反应中的抑制物，通过旁路途径治疗出血。有两种类型的旁路制剂：活化因子Ⅶ和活化四因子凝血酶原复合体浓缩物（aPCC），后者含活化的因子Ⅱ、Ⅶ、Ⅸ和X。可使用Bethesda法来检测抑制物滴度；能使正常血浆FⅧ/FⅨ活性减少50%的FⅧ/FⅨ抑制物的含量被定义为1个Bethesda单位（BU）。高滴度抑制物（>5 BU）可完全中和输注的因子浓缩物的活性，而低滴度抑制物可通过使用更大剂量的因子来抵消其抑制作用，但有增加抑制物滴度水平的风险。凝血因子抑制物可暂时存在，也可永久存在，有时可通过诱导免疫耐受来清除抑制物，即频繁输注大剂量凝血因子使者对该因子脱敏。存在凝血因子抑制物的患者病情更严重，对现有治疗的反应较差。凝血因子抑制物的存在使治疗费用更加昂贵。

许多血友病患者在20世纪80—90年代因输注受污染的血液和凝血因子制品而感染HIV和肝炎病毒，这些感染所致的后遗症至今仍困扰着患者，这并不是历史上的一件小事。事实上，很大一部分血友病患者死于这些感染所致的并发症。20世纪90年代，重组凝血因子制品问世，尽管通过病毒检测和灭活程序，血浆源性凝血因子制品已变得更加安全，但大多数患者仍选择使用重组凝血因子制剂。此外，一项大型随机对照试验表明，与重组凝血因子制剂相比，血浆源性凝血因子制品所致的凝血因子抑制物生成更少，但大多数患者仍选择使用重组凝血因子制品。

针对血友病的新治疗方法正在迅速发展，包括丙型肝炎的治愈性疗法、艾美赛珠单抗及其他研发中的新药，通过病毒载体将凝血因子DNA注入肝内的基因治疗也即将到来。基因治疗在多项研究中初见成效，并已进入Ⅲ期临床试验，预计在未来几年将会获得更广泛的应用批准。

血友病C

血友病C是指因子Ⅺ缺乏。虽然因子Ⅺ在凝血级联反应中位于因子Ⅸ上游，但因子Ⅺ缺乏与血友病A和血友病B有很大差异。首先，血友病C的出血多见于皮肤和黏膜，与血小板和vWF相关疾病类似。其次，血友病C的出血风险与凝血因子活性水平并不平行，通常是轻度出血。例如，一些因子Ⅺ活性为零的患者也很少出血。确定出血风险的最佳依据是患者的出血史；因此，是否需要在手术前进行凝血因子替代治疗取决于患者是否有出血倾向。在美国，因子Ⅺ替代治疗选择新鲜冰冻血浆（FFP）。有些国家可使用因子Ⅺ浓缩物。血友病C是常染色体隐性遗传病，常见于阿什肯纳兹犹太人。

其他先天性凝血因子缺陷

任何凝血因子都可能发生缺陷。因子Ⅴ缺乏症的患者通常缺乏血浆因子Ⅴ和血小板因子Ⅴ，其关节和肌肉出血表现与血友病患者相似。部分血浆因子Ⅴ缺乏的患者并无症状，直到他们面临手术或创伤，目前认为这些患者的血小板因子Ⅴ水平是正常的。遗传性联合因子缺乏的患者比较罕见，如因子Ⅴ和Ⅷ联合缺乏症。部分因子缺乏症可通过特定的因子浓缩物进行治疗，如因子Ⅶa、Ⅹ和ⅩⅢ。在一些国家，如果没有专门的因子浓缩物，也可用FFP进行治疗。

在新生儿中，因子ⅩⅢ缺乏症表现为晚期脐带残端出血或颅内出血。出血虽然有延迟，但很严重。因子ⅩⅢ缺乏不影响PT或APTT。通过筛查发现血凝块在尿素中的溶解度增加可进行诊断；如果血凝块溶解异常迅速，则应进行酶联免疫吸附试验，以精准测定因子ⅩⅢ的水平。因子ⅩⅢ缺乏症可用因子ⅩⅢ浓缩物或冷沉淀进行治疗。由于因子ⅩⅢ的半衰期很长，对严重缺乏的预防性治疗仅需单剂量给药，每3～4周给药1次。

纤维蛋白原（因子Ⅰ）在血管损伤部位作为血小板黏附聚集物中血小板受体GPⅡb/Ⅲa的桥接配体来发挥作用。纤维蛋白原在被凝血酶（因子Ⅱa）激活后形成纤维蛋白凝块，在凝血级联反应的最后步骤中也发挥作用。由于具有这种双重作用，当存在纤维蛋白原缺陷时，可导致不同的出血表型，包括浅表和深部出血。先天性纤维蛋白原异常包括纤维蛋白原水平低（低纤维蛋白原血症）、纤维蛋白原缺乏（纤维蛋白原缺乏血症）和纤维蛋白原功能异常（异常纤维蛋白原血症）。实验室检查可进行诊断，包括筛查试验、纤维蛋白原水平检测，以及用于测定纤维蛋白原功能的凝血酶时间等。蛇毒凝血酶时间异常也可确诊异常纤维蛋白原血症；该检测不受肝素影响（肝素可干扰凝血酶时间）。纤维蛋白原异常时PT和APTT延长。纤维蛋白原浓缩物可用于替代治疗，如果不可用，与FFP相比，冷沉淀可提供高浓度的纤维蛋白原。

获得性凝血因子抑制物

获得性凝血因子抑制物可发生于上述的先天性血友病中（见上文"血友病A和血友病B"），但也可见于出生时凝血系统正常的个体。获得性因子Ⅷ抑制物最常见，其与妊娠、自身免疫病和恶性肿瘤，特别是

The diagnosis of an acquired inhibitor can be made by laboratory techniques similar to those detailed for patients with congenital hemophilia. A mixing study can be a critical piece to the evaluation. It mixes control plasma with patient plasma, correcting any deficiencies unless an inhibitor is present since the inhibitor will also block the factor in the control plasma. For the treatment of bleeding, patients with acquired inhibitors to factors VIII or IX are administered factor VIIa or aPCC to promote hemostasis by bypassing the inhibitor. Rituximab, an anti-CD20 agent, has become the mainstay for successful treatment along with steroids and should be started as soon as possible to eradicate the inhibitor.

Acquired factor X deficiency can occur in patients with amyloidosis, a condition in which the abnormal circulating light chains adsorb and clear factor X, producing low levels and severe bleeding.

Vitamin K Deficiency

Bleeding in inpatients and outpatients who are severely ill may be caused by acquired coagulation factor deficiencies from vitamin K deficiency. Because vitamin K is fat-soluble, biliary tract disease can interfere with its absorption. Antibiotics can sterilize the gut and reduce bacterial sources of vitamin K. Other drugs such as cholestyramine directly block vitamin K absorption. Vitamin K deficiency also may reflect poor nutritional status due to malabsorption, chronic disease, or reduced oral intake in patients who are acutely or chronically ill.

Factors II, VII, IX, and X are vitamin K–dependent procoagulant factors and proteins C and S are the natural vitamin K-dependent anticoagulants. In addition to disease-associated vitamin K deficiency, the anticoagulant warfarin blocks vitamin K–dependent γ-carboxylation of factors II, VII, IX, and X and causes an acute decrease in functional factor VII levels because factor VII has the shortest half-life (4-6 hours) of all vitamin K–dependent factors in vivo. Individuals who experience bleeding while on warfarin may be treated with vitamin K or, for life-threatening bleeding, a 4-factor PCC or FFP infusion.

Dilutional Coagulopathy

As with platelets, coagulation factors can be depleted through the dilutional effects of a pure red blood cell transfusion or with the administration of massive amounts of volume expanders or saline solutions. For every 10 units of red cells acutely transfused, there is a concomitant increase in the international normalized ratio (INR) to greater than 2. Acute bleeding and trauma can also lead to consumption of circulating coagulation factors.

In the setting of trauma, it is important to maintain adequate coagulation factor activity through plasma transfusions. Evidence from the trauma literature suggests that transfusion ratios of red cells to plasma should approach 1:1 to optimize hemostasis. However, even this may not fully restore depleted coagulation factors. The effects of dilutional coagulopathy should be monitored by repeated testing of PT and aPTT and supported with a liberal plasma transfusion strategy. As described above (see "Standard Platelet Therapy" section), caregivers must also be vigilant about repletion of platelets.

Liver Disease

Unlike patients with vitamin K deficiency or those receiving warfarin, patients with liver disease have low levels of most factors, not just the vitamin K–dependent factors. The exception is factor VIII. Factor VIII levels are usually normal with liver disease because factor VIII is produced in endothelial cells and megakaryocytes. Seemingly in contrast to this, factor VIII levels in hemophilia A patients normalize after liver transplant because factor VIII is synthesized in endothelial cells within the transplanted liver. If factor VIII levels are decreased in patients with liver disease, consideration should be given to superimposed DIC.

Evaluating a prolonged PT, measurement of factor VII and a non–vitamin K–dependent factor, such as factor V, is useful. In vitamin K deficiency, the level of factor VII is low, and that of factor V is normal; levels of both factors are low in patients with generalized liver disease. The PT is a sensitive measure of liver function and becomes prolonged in patients with even mild liver disorders; elevation precedes a significant decrease in the albumin or prealbumin levels and is usually coincident with transaminase changes. In patients with mild to moderate liver disease, the PT is prolonged, but the aPTT usually remains within the normal range. In severe liver disease, the PT becomes even more prolonged, and the aPTT also becomes abnormal.

Other causes of bleeding in liver disease include associated DIC, inhibition of platelet function and production, removal of platelets from hypersplenism, and increased levels of tissue plasminogen activator. Treatment of bleeding associated with liver disease is based primarily on replacement of coagulation factors by plasma transfusions, although they only temporarily correct abnormalities. Liver transplantation is the only definitive treatment for these synthetic defects.

Acquired Fibrinogen Loss or Defects

Congenital fibrinogen disorders were described earlier, but more common are acquired causes such as DIC, causing a consumption of fibrinogen, and liver disease, where defects in post-translational modification of fibrinogen lead to dysfunction or dysfibrinogenemia. The abnormal fibrinogen molecules cannot undergo normal cross-linking or polymerization, resulting in bleeding.

BLEEDING IN PATIENTS WITH NORMAL LABORATORY VALUES

Sometimes confirmatory testing of a bleeding disorder can be elusive. Bleeding diathesis from connective tissue disease and vascular causes may have normal coagulation tests. Vitamin C deficiency can lead to bleeding through an acquired connective tissue disease (scurvy). Low VWF and mild deficiencies of clotting factors may not prolong PT and aPTT. Factor XIII deficiency does not affect PT, aPTT, and other tests. Tests of fibrinolysis (plasminogen activator inhibitor-1, alpha-2 antiplasmin, plasminogen, and tissue plasminogen activator) may find rare causes of bleeding. Often cases with significant bleeding histories remain unsolved.

Plasma and Coagulation Factor Transfusion Therapy

For patients with one or multiple defects in coagulation proteins, there are several options for replacement therapy. The most widely used product for replacement of coagulation factors is FFP. It is collected from the whole blood of healthy donors and is frozen within 8 hours of collection. It contains normal (i.e., therapeutic) levels of all coagulation factors necessary to maintain hemostasis. FFP is an excellent choice for replacement of coagulation factors for many conditions, including liver failure and deficiencies of factors II, V, X, and XI.

FFP is commonly used with vitamin K therapy for the reversal of warfarin before invasive procedures or for the onset of bleeding. The appropriate dose of FFP is weight based and does not depend on the extent of prolongation in coagulation studies alone. Administration of FFP at 10 to 15 mL/kg should be sufficient to replace deficient coagulation factors and correct abnormal coagulation values. Assuming a volume of about 200 mL per unit of FFP, a reasonable dose for a 70-kg individual is 4 units of FFP. Administration is time sensitive because coagulation factors degrade at standard half-lives on infusion.

淋巴增殖性疾病有关。部分为特发性。获得性凝血因子抑制物的产生机制目前仍不清楚。

诊断获得性抑制物可通过与先天性血友病患者类似的实验室检查。混合试验在诊断评估中非常关键。它将对照血浆与患者血浆混合，如果不存在抑制物，则凝血因子缺陷可被纠正，如果存在抑制物，则不能被纠正，因为抑制物也会抑制对照血浆中的凝血因子。对于有获得性因子Ⅷ或Ⅸ抑制物的患者，可输注因子Ⅶa或aPCC，以绕过抑制物通过旁路途径止血。利妥昔单抗（一种抗CD20药物）联用类固醇已成为主要治疗手段，且应尽快开始使用，以清除抑制物。

获得性因子X缺乏症可发生于淀粉样变性患者，在这种情况下，循环中异常的轻链可吸附并清除因子X，导致因子X水平降低和严重出血。

维生素K缺乏症

出血严重的住院和门诊患者可能由维生素K缺乏引起的获得性凝血因子缺乏所致。由于维生素K为脂溶性，胆道疾病会影响其吸收。抗生素可通过杀灭肠道菌群来减少细菌来源的维生素K。其他药物（如考来烯胺）可直接抑制维生素K的吸收。吸收不良、慢性疾病或急慢性疾病患者饮食量减少引起的营养状况差也可导致维生素K缺乏。

因子Ⅱ、Ⅶ、Ⅸ和X是维生素K依赖性促凝血因子，蛋白C和S是天然的维生素K依赖性抗凝剂。除了与疾病相关的维生素K缺乏外，抗凝药物华法林可阻断维生素K依赖性因子Ⅱ、Ⅶ、Ⅸ和X的γ-羧化，此外，由于因子Ⅶ在体内所有维生素K依赖性因子中的半衰期最短（4~6 h），华法林还可导致功能性因子Ⅶ水平急性下降。服用华法林期间发生出血的患者可使用维生素K治疗，对于危及生命的出血，可输注四因子凝血酶原复合体浓缩物（4F-PCC）或FFP。

稀释性凝血功能障碍

与血小板相同，凝血因子的作用可能因单纯红细胞输注或输注大量扩容液体或生理盐水的稀释作用而被消除。快速输注10 U的红细胞可导致国际标准化比值（INR）＞2。急性出血和创伤也可导致循环凝血因子消耗。

在创伤情况下，通过输注血浆维持足够的凝血因子活性很重要。创伤相关研究证据表明，红细胞与血浆的输注比例接近1:1时止血效果最佳。但是，即使这样也不能完全恢复被耗竭的凝血因子。应通过反复检测PT和APTT来监测稀释性凝血功能障碍的影响，并灵活调整血浆输注策略。如上所述（见上文"标准血小板治疗"），医务人员必须注意对血小板的补充。

肝病

与维生素K缺乏症或接受华法林治疗的患者不同，肝病患者的大多数凝血因子水平均较低，而不仅是维生素K依赖性因子。但是，因子Ⅷ是个例外。由于因子Ⅷ在内皮细胞和巨核细胞中产生，肝病患者的因子Ⅷ水平通常正常。血友病A患者的因子Ⅷ水平在肝移植后可恢复正常，因为移植肝的内皮细胞可合成因子Ⅷ。如果肝病患者的因子Ⅷ水平降低，应考虑合并DIC。

诊断PT延长的病因时，检测因子Ⅶ和非维生素K依赖性因子（如因子Ⅴ）是有帮助的。维生素K缺乏时，因子Ⅶ水平降低，而因子Ⅴ水平正常；肝病患者两者水平均降低。PT是衡量肝功能的敏感指标，即使是轻度肝病患者也会出现PT延长；PT延长先于白蛋白或前白蛋白水平的显著降低，通常与转氨酶的改变同时发生。轻中度肝病患者PT延长，但APTT通常在正常范围内。严重肝病患者的PT会进一步延长，APTT也会出现异常。

肝病引起出血的其他原因包括相关的DIC、血小板功能和生成受抑制、脾功能亢进导致血小板清除、组织纤溶酶原激活物增加。肝病相关出血的治疗基本依赖于输注血浆进行凝血因子替代治疗，但这只能暂时缓解病情。肝移植才是彻底治疗这些合成缺陷的唯一方法。

获得性纤维蛋白原缺失或缺陷

先天性纤维蛋白原异常已在上文进行了介绍，但纤维蛋白原缺失或缺陷的获得性病因更常见，如DIC（导致纤维蛋白原消耗）和肝病（引起纤维蛋白原翻译后修饰缺陷，导致纤维蛋白原功能障碍或异常纤维蛋白原血症）。异常的纤维蛋白原分子不能进行正常的交联或聚合，从而导致出血。

实验室指标正常的出血

部分出血性疾病并不表现出任何确诊性实验室检查指标的异常。在结缔组织病和血管原因引起的出血倾向中，凝血功能检查可能正常。维生素C缺乏可通过导致获得性结缔组织病（坏血病）而引起出血。低vWF水平和凝血因子轻度缺乏可能不会导致PT和APTT延长。因子XIII缺乏不会影响PT、APTT和其他检查结果。纤维蛋白溶解相关检测［包括纤溶酶原激活物抑制物-1（PAI-1）、α_2-纤溶酶抑制物、纤溶酶原和组织纤溶酶原激活物］可能发现罕见的出血原因。实验室指标正常但有明显出血史的病例仍有待解决。

血浆及凝血因子输注治疗

对于有1种或多种凝血蛋白缺陷的患者，目前有多种替代治疗方案。最常用的凝血因子替代制品是FFP。FFP是从健康献血者的全血中采集，并在采集后8 h内冷冻，含有正常（治疗）水平的、维持止血所需的所有凝血因子。在很多情况下，FFP是替代凝血因子的最佳选择，包括肝衰竭及缺乏因子Ⅱ、Ⅴ、Ⅹ和Ⅺ。

在有创性操作前或出血时，FFP通常与维生素K联用，以逆转华法林的作用。FFP的合适剂量根据患者体重而定，而不是根据凝血指标的延长程度。10~15 ml/kg的FFP足以替代凝血因子缺乏，纠正凝血指标异常。假设每个单位FFP的体积约为200 ml，那么对于70 kg的患者，合理的剂量是4 U FFP。由于凝血因子在输注过程中

FFP should be provided immediately before an intended procedure to ensure adequate hemostasis.

In some cases, patients may not be able to tolerate the infusion of the large volume of FFP required to reverse coagulopathic states. Prothrombin complex concentrate (PCC) offers quick reversal of prolonged PT and aPTT without the need for large volumes of FFP. Four-factor PCC is a concentrated, lyophilized, human-derived concentrate containing factors II, VII, IX, and X that can be reconstituted in small volumes and provided by intravenous bolus injection. A 4-factor PCC was approved for clinical use in 2013 by the U.S. Food and Drug Administration (FDA). A variant PCC (FEIBA) containing activated factors II, VII, IX, and X is used as a bypass agent to treat bleeding in the setting of an inhibitor and is administered in doses of 50 to 100 U/kg every 8 to 12 hours.

Vitamin K can be given in addition to plasma infusion or factor concentrates. Oral or parenteral replacement of vitamin K (1 to 10 mg/day for 1 to 3 days) restores coagulation factor synthesis in patients with normal liver function and vitamin K deficiency.

For patients with hemophilia A or B, multiple virally inactivated, human-derived or recombinant factor VIII and IX concentrates are available (see "Hemophilia A and B"). Patients with severe hemophilia often infuse themselves with prophylactic factor on a regular basis (25-50 U/kg three times per week for hemophilia A; 50-100 U/kg twice per week for hemophilia B) and boost their dose or frequency of infusion when they sense internal bleeding, sustain trauma, or undergo dental procedures. Patients with mild hemophilia A may not need factor infusions for minor surgery. Their disease is often managed with DDAVP (0.3 µg/kg) or antifibrinolytic agents such as tranexamic acid 1300 mg three times a day or ε-aminocaproic acid 4 g every 4 to 6 hours.

Most patients with hemophilia require factor infusions prophylactically or at times of surgery or trauma. Factor VIII products are infused every 8 to 12 hours, and 1 U/kg of factor VIII concentrate raises plasma factor VIII activity by 2%; 50 U/kg of factor VIII theoretically yields 100% factor VIII activity in a patient with severe hemophilia A. Factor IX has a longer half-life and is infused every 18 to 24 hours; factor IX requires 1 U/kg for a 1% increase in factor IX activity (i.e., 100 U/kg for 100% activity). Major surgery in patients with hemophilia requires intensive factor therapy to achieve normal factor levels (>80%) in the intraoperative period and the early postoperative period to prevent wound hematoma formation. The dose of factors is adjusted downward from this intensity, depending on the severity of the insult, the patient's response to previous factor infusions, and whether factor inhibitors have developed.

Hemophilia patients with inhibitors need bypass agents, allowing activation of the extrinsic and common pathways of the clotting cascade. Activated 4-factor PCC is given at doses of 50 to 100 U/kg every 6 to 12 hours.

Another widely used bypass agent is activated factor VII (factor VIIa), a recombinant factor protein administered at 90 µg/kg every 2 hours until the bleeding is controlled. This agent is used to control bleeding in patients with hemophilia inhibitors, acquired hemophilia, congenital factor VII deficiency, and Glanzmann thrombasthenia. It has also been used successfully in Bernard-Soulier syndrome.

Several virally inactivated plasma-derived VWF concentrate products and one recombinant VWF are available. The plasma-derived VWF products also contain factor VIII and are particularly useful for bleeding or prophylaxis in moderate to severe VWD when factor VIII levels are low. Recombinant VWF has no factor VIII, so it would need additional factor VIII infused if factor VIII levels were low, as can happen in VWD.

Cryoprecipitate Transfusion Therapy

Cryoprecipitate is an often overlooked but important blood product for the treatment of a variety of bleeding disorders. It is prepared by thawing frozen plasma and removing the precipitated portion. It contains a narrow array of coagulation factors, but fibrinogen, factor VIII, VWF, and factor XIII occur in high concentrations. A major advantage of cryoprecipitate is that the average single unit is only 10 to 20 mL.

Based on its contents and small volume, cryoprecipitate is useful for the replacement of fibrinogen in DIC or in patients with hypofibrinogenemia or dysfibrinogenemia. The product may be helpful for isolated factor XIII deficiency or factor XIII consumption in DIC. Mounting evidence suggests that the VWF and factor VIII in cryoprecipitate can be used to overcome bleeding in uremia by enhancing the adhesive properties of circulating platelets.

Cryoprecipitate is most frequently administered for hypofibrinogenemia, and appropriate dosing should take into account a patient's total plasma volume, baseline fibrinogen levels, and goal fibrinogen levels. For most bleeding associated with hypofibrinogenemia, a goal fibrinogen of more than 100 mg/dL is reasonable. For a 70-kg adult with a fibrinogen level less than 100 mg/dL, a 10-unit pool (total volume of about 150 to 200 mL) should be sufficient to provide adequate fibrinogen. For more complex dosage protocols, such as for children, obese patients, or those with extreme hypofibrinogenemia, consultation with the blood bank is strongly recommended for specific calculations.

PROSPECTUS FOR THE FUTURE

Novel modalities continue to be developed for the diagnosis of patients with bleeding disorders. For instance, assays measuring thrombin generation, thromboelastography (TEG), and rotational thromboelastometry (ROTEM) offer a quantitative view of coagulation that may provide greater insight into the source of abnormal bleeding than current tests. Alternatives and improvements in transfusion are also being developed, including cells harvested from induced progenitor cells that can be customized for specific needs. Progress continues to be made in the development and application of novel therapies for hemophilia. Finally, gene therapy and gene editing portend an exciting shift in hematology and medical care, in general.

会以标准半衰期降解，故输注具有时效性。因此在进行预期操作时，应立即输注FFP以确保充分止血。

在某些情况下，患者可能无法耐受用于逆转凝血障碍的大剂量FFP输注。凝血酶原复合体浓缩物（PCC）可快速纠正PT和APTT延长，无须输注大量FFP。4F-PCC是一种浓缩冻干人源浓缩物，含有因子Ⅱ、Ⅶ、Ⅸ和Ⅹ，可溶于少量液体后静脉输注。2013年FDA批准4F-PCC用于临床。PCC的一种变体（FEIBA）含有活化因子Ⅱ、Ⅶ、Ⅸ和Ⅹ，可作为旁路制剂在有抑制物存在的情况下治疗出血，给药剂量为50～100 U/kg，每8～12 h 1次。

除输注血浆或因子浓缩物外，还可给予维生素K。对于肝功能正常但维生素K缺乏的患者，口服或肠外补充维生素K（1～10 mg/d，持续1～3天）可恢复凝血因子合成。

对于血友病A或血友病B患者，多种病毒灭活的人源性或重组因子Ⅷ和Ⅸ浓缩物可供选择（见上文"血友病A和血友病B"）。重度血友病患者常定期自行注射凝血因子进行预防性治疗（血友病A患者的剂量为25～50 U/kg，每周3次；血友病B患者的剂量为50～100 U/kg，每周2次），当出现内出血、遭受创伤或进行牙科手术时，需增加注射剂量或频率。轻度血友病A患者在小手术时可能不需要输注凝血因子，常可使用DDAVP（0.3 μg/kg）或抗纤溶药物，如氨甲环酸（1300 mg，3次/日）或ε-氨基己酸（4 g，每4～6 h 1次）。

大多数血友病患者需要预防性输注或在手术或创伤时输注凝血因子。1 U/kg因子Ⅷ浓缩物（每8～12 h 1次）可使血浆因子Ⅷ活性提高2%；在重度血友病A患者中，50 U/kg因子Ⅷ理论上可产生100%的因子Ⅷ活性。因子Ⅸ的半衰期较长，每18～24 h输注1次；1 U/kg因子Ⅸ能使血浆因子Ⅸ活性提高1%（即100 U/kg才能使活性达到100%）。血友病患者进行大手术时需要在术中和术后早期进行凝血因子强化治疗，使血浆凝血因子达到正常水平（>80%），以防止形成伤口血肿。根据损伤的严重程度、患者对既往输注的反应及是否产生凝血因子抑制物，凝血因子的剂量在上述给药强度的基础上进行下调。

有抑制物的血友病患者需要使用旁路药物，从而激活凝血级联反应中的外源性凝血途径和共同途径。活化4F-PCC的剂量为50～100 U/kg，每6～12 h 1次。

另一种广泛使用的旁路制剂是活化因子Ⅶ（因子Ⅶa），它是一种重组的凝血因子蛋白，使用方法为90 μg/kg，每2 h 1次，直到出血得到控制。该药可用于血友病伴抑制物、获得性血友病、先天性因子Ⅶ缺乏症和格兰茨曼血小板功能不全患者，以控制出血。它也被成功用于治疗巨血小板综合征。

目前已有多种病毒灭活的血浆源性vWF浓缩物制品和1种重组vWF。血浆源性vWF制品也含有因子Ⅷ，尤其适用于治疗因子Ⅷ水平较低的中重度vWD患者的出血或预防性治疗。重组vWF不含因子Ⅷ，因此因子Ⅷ水平较低的患者（如vWD）需要额外输注因子Ⅷ。

冷沉淀输注治疗

冷沉淀是一种经常被忽视的血液制品，但其对多种出血性疾病的治疗很重要。它是通过将冰冻血浆解冻并除去沉淀之后制备而成，包含少数凝血因子，但富含纤维蛋白原、因子Ⅷ、vWF及因子ⅩⅢ。冷沉淀的主要优势在于平均每个单位只有10～20 ml。

基于冷沉淀的成分和小体积，它可被用于DIC或低纤维蛋白原血症或异常纤维蛋白原血症患者的纤维蛋白原替代治疗。冷沉淀还可治疗单纯因子ⅩⅢ缺乏或DIC所致的因子ⅩⅢ消耗。大量证据表明，冷沉淀中的vWF和因子Ⅷ可通过增加循环血小板的黏附性来缓解尿毒症患者的出血症状。

冷沉淀最常用于治疗低纤维蛋白原血症，其剂量应根据患者的血浆总量、纤维蛋白原基线水平和目标纤维蛋白原水平而定。对于大多数与低纤维蛋白原血症相关的出血，目标纤维蛋白原>100 mg/dl是合理的。对于一位纤维蛋白原<100 mg/dl且体重为70 kg的成人，10 U冷沉淀（总体积为150～200 ml）能提供足够的纤维蛋白原。对于复杂情况下的剂量方案，如儿童、肥胖症或极端低纤维蛋白原血症患者，强烈建议咨询血库，以进行更加具体的剂量计算。

未来展望

诊断出血性疾病的新方法仍在持续发展。例如，与目前已有的检测方法相比，测定凝血酶生成的检测方法、血栓弹力图（TEG）和旋转式血栓弹力图（ROTEM）为理解异常出血的病因提供了更深入和广阔的视角。输血的新方法及其改良方案也正在研究中，包括从诱导祖细胞中获取具有特定功能的细胞。血友病新型治疗的开发和应用也在不断取得进展。此外，基因治疗和基因编辑的发展预示着血液学和医疗领域将发生令人振奋的转变。

SUGGESTED READINGS

Altomare I, Wasser J, Pullarkat V: Bleeding and mortality outcomes in ITP clinical trials: a review of thrombopoietin mimetics data, Am J Hematol 87:984–987, 2012.

Hayward CP, Moffat KA, Liu Y: Laboratory investigations for bleeding disorders, Semin Thromb Hemost 38:742–752, 2012.

Hod E, Schwartz J: Platelet transfusion refractoriness, Br J Haematol 142:348–360, 2008.

Kearon C, Akl EA, Ornelas J, et al: Antithrombotic therapy for VTE disease, ed 10, American College of Chest Physicians Guideline and Expert Panel Report, Chest 149:315–352, 2016.

Levy JH, Greenberg C: Biology of factor XIII and clinical manifestations of factor XIII deficiency, Transfusion 53:1120–1131, 2013.

Mahlangu J, Oldenburg J, Paz-Priel I, et al: Emicizumab prophylaxis in patients who have hemophilia A without inhibitors, N Engl J Med 379:811–822, 2018.

Mannucci PM: New therapies for von Willebrand disease, Hematology Am Soc Hematol Educ Program 590–595, 2019.

Menegatti M, Biguzzi E, Peyvandi F: Management of rare acquired bleeding disorders, Hematology Am Soc Hematol Educ Program 80–87, 2019.

Roback JD, Caldwell S, Carson J, et al: Evidence-based practice guidelines for plasma transfusion, Transfusion 50:1227–1239, 2010.

Rydz N, James PD: Why is my patient bleeding or bruising?, Hematol Oncol Clin North Am 26:321–344, viii, 2012.

Seligsohn U: Treatment of inherited platelet disorders, Haemophilia 18(Suppl 4):161–165, 2012.

Sharma R, Haberichter SL: New advances in the diagnosis of von Willebrand disease, Hematology Am Soc Hematol Educ Program 596–600, 2019.

Wada H, Matsumoto T, Hatada T: Diagnostic criteria and laboratory tests for disseminated intravascular coagulation, Expert Rev Hematol 5:643–652, 2012.

Weyand AC, Pipe SW: New therapies in hemophilia, Blood 133:389–398, 2019.

Winkelhorst D, Murphy MF, Greinacher A, et al.: Antenatal management in fetal and neonatal alloimmune thrombocytopenia: a systematic review, Blood 129:1538–1547, 2017.

推荐阅读

Altomare I, Wasser J, Pullarkat V: Bleeding and mortality outcomes in ITP clinical trials: a review of thrombopoietin mimetics data, Am J Hematol 87:984–987, 2012.

Hayward CP, Moffat KA, Liu Y: Laboratory investigations for bleeding disorders, Semin Thromb Hemost 38:742–752, 2012.

Hod E, Schwartz J: Platelet transfusion refractoriness, Br J Haematol 142:348–360, 2008.

Kearon C, Akl EA, Ornelas J, et al: Antithrombotic therapy for VTE disease, ed 10, American College of Chest Physicians Guideline and Expert Panel Report, Chest 149:315–352, 2016.

Levy JH, Greenberg C: Biology of factor XIII and clinical manifestations of factor XIII deficiency, Transfusion 53:1120–1131, 2013.

Mahlangu J, Oldenburg J, Paz-Priel I, et al: Emicizumab prophylaxis in patients who have hemophilia A without inhibitors, N Engl J Med 379:811–822, 2018.

Mannucci PM: New therapies for von Willebrand disease, Hematology Am Soc Hematol Educ Program 590–595, 2019.

Menegatti M, Biguzzi E, Peyvandi F: Management of rare acquired bleeding disorders, Hematology Am Soc Hematol Educ Program 80–87, 2019.

Roback JD, Caldwell S, Carson J, et al: Evidence-based practice guidelines for plasma transfusion, Transfusion 50:1227–1239, 2010.

Rydz N, James PD: Why is my patient bleeding or bruising?, Hematol Oncol Clin North Am 26:321–344, viii, 2012.

Seligsohn U: Treatment of inherited platelet disorders, Haemophilia 18(Suppl 4):161–165, 2012.

Sharma R, Haberichter SL: New advances in the diagnosis of von Willebrand disease, Hematology Am Soc Hematol Educ Program 596–600, 2019.

Wada H, Matsumoto T, Hatada T: Diagnostic criteria and laboratory tests for disseminated intravascular coagulation, Expert Rev Hematol 5:643–652, 2012.

Weyand AC, Pipe SW: New therapies in hemophilia, Blood 133:389–398, 2019.

Winkelhorst D, Murphy MF, Greinacher A, et al.: Antenatal management in fetal and neonatal alloimmune thrombocytopenia: a systematic review, Blood 129:1538–1547, 2017.

Disorders of Hemostasis: Thrombosis

Rebecca Zon, Nathan T. Connell

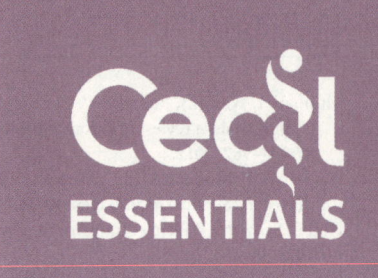

PATHOLOGY OF THROMBOSIS

The Virchow triad defines the pathologic mechanisms underlying thrombosis: diminished blood flow, damage to the vascular wall, and an imbalance favoring procoagulant over anticoagulant factors. The first two factors are clearly localized to specific vascular beds; although the last element of the triad may be systemic, data show at least partial regulation of the hemostatic balance by anatomic region. For example, congenital deficiency of antithrombin, protein C, or protein S typically leads to venous thromboembolism (VTE) of the lower extremities. In contrast, the inherited hypercoagulable disorders associated with the factor V Leiden and prothrombin G20210A mutations not only produce lower extremity VTE but also are associated with thrombosis of the cerebral veins and sinuses.

This hemostatic regulation in vascular tissues is mediated by multiple factors that include (1) microenvironmental signals, such as shear stress resulting from turbulence in the disrupted flow of damaged vessels, that affect endothelial cell (EC) expression of thrombomodulin, tissue factor, and nitric oxide synthase as well as platelet activation; (2) EC subtype–specific signaling (e.g., shear stress upregulates aortic, but not pulmonary artery, nitric oxide synthase); (3) differences in EC transcriptional regulation of proteins such as von Willebrand factor (VWF) and its cleaving protease, ADAMTS13; and (4) the increasingly appreciated important link between inflammation and thrombosis that is mediated in both physiologies by selectin and integrin ligands.

Atherothrombosis

This section briefly discusses hematologic factors that predispose to thrombosis in the setting of atherosclerotic plaque (atherothrombosis); the pathophysiologic mechanisms of atherogenesis are discussed in "Cardiovascular Disease" Chapter 7.

Atherothrombosis and Fibrinolysis

In addition to EC-directed regulation of hemostasis, the interaction of EC with the fibrinolytic system is important in the development of atherothrombotic disease because it affects the degree of clot propagation. The breakdown of stable fibrin polymers into fibrin split products, including the D-dimer segments that are routinely measured in the laboratory to detect recent thrombosis, is mediated by plasmin. Plasmin is converted from its inactive form, plasminogen, by tissue-type plasminogen activator (t-PA), the activity of which is regulated by plasminogen activator inhibitor-1 (PAI-1). Abnormal levels of both t-PA and PAI-1 are epidemiologically associated with an increased risk for arterial thrombosis, but the degree to which absolute levels contribute to arterial thrombosis remains controversial. For this reason, the current clinical utility of t-PA and PAI-1 measurements is limited.

There is a correlation between higher PAI-1 levels and atherosclerotic disease, which is possibly due to the fact that PAI-1 is markedly increased in generalized inflammation and there is known thrombosis-inflammation interplay. This is especially prominent in patients with type 2 diabetes with acute myocardial infarction and stroke. Elevated PAI-1 levels systemically may prevent thrombi removal from vessels, whereas locally it contributes to increased fibrin deposition in the lumen of the vessels. Currently there are agents that indirectly decrease PAI-1 levels, including angiotensin-converting enzyme (ACE) inhibitors and diabetes medications (including thiazolidinediones and metformin). The first PAI-1 antagonist, tiplaxtinin, has been studied in experimental models and was found to decrease VTE and atherosclerosis, although the clinical trial was discontinued given unfavorable risk-benefit outcomes. Also, meta-analyses have demonstrated PAI-1 4G/5G polymorphisms represent a risk candidate locus for higher VTE risk, which is even further heightened in patients with genetic thrombophilic disorders.

Hyperhomocysteinemia in Arterial Disease

Increased levels of plasma homocysteine (HCY) are linked to atherothrombosis. The rare congenital syndromes (e.g., cystathionine β-synthase deficiency) that are characterized by homocystinuria and hyperhomocysteinemia are associated with both VTE and premature atherosclerosis. Elevated HCY induces EC dysfunction and apoptosis, triggering normal coagulation pathways designed to respond to EC damage but without the corresponding upregulation of EC-dependent anticoagulant function (e.g., activated protein C [APC]). Even moderate elevations in HCY may thus contribute to coronary, peripheral, and cerebral arterial disease. Mildly elevated HCY levels are associated with the thermolabile form of the methylene tetrahydrofolate reductase (MTHFR) enzyme, which results from a polymorphism (C677T) in the coding region of the MTHFR binding site. This isoform occurs in 30% to 40% of the general population and introduces a higher set point for regulation of HCY concentration (the substrate for MTHFR), particularly when a relative folate deficiency exists. In fact, deficiency of any of the vitamin cofactors of HCY metabolism (folate, vitamin B_6, and vitamin B_{12}) may lead to mild hyperhomocysteinemia.

Reduction in HCY levels by supplementation with vitamin B_6, vitamin B_{12}, and folate is probably the most effective means of reducing modest HCY elevations, but such supplementation and ultimately lower HCY levels does not decrease atherothrombotic risk, regardless of the cause of hyperhomocysteinemia or the presence of the MTHFR polymorphism. Therefore, the origin of the connection between high HCY and thrombosis remains incomplete, and the search for associated factors that link HCY and hypercoagulability continues.

止血障碍：血栓形成

董焕 译　杨仁池　张磊 审校　王建祥 通审

血栓形成的病理学

Virchow 三要素定义了血栓形成的病理学机制，即血流淤滞、血管壁损伤及促凝因素与抗凝因素失衡。其中，前两个要素可定位于特定的血管床；最后一个要素可能是全身性的，但数据显示解剖区域至少可部分调节止血平衡。例如，先天性缺乏抗凝血酶、蛋白 C、蛋白 S 通常可导致下肢静脉血栓栓塞（VTE）。相反，遗传性高凝性疾病伴有因子 V Leiden 突变及凝血酶原 G20210A 突变不仅会导致下肢 VTE，还与大脑静脉及静脉窦血栓形成相关。

这种血管组织的止血调节主要由以下因素介导：①微环境信号，如血管损伤形成血液湍流所产生的剪切应力，其影响内皮细胞（EC）表达凝血调节蛋白、组织因子及一氧化氮合成酶和血小板活化；②EC 亚型特异性信号转导，如剪切应力可上调主动脉（而不是肺动脉）一氧化氮合成酶水平；③EC 对蛋白质转录的差异性调控，如血管性血友病因子（vWF）及其裂解蛋白酶 ADAMTS13；④炎症与血栓之间的重要联系，两者均由选择素和整合素配体介导。

动脉粥样硬化血栓形成

下文将简要讨论动脉粥样硬化斑块易形成血栓的血液学因素（动脉粥样硬化血栓形成）；动脉粥样硬化形成的病理生理学机制见《心血管疾病分册》第 7 章。

动脉粥样硬化血栓形成和纤维蛋白溶解

除了 EC 介导的止血调节机制外，EC 与纤维蛋白溶解系统之间的相互作用在动脉粥样硬化血栓形成性疾病的发生中发挥重要作用，因其影响着血凝块扩增的程度。纤溶酶介导稳定的纤维蛋白聚合物降解为纤维蛋白降解产物，包括实验室常规检测的 D- 二聚体，其是近期血栓形成的相关指标。组织纤溶酶原激活物（t-PA）将无活性的纤溶酶原转化为纤溶酶，其活性受纤溶酶原激活物抑制物 -1（PAI-1）的调节。在流行病学上，t-PA 和 PAI-1 水平异常与动脉血栓形成的风险增加相关，但其绝对水平会在多大程度上导致动脉血栓形成仍存在争议。因此，目前 t-PA 和 PAI-1 检测的临床应用有限。

PAI-1 水平升高与动脉粥样硬化性疾病的发生相关，这可能是由于在全身性炎症中 PAI-1 水平显著升高，且已知血栓形成和炎症反应之间存在相互作用。这在 2 型糖尿病合并急性心肌梗死和脑卒中的患者中尤为突出。全身 PAI-1 水平升高可能会阻止血栓从血管中清除，而局部 PAI-1 水平升高则会增加血管腔内的纤维蛋白沉积。目前，可间接降低 PAI-1 水平的药物包括血管紧张素转换酶抑制剂（ACEI）和糖尿病治疗药物（包括噻唑烷二酮类和二甲双胍），其中第一种 PAI-1 拮抗剂替普沙汀已在实验动物模型中进行了研究，结果发现其可减少 VTE 和动脉粥样硬化，但其临床试验因风险效益不佳而被终止。此外，荟萃分析显示 PAI-1 的 4G/5G 多态性是更高 VTE 风险的候选位点，在遗传性血栓疾病患者中这种风险会进一步升高。

高同型半胱氨酸血症在动脉疾病中的作用

血浆同型半胱氨酸（HCY）水平升高与动脉粥样硬化血栓形成相关。以同型半胱氨酸尿症和高同型半胱氨酸血症为特征的罕见先天性综合征（如胱硫醚 β- 合酶缺乏症）与 VTE 和早期动脉粥样硬化血栓形成相关。HCY 水平升高可导致 EC 功能障碍和凋亡，EC 损伤触发正常的凝血途径，但没有上调 EC 依赖性抗凝血功能[如活化蛋白 C（APC）]。因此，即使 HCY 水平中度升高亦可导致冠状动脉、外周动脉和脑动脉疾病。HCY 水平轻度升高与不耐热型亚甲基四氢叶酸还原酶（MTHFR）相关，而后者由 MTHFR 结合位点编码区的多态性（C677T）引起。30%～40% 的普通人群中存在该亚型，该亚型调节 HCY 浓度（MTHFR 的底物）的阈值更高，尤其是在叶酸相对缺乏时。事实上，调节 HCY 代谢的任何一种维生素辅因子（叶酸、维生素 B_6 和维生素 B_{12}）的缺乏均可能导致轻度高同型半胱氨酸血症。

补充维生素 B_6、维生素 B_{12} 和叶酸以降低 HCY 水平可能是治疗轻度 HCY 水平升高最有效的方法，但无论引起高同型半胱氨酸血症的原因是什么或是否存在 MTHFR 多态性，这种治疗方法都不会降低动脉粥样硬化血栓形成的风险。因此，高 HCY 水平和血栓形成之间的关系尚未完全明确，探究 HCY 与高凝状态关联的相关因素的研究仍在继续。

TABLE 8.1 Antiplatelet Therapies

Inhibitors of Cyclooxygenase
Aspirin
Nonaspirin NSAIDs (not COX2 selective)

P2Y12 Antagonists
Prasugrel
Ticagrelor
Clopidogrel

Phosphodiesterase Inhibitors
Dipyridamole
Prostacyclin

GPIIB/IIIA Blockers
Abciximab
Integrilin
Tirofiban

COX2, Cyclooxygenase 2; *GPIIb/IIIa*, glycoprotein IIb/IIIa complex; *NSAIDs*, nonsteroidal anti-inflammatory drugs.

Role of Platelets in Atherothrombosis

Although EC-associated abnormalities clearly influence hemostasis, platelet activation and adhesion are also critical to the development of atherothrombosis, especially in patients with acute coronary syndrome or ischemic stroke. Antiplatelet therapies are the primary modalities for maintaining short- and long-term patency in arteries, especially after coronary revascularization. Antiplatelet therapy can be targeted against specific platelet functions, including cyclooxygenase-mediated formation of thromboxane A_2, interaction of adenosine diphosphate (ADP) with its platelet receptor, and binding of the glycoprotein IIb/IIIa complex (GPIIb/IIIa) to fibrinogen for aggregation (Table 8.1).

Aspirin has long been a mainstay in the treatment of myocardial infarction, angina, and stroke because of its irreversible inhibition of platelet cyclooxygenase, a process that blocks the release of thromboxane A_2. Aspirin effectively prevents platelet aggregation over the lifetime of a platelet (7 to 10 days); however, aspirin is usually unable to inhibit platelet activation, secretion, and aggregation by thrombin or other strong agonists such as collagen. Therefore, blockade of other platelet activation pathways is important for patients who are at risk for arterial thrombosis.

Some drugs used to treat stroke or coronary disease (i.e., clopidogrel and prasugrel) specifically block platelet P2Y12, the ADP receptor, from interaction with ADP in the clot milieu, thereby decreasing platelet recruitment by preventing locally released ADP from activating additional platelets.

The CHANCE Trial (2013) and POINT Trial (2018) have shown reduced 90-day stroke risk with the combination of ASA/clopidogrel compared with ASA alone, although results are conflicting between the trials about increased bleeding risk with dual antiplatelet therapy (DAPT). In symptomatic peripheral arterial disease (PAD), where there is poor flow in the extremities due to atherosclerotic plaque, there are benefits with using clopidogrel compared to aspirin (demonstrated by the CAPRIE Trial 1996) but no additional benefit to using both clopidogrel and aspirin together as compared to clopidogrel monotherapy (demonstrated by the MATCH Trial 2004).

Antiplatelet therapy with aspirin and a P2Y12 inhibitor (clopidogrel, prasugrel, or ticagrelor) also reduces the risk of stent thrombosis and subsequent cardiovascular events after percutaneous coronary intervention and should be administered for at least 12 months unless the patient is at high risk for bleeding. The PLATO Trial (2009) showed, in acute coronary syndrome, prasugrel and ticagrelor further reduce cardiovascular ischemic events compared with clopidogrel, although they are associated with higher bleeding risk. This effect occurs because drug interactions and variant cytochrome genotypes do not significantly affect production of the active metabolites of prasugrel and ticagrelor; the result is greater and more rapid inhibition of P2Y12 receptor–mediated platelet aggregation in most patients. The EUCLID Trial showed that in PAD, there was no improvement with ticagrelor compared to clopidogrel in terms of cardiovascular death, myocardial infarction, or stroke.

Despite its wide use, a significant proportion (up to one third) of patients demonstrate functional platelet resistance to clopidogrel. Under such circumstances, clopidogrel is poorly metabolized to its active form because of the presence of polymorphisms in the cytochrome P-450 gene, *CYP2C19*, that cause loss of function. The more potent inhibitor, prasugrel, is not affected by cytochrome P-450 genotypes, although nongenetic factors such as platelet turnover, absorption, and compliance also play important roles in response variability.

A third avenue for blocking platelet activation targets GPIIb/IIIa, the primary platelet receptor for binding to fibrinogen and VWF. Abciximab, a modified monoclonal antibody, prevents GPIIb/IIIa from binding to fibrinogen and blocks platelet aggregation after angioplasty, stent placement, or pharmacologic thrombolysis. Abciximab has been shown to reduce the incidence of recurrent acute ischemic events after percutaneous coronary revascularization in patients with myocardial infarction or unstable angina, mainly by decreasing the incidence of platelet-mediated thrombosis within the infarct-related vessel during and after the procedure. Other GPIIb/IIIa blockers, including eptifibatide (Integrilin) and tirofiban (Aggrastat), interfere with the GPIIb/IIIa arginine-glycine-aspartate (RGD) binding sites; they are used acutely for parenteral administration in patients with acute coronary syndrome or to maintain coronary patency after percutaneous coronary intervention. Thrombocytopenia is an uncommon (<2%) complication of all the GPIIb/IIIa inhibitors; it is most likely related to exposure of neoepitopes on the receptor and immune-mediated platelet destruction. Clearance of the drug typically resolves the thrombocytopenia within 1 week. Platelet transfusion should be considered only if there is significant thrombocytopenic bleeding because of the higher incidence of stent thrombosis after stent implantation with platelet transfusion.

Additional novel strategies for mediating platelet activity include inhibition of cyclic nucleotide phosphodiesterases (e.g., dipyridamole, cilostazol) and blockade of proteinase-activated receptor 1 (PAR-1). Phosphodiesterase inhibitors most likely have multiple mechanisms of action. They result in decreased signal transduction within platelets, which impairs their responsiveness. PAR-1 is one of two principal recognized targets for thrombin stimulation of platelets, the other being PAR-4. The potential benefit of adding phosphodiesterase or PAR-1 inhibitors to aspirin and/or clopidogrel (e.g., prevention of restenosis in atherothrombosis) is being evaluated. As shown in ESPS-2 (1996) and ESPRIT (2006), aspirin/dipyridamole outperformed aspirin alone in secondary prevention of ischemic strokes—current guidelines recommended either aspirin monotherapy or aspirin/dipyridamole as secondary prevention for ischemic stroke. Additionally, for recent stroke, there appears to be no difference in recurrence rates of ischemic stroke when comparing aspirin/dipyridamole to clopidogrel, as shown in the PRoFESS Trial (2008). Currently, either of these options or aspirin monotherapy is recommended after noncardioembolic ischemic stroke; aspirin in combination with clopidogrel is not recommended given increased bleeding risk (POINT Trial 2018).

表 8.1　抗血小板治疗
环氧合酶（COX）抑制剂
阿司匹林
非阿司匹林类 NSAID（非选择性抑制 COX-2）
P2Y12 拮抗剂
普拉格雷
替格瑞洛
氯吡格雷
磷酸二酯酶抑制剂
双嘧达莫
前列环素
GP Ⅱb/Ⅲa 抑制剂
阿昔单抗
依替巴肽
替罗非班

COX-2，环氧合酶 2；GP Ⅱb/Ⅲa，糖蛋白 Ⅱb/Ⅲa 复合物；NSAID，非甾体抗炎药。

血小板在动脉粥样硬化血栓形成中的作用

虽然 EC 相关异常可影响止血，但血小板的活化和黏附也是动脉粥样硬化血栓形成的关键环节，在急性冠脉综合征或缺血性脑卒中的患者中更是如此。抗血小板治疗是维持动脉短期和长期通畅的主要方式，尤其是在冠状动脉血运重建后。抗血小板治疗可针对血小板特定的功能，包括环氧合酶（COX）介导的血栓烷 A_2 形成、腺苷二磷酸（ADP）与其血小板受体的相互作用，以及糖蛋白 Ⅱb/Ⅲa 复合物（GP Ⅱb/Ⅲa）与纤维蛋白原结合引起的血小板聚集（表 8.1）。

阿司匹林长期以来一直是心肌梗死、心绞痛和卒中的主要治疗药物，因为它不可逆地抑制血小板 COX，进而阻断血栓素 A_2 释放。阿司匹林能在血小板的寿命周期内（7～10 天）有效阻止血小板聚集；然而，阿司匹林通常不能抑制凝血酶和其他强效激动剂（如胶原蛋白）诱导的血小板活化、分泌和聚集。因此，阻断血小板活化的其他途径对于有动脉血栓形成风险的患者很重要。

一些用于治疗卒中或冠状动脉疾病的药物（如氯吡格雷和普拉格雷）可特异性地阻断血小板 P2Y12（ADP 受体）与血栓环境中 ADP 的相互作用，通过抑制血栓局部释放的 ADP 来激活更多的血小板，从而减少血小板募集。

CHANCE 试验（2013 年）和 POINT 试验（2018 年）显示，与单用阿司匹林相比，阿司匹林联用氯吡格雷可降低 90 天时的卒中风险，尽管两项试验关于双重抗血小板治疗（DAPT）增加出血风险的结果并不一致。在症状性外周动脉疾病（PAD）中，动脉粥样硬化斑块可导致四肢血流不畅，与阿司匹林相比，使用氯吡格雷的获益更大（经 1996 年 CAPRIE 试验证实），但与氯吡格雷单药治疗相比，氯吡格雷联用阿司匹林没有额外的益处（经 2004 年 MATCH 试验证实）。

联合使用阿司匹林和 P2Y12 拮抗剂（氯吡格雷、普拉格雷或替格瑞洛）的抗血小板治疗降低了经皮冠状动脉介入治疗（PCI）后支架内血栓形成和后续心血管事件的风险，应至少用药维持 12 个月，除非患者的出血风险高。PLATO 试验（2009 年）显示，在急性冠脉综合征中，与氯吡格雷相比，普拉格雷和替格瑞洛可进一步减少心血管缺血事件，尽管它们与更高的出血风险相关。这种效应是因为药物相互作用和细胞色素基因型变异不会显著影响普拉格雷和替格瑞洛活性代谢产物的生成；在大多数患者中它们更有效且迅速地抑制了 P2Y12 受体介导的血小板聚集。EUCLID 试验表明，在 PAD 中，与氯吡格雷相比，替格瑞洛在心血管死亡、心肌梗死或卒中方面没有改善。

尽管氯吡格雷已被广泛使用，但有很大一部分患者（高达 1/3）对其耐药。这是因为这些患者的细胞色素 P450 基因（*CYP2C19*）多态性导致其失去功能，使氯吡格雷很少代谢为其活性形式。更强效的普拉格雷不受细胞色素 P450 基因型的影响，但非遗传因素（如血小板更新率、药物吸收和患者依从性）对疗效起重要作用。

阻断血小板活化的第三种途径是靶向 GP Ⅱb/Ⅲa，它是血小板与纤维蛋白原和 vWF 结合的主要受体。阿昔单抗是一种修饰的单克隆抗体，可防止血小板的 GP Ⅱb/Ⅲa 与纤维蛋白原结合，并在血管成形术后、支架置入术后或药物溶栓后阻断血小板聚集。研究显示，在心肌梗死或不稳定型心绞痛患者中，阿昔单抗可降低经皮冠状动脉血运重建后的急性缺血事件复发率，它主要降低术中和术后梗死相关血管内血小板介导的血栓形成的发生率。其他 GP Ⅱb/Ⅲa 抑制剂（如依替巴肽和替罗非班）通过干扰 GP Ⅱb/Ⅲa 的精氨酸-甘氨酸-天冬氨酸（RGD）结合位点发挥作用。它们可用于急性冠脉综合征患者的急性静脉给药或用于经皮冠状动脉介入术后保持冠状动脉通畅。血小板减少症是所有 GP Ⅱb/Ⅲa 抑制剂的少见并发症（<2%），很可能与受体新表位的暴露及免疫介导的血小板破坏有关。随着药物的清除，血小板计数通常在 1 周内逐渐恢复正常。输注血小板仅用于严重血小板减少导致出血时，因其与支架置入术后支架内血栓形成的发生率升高相关。

其他抑制血小板活性的新策略包括抑制环核苷酸磷酸二酯酶（如双嘧达莫、西洛他唑）和阻断蛋白酶激活受体 1（PAR-1）。磷酸二酯酶抑制剂很可能具有多种作用机制，可导致血小板内信号转导减少，从而减弱其反应性。PAR-1 和 PAR-4 是凝血酶激活血小板的两个主要靶点。目前还在评估磷酸二酯酶抑制剂或 PAR-1 抑制剂联合阿司匹林和（或）氯吡格雷的潜在效用（如预防动脉粥样硬化血栓形成中的再狭窄）。ESPS-2 试验（1996 年）和 ESPRIT 试验（2006 年）显示，在缺血性卒中的二级预防方面，阿司匹林/双嘧达莫优于单用阿司匹林，当前指南建议将阿司匹林单药治疗或阿司匹林/双嘧达莫联合治疗作为缺血性卒中的二级预防。此外，PRoFESS 试验（2008 年）表明，对于新近出现的卒中，阿司匹林/双嘧达莫组和氯吡格雷组的缺血性卒中复发率似乎没有差异。目前，非心源性血栓性缺血性卒中后推荐使用上述方法或阿司匹林单药治疗；考虑到出血风险增加，不建议阿司匹林与氯吡格雷联合使用（2018 年 POINT 试验）。

TABLE 8.2 Prevalence and Thrombotic Relative Risk Associations of Laboratory Findings[a]

Prevalence in General Population	Venous RR	Arterial RR
Hyperhomocysteinemia (25%)	1-2	1.16
Activated protein C resistance (5%)		
Heterozygous FVL	7	1
Homozygous FVL	20-80	
Prothrombin G20210A mutation (1-2%)		
Heterozygous	2-5	1
Homozygous	>5	1
Platelet GPIIb/IIIa HPA-Ib homozygosity (2-3%)		4 (MI in men)
Protein C deficiency (0.2-0.5%)	7	1
Protein S deficiency (0.1%)	8.5	1
AT deficiency (0.02-0.05%)	8	1
Dysfibrinogenemia (rare)	≈1	1.5

AT, Antithrombin; *FVL*, factor V Leiden; *GPIIb/IIIa*, glycoprotein IIb/IIIa complex; *HPA-1b*, human platelet antigen-1b; *MI*, myocardial infarction; *RR*, relative risk.
[a]Data on prevalence and relative risk vary widely, often with conflicting results. This information represents an interpretation of data collected from various sources, mainly meta-analyses.

When using platelet inhibitors, physicians and patients must also consider the risk of bleeding if they are on anticoagulation therapy. RE-DUAL (2017) and WOEST (2013) concluded that in patients on anticoagulation prior to percutaneous coronary intervention (PCI) it is recommended to use additionally only clopidogrel rather than ASA/clopidogrel after PCI given the increased bleeding risk with triple therapy.

Venous Thromboembolism: Inherited Risk Factors

The balance between thrombin formation and anticoagulant pathways has been extensively studied in patients with inherited deficiencies of naturally occurring anticoagulants (Table 8.2). These patients are predisposed to VTE, which includes deep vein thrombosis (DVT) and pulmonary embolism (PE).

Factor V Leiden

The most common inherited disorder leading to VTE is the factor V Leiden (FVL) mutation although it remains a fairly weak risk factor for VTE overall. About 5% of individuals of European ancestry are heterozygous for FVL. The FVL mutation increases VTE risk by decreasing the susceptibility of factor Va to APC-mediated inactivation and by impairing the APC-cofactor activity of factor V in factor VIIIa inactivation, all of which lead to increased thrombin generation. APC resistance can be demonstrated by specialized clotting tests in which the addition of APC fails to inhibit thrombin generation. About one fourth of patients with their first VTE are heterozygous for FVL, and this percentage increases to almost 60% among those with recurrent VTE or a strong family history of VTE.

Heterozygous FVL mutation conveys a 7-fold increased risk for VTE. However, at 50 years of age, only 25% of persons with heterozygous FVL mutation have had VTE, compared with much higher percentages in other inherited thrombophilias. It is with concomitant *acquired* risk factors such as immobilization, pregnancy, or oral contraceptive use that the risk for VTE in persons with FVL mutation becomes more significant. The prothrombin G20210A mutation demonstrates a synergistic effect with FVL mutation, but the MTHFR mutation does not. Homozygous FVL mutation individuals have a 20- to 80-fold increased risk for VTE. APC resistance *without* the FVL mutation occurs rarely. Factor V Cambridge mutation, although much less common than FVL mutation, has a similar mutation at an APC cleavage site (Arg306) and is associated with APC resistance and thrombosis. Other minor alleles of factor V, including the 6755 A/G (D2194G) R2 haplotype, may enhance APC resistance. When this haplotype is on a different chromosome than the FVL mutation, it diminishes normal factor V transcription and increases the ratio of FVL to normal factor V.

Prothrombin G20210A

Another mutation associated with inherited thrombophilia is the prothrombin G20210A mutation, which occurs in the 3′-untranslated region of the prothrombin gene. This mutation leads to higher than normal prothrombin levels and a 2-fold increased risk for VTE. The heterozygous mutation is present in about 3% of European-derived populations but is identified in about 15% of patients with VTE. Patients homozygous for prothrombin G20210A are rare, but their relative risk for VTE is thought to be about 10-fold. Exactly how the prothrombin mutation affects thrombus development has not been fully defined, but changes in polyadenylation of the prothrombin messenger RNA (mRNA) during transcription appear to be involved. The distribution of circulating prothrombin levels overlaps significantly between those with and without the mutation, so Factor II levels are not helpful in diagnosing the condition. Diagnosis of the G20210A genotype is made by examination of the patient's DNA for this specific mutation; no screening or functional assays are available.

Inherited Deficiency of Natural Anticoagulants

Deficiencies in the natural anticoagulant proteins (antithrombin, protein C, and protein S) are less common than FVL or prothrombin G20210A, but they are more likely to produce symptomatic VTE at an earlier age. Only about one half of the cases of VTE occurring in patients with these deficiencies are associated with acquired risk factors such as pregnancy, surgery, or immobilization. Deficiencies of antithrombin, protein C, or protein S are detected by functional or antigenic assays because some mutations cause a quantitative decrease in the factor, whereas others produce a dysfunctional protein. Many gene mutations have been associated with these deficiencies, but none is predominant. Deficiencies of antithrombin (AT), protein C, and protein S in the aggregate account for fewer than 5% to 10% of all patients with VTE.

Antithrombin is a naturally occurring anticoagulant that complexes with endogenous heparin sulfates to inhibit both formed thrombin and factor Xa. Heterozygous antithrombin deficiency leads to antithrombin activity levels less than 70% of normal and a 20-fold increase in the risk for VTE; VTE usually occurs by the age of 25 years in 50% of such patients. More than 200 associated mutations are known. Homozygous mutations are very rare, likely because of lethality *in utero*.

Acquired causes of antithrombin deficiency are more common. Because antithrombin has a low molecular weight, it is lost in the proteinuria of nephrotic syndrome. Acquired antithrombin deficiency is common in patients receiving asparaginase therapy for acute lymphocytic leukemia and may also be associated with severe hepatic veno-occlusive disease after stem cell transplantation; antithrombin and protein C may be excessively consumed in the damaged hepatic microvasculature. Low levels of antithrombin are also associated with poorer outcomes in severely ill patients. Successful treatment of symptomatic patients with heterozygous antithrombin deficiency has included short-term replacement with fresh-frozen plasma or recombinant AT protein, usually coupled with unfractionated heparin (UFH) anticoagulation; long-term therapy for congenitally deficient

表 8.2 实验室检查的阳性率及血栓事件相关风险 [a]

普通人群的患病率	静脉血栓 RR	动脉血栓 RR
高同型半胱氨酸血症（25%）	1～2	1.16
活化蛋白 C 抵抗（5%）		
FVL 杂合子	7	1
FVL 纯合子	20～80	1
凝血酶原 G20210A 突变（1%）		
杂合子	2～5	1
纯合子	>5	1
血小板 GPⅡbⅢa HPA-1b 纯合子（2%～3%）		4（男性发生心肌梗死）
蛋白 C 缺陷（0.2%～0.5%）	7	1
蛋白 S 缺陷（0.1%）	8.5	1
AT 缺陷（0.02%～0.05%）	8	1
异常纤维蛋白原血症（罕见）	≈1	1.5

AT，抗凝血酶；FVL，因子 V Leiden；GPⅡb/Ⅲa，糖蛋白Ⅱb/Ⅲa复合物；HPA-1b，人类血小板抗原 -1b；RR，相对危险度。

[a] 不同研究关于患病率和相对危险度的数据差异很大，通常有相互矛盾的结果。该表综合了不同研究的数据，主要是来自荟萃分析。

在使用血小板抑制剂时，医生和患者必须考虑抗凝治疗时出血的风险。RE-DUAL 试验（2017 年）和 WOEST 试验（2013 年）的结论是对于在 PCI 前接受抗凝治疗的患者，鉴于三联治疗的出血风险增加，建议在 PCI 后仅使用氯吡格雷，而不是阿司匹林联用氯吡格雷。

静脉血栓栓塞：遗传性危险因素

凝血酶形成和抗凝血途径之间的平衡已在先天性抗凝物质缺陷的患者中进行了广泛研究（表 8.2）。这些患者易患 VTE，包括深静脉血栓形成（DVT）和肺栓塞（PE）。

因子 V Leiden 突变

导致 VTE 的最常见的遗传病是因子 V Leiden（FVL）突变，但总体而言，它仍然是 VTE 的一个相当弱的危险因素。欧裔人群 FVL 杂合子的检出率约为 5%。FVL 突变可降低因子 Va 对 APC 介导失活的易感性，并损害因子 V 在因子Ⅷa 失活过程中的 APC 辅因子活性，所有这些均会导致凝血酶生成增加，从而增加 VTE 风险。APC 抵抗可通过特异性凝血试验加以证实，试验中可见增加 APC 不能抑制凝血酶生成。在首次发生 VTE 的患者中，约 1/4 是 FVL 杂合子，而在复发性 VTE 或有较强 VTE 家族史的患者中，该比例增加至约 60%。

FVL 杂合子可使 VTE 的风险增加 7 倍。然而，只有 25% 的 FVL 杂合子患者在 50 岁时发生 VTE，而其他遗传性易栓症的 VTE 发生率更高。若同时存在获得性危险因素，如制动、妊娠或口服避孕药，FVL 突变患者的 VTE 风险更高。目前已证实凝血酶原 G20210A 突变与 FVL 突变具有协同作用，而与 *MTHFR* 突变无协同作用。FVL 纯合子发生 VTE 的风险增加 20～80 倍。无 FVL 突变的 APC 抵抗极少见。虽然因子 V Cambridge 突变比 FVL 突变更少见，但其在 APC 的切割位点（Arg306）具有相似的突变，并与 APC 抵抗和血栓形成有关。因子 V 的其他次要等位基因，包括 6755A/G（D2194G）R2 单体型，可能增强 APC 抵抗。当该单体型与 FVL 突变位于不同的染色体上时，可减少正常因子 V 的转录，使 FVL 与正常因子 V 的比例增大。

凝血酶原 G20210A

与遗传性易栓症相关的另一种突变是凝血酶原 G20210A 突变，该突变发生在凝血酶原基因的 3′- 非翻译区。这种突变导致凝血酶原水平高于正常，使发生 VTE 的风险增加 2 倍。在欧裔人群中杂合子约占 3%，但在 VTE 患者中约占 15%。凝血酶原 G20210A 突变纯合子很罕见，但其发生 VTE 的相对风险约增加 10 倍。凝血酶原突变影响血栓发生的机制尚未完全明确，但凝血酶原信使 RNA（mRNA）在转录过程中的多聚腺苷酸化改变可能与此有关。循环凝血酶原水平在携带和未携带突变的个体之间存在明显重叠，因此检测因子Ⅱ水平对诊断没有帮助。G20210A 基因型的诊断可通过检测患者 DNA 中的这种特异性突变；目前尚无可用于筛查或功能测定的试验。

天然抗凝剂的遗传性缺陷

虽然天然抗凝蛋白（抗凝血酶、蛋白 C 和蛋白 S）缺陷较 FVL 或凝血酶原 G20210A 少见，但它们更可能导致年轻人群发生有症状的 VTE。这些天然抗凝蛋白缺陷的患者发生 VTE 时，仅 1/2 伴有获得性血栓危险因素（如妊娠、手术或制动）。通过功能测定或抗原测定可检测抗凝血酶、蛋白 C 或蛋白 S 缺陷，因为部分突变可引起抗凝蛋白含量减少，而其他突变可导致蛋白质功能障碍。目前已发现许多基因突变与这些抗凝蛋白缺陷有关，但尚未发现某个基因起主导作用。总体而言，在所有 VTE 患者中，抗凝血酶（AT）、蛋白 C 和蛋白 S 缺陷的占比不足 5%～10%。

AT 是一种天然存在的抗凝剂，可与内源性硫酸肝素形成复合物，从而抑制已形成的凝血酶和因子 Xa 活性。杂合突变所致抗凝血酶缺陷的患者抗凝血酶的活性低于正常水平的 70%，发生 VTE 的风险增加 20 倍。这类患者中 50% 在 25 岁时发生 VTE。已知的相关基因突变超过 200 种。纯合突变非常罕见，可能是因为这些患儿会在宫内死亡。

获得性抗凝血酶缺乏症更为常见。由于抗凝血酶分子量小，可随肾病综合征患者的蛋白尿而丢失。获得性 AT 缺陷常见于接受天冬酰胺酶治疗的急性淋巴细胞白血病患者，也可能与造血干细胞移植术后发生严重肝静脉闭塞性疾病相关；抗凝血酶和蛋白 C 可能在受损的肝微血管系统中过度消耗。抗凝血酶水平低也与危重症患者的不良结局相关。成功治疗症状性抗凝血酶缺陷杂合子患者的措施包括新鲜冰冻血浆或重组 AT 的短期替代治疗，常联用普通肝素（UFH）；先天

patients has consisted primarily of warfarin although the direct oral anticoagulants have become increasingly popular due to their lack of requiring functional antithrombin activity in order to cause an anticoagulant effect.

The complex of thrombin and thrombomodulin on the EC surface activates protein C; APC coupled with its cofactor, protein S, cleaves and inactivates factors Va and VIIIa. These actions downregulate the prothrombinase and tenase complexes, respectively, to slow the rate of thrombin generation. Like antithrombin deficiency, heterozygous protein C and protein S deficiencies are observed with venous, and occasionally arterial, thrombosis in younger patients (median age at occurrence, 20 to 40 years).

The rare homozygous protein C deficiency manifests in the neonate as *purpura fulminans* with widespread VTE and skin necrosis. A similar clinical presentation has been reported in heterozygous protein C–deficient adults after institution of warfarin therapy without simultaneous heparinization; this is called *warfarin-induced skin necrosis*. About one third of these patients are deficient in protein C on a hereditary basis, whereas the rest appear to have acquired protein C deficiency, possibly associated with vitamin K deficiency. Warfarin is a vitamin K antagonist that inhibits production of vitamin K–dependent protein C synthesis; and because of its short half-life, protein C levels rapidly fall before a decline in the levels of the procoagulant factors II, IX, and X. This imbalance shortly after starting warfarin favors a procoagulant state and may result in widespread microvascular thrombosis. Therefore, patients with active VTE should be fully anticoagulated with UFH or low-molecular-weight heparin (LMWH) before concurrent warfarin therapy is begun. UFH/LMWH should be continued for at least 48 hours, warfarin has a full therapeutic effect.

Inherited deficiency of protein S has similarly been implicated in warfarin-induced skin necrosis. Protein S deficiency is commonly acquired in acute illness. Protein S circulates in a free form and is bound by complement 4b (C4b)-binding protein; only free protein S is active as a cofactor for protein C. Because C4b-binding protein is an acute phase reactant, its increase with severe illness can decrease the level of free protein S. A similar effect is seen in normal pregnancy.

Short-term therapy for homozygous protein C deficiency or for doubly heterozygous protein C or S deficiency, especially in the setting of neonatal purpura fulminans, has included plasma or protein C concentrate with full-dose UFH anticoagulation. Functional and antigenic levels of antithrombin, protein S, and protein C can be assessed to define whether functional deficiency is caused by a dysfunctional protein or by diminished synthesis. As with AT deficiency, initial heparin therapy followed by long-term treatment with warfarin has been successful in heterozygous protein C or S deficiency. As expected, both protein C and protein S levels are decreased during warfarin therapy; therefore, for adequate evaluation of protein C and S, the patient must not be taking warfarin when tested.

Venous Thrombosis: Acquired Risk Factors
Surgery and Medical Hospitalization
Medical and surgical illnesses convey increased thrombotic risk; these *acquired* risk factors are well accepted, even though the pathophysiologic features favoring thrombosis may be uncertain (Table 8.3). Stasis of blood flow is a clear risk factor for thrombus formation (e.g., VTE in immobilized inpatients). Other high-risk situations, including surgery (especially orthopedic) and trauma, are similarly associated with immobilization and stasis of lower extremity blood flow. When evidence of thrombosis is thoroughly sought, both surgery and trauma can be shown to be associated with extremely high (>50%) incidences of VTE. Fat embolism and tissue damage may also contribute to the risk for VTE with surgery and trauma, particularly in closed head injuries that result in massive tissue factor release. Prophylactic inferior vena cava (IVC) filters are often placed in trauma patients to protect against PE, especially in high-risk patients for whom anticoagulation is contraindicated because of the increased risk for bleeding, but there remains a high risk for thrombus formation proximal to the filter with subsequent pulmonary embolism. IVC filters should be removed as soon as patients may be safely anticoagulated.

All hospitalized medical patients should be considered for venous thromboprophylaxis with UFH or LMWH. Factors that increase bleeding risk that argue against anticoagulation include thrombocytopenia (typically a platelet count <50,000), coagulopathy (with or without liver disease), and recent hemorrhage. Risk factors that warrant aggressive prophylaxis include malignancy, prior VTE, immobilization, and thrombophilic conditions.

Pregnancy and Fetal Loss
Pregnancy is a hypercoagulable state associated with venous stasis; the risk for VTE during pregnancy and in the postpartum period for women with identified thrombophilia is about 5-fold higher than it is for nonpregnant women. Pregnancy increases procoagulant proteins, including fibrinogen, VWF, and factors VII, VIII, and X, and decreases natural anticoagulants such as protein S and antithrombin as well as fibrinolytic inhibitors such as PAI-1 and thrombin activator fibrinolysis inhibitor (TAFI). VTE can occur at any time during pregnancy or the puerperium. The risk of postpartum VTE is significantly higher in women with any of the following conditions: stillbirth, pre-term delivery, obstetric hemorrhage, caesarean procedure, medical comorbidities, or a pre-pregnancy body mass index greater than 30 kg/m².

Inherited maternal thrombophilia can compound the procoagulant state of pregnancy and predispose to both fetal loss and VTE in the mother. The principal inherited associated risk factors for fetal loss are FVL mutation, the G20210A prothrombin mutation, antithrombin deficiency, and protein C or protein S deficiency. The relative risk for fetal loss is markedly higher in those mothers with a history of prior

TABLE 8.3 Acquired Risk Factors for Thrombosis

Medical and Surgical Illnesses
Antiphospholipid antibody, lupus anticoagulant
Artificial heart valves
Atrial fibrillation (nonvalvular)
Congestive heart failure
Hemolytic anemias (autoimmune hemolysis, sickle cell, thrombotic thrombocytopenic purpura, paroxysmal nocturnal hemoglobinuria)
Hyperlipidemia
Immobilization
Malignancy
Myeloproliferative disorders with thrombocytosis
Nephrotic syndrome
Orthopedic procedures
Pregnancy
Trauma, fat embolism

Medications
Heparin-induced thrombocytopenia
Oral contraceptives, hormone replacement therapy
Prothrombin complex concentrates

性缺陷患者的长期治疗主要是华法林，但直接口服抗凝剂（DOAC）的应用越来越广泛，因其无须功能性抗凝血酶活性即可发挥抗凝作用。

凝血酶和凝血调节蛋白在 EC 表面形成复合物来激活蛋白 C；APC 与其辅因子蛋白 S 偶联，剪切和灭活因子 Ⅴa 和 Ⅷa，进而分别下调凝血酶原酶及因子 X 酶复合物，以减慢凝血酶产生的速度。与抗凝血酶缺乏症相同，蛋白 C 和蛋白 S 缺陷的杂合子可导致年轻患者（中位发病年龄为 20 ~ 40 岁）发生静脉血栓，偶可发生动脉血栓。

罕见的纯合子蛋白 C 缺陷在新生儿中可出现暴发性紫癜伴广泛 VTE 和皮肤坏死。在杂合子蛋白 C 缺陷的成人患者中，若开始华法林治疗时未同时进行肝素抗凝，可出现类似的临床表现，即"华法林诱导的皮肤坏死"。这些患者中约 1/3 存在遗传性蛋白 C 缺陷，而其余患者存在获得性蛋白 C 缺陷，这可能与维生素 K 缺乏有关。华法林是一种维生素 K 抑制剂，抑制维生素 K 依赖的蛋白 C 的合成；由于蛋白 C 的半衰期较短，其水平会在因子 Ⅱ、Ⅸ 和 X 水平降低前迅速下降。在华法林治疗早期，这种失衡倾向于促凝状态，可导致广泛的微血管血栓形成。因此，活动性 VTE 患者在开始华法林治疗之前应使用 UFH 或低分子量肝素（LMWH）充分抗凝，并持续使用至华法林治疗开始后至少 48 h。

遗传性蛋白 S 缺陷同样与华法林诱导的皮肤坏死有关。蛋白质 S 缺陷通常发生在急性疾病中。蛋白 S 以游离形式循环，并与补体 4b（C4b）结合蛋白结合；只有游离的蛋白 S 才具有活性，并作为蛋白 C 的辅因子。由于 C4b 结合蛋白是急性期反应蛋白，因此疾病危重时 C4b 结合蛋白增多，使游离蛋白 S 水平降低。在正常妊娠中亦可观察到类似情况。

纯合子蛋白 C 缺陷或双重杂合子蛋白 C 或 S 缺陷的短期治疗（尤其是新生儿暴发性紫癜）包括补充血浆或蛋白 C 浓缩物联合足量 UFH 抗凝。可通过测定 AT、蛋白 S 和蛋白 C 活性及抗原水平来判断功能缺陷的原因是功能障碍还是合成减少。与抗凝血酶缺乏症一样，初始肝素治疗后序贯华法林的长期治疗已在杂合子蛋白 C 或 S 缺陷患者中取得成功。正如预期，华法林治疗期间蛋白 C 和蛋白 S 水平均降低。因此，为了充分评估蛋白 C 和蛋白 S，患者在检测时需暂停服用华法林。

静脉血栓形成：获得性危险因素
手术和住院

一些内科及外科疾病可增加血栓风险；虽然其有利于血栓形成的病理生理学特点尚不明确，但这些获得性危险因素已得到公认（表 8.3）。血流淤滞是明确的血栓形成危险因素（如长期制动的住院患者易发生 VTE）。其他高风险情况［包括手术（特别是骨科手术）和创伤］也与下肢制动和血流淤滞相关。在彻底

表 8.3　血栓形成的获得性危险因素

内科和外科疾病
抗磷脂抗体、狼疮抗凝物
人工心脏瓣膜
心房颤动（非瓣膜性）
充血性心力衰竭
溶血性贫血（自身免疫性溶血性贫血、镰状细胞贫血、血栓性血小板减少性紫癜、阵发性睡眠性血红蛋白尿症）
高脂血症
制动
恶性肿瘤
伴血小板增多的骨髓增生性疾病
肾病综合征
骨科手术
妊娠
创伤、脂肪栓塞

药物因素
肝素诱导的血小板减少症
口服避孕药、激素替代治疗
凝血酶原复合物浓缩物

寻找血栓形成的证据时，手术和创伤均与极高的 VTE 发生率（> 50%）相关。脂肪栓塞和组织损伤也可能增加手术和创伤后发生 VTE 的风险，特别是释放大量组织因子的闭合性头部损伤。创伤患者常预防性放置下腔静脉（IVC）滤器以防止发生 PE，尤其是对于因出血风险增加而有抗凝禁忌的血栓高危患者，但滤器近端血栓形成及后续发生肺血栓的风险仍然很高。一旦患者可以安全地接受抗凝治疗，应立即移除 IVC 滤器。

所有住院患者均应考虑是否需要使用 UFH 或 LMWH 预防静脉血栓。若患者同时存在增加出血风险的因素，包括血小板减少症（通常血小板计数 < 50 000/μl）、凝血功能障碍（伴或不伴肝病）及新发出血，不应予抗凝治疗。需积极进行预防性抗凝治疗的疾病包括恶性肿瘤、既往发生 VTE、制动和血栓性疾病。

妊娠和流产

妊娠女性存在与静脉淤滞相关的高凝状态，妊娠期和产后期女性比非妊娠期女性发生易栓症的风险高约 5 倍。妊娠可升高促凝血蛋白的水平，包括纤维蛋白原、vWF，以及因子 Ⅶ、Ⅷ 和 X，同时降低天然抗凝剂的水平，如蛋白 S、AT 及纤维蛋白溶解抑制剂［如 PAI-1 和凝血酶活化纤维蛋白溶解抑制物（TAFI）］。妊娠期或产褥期的任何时间均可能发生 VTE。合并以下任何一种情况的女性在产后发生 VTE 的风险更高：死产、早产、产后出血、剖宫产、存在合并症或妊娠前体重指数 > 30 kg/m²。

母体血栓形成倾向可使妊娠的促凝状态复杂化，使母体易发生流产和 VTE。流产的遗传性危险因素包括 FVL 突变、凝血酶原 G20210A 突变、AT 缺陷、蛋白 C 或蛋白 S 缺陷。既往有 VTE 病史的孕妇发生流产的相对风险显著升高，尽管这种特定的风险似乎仅限

VTE, although this particular risk appears to be restricted to the period after 9 weeks' gestation. In fact, inherited thrombophilia may be protective against fetal loss during the first 9 weeks, possibly by limiting oxygen toxicity to the early embryo. Therefore, recommended indications for evaluating the inherited thrombophilia risk in women seeking to become pregnant are a history of VTE or recurrent fetal loss after 9 weeks of gestation when no other specific cause (e.g., antiphospholipid syndrome) can be identified. Both antithrombin deficiency and hyperhomocysteinemia have also been associated with placental abruption.

In the absence of an identified inherited thrombophilia or a diagnosis of antiphospholipid syndrome (discussed later), no role has been identified for prophylactic anticoagulant therapy with recurrent pregnancy loss although prophylactic aspirin is increasingly used in many women with high-risk pregnancy.

Oral Contraceptives and Hormone Replacement

Estrogen-containing oral contraceptive use conveys an increased risk for VTE, and a similar increased risk is seen early after institution of hormone replacement therapy in postmenopausal women. Concomitant heterozygosity for FVL mutation synergistically increases the risk for VTE in women who take estrogen-based oral contraceptives or hormone replacement therapy. Cigarette use in women using oral contraceptives also increases the risk of thrombosis, possibly through increased platelet reactivity mediated by increased thromboxane synthesis. On the arterial side, epidemiologic evidence clearly points to smoking as the main cardiovascular risk factor. Paradoxically, most data suggest a protective role for hormone replacement therapy in cardiovascular disease. As discussed previously, acquired APC resistance and decreases in the levels of both free and functional protein S occur with oral contraceptive use.

VTE in Malignancy

VTE is the second leading cause of death in malignancy. VTE occurs in a wide spectrum of malignancies, including mucin-producing malignancies (i.e., pancreatic, gastric, ovarian), gastrointestinal, lung, breast, lymphoma, and more. Interestingly, the part of the Virchow triad that is most affected can vary; for example, adenocarcinoma is known to increase hypercoagulability, whereas lymphoma can lead to VTE through compression of blood vessels and thus blood flow stasis.

When idiopathic VTE occurs in a cancer-free individual, an intensive work-up to find an occult malignancy is not necessarily warranted and has not been shown to improve subsequent cancer-related morbidity or mortality, as shown in the SOME Trial (2015). However, once a cancer diagnosis is established in patients with prior VTE, they are at increased risk for subsequent VTE events, especially if the FVL or G20210A prothrombin mutation is present. LMWH prophylaxis after malignancy-associated VTE achieves superior prevention compared to warfarin, possibly because of better maintenance of an anticoagulated state. Direct oral anticoagulants (DOACs) are being increasingly used given numerous recent clinical trials (see section "Therapy for VTE in Malignancy").

In the special case of myeloproliferative disorders (e.g., essential thrombocythemia), abnormal platelet physiologic mechanisms causing hyperaggregation are often present and require platelet-specific inhibition (see "Hypercoagulability and Platelet Disorders").

Other Prothrombotic Disease States

As described earlier, thrombosis in nephrotic syndrome is associated with loss of antithrombin through the kidneys. Hemolysis is a general prothrombotic state that appears to be mediated through blood cell destruction, perhaps through increased exposure to procoagulant membrane phospholipids; hemolysis with thromboembolic complications has been observed in patients who have artificial heart valves, sickle cell disease, and other hemolytic anemias, including Coombs-positive autoimmune hemolytic anemia. In the case of paroxysmal nocturnal hemoglobinuria (PNH), complement activation may directly mediate platelet activation, and therapy with the complement inhibitor eculizumab has significantly decreased the rate of thromboembolic disease in PNH.

Platelet activation and clearance appear to be the primary prothrombotic manifestations of heparin-induced thrombocytopenia (HIT) and thrombotic thrombocytopenic purpura (TTP).

Additionally, chronic disseminated intravascular coagulation (DIC) is classically associated with certain malignancies such as mucinous adenocarcinoma and promyelocytic leukemia. In that setting, known as Trousseau syndrome, there is an increased risk in malignancy for VTE that is not related to DIC.

Antiphospholipid Antibody Syndrome

Another acquired prothrombotic disorder is the antiphospholipid antibody syndrome (APS). APS is a primary disorder, unlike the occasional association of lupus anticoagulant or antiphospholipid antibodies with other autoimmune diseases such as systemic lupus erythematosus (SLE). The etiologic connection with SLE has not been fully defined, but replacement of the host immune system after hematopoietic stem cell transplantation for refractory SLE has the potential to eradicate the lupus anticoagulant and thromboembolic risk. All of the manifestations of APS are related to hypercoagulability, including recurrent venous or arterial thrombosis, thrombocytopenia caused by microcirculatory platelet clearance, and recurrent fetal loss resulting from placental vascular insufficiency. Serologic markers of APS include *anticardiolipin antibodies, anti–β_2-glycoprotein I antibodies*, and *lupus anticoagulants*. The Sydney Consensus Criteria for Antiphospholipid Syndrome (also known as the revised Sapporo criteria) are the current standard for diagnosis of APS. Diagnosis requires both the clinical criterion of radiologically or pathologically confirmed thrombosis or thrombosis-related fetal loss and the laboratory criterion of positive tests on two or more occasions at least 12 weeks apart. Anticardiolipin and anti-glycoprotein antibodies are detected by enzyme-linked immunosorbent assay (ELISA), whereas lupus anticoagulants are defined by correction of prolonged phospholipid-dependent clotting tests (most commonly hexagonal phase partial thromboplastin time [PTT] or Russell viper venom clotting time), with addition of excess phospholipid. Therefore, *lupus anticoagulant* is a misnomer; its presence predisposes the patient to clotting rather than to bleeding, and the risk for thrombosis is highest when a lupus anticoagulant is detectable. Another misleading aspect of this nomenclature is that phospholipid-reactive antibodies are actually directed against phospholipid-binding proteins in plasma (e.g., β_2-glycoprotein I antibody, annexin V, prothrombin). Anti–β_2-glycoprotein I antibody is detected by immunoassay, and high titers of this marker are also correlated with thromboembolic risk.

In patients with recurrent pregnancy loss in the context of APS, LMWH during pregnancy can help reduce further miscarriages.

Hypercoagulability and Platelet Disorders

Essential thrombocythemia and polycythemia vera are clonal myeloproliferative disorders commonly associated with somatic mutations in the *JAK2* gene. In essential thrombocythemia, mutations are also found in CALR and MPL in those negative for *JAK2* mutations. They are wholly (essential thrombocythemia) or partially (polycythemia vera) characterized by thrombocytosis, and patients with these disorders are at increased risk for thrombosis. Platelet aggregometry in these disorders often shows abnormal

于妊娠第 9 周后。事实上，在妊娠期前 9 周，遗传性易栓症可能通过限制早期胚胎的氧化损伤而防止孕妇发生流产。因此，建议对以下备孕女性进行遗传性易栓症风险评估：既往有 VTE 病史或反复在妊娠第 9 周后流产且未发现特定原因（如抗磷脂综合征）。抗凝血酶缺乏症和高同型半胱氨酸血症也与胎盘早剥相关。

尽管越来越多的高危妊娠女性预防性使用阿司匹林，但对于习惯性流产的孕妇，若未确诊遗传性易栓症或抗磷脂综合征（见下文），则不需要预防性抗凝治疗。

口服避孕药和激素替代治疗

使用含有雌激素的口服避孕药会增加 VTE 风险，绝经后女性在接受激素替代治疗的早期也会增加 VTE 风险。若使用口服避孕药或激素替代治疗的女性同时存在杂合子 FVL 突变，则可协同增加 VTE 发生的风险。在使用口服避孕药的女性中，吸烟可增加血栓形成的风险，这可能是由于吸烟增加血栓素合成，进而增加了血小板反应性。在动脉系统中，流行病学证据已明确指出吸烟是心血管疾病的主要危险因素。矛盾的是，大多数数据表明激素替代治疗在心血管疾病中起保护作用。如前所述，口服避孕药可导致获得性 APC 抵抗和游离及功能性蛋白 S 水平降低。

恶性肿瘤中的 VTE

VTE 是恶性肿瘤的第二大致死原因。VTE 可发生于多种恶性肿瘤中，包括产生黏蛋白的恶性肿瘤（如胰腺癌、胃癌、卵巢癌），胃肠道恶性肿瘤、肺癌、乳腺癌、淋巴瘤等。不同肿瘤中 Virchow 三要素最受影响的部分可能有所不同；例如，腺癌会促进高凝状态，而淋巴瘤可通过压迫血管导致血流淤滞而引起 VTE。

当特发性 VTE 发生在未患癌症的个体时，SOME 试验（2015 年）表明，进一步筛查隐匿性恶性肿瘤并不是必需的，且不会改善随后的癌症相关患病率或死亡率。然而，既往有 VTE 病史的患者一旦确诊恶性肿瘤，则后续 VTE 事件的风险增加，特别是同时存在 FVL 突变或凝血酶原 G20210A 突变时。与华法林相比，LMWH 可以更好地预防恶性肿瘤相关性 VTE，这可能是因为 LMWH 可以更好地维持抗凝状态。基于近期大量临床试验数据，DOAC 的使用越来越广泛（见下文"恶性肿瘤中 VTE 的治疗"）。

骨髓增生性疾病（如原发性血小板增多症）患者通常存在引起高聚集性的异常血小板生理学机制，需要特异性抑制血小板（见下文"高凝状态和血小板疾病"）。

其他血栓前疾病状态

如前所述，肾病综合征中的血栓形成与经肾丢失 AT 有关。溶血是一种由血细胞破坏介导的全身血栓前状态，这可能与溶血过程增加了促凝血的膜磷脂暴露有关；有人工心脏瓣膜、镰状细胞贫血和其他溶血性贫血（包括 Coombs 试验阳性的自身免疫性溶血性贫血）的患者可出现溶血合并血栓栓塞并发症。在阵发性睡眠性血红蛋白尿症（PNH）中，补体激活可直接介导血小板活化，因此应用补体抑制剂依库珠单抗可显著降低 PNH 中血栓栓塞性疾病的发生率。

血小板活化和清除增加似乎是肝素诱导的血小板减少症（HIT）和血栓性血小板减少性紫癜（TTP）的主要血栓前表现。

此外，慢性弥散性血管内凝血（DIC）与某些恶性肿瘤（如黏液腺癌和急性早幼粒细胞白血病）相关。然而，Trousseau 综合征的 VTE 发生风险增加与 DIC 无关。

抗磷脂综合征

另一种获得性血栓前疾病是抗磷脂综合征（APS）。APS 是一种原发性疾病，不同于有时伴有狼疮抗凝物或抗磷脂抗体的其他自身免疫病［如系统性红斑狼疮（SLE）］。APS 与 SLE 的病因学关联尚不明确，但难治性 SLE 患者通过造血干细胞移植来替代宿主免疫系统可能清除狼疮抗凝物和血栓栓塞风险。APS 的所有表现都与高凝状态相关，包括复发性静脉或动脉血栓形成、由微循环血小板清除引起的血小板减少、由胎盘血管功能不全引起的习惯性流产。APS 的血清标志物包括抗心磷脂抗体、抗 β_2 糖蛋白 I 抗体和狼疮抗凝物。APS 悉尼共识标准（又称修订版札幌标准）是目前 APS 的诊断标准。诊断需同时具备临床标准和实验室标准，临床标准包括需要影像学或病理学证实的血栓形成或血栓形成相关流产，实验室标准即相隔至少 12 周检测≥ 2 次血清标志物阳性。可通过酶联免疫吸附试验（ELISA）检测抗心磷脂抗体和抗 β_2 糖蛋白 I 抗体，通过加入过量磷脂纠正磷脂依赖的凝血试验结果［最常用活化部分凝血活酶时间（APTT）或蝰蛇毒凝血时间］来检测狼疮抗凝物。因此，狼疮抗凝物是一个误称，它的存在会使患者倾向于凝血而不是出血，当可检测到狼疮抗凝物时，血栓形成的风险最高。另一个误导性命名是磷脂反应性抗体，这些抗体实际上是针对血浆中的磷脂结合蛋白，如抗 β_2 糖蛋白 I 抗体、膜联蛋白 V 和凝血酶原。免疫分析可测定抗 β_2 糖蛋白 I 抗体，该标志物的高滴度也与血栓栓塞风险高相关。

在 APS 合并习惯性流产的患者中，妊娠期应用 LMWH 可减少流产风险。

高凝状态和血小板疾病

原发性血小板增多症和真性红细胞增多症是与 JAK2 基因体细胞突变相关的克隆性骨髓增生性疾病。在原发性血小板增多症中，JAK2 基因突变阴性患者的 CALR 和 MPL 基因可发生突变。所有原发性血小板增多症或部分真性红细胞增多症均以血小板增多为特征，且这些患者的血栓形成风险增加。患者通常存在血小板聚集异常，特别是肾上腺素和 ADP 诱导的血小板聚

responses, especially to epinephrine and ADP; however, the abnormal aggregation does not correspond to either bleeding or thrombosis risk. Patients with polycythemia vera in particular have a high incidence of thrombosis in the mesenteric, portal, and hepatic venous circulation.

Thrombotic complications, both arterial and venous, occur in essential thrombocythemia, even in young patients. The risk of arterial thrombosis in essential thrombocythemia (and probably also in primary myelofibrosis and polycythemia vera) is most increased by a history of previous thrombosis or the presence of the *JAK2* V617F mutation. Therefore, prophylaxis with low-dose aspirin is probably justified in patients with high-risk essential thrombocythemia and other myeloproliferative disorders.

Increased platelet turnover in thrombocytosis is also associated with thromboembolic complications, but this does not necessarily involve high platelet counts, as has been demonstrated by radioactive platelet survival studies and an increase in reticulated (young) platelets in thrombotic essential thrombocytopenia. Moreover, successful treatment of symptomatic patients with aspirin increases platelet survival by decreasing platelet clearance. Concomitant therapy to prevent thrombotic complications of thrombocytosis includes lowering the platelet count with hydroxyurea, pegylated alpha interferon or anagrelide. Evidence suggests that patients with essential thrombocythemia who are at high risk for thrombosis (prior thrombosis or over age 60) are most effectively treated with the combination of hydroxyurea and low-dose aspirin. Patients with reactive (secondary) thrombocytosis resulting from iron deficiency anemia, chronic infection, or rheumatoid arthritis do not generally have increased thrombotic risk and do not require aspirin prophylaxis.

Heparin-Induced Thrombocytopenia

HIT must be distinguished from other drug-induced forms of immune thrombocytopenia because of its potentially catastrophic *thrombotic* complications and its unique pathophysiologic features. Almost 25% of patients who are exposed to UFH develop antibodies (detected by ELISA) that recognize the complex of heparin and platelet factor 4 (PF4), the latter being released from activated platelets, although most will not develop the clinical syndrome of HIT. When such patients receive heparin again, between 5% and 10% develop HIT, most with platelet counts between 50,000 and 100,000/μL. HIT rarely occurs in patients who have not been previously exposed to heparin (0.3% incidence).

Surgery is a specific risk factor for HIT; the incidence of HIT in surgical patients is about 2.6%, compared with 1.7% in medical patients. HIT antibodies occur with high frequency in patients undergoing either cardiac surgery with cardiopulmonary bypass or an orthopedic procedure such as hip replacement. The incidence of HIT in patients who have received only LMWH is far lower, only about one tenth the rate seen with UFH. However, the mechanism of thrombocytopenia for both UFH and LMWH appears to be similar: Platelet Fc-receptor binding of the heparin-PF4 antibody complex causes signal transduction and platelet activation with enhanced thrombin generation on the platelet surface.

The diagnosis is predominantly clinical (e.g., using the 4Ts algorithm for scoring HIT—magnitude of *t*hrombocytopenia, *t*iming of platelet fall, *t*hrombotic sequelae, and ruling out *o*ther causes of thrombocytopenia), but the rapid ELISA test will detect heparin-PF4 antibodies in serum. The main drawback of ELISA is that it does not indicate whether the antibody complex is a functional activator of platelets; therefore, it is sensitive but not specific for HIT. The serotonin release assay is the functional test for HIT; it detects platelet activation after exposure to serum antibody in the presence of a therapeutic heparin level. However, a low probability for HIT based on the 4Ts score can be used to exclude the HIT diagnosis.

The thrombin-based procoagulant response in HIT incorporates platelets into microcirculatory clots, leading to thrombocytopenia; about 30% of HIT patients have overt thromboembolic complications, which can be severe or life-threatening. Thromboembolic events can occur before, concurrent with, and after development of thrombocytopenia in HIT, with about equal frequency. Although thrombosis is more frequent in patients with both HIT and concomitant cardiovascular disease and in those receiving full-dose heparin, any heparin dose (even intravenous catheter heparin flushes) can result in thrombosis in HIT. Arterial and venous thromboembolic disease can occur even weeks after heparin has been discontinued, an effect perhaps mediated by EC glycosaminoglycan binding to PF4, which serves as a target for circulating HIT antibodies.

Discontinuation of all heparin is critical; moreover, although the antibody may have been induced by treatment with UFH, more than 80% of these antibodies cross-react with LMWH. Therefore, the preferred therapy for short-term anticoagulation in patients with HIT is a direct thrombin inhibitor (DTI), such as argatroban or bivalirudin, which is not a target for the heparin-PF4 antibodies. Indeed, because the event rate for subsequent thrombosis, limb amputation, and death is increased in patients with HIT even if they do not have thrombosis at presentation, DTI therapy is mandated after discontinuation of heparin. The choice of DTI may be dictated by other clinical conditions; for example, renal insufficiency slows bivalirudin clearance, increasing bleeding risk, whereas argatroban is cleared by hepatic metabolism. For patients who develop HIT after warfarin has already been started, in addition to substituting a DTI, one should administer vitamin K to correct protein C levels. Although it has not been approved by the US Food and Drug Administration (FDA) for this clinical scenario, the synthetic pentasaccharide indirect Xa inhibitor fondaparinux has the advantages of once-daily subcutaneous administration without need for laboratory monitoring and of having no effect on the International Normalized Ratio (INR). DOACs are also an attractive option for treatment with clinical trials ongoing to determine safety and efficacy.

DTI therapy should be continued until the platelet count is higher than 100,000 to 150,000/μL. Warfarin can then be added, and the two therapies should overlap for at least 5 days with the INR at a therapeutic level for at least 48 hours. Because DTIs prolong the INR, a therapeutic warfarin level after 5 days may result in a supratherapeutic INR (usually >4); gradual downward titration of the DTI as the INR increases is a logical management strategy. Once DTIs are stopped, it is essential to repeat the INR measurement after 4 to 6 hours to confirm that it remains within the therapeutic range.

If there is no thrombosis with HIT, the total duration of anticoagulation should be at least 4 weeks; if thrombosis is present, anticoagulation should be continued for 3 to 6 months. Warfarin should never be used as initial therapy to treat HIT, and it should not later be instituted without simultaneous DTI coverage because it may induce acquired protein C deficiency leading to venous limb gangrene. One hallmark of protein C depletion in HIT is a sudden rise in the INR (to >3.5) after a single warfarin dose; in that circumstance, warfarin should be discontinued and the patient repleted with vitamin K. Patients with a history of HIT who need surgery requiring cardiopulmonary bypass can be safely reexposed to brief systemic UFH if ELISA testing is negative for the antibody at least 100 days after the previous UFH exposure.

集。然而，异常血小板聚集与出血或血栓形成的风险并不相关。真性红细胞增多症患者的肠系膜静脉、门静脉和肝静脉血栓的发生率尤其高。

原发性血小板增多症患者可发生动脉和静脉血栓性并发症，即使是年轻患者。既往血栓病史或存在 JAK2 V617F 突变会显著增加原发性血小板增多症患者（也可能包括原发性骨髓纤维化和真性红细胞增多症的患者）动脉血栓形成的风险。因此，在血栓形成高风险的原发性血小板增多症和其他骨髓增生性疾病患者中，预防性使用低剂量阿司匹林可能是合理的。

在血小板增多症中，血小板更新率增加也与血栓栓塞性并发症相关，但与血小板计数增多不一定相关，放射性血小板寿命试验和血栓性原发性血小板减少症中网织（新生成的）血小板增加证明了这一点。此外，阿司匹林可治疗有症状的患者是通过减少血小板清除，从而延长了血小板寿命。预防血小板增多症患者出现血栓性并发症的治疗方法还包括应用羟基脲、聚乙二醇干扰素α、阿那格雷，以降低血小板计数。有证据表明，对于血栓形成高风险（既往血栓史或年龄 > 60 岁）的原发性血小板增多症患者，最有效的治疗是联用羟基脲和低剂量阿司匹林。由缺铁性贫血、慢性感染、类风湿关节炎引起的反应性（继发性）血小板增多症患者的血栓形成风险通常不增加，无须预防性应用阿司匹林。

肝素诱导的血小板减少症

HIT 必须与其他药物诱导的免疫性血小板减少症相鉴别，因为它可能导致灾难性血栓性并发症且具有独特的病理生理学特征。近 25% 应用 UFH 的患者会产生能识别肝素和血小板因子 4（PF4）复合物的抗体（可通过 ELISA 检测），PF4 从活化的血小板中释放，但大多数患者不会发展为 HIT 的临床综合征。当这些患者再次应用肝素时，5%～10% 的患者可能发生 HIT，其血小板计数多为 50 000～100 000/μl。极少数情况下，HIT 可发生在既往没有接触过肝素的患者中（发生率为 0.3%）。

手术是 HIT 的特异性危险因素。外科手术患者的 HIT 发生率约为 2.6%，内科患者为 1.7%。在进行体外循环心脏手术或髋关节置换术等骨科手术的患者中，HIT 抗体的检出率较高。在仅应用 LMWH 的患者中，HIT 的发生率显著降低，仅为应用 UFH 患者的约 1/10。然而，UFH 和 LMWH 引起血小板减少症的机制是相似的：肝素 -PF4 抗体复合物与血小板 Fc 受体结合，引起信号转导和血小板活化，在血小板表面增加凝血酶的产生。

HIT 的诊断主要根据临床表现[如使用 "4T" 积分标准，包括血小板减少（thrombocytopenia）的程度、血小板减少的时间（timing）、血栓性并发症（thrombotic sequelae）和排除血小板减少症的其他原因（other causes）]，但可通过快速 ELISA 检测血清中的肝素 -PF4 抗体。ELISA 的主要缺点是不能提示抗体复合物是否是血小板的功能性激活剂，因此对 HIT 敏感但不特异。5- 羟色胺释放试验是 HIT 的功能测定试验，可在肝素达到治疗水平时检测暴露于血清抗体后的血小板活化。然而，"4T" 积分呈低风险可用于排除 HIT 诊断。

在 HIT 中，基于凝血酶的促凝反应将血小板结合到微循环血凝块中，导致血小板减少；约 30% 的 HIT 患者会发生明显的血栓栓塞性并发症，甚至是严重或危及生命的血栓栓塞。在 HIT 中，血栓栓塞事件可发生在血小板减少之前、同时和之后，且各阶段的发生率相同。虽然血栓形成在 HIT 合并心血管疾病及接受足量肝素治疗的患者中更为常见，但任何剂量的肝素（甚至肝素冲管）都可能导致血栓形成。动静脉血栓栓塞性疾病甚至可以发生在停用肝素后数周，这种作用可能由 EC 糖胺聚糖结合 PF4 介导，PF4 是循环 HIT 抗体的靶点。

停用所有类型的肝素是治疗 HIT 的关键。此外，尽管抗体可能由 UFH 诱导生成，但超过 80% 的抗体与 LMWH 有交叉反应。因此，HIT 患者短期抗凝治疗的首选是直接凝血酶抑制剂（DTI），如阿加曲班或比伐卢定，二者不是肝素 -PF4 抗体的靶点。事实上，由于 HIT 患者后续血栓形成、截肢和死亡的发生率升高，即使目前没有血栓形成，在停用肝素后也应使用 DTI。DTI 的选择可根据其他临床情况，如肾功能不全患者的比伐卢定清除率降低，出血风险增加，而阿加曲班可通过肝代谢清除。已经开始使用华法林的患者发生 HIT 时，除应用 DTI 替代外，还应使用维生素 K 以纠正蛋白 C 水平。虽然 FDA 尚未批准用于治疗 HIT，但人工合成的因子 Xa 抑制剂磺达肝素具有每日 1 次皮下给药的优点，无须实验室监测且不影响国际标准化比值（INR）。DOAC 也是有前景的治疗选择，有关其安全性和有效性的临床试验正在进行中。

DTI 应持续使用直至血小板计数 > 100 000～150 000/μl。随后可加用华法林，两种药物应重叠使用至少 5 天，直至 INR 达到治疗水平至少 48 h。由于 DTI 可升高 INR，重叠华法林治疗 5 天后可导致 INR 超标（通常 > 4）。随着 INR 的升高，可逐渐减少 DTI 的使用剂量。一旦停用 DTI，必须在 4～6 h 后复查 INR，以确认其在治疗目标范围内。

如果 HIT 患者未出现血栓形成，抗凝治疗的总疗程为 4 周；如果存在血栓形成，抗凝治疗的总疗程应持续 3～6 个月。华法林不应作为 HIT 的初始治疗，在无皮下注射 DTI 的情况下也不应单独使用华法林，因为它可能诱导获得性蛋白 C 缺陷，导致静脉性肢体坏疽。HIT 中蛋白 C 耗竭的标志是在单次华法林剂量后 INR 突然升高（> 3.5）。在这种情况下，患者应停用华法林，并补充维生素 K。既往有 HIT 病史的患者，若因手术需行体外循环时，如果距离上次使用 UFH 至少 100 天后 ELISA 检测抗体为阴性，则可以短期安全使用 UFH。

Thrombotic Thrombocytopenic Purpura

Another cause of thrombocytopenia resulting from platelet activation and clearance is TTP. In patients with congenital or familial TTP, mutations in the VWF-cleaving protease, ADAMTS13 (*a disintegrin and metalloproteinase with thrombospondin type 1 motif, member 13*), abrogate its activity. Patients with acquired TTP usually have an antibody that blocks the normal function of VWF-cleaving protease to less than 10% of normal. Ultralarge VWF multimers released by EC normally anchor to EC through P-selectin and form long strings that adhere and aggregate platelets in the microcirculation. ADAMTS13 downregulates the size of these multimers by docking to the A1/A3 VWF domains and cleaving within the A2 site. Deficient cleaving protease function in TTP leads to an increase in the larger, highest-molecular-weight VWF multimers, which are most effective in anchoring and activating platelets. These, in turn, cause increased platelet adhesion and clearance *without* activating the coagulation cascade. Therefore, both the prothrombin time (PT) and the PTT are normal in TTP, unlike the case in DIC.

TTP after chemotherapy (mitomycin C) or in association with pregnancy, stem cell transplantation, lupus, or HIV infection appears to have a similar pathogenic mechanism of thrombosis. Thrombocytopenia (often severe) is accompanied by microangiopathy with schistocytes on smear and increased serum lactate dehydrogenase. Microvascular occlusions in multiple organs cause symptoms, especially in the kidney and brain. The classic pentad (fever, thrombocytopenia, microangiopathic hemolysis, neurologic symptoms, and renal insufficiency) is present in fewer than 5% of patients with TTP. The diagnosis is typically made based on the clinical assessment of thrombocytopenia and microangiopathic hemolytic anemia; assays for ADAMTS13 activity and inhibitor do not have a rapid turnaround time in most laboratories. Clinical prediction scores (e.g., the PLAMIC score) are helpful as an additional piece of clinical information in the decision to initiate treatment for TTP but cannot be used on their own to exclude TTP. In validation studies, some patients ultimately found to have an ADAMTS13 activity level, less than 10% were noted to have low PLASMIC scores.

Treatment of familial TTP is based on replenishment of cleaving protease activity with plasma transfusion; acquired TTP additionally requires removal of the antibody. The latter is accomplished by therapeutic plasma exchange, whereby patient plasma is removed (plasmapheresis) and replaced with fresh-frozen plasma, which often has been made "cryo-poor" to reduce ultralarge VWF multimers in transfused plasma. Corticosteroids are often administered simultaneously, but any added benefit to plasma exchange remains unclear. Platelet transfusions are relatively contraindicated in TTP because of the risk of thrombosis, and they should not be given for thrombocytopenia in the absence of significant bleeding. When plasma exchange fails to remit acquired TTP or when early relapse occurs, immunosuppressive therapy with anti-CD20 may be successful and data suggest that early rituximab will reduce the risk of relapse. The mortality rate associated with severe TTP (defined as undetectable ADAMTS-13 activity) is still significant, almost 10% at 18 months after therapy with plasma exchange. Replacement of ADAMTS-13, which is present in fresh-frozen plasma and in cryoprecipitate, is a potential treatment. Clinical trials have shown the anti-VWF therapy caplacizumab to have benefit in reducing the number of days of plasma exchange needed to achieve a normal platelet count and also reductions in mortality, although with increasing bleeding risk. The ideal subset of patients to receive caplacizumab in conjunction with other therapies for TTP remains to be defined. Caplacizumab does not address the underlying autoantibody causing ADAMTS13 deficiency and use of rituximab for inhibitor eradication is most likely to be beneficial in patients receiving caplacizumab therapy.

The *hemolytic-uremic syndrome* (HUS) is part of the TTP spectrum of disease and also is associated with microvascular platelet thrombi. However, the hemolytic anemia and renal failure of HUS are not usually accompanied by neurologic impairment, and HUS usually does not produce the same degree of thrombocytopenia or microangiopathy as TTP. Moreover, fewer than 3% of HUS cases are associated with any decrease in VWF-cleaving protease activity. Unlike TTP, HUS is usually diagnosed in children (and less commonly in adults) who have hemorrhagic colitis caused by Shiga-like, toxin-producing bacteria, especially the *Escherichia coli* O157:H7 serotype. Atypical HUS (i.e., without diarrhea or Shiga-like toxin) is rarely associated with other bacterial infections or with complement dysregulation due to mutations or polymorphisms in factors H, I, and B. These mutations increase platelet activation through complement (C3) deposition on the platelet surface. Atypical HUS cases are those that are clinically consistent with HUS but are not associated with toxin-producing bacteria. Some HUS cases, particularly atypical forms, may temporarily respond to plasma exchange along with maintenance hemodialysis until renal function recovers. Data support use of the anti-C5a complement therapy eculizumab to prevent the complement-mediated damage associated with this disease. More recently, a modified form of eculizumab with a longer half-life, ravulizumab, has been approved to treat atypical HUS, allowing patients longer intervals between therapeutic infusions.

CLINICAL EVALUATION OF THROMBOSIS

The approach to patients with thromboembolism is defined by the clinical history, results of laboratory studies, and even physical findings. Events that trigger VTE disease include immobilization, orthopedic and other surgical procedures, use of oral contraceptives, and pregnancy. VTE that is recurrent (thrombophilia) may manifest at an early age or at unusual thrombotic sites (e.g., cerebral vessels) and may be accompanied by a family history of VTE, suggesting an inherited disorder. Acquired VTE risk may be associated with systemic disorders such as hemolysis (e.g., PNH, autoimmune hemolytic anemia), collagen vascular disorders (e.g., lupus), or various malignant diseases (e.g., adenocarcinoma). In contrast, arterial thromboembolic disease is more commonly superimposed on ruptured atherosclerotic plaque (e.g., coronary artery disease) or on atheroembolic disorders (e.g., ischemic stroke, peripheral arterial disease). Arterial vascular disease is mainly associated with metabolic risk factors including hypertension, hypercholesterolemia, and diabetes. The clinical approach to thrombotic disease is tailored to the location of the disease (arterial vs. venous and the specific vascular bed) and whether there are abnormalities of the vascular endothelium, platelets, or soluble coagulation factors that predispose the patient to thromboembolic risk.

Laboratory Diagnostics

Recurrent VTE is a strong indication for laboratory testing for causes of thrombophilia, especially in patients younger than 50 years of age, in those with unexplained VTE, and in those with a first-degree family history of VTE. Any risk factors that may predispose these individuals to recurrence must be defined, as well as any inherited disorders that may necessitate family counseling or avoidance of additional environmental risks. The current work-up for VTE thrombophilia includes the following: (1) APC resistance, (2) genotyping for prothrombin G20210A, (3) lupus anticoagulant assay and anti-cardiolipin and anti–β_2-glycoprotein I antibody serologies, (4) functional AT and protein C levels, and (5) free protein S (Table 8.4).

血栓性血小板减少性紫癜

血小板活化和清除增加导致血小板减少的另一个病因是血栓性血小板减少性紫癜（TTP）。在先天性或家族性TTP患者中，vWF裂解蛋白酶ADAMTS13（一种具有血小板应答蛋白1型基序的去整合素和金属蛋白酶家族成员13）基因突变可使其失活。获得性TTP患者通常存在能阻断vWF裂解蛋白酶正常功能的抗体，其活性小于正常的10%。EC释放的超大分子量vWF多聚体可通过P选择素锚定到EC表面，形成长链，黏附和聚集微循环中的血小板。ADAMTS13通过对接到A1/A3 vWF结构域并在A2位点内切割，从而下调多聚体的大小。在TTP中，裂解蛋白酶功能缺陷导致超大分子量vWF多聚体增多，而后者可有效锚定和激活血小板。上述过程会导致血小板黏附和清除增加，但不激活凝血级联反应。因此，不同于DIC，TTP患者的凝血酶原时间（PT）和APTT正常。

化疗（丝裂霉素C）后TTP，或与妊娠、干细胞移植、狼疮或HIV感染有关的TTP似乎具有类似的血栓形成机制。血小板减少（通常为重度）常伴有微血管病变，如外周血涂片见破碎红细胞、血清乳酸脱氢酶水平升高。多个器官（特别是肾和脑）的微血管闭塞可引起临床症状。不足5%的TTP患者可表现为经典五联征（发热、血小板减少、微血管病性溶血性贫血、神经系统症状和肾功能不全）。TTP的诊断通常基于对血小板减少症和微血管病性溶血性贫血的临床评估，而大多数实验室对ADAMTS13活性和抑制物的检测周期较长。临床预测评分（如PLAMIC评分）在决定启动TTP治疗方面可提供额外的临床信息，但不能仅依靠此评分来排除TTP。在验证试验中，一些最终发现ADAMTS13活性水平减低的TTP患者中仍有不足10%的PLASMIC评分较低。

遗传性TTP的治疗主要是输注血浆以补充裂解蛋白酶活性，而获得性TTP还需要去除抗体。后者可通过血浆置换以去除患者血浆（血浆单采术）并用新鲜冰冻血浆代替，这种血浆通常被制成"乏冷沉淀"血浆，以减少输入血浆中的超大分子量vWF多聚体。通常需同时使用皮质类固醇，但其是否对血浆置换有额外益处仍不明确。TTP是血小板输注的相对禁忌证，在没有明显出血的情况下，不应输注血小板，因为存在血栓形成的风险。当血浆置换效果差或发生早期复发时，使用抗CD20的免疫抑制治疗可能有效，数据表明早期使用利妥昔单抗能降低复发风险。重度TTP（定义为无法测出ADAMTS13活性）相关的死亡率仍然很高，血浆置换治疗后18个月的死亡率近10%。使用新鲜冰冻血浆和冷沉淀替代ADAMTS13是一种潜在的治疗方法。临床试验表明，尽管抗vWF治疗卡普赛珠单抗会增加出血风险，但该药有利于减少为纠正血小板计数所需的血浆置换天数，并降低死亡率。卡普赛珠单抗联合其他治疗的理想TTP患者亚群仍有待确定。卡普赛珠单抗无法解决导致ADAMTS13缺乏的潜在自身抗体，对于接受卡普赛珠单抗治疗的患者，使用利妥昔单抗清除体内抑制性抗体最有可能获益。

溶血性尿毒综合征（HUS）是TTP疾病谱的一部分，且与微血管病性血小板血栓相关。然而，HUS的溶血性贫血和肾衰竭通常不伴有神经系统损害，且HUS引起的血小板减少或微血管病变的程度与TTP不同。此外，不足3%的HUS患者与vWF裂解蛋白酶活性降低相关。与TTP不同，HUS主要见于儿童（成人不常见），患者可出现由产生志贺样毒素的细菌（特别是大肠埃希菌O157：H7血清型）引起的出血性结肠炎。非典型HUS（即无腹泻或志贺样毒素）很少与其他细菌感染相关，多与因子H、I和B的突变或基因多态性引起的补体失调相关。这些突变使补体（C3）沉积在血小板表面，从而增加血小板活化。非典型HUS在临床上与HUS表现一致，但与产毒素细菌无关。一些HUS病例（特别是非典型HUS）对血浆置换联合维持性血液透析治疗有应答，且可持续至肾功能恢复。数据表明，抗C5a补体治疗药物依库珠单抗有助于预防该病中补体介导的损伤。近年来，半衰期更长、给药间隔更长的改良版依库珠单抗——雷夫利珠单抗，已被批准用于治疗非典型HUS。

血栓形成的临床评估

血栓栓塞患者的接诊包括临床病史、实验室检查及体格检查。诱发VTE疾病的事件包括制动、骨科或外科手术操作、使用口服避孕药和妊娠。复发性VTE（易栓症）见于年轻患者或少见部位（如脑血管），且伴有VTE家族史，提示遗传性疾病。获得性VTE风险可能与全身性疾病相关，如溶血（如PNH、自身免疫性溶血性贫血），胶原血管疾病（如狼疮）或各种恶性疾病（如腺癌）。相反，动脉血栓栓塞性疾病更常在破裂的动脉粥样硬化斑块（如冠状动脉疾病）或动脉粥样硬化性疾病（如缺血性卒中、外周动脉疾病）的基础上发生。动脉血管疾病主要与代谢性危险因素相关，包括高血压、高胆固醇血症和糖尿病。临床接诊血栓性疾病需基于疾病发生的位置［动脉、静脉和（或）特定血管床］及是否存在易导致血栓栓塞风险的血管内皮、血小板或可溶性凝血因子异常。

实验室诊断

复发性VTE是实验室筛查易栓症病因的强指征，尤其是年龄<50岁、不明原因VTE和具有VTE一级亲属家族史的患者。必须明确所有易导致血栓复发的危险因素，以及任何一种可能需要家庭咨询或避免额外环境风险的遗传病。目前易栓症患者需完善以下检查：①APC抵抗；②凝血酶原G20210A的基因分型；③狼疮抗凝物、抗心磷脂抗体和抗β₂糖蛋白I抗体血清学检查；④AT功能和蛋白C水平；⑤游离蛋白S（表8.4）。FVL突变的基

TABLE 8.4 Laboratory Evaluation of Venous Thrombosis
Activated protein C resistance, factor V Leiden
Lupus anticoagulant
Anticardiolipin, anti–β_2-glycoprotein I antibody serology
Homocysteine level: fasting or after methionine load
Prothrombin G20210A mutation
Antithrombin activity
Protein C activity
Free protein S level
Paroxysmal nocturnal hemoglobinuria (select patients)
Myeloproliferative disorders (in select patients)

Genotyping for the FVL mutation can substitute for APC resistance and also determines whether the patient is heterozygous or homozygous, although it may miss rare variants of APC resistance. Patients need to be off of warfarin during these tests and they should not be performed during the acute episode, given the changes in protein levels during these instances.

The utility of laboratory testing in the setting of atherothrombosis and arterial thromboembolism is unclear. In the setting of a myeloproliferative disorder, the use of hydroxyurea and/or aspirin therapy may be justified by platelet count and platelet function testing, but typically risk prediction models based on age and prior thrombosis are used to guide management decisions. In patients with unusual or recurrent arterial disease, other assays can be justified, including testing for t-PA and PAI-1 levels and for dysfibrinogenemia (thrombin time and antigen activity ratio), all of which should be performed in consultation with specialists in hemostasis.

THERAPY FOR VENOUS THROMBOEMBOLISM

Once VTE has been diagnosed, immediate therapy is required. In most patients, anticoagulation options include heparin, LMWH, or the newer direct oral anticoagulants (DOACs) (i.e., apixaban, rivaroxaban) initially and then warfarin or DOACs thereafter. The DOACs edoxaban and dabigatran require initial parenteral anticoagulation prior to use of the DOAC, but apixaban and rivaroxaban may be started as initial therapy with higher doses. Thrombolytic therapy is indicated for patients with extensive proximal venous clots or PE. IVC filters are used in patients with contraindications to anticoagulation, complications of anticoagulation (usually active bleeding), or failure of anticoagulation (recurrent PE). IVC filters clearly decrease the incidence of early PE, but their use is also associated with thrombosis at the insertion site and late complications of IVC thrombosis as well as a 10% to 20% incidence of postphlebitic syndrome. In patients who may be safely anticoagulated, IVC filters do not reduce the risk of pulmonary embolism and appear to be associated with a higher risk of PE. Temporary IVC filters are often used in trauma patients and appear to be most efficacious when they are placed for fewer than 7 to 10 days.

UFH is often the anticoagulation therapy of choice for many inpatients because of its short half-life and reversibility, but LMWH is increasingly used for this indication. UFH is begun as a bolus intravenous infusion of 80 U/kg, followed by a continuous infusion of 18 U/kg/hour; UFH doses in excess of 30,000 U/day have been shown to be most efficacious at preventing recurrent VTE. UFH is monitored by the PTT, and the therapeutic PTT range determined by each hospital corresponds to anti-Xa levels of 0.3 to 0.7 U/mL. Many hospitals have established protocols for adjustment of UFH infusion based on the patient's weight and PTT monitoring.

UFH should be continued for at least 5 days (longer in patients with extensive clots) and may be discontinued after the patient has been fully anticoagulated with warfarin (INR ≥2 for 2 consecutive days). Some patients receiving large doses of heparin (usually >40,000 U/day) do not develop a therapeutic PTT. This heparin resistance can be caused by a variety of mechanisms, including increased heparin-binding proteins, counteracting medications (e.g., protamine), and decreased antithrombin. An *apparent* heparin resistance is often seen in patients with coexistent inflammatory disease with high plasma levels of factor VIII and fibrinogen; direct monitoring of anti-Xa levels is indicated. It is important to remember that the anti-Xa level is a measurement of anticoagulant level in the blood but is not a direct measure of the anticoagulant effect present. Some patients may require a higher anti-Xa level in order to achieve therapeutic anticoagulation.

LMWH is an excellent alternative to UFH in the treatment of thromboembolism and acute coronary events. The small controlled-size elements of LMWH stimulate antithrombin activity that is more restricted to factor Xa compared with UFH, which has effects on thrombin, factor IX, and factor XI, in addition to others. The practical advantages of LMWH over UFH include increased plasma half-life, more predictable dose response allowing for intermittent fixed dosing, a lower *de novo* incidence of HIT (10% to 20% of the rate for UFH), and significantly reduced monitoring requirements. LMWH levels are prolonged in renal failure and in those circumstances may need to be monitored and adjusted based on anti-Xa levels. Peak anti-Xa levels (0.5 to 1 U/mL for twice-daily dosing and 1 to 2 U/mL for once-daily dosing) typically occur between 3 and 5 hours after subcutaneous LMWH injection. As with UFH, switching from LMWH to warfarin for long-term management can be accomplished after therapeutic INR values have been present for at least 2 days.

Supratherapeutic INR levels commonly occur with warfarin therapy, with or without bleeding. In patients with moderately elevated INR values (>5) and little or no bleeding, temporary discontinuation of warfarin and reinstitution of the drug at a lower maintenance dose may be sufficient. Patients with higher INR values (5 to 9) who are without serious bleeding should have warfarin withheld and should receive low doses (1 to 2.5 mg/day) of oral vitamin K to reach therapeutic INR levels; parenteral vitamin K may be given if gastrointestinal function is problematic. If serious active bleeding occurs with high INR values, especially if surgery is required to correct the bleeding, a combination of vitamin K and transfusion of plasma (see Chapter 7) will rapidly correct the INR. The INR can become elevated as a result of concurrent use of drugs that increase free warfarin levels (Table 8.5). Whenever bleeding occurs as a complication of anticoagulation, serious consideration must be given to future bleeding risks and to whether the patient requires placement of a filter for prophylaxis.

Recently, DOACs have been used with increased frequency because their efficacy and safety have now been evaluated in many circumstances. For patients with acute DVT, the initial anticoagulation (within the first week or two) options include: oral factor Xa inhibitors rivaroxaban or apixaban (in addition to the previously mentioned LMWH, subcutaneous fondaparinux, or unfractionated heparin). The decision of which agent to use is based on risk of bleeding, clinician comfort, patient comorbidities, and cost. The doses are: rivaroxaban 15 mg twice daily for 21 days then 20 mg daily; apixaban 10 mg twice daily for 7 days then 5 mg twice daily. For long-term, maintenance therapy, the DOACs approved are: direct factor Xa inhibitors (rivaroxaban, apixaban, edoxaban), thrombin inhibitors (dabigatran); as mentioned, warfarin, LMWH and fondaparinux can also be used for

表 8.4　静脉血栓形成相关的实验室评估
活化蛋白 C 抵抗、因子 V Leiden
狼疮抗凝物
血清抗心磷脂抗体、抗 β₂ 糖蛋白 I 抗体
同型半胱氨酸检测：禁食及甲硫氨酸负荷后
凝血酶原 G20210A 突变
抗凝血酶活性
蛋白 C 活性
游离蛋白 S 水平
阵发性睡眠性血红蛋白尿症（部分患者）
骨髓增生性疾病（部分患者）

因分型可替代 APC 抵抗检测，并能确定患者是杂合子还是纯合子，尽管其可能漏诊 APC 抵抗的罕见变异型。在进行这些检测时，患者需停用华法林，且不应在急性发作期检测，因为此时蛋白质水平会发生改变。

实验室检查在动脉粥样硬化血栓形成和动脉血栓栓塞中的用途尚不清楚。在骨髓增生性疾病中，血小板计数和血小板功能可为羟基脲和（或）阿司匹林的使用提供依据，但通常使用基于年龄和既往血栓史的风险预测模型来指导管理决策。对于少见或复发性动脉疾病患者，可进行的其他检测包括 t-PA 和 PAI-1 水平检测、异常纤维蛋白原血症相关检查（凝血酶时间和抗原活性比），所有检测均应咨询出凝血专家。

静脉血栓栓塞的治疗

一旦诊断 VTE，需立即治疗。大多数患者的初始抗凝治疗选择包括肝素、LMWH 或 DOAC（如阿哌沙班和利伐沙班），随后使用华法林或 DOAC。在 DOAC 中，艾多沙班和达比加群在使用前需要先进行肠外抗凝，但阿哌沙班和利伐沙班可予大剂量作为初始治疗。溶栓治疗适用于大面积近端静脉血栓或 PE 患者。IVC 滤器可用于存在抗凝血禁忌证、有抗凝并发症（通常为活动性出血）或抗凝失败（复发性 PE）的患者。IVC 滤器可明显降低早期 PE 的发生率，但也与置入部位血栓形成、远期 IVC 血栓并发症及静脉炎后综合征（10%～20%）相关。在可以安全抗凝的患者中，IVC 滤器不能降低肺栓塞的风险，且似乎与较高的 PE 风险相关。临时 IVC 滤器通常用于创伤患者，放置时间少于 7～10 天时似乎疗效最佳。

UFH 的半衰期短，其作用具有可逆性，故通常作为住院患者的首选抗凝治疗，但 LMWH 在这类患者中的使用已越来越广泛。UFH 的起始剂量为单剂注射 80 U/kg，之后按 18 U/(kg·h) 持续输注；UFH > 30 000 U/d 对于预防复发性 VTE 最有效。使用 UFH 时需监测 APTT，各个医院根据其抗 Xa 水平确定 APTT 的治疗范围，相当于 0.3～0.7 U/ml。许多医院都制订了基于患者体重和 APTT 监测来调整 UFH 输注的方案。

UFH 应持续使用至少 5 天（广泛血栓形成的患者使用时间应更长），在华法林充分抗凝（连续 2 天 INR ≥ 2）后可停用。部分接受大剂量肝素（通常 > 40 000 U/d）治疗的患者，APTT 仍无法达到治疗范围。这种肝素抵抗由多种机制引起，包括肝素结合蛋白增加、存在中和药物（如鱼精蛋白）和 AT 活性降低。明显的肝素抵抗常见于同时存在炎症性疾病且血浆中因子 Ⅷ 和纤维蛋白原水平较高的患者，建议直接监测抗因子 Xa 水平。需注意，抗因子 Xa 水平是检测血液中的抗凝剂水平，而不是直接检测当前的抗凝效果。部分患者可能需要更高的抗因子 Xa 水平以达到抗凝治疗的效果。

在治疗血栓栓塞和急性冠状动脉事件时，LMWH 是 UFH 的最佳替代药物。LMWH 的小分子量成分可激活 AT，且这种活性更局限于因子 Xa，而 UFH 对凝血酶、因子 Ⅸ 和 Ⅺ 及其他因子均有影响。与 UFH 相比，LMWH 的优点包括血浆半衰期长，具有更佳的剂量反应预测，允许间歇性固定剂量给药，新发 HIT 的发生率更低（为 UFH 的 10%～20%），且监测需求显著减小。在肾衰竭患者中，LMWH 持续时间延长，可能需要根据抗 Xa 水平进行监测和调整药物剂量。抗 Xa 活性通常在皮下注射 LMWH 后 3～5 h 达峰（每日 2 次给药时为 0.5～1 U/ml，每日 1 次给药时为 1～2 U/ml）。与 UFH 相同，在 LMWH 序贯华法林作为长期抗凝治疗时，两者需重叠使用直至 INR 达标至少 2 天后才可停用 LMWH。

INR 超治疗水平通常发生在华法林治疗中，患者可有出血表现或无出血。对于 INR 中度升高（> 5）且出血很少或无出血的患者，暂停华法林并以较低的维持剂量重新用药即可。INR 较高（5～9）且无严重出血的患者应停用华法林，并接受小剂量（1～2.5 mg/d）口服维生素 K，以达到 INR 治疗水平；如果有胃肠功能问题，可肠外给予维生素 K。如果发生严重的活动性出血且 INR 较高，尤其是需要手术纠正出血的患者，维生素 K 联合血浆输注（见第 7 章）可迅速纠正 INR。同时使用增加游离华法林水平的药物会导致 INR 升高（表 8.6）[译者注：原文（Table 8.5）有误]。当抗凝过程中出现出血并发症时，需认真评估未来的出血风险及患者是否需要放置滤器以进行预防。

近年来，DOAC 的使用频率增加，因其有效性和安全性已在许多情况下得到评估。对于急性 DVT 患者，最初的抗凝治疗（前 1～2 周内）包括口服因子 Xa 抑制剂利伐沙班或阿哌沙班（除 LMWH、皮下注射磺达肝素或 UFH 外）。以上药物选择需基于出血风险、临床医师用药倾向、患者合并症和费用来决定。具体剂量：利伐沙班初始剂量 15 mg，2 次/日，共 21 天，之后为 20 mg/d；阿哌沙班 10 mg，2 次/日，连用 7 天，之后为 5 mg，2 次/日。对于长期维持治疗，已被批准的 DOAC 包括直接 Xa 因子抑制剂（利伐沙班、阿哌沙班、艾多沙班）和凝血酶抑制剂（达比加群）；如前所述，华法林、LMWH 和磺达肝素也可用于长期治疗。具体剂量：达比加群 150 mg，2 次/日［若肌酐

TABLE 8.5	Guidelines for Duration of Prophylactic Anticoagulation After VTE
Condition	Duration of Therapy
Distal or superficial vein thrombus	3-12 wk
First Proximal VTE	
No risk factors	3-6 mo[a]
Correctable risk factor (e.g., surgery, trauma)	3-6 mo
Malignancy	Long-term[b]
Antiphospholipid syndrome	Long-term
Inherited risk factor[c]	>6 mo
Recurrent VTE/PE	Lifelong

PE, Pulmonary embolism; VTE, venous thromboembolism (includes deep vein thrombosis, pulmonary embolism, and sinus or cerebral thrombosis).
[a]Evaluation of D-dimer after 3-6 mo may assist in the decision to stop prophylaxis.
[b]Long-term therapy must be adjusted individually according to presence of other diseases, risks for bleeding, presence of transient risk factors, and ease of compliance.
[c]Inherited risk factors include factor V Leiden; prothrombin 20210A; deficiencies of antithrombin, protein C, or protein S.

long-term therapy. Dosing is as follows: dabigatran 150 mg BID (needs renal dose adjustment 75 mg BID if CrCl 15-30), edoxaban (after acute phase parenteral anticoagulation). DOACs are not recommended with severe renal impairment. However, apixaban can be dose adjusted for renal impairment and other variables. If creatinine is greater than 1.5, age older than 80, or weight 60 kg or less, decrease apixaban dosing to 2.5 mg orally twice daily. RE-COVER (2009) demonstrated, in patients with acute VTE, the oral direct thrombin inhibitor, dabigatran, was found to be as effective as warfarin for reducing recurrence risk and is associated with less bleeding. The benefit is that the DOACs have less variability in therapeutic range compared with warfarin and patients do not need to have blood drawn for INR checks when on the DOACs, as they have to do on warfarin.

In summary, based on the most recent American College of Client Physicians (ACCP) Antithrombotic Therapy for VTE Disease Guidelines (2016), DVT of the leg or PE without cancer, dabigatran, rivaroxaban, apixaban, or edoxaban is preferred over vitamin K antagonist therapies as treatment for the 3 months of maintenance therapy.

The treatment duration varies based on unprovoked or provoked DVT, location of clot, and initial or recurrent DVT. For most patients with a first episode of DVT (provoked and unprovoked, proximal and distal), treatment should be for 3 months. If proximal DVT or PE and low/moderate bleeding risk, this should be extended beyond 3 months. In patients with recurrent VTE, regardless of bleeding risk, the duration should be greater than 3 months and depending on risk factors of bleeding and patient comorbidities, indefinite anticoagulation may be recommended. The duration of therapy greater than 3 months has not been fully specified and will vary on a case-to-case basis. For patients who have received at least 6 to 12 months of anticoagulant therapy and have clinical equipoise to continue anticoagulation, low-dose rivaroxaban (10 mg once daily) or apixaban (2.5 mg twice daily) is safe and effective to reduce VTE risk with little to no increased bleeding risk as shown in the EINSTEIN Choice and AMPLIFY-EXT trials, respectively.

After stopping anticoagulation for unprovoked proximal DVT or PE, guidelines suggest aspirin over no aspirin to prevent recurrent DVT in patients with no contraindication to aspirin but in whom anticoagulant is not continued.

Therapy for VTE in Malignancy

In patients with malignancy, LMWH is preferred to warfarin. Based on the CLOT trial in 2003, dalteparin (LMWH) had a lower recurrent VTE risk without increasing bleeding risks or deaths compared to warfarin. These were confirmed in the 2006 LITE and ONCENOX trials. The Hokusai VTE Cancer Trial (2018) demonstrated that in patients with VTE and malignancy edoxaban was noninferior to dalteparin for recurrent VTE in an open label study but had higher bleeding risk. For specific malignancies, such as gastrointestinal cancer, LMWH is preferred to edoxaban for long-term anticoagulation (see Raskob 2017). Additionally, some studies recommend not using edoxaban if the CrCl is greater than 95, although the data for avoiding this medication in VTE are not clear. The SELECT-D pilot trial compared rivaroxaban to dalteparin in cancer-associated VTE and showed a decreased rate of recurrent VTE in the rivaroxaban group compared to dalteparin but an increased rate of non-major bleeding. There are multiple current trials studying apixaban versus dalteparin for patients with malignancy-associated VTE: the Caravaggio Trial is ongoing, and preliminary results for ADAM-VTE suggest low bleeding risk and low VTE recurrence rates.

In summary, based on the most recent ACCP Antithrombotic Therapy for VTE Guidelines (2016), for patients with cancer-associated VTE, as therapy for the first 3 months, LMWH is recommended over other agents whereas ASCO guidelines suggest DOACs may be used as first-line therapy. As mentioned previously, duration of therapy for VTE depends on cancer type (clotting and bleeding risks) and treatment plan for the malignancy.

Given known interactions and lack of safety data, DOACs should not be prescribed for patients on dual P-glycoprotein and strong CYP3A inhibitors, including medications such as carbamazepine, phenytoin, ketoconazole, ritonavir, rifampin, and more. Certain antibiotics (i.e., erythromycin or clarithromycin) may increase levels of DOACs, especially in individuals with renal dysfunction.

Prophylaxis of VTE

Even with the advent of the DOACs, both warfarin and LMWH are often used for treatment of VTE. Warfarin should be begun during the first 24 hours after presentation with VTE, concurrent with heparin treatment. The PT is prolonged within hours by warfarin because of a rapid decrease in factor VII levels; however, therapeutic warfarin anticoagulation does not occur until other vitamin K–dependent factors (II, IX, and X) also decrease. Therapeutic warfarin anticoagulation is usually achieved within 4 to 5 days with adequate warfarin dosing; UFH or LMWH may be discontinued after the INR has been greater than 2 for at least 2 consecutive days. One long-standing problem with warfarin anticoagulation is the interindividual variability in INR response; at least 50% of this variability in sensitivity to warfarin may be explained by polymorphisms in the *CYP2C9* and *VKORC1* genes. Although these have been incorporated into models for predicting safe and therapeutic warfarin dosing, most clinicians simply begin dosing and adjust therapy as needed based on periodic monitoring.

The therapeutic INR range depends on the condition predisposing the patient to thromboembolism. Prophylaxis after uncomplicated VTE in a patient without known risk factors requires an INR between 2 and 3; in contrast, warfarin prophylaxis for patients with APS and recurrent VTE may require INR values as high as 3 to 4 (Table 8.6).

The duration of warfarin or LMWH prophylaxis varies depending on the circumstances of the VTE, the risk for bleeding, and the potential for recurrence. In general, the longer the period of anticoagulation with warfarin, the less the chance of recurrence. Short-term warfarin (6 weeks) is less effective at preventing recurrence than longer courses (6 months). Patients with definite transient risk factors such

表 8.5　VTE 后预防性抗凝治疗疗程的指南建议

临床情况	治疗疗程
远端或浅表的静脉血栓	3～12 周
初发的近端 VTE	
无危险因素	3～6 个月 [a]
可纠正的危险因素（如手术、创伤）	3～6 个月
恶性肿瘤	长期 [b]
抗磷脂综合征	长期
遗传性危险因素 [c]	＞6 个月
复发性 VTE/PE	终身

PE，肺栓塞；VTE，静脉血栓栓塞（包括深静脉血栓形成、肺栓塞、静脉窦血栓形成及脑血栓形成）。

[a] 3～6 个月后评估 D-二聚体有助于决定是否停止预防性治疗。
[b] 长期抗凝治疗必须根据其他合并症、出血风险、暂时性的危险因素、依从性来进行个体化调整。
[c] 遗传性危险因素包括因子 V Leiden 突变、凝血酶 G20210A 突变、抗凝血酶缺陷、蛋白 C 缺陷、蛋白 S 缺陷。

清除率（CrCl）为 15～30 ml/min，需要调整剂量为 5 mg，2 次/日］；艾多沙班（急性期肠外抗凝后使用）。在严重肾功能不全的情况下，不建议使用 DOAC。但是，阿哌沙班可根据肾损害和其他因素调整用药剂量：如果肌酐＞1.5 mg/dl、年龄＞80 岁或体重≤60 kg，需将阿哌沙班剂量减少至口服 2.5 mg，2 次/日。RE-COVER 试验（2009 年）表明，在急性 VTE 患者中，达比加群在降低复发风险方面与华法林同样有效，且出血更少。与华法林相比，DOAC 的治疗范围变异性较小，在使用时无须抽血行 INR 检测。

总之，根据美国胸科医师协会（ACCP）静脉血栓栓塞性疾病抗血栓治疗指南（2016 年），对于发生在下肢的 DVT 或未患癌症的 PE 患者，在 3 个月的维持治疗中，达比加群、利伐沙班、阿哌沙班或艾多沙班比维生素 K 拮抗剂疗效更好。

治疗持续时间取决于有无 DVT 诱因、血栓位置及初发或复发血栓。大多数初发 DVT 患者（无论有无诱因或近端及远端血栓）应持续治疗 3 个月。如果为近端 DVT 或 PE，且出血风险为低危/中危，则应延长至 3 个月以上。对于复发性 VTE 患者，无论出血风险如何，应持续治疗 3 个月以上，具体时间根据出血危险因素和患者合并症确定，甚至可能建议终身抗凝。3 个月以上的治疗持续时间尚未完全确定，需视具体情况而定。对于接受抗凝治疗至少 6～12 个月且临床稳定的患者，EINSTEIN Choice 试验和 AMPLIFY-EXT 试验结果分别提示低剂量利伐沙班（10 mg，1 次/日）或阿哌沙班（2.5 mg，2 次/日）可以安全有效地降低 VTE 风险，且几乎不会增加出血风险。

对于无诱因的近端 DVT 或 PE 停止抗凝后，指南建议在没有阿司匹林禁忌证且未继续使用抗凝剂的患者中使用阿司匹林，以预防 DVT 复发。

恶性肿瘤中 VTE 的治疗

在恶性肿瘤患者中，LMWH 的疗效优于华法林。根据 2003 年的 CLOT 试验，与华法林相比，达肝素（LMWH）具有较低的 VTE 复发风险，且不会增加出血风险或死亡。这些结果在 2006 年的 LITE 试验和 ONCENOX 试验中得到了证实。Hokusai VTE 癌症试验（2018 年）显示，在开放标签研究中，对于恶性肿瘤合并 VTE 的患者，艾多沙班对复发性 VTE 的疗效不逊于达肝素，但出血风险更高。对于特定的恶性肿瘤（如胃肠癌），LMWH 比艾多沙班更适用于长期抗凝治疗（见 Raskob 2017）。此外，一些研究建议，如果 CrCl＞95 ml/min，则不应使用艾多沙班，但在 VTE 中避免使用此药的数据尚不清楚。SELECT-D 预试验对利伐沙班和达肝素治疗癌症相关 VTE 进行了比较，结果显示利伐沙班组的 VTE 发生率低于达肝素组，但非严重出血的发生率增加。目前有多项试验对比了阿哌沙班与达肝素治疗恶性肿瘤相关 VTE 患者的疗效：Caravaggio 试验正在进行中，ADAM-VTE 试验的初步结果表明阿哌沙班组的出血风险低且 VTE 复发率低。

综上，根据 ACCP 静脉血栓栓塞性疾病抗血栓治疗指南（2016 年），对于癌症相关 VTE 患者，最初 3 个月的治疗推荐 LMWH 而非其他药物，而美国临床肿瘤学会（ASCO）指南建议可将 DOAC 作为一线治疗。如前所述，VTE 的治疗持续时间取决于癌症类型（凝血与出血风险）及恶性肿瘤的治疗计划。

鉴于已知的相互作用且缺乏安全性数据，DOAC 不应与 P 糖蛋白和强效 CYP3A 抑制剂（如卡马西平、苯妥英、酮康唑、利托那韦、利福平）等药物同时服用。某些抗生素（如红霉素或克拉霉素）可能增加 DOAC 的血药浓度，特别是在肾功能不全的个体中。

VTE 的预防性治疗

尽管有了 DOAC，华法林和 LMWH 仍然常被用于治疗 VTE。华法林应在有 VTE 表现后的最初 24 h 内开始使用，同时配合肝素治疗。华法林可通过迅速降低 FⅦ 水平使凝血时间（PT）在数小时内延长；然而，只有当其他维生素 K 依赖性凝血因子（Ⅱ、Ⅸ和Ⅹ）水平也降低时，才能达到华法林的治疗性抗凝效果。华法林的治疗性抗凝水平通常可在足量治疗 4～5 天内达到；当连续 2 天 INR＞2 时，可停用 UFH 或 LMWH。华法林抗凝治疗的一个长期存在的问题是 INR 反应的个体差异，在这种对华法林敏感性的差异中，至少有 50% 可通过 *CYP2C9* 和 *VKORC1* 基因多态性来解释。虽然这些基因多态性已被纳入预测华法林安全性和治疗剂量的模型中，但大多数临床医师只是简单地开始给药并根据定期监测结果按需调整治疗。

INR 的治疗范围取决于患者易患血栓栓塞的情况。无已知危险因素且无并发症的 VTE 的预防性治疗需使 INR 维持在 2～3；相比之下，对于具有 APS 和复发性 VTE 的患者，华法林预防性治疗可能需要 INR 高达 3～4（表 8.7）[译者注：原文（Table 8.6）有误]。

华法林或 LMWH 预防性治疗的持续时间取决于 VTE 的具体临床情况、出血风险和复发可能性。一般情况下，使用华法林的抗凝时间越长，复发的可能性越小。与华法林长期治疗（6 个月）相比，短期治疗

TABLE 8.6 Drugs That Affect Warfarin Levels
Increased Warfarin Levels: Prolonged INR
↓ Warfarin clearance
Disulfiram
Metronidazole
Trimethoprim-sulfamethoxazole
↓ Warfarin-protein binding
Phenylbutazone
↑ Vitamin K turnover
Clofibrate
Decreased Warfarin Levels: Subtherapeutic INR
↑ Hepatic metabolism of warfarin
Barbiturates
Rifampin
↓ Warfarin absorption
Cholestyramine

↑, Increased; ↓, decreased; *INR*, international normalized ratio.

TABLE 8.7 Therapeutic International Normalized Ratio (INR) Ranges for Warfarin	
Patient Subgroup	INR Range
Venous Thrombosis	
Treatment	2.0-3.0
Prophylaxis	1.5-2.5
Artificial Heart Valves	
Tissue	2.0-2.5
Mechanical	3.0-4.0
Atrial Fibrillation (Nonvalvular)	
Prophylaxis	1.5-2.5
Lupus Anticoagulant	
Treatment, prophylaxis	2.0-3.0
Refractory thromboembolism	3.0-4.0

as orthopedic surgery have low recurrence rates, even with short-term therapy; still, prolonged thromboprophylaxis (>21 days) after total hip replacement is more efficacious than shorter therapy (7 to 10 days). It is not clear that oral Xa inhibitors and dabigatran provide any additional benefit over LMWH for thromboprophylaxis after total hip or knee replacement (Table 8.7).

Additionally, DOACs have been studied as thromboprophylaxis in specific patient settings. The MARINER trial evaluated patients who were discharged after medical illness with increased risk of VTE and showed that rivaroxaban 10 mg by mouth daily for 45 days after discharge did not reduce VTE or VTE mortality compared with placebo.

In contrast, patients with "unprovoked" VTE (i.e., outside the setting of trauma, surgery, immobilization, pregnancy, or cancer) have significant recurrence rates, even after 3 to 6 months of warfarin therapy. Because the risk for recurrence in patients with unprovoked proximal VTE or PE is relatively low when D-dimer levels are normal 3 weeks after cessation of anticoagulation, this measure may help providers decide whether anticoagulation past 3 to 6 months is necessary.

Given increased risk of recurrence in patients without reversible risk factors for VTE, extended-duration anticoagulation is sometimes warranted. Two studies evaluated using aspirin 100 mg versus placebo after anticoagulation therapy for unprovoked VTE. ASPIRE 2012 found a nonsignificant trend towards fewer recurrent VTE events and a nonsignificant trend towards higher bleeding risk, whereas WARFASA 2012 found statistically significant demonstration of fewer VTE recurrences without differences in major bleeding. There is thought that the trials differ in outcomes due to ASPIRE's lack of enrollment for prespecified power, differences in inclusion criteria, and that only two thirds of ASPIRE patients had received 6 or more months of anticoagulation prior to initiation of aspirin.

Furthermore, the EINSTEIN-CHOICE Trial demonstrated that, in patients with VTE who have completed 6 to 12 months of anticoagulation, there was reduced risk of recurrent VTE without significant bleeding when using both 10 or 20 mg/day of rivaroxaban compared to aspirin 100 mg/day. In AMPLIFY-EXT, another oral factor Xa inhibitor, apixaban, was studied for extended anticoagulation at doses of 5 mg (treatment) or 2.5 mg (prophylactic) and was found to have statistically decreased number of recurrent VTE and no increased bleeding risk compared to placebo.

Thus, current management for an unprovoked acute VTE includes use of either rivaroxaban or apixaban for the initial 6 months of therapy followed by a dose reduction in either agent. For patients with a provoked VTE, initial anticoagulation practice is the same, but anticoagulation may be stopped 3 months after the provoking risk factor has resolved.

Evidence also indicates that inherited hypercoagulable disorders (e.g., FVL mutation) probably confer a lifelong increased risk for VTE or PE, but whether the index VTE was provoked or unprovoked determines length of therapy. Some studies have shown that the bleeding risks incurred by long-term, low-intensity warfarin use are favorably balanced by the decreased incidence of recurrent thrombosis. Therefore, the presence of inherited thrombophilia may warrant continuation of anticoagulation for a longer period, depending on the patient's other medical illnesses and whether transient circumstances may have predisposed the patient to VTE. Patients who develop recurrent VTE after discontinuation of anticoagulation should receive long-term anticoagulation regardless of whether they have a defined cause of thrombophilia. Patients with APS and a first episode of VTE are at very high risk for recurrent VTE (up to 50% per year) after anticoagulation is discontinued, clearly supporting the rationale of testing for antiphospholipid. Table 8.8 suggests broad guidelines for the duration of warfarin therapy in specific patient subgroups. Because warfarin is a teratogen, effective contraception should be used concurrently in women of childbearing age.

Prophylaxis for VTE in Orthopedic Surgeries

RECORD1 and RECORD3 (both published 2008) demonstrated improved efficacy of short-course rivaroxaban over short-course enoxaparin in prevention of VTE after hip and knee replacements, respectively, without increased bleeding risk. RECORD2 (2008) demonstrated that extended-course rivaroxaban was more effective in preventing VTE than short-course enoxaparin without increasing bleeding rates following hip replacement.

Prophylactic Anticoagulation in Hospitalized Medically Ill Patients

MEDENOX, PREVENT, and ARTEMIS demonstrated promise of in-hospital thromboprophylaxis with LMWH with a relative risk reduction of 45% to 63% compared to placebo. In acutely medically ill hospitalized patients, MAGELLAN (2013) demonstrated short-course rivaroxaban (10 mg daily for 10 days) is noninferior to short-course

表 8.6 影响华法林水平的药物
升高华法林水平：INR 升高
华法林清除率降低
双硫仑
甲硝唑
复方磺胺甲噁唑
华法林蛋白结合率降低
保泰松
维生素 K 转化增加
氯贝丁酯
降低华法林水平：INR 未达标
华法林肝代谢增加
巴比妥类药物
利福平
华法林吸收减少
考来烯胺

INR，国际标准化比值。

表 8.7 华法林抗凝治疗的 INR 预期范围	
患者亚组	INR 的范围
静脉血栓形成	
治疗	2.0～3.0
预防性治疗	1.5～2.5
人工心脏瓣膜	
生物瓣膜	2.0～2.5
机械瓣膜	3.0～4.0
心房颤动（非瓣膜性）	
预防性治疗	1.5～2.5
狼疮抗凝物	
治疗及预防性治疗	2.0～3.0
复发性血栓栓塞	3.0～4.0

（6 周）预防血栓复发的效果较差。具有明确的暂时性危险因素（如骨科手术）的患者血栓复发率较低，即使仅接受短期治疗。尽管如此，全髋关节置换术后行长期血栓预防性治疗（>21 天）比短期治疗（7～10 天）更有效。目前尚不清楚口服因子 X a 抑制剂和达比加群在预防全髋关节或膝关节置换术后血栓预防方面是否比使用 LMWH 有更多获益（表 8.8）[译者注：原文（Table 8.7）有误]。

此外，DOAC 已被研究用于特定患者群体的血栓预防。MARINER 试验评估了出院时 VTE 风险增加的患者，结果显示，与安慰剂相比，出院后 45 天中每天口服利伐沙班 10 mg 并不能降低 VTE 发生率及其死亡率。

"无诱因"（即无创伤、手术、制动、妊娠或癌症等情况）VTE 患者的复发率很高，即使接受了 3～6 个月的华法林治疗。在停止抗凝治疗 3 周后，若 D- 二聚体水平正常，则无诱因的近端 VTE 或 PE 患者的血栓复发风险相对较低，因此检测 D- 二聚体可能有助于医生决定是否需要将抗凝治疗延长至 3～6 个月以上。

考虑到没有可逆性危险因素的 VTE 患者的复发风险增加，延长抗凝时间有时是必要的。两项研究评估了无诱因 VTE 患者抗凝治疗后使用 100 mg 阿司匹林与安慰剂的效果。ASPIRE 2012 试验显示，阿司匹林组 VTE 复发事件减少的趋势不明显，出血风险增加的趋势也不明显；WARFASA 2012 试验显示，使用阿司匹林可显著减少 VTE 复发，且在严重出血方面没有差异。有观点认为这两项试验的结果不同是由于 ASPIRE 试验入组人数未能达到预设的统计检验功效、纳入标准不同，且 ASPIRE 试验的患者中只有 2/3 在开始使用阿司匹林前接受了 6 个月或更长时间的抗凝治疗。

此外，EINSTEIN-CHOICE 试验表明，对于已完成 6～12 个月抗凝治疗的 VTE 患者，与 100 mg/d 阿司匹林相比，10 mg/d 或 20 mg/d 利伐沙班可降低复发性 VTE 的风险，且不会显著增加出血风险。AMPLIFY-EXT 试验对另一种口服因子 X a 抑制剂阿哌沙班 [5 mg/d（治疗剂量）或 2.5 mg/d（预防剂量）] 长期抗凝进行了研究，结果显示，与安慰剂相比，阿哌沙班能显著减少复发性 VTE 且不增加出血风险。

因此，急性无诱因 VTE 的当前治疗包括在最初的 6 个月治疗中使用利伐沙班或阿哌沙班，随后减少药物剂量。对于有诱因的 VTE 患者，初始抗凝治疗相同，但在诱发因素消除后 3 个月可停止抗凝治疗。

有证据表明，遗传性高凝状态（如 FVL 突变）可能会终身增加 VTE 或 PE 的风险，但是否存在 VTE 诱因决定了治疗时间的长短。部分研究显示，长期低强度应用华法林所带来的出血风险与复发性血栓的减少相平衡。因此，遗传性易栓症可能需要更长的华法林抗凝治疗时间，这取决于患者的合并症及是否处于易诱发 VTE 的环境。无论是否有明确的易栓症病因，停止抗凝治疗后复发的 VTE 患者均应接受长期抗凝治疗。患有 APS 且首次发生 VTE 的患者在停止抗凝治疗后 VTE 复发的风险非常高（每年高达 50%），因此应进行抗磷脂抗体检测。表 8.5 提供了特定患者人群华法林治疗持续时间的大体指导原则。由于华法林是致畸剂，育龄期女性应同时采用有效的避孕措施。

骨科手术中 VTE 的预防

RECORD1 试验和 RECORD3 试验（均发表于 2008 年）表明，在髋关节和膝关节置换术后，短疗程利伐沙班在预防 VTE 方面比短疗程依诺肝素更有效，且未增加出血风险。RECORD2 试验（2008 年）则表明，在髋关节置换术后，长疗程利伐沙班在预防 VTE 方面比依诺肝素短疗程应用更有效，且未升高出血发生率。

内科住院患者的预防性抗凝治疗

MEDENOX 试验、PREVENT 试验和 ARTEMIS 试验展示了院内使用 LMWH 预防血栓的应用前景，与安慰剂相比，使用 LMWH 的血栓相对风险降低了 45%～63%。MAGELLAN 试验（2013 年）显示，在因急性内科疾病住院的患者中，尽管采用短疗程利伐沙班（10 mg/d，持续 10 天）增加了出血风险，但其

TABLE 8.8	Direct Oral Anticoagulants (DOAC) and Their Indications
DOAC	Indications
Dabigatran	Direct thrombin inhibitor for nonvalvular atrial fibrillation (to prevent stroke and non-CNS embolism); VTE as maintenance therapy (after initial therapy); VTE prophylaxis of VTE after hip replacement
Rivaroxaban	Anti-Xa for nonvalvular atrial fibrillation (to prevent stroke and non-CNS embolism); treatment of VTE and subsequent prophylaxis; and VTE prophylaxis of VTE after hip or knee replacement
Apixaban	Anti-Xa for nonvalvular atrial fibrillation (to prevent stroke and non-CNS embolism); VTE as initial therapy or maintenance therapy; VTE prophylaxis of VTE after hip or knee replacement
Edoxaban	Anti-Xa for prevention of VTE as maintenance therapy (after initial therapy); prevention of embolism in atrial fibrillation; has been studied for treatment of VTE in patients with malignancy and is noninferior to dalteparin (a LMWH) with an increased bleeding risk

CNS, Central nervous system; *VTE*, venous thromboembolism; *Xa*, activated factor X.

enoxaparin (40 mg daily for 10 days) in preventing VTE, although it increases risk of bleeding. Extended rivaroxaban (10 mg daily for 35 ± 4 days) was also found to be superior to short-course enoxaparin for prevention of VTE and its complications but also had increased bleeding risk.

The APEX trial studied acutely ill medical patients and showed that extended-duration betrixaban for 35 to 42 days did not reduce the primary end point of asymptomatic proximal clot or symptomatic VTE compared to standard enoxaparin for 6 to 14 days.

Prophylactic Anticoagulation in High-Risk Patients With Malignancy in the Ambulatory Setting

The CASSINI trial evaluated ambulatory cancer patients at high risk for thromboembolism (Khorana score ≥2) and whether low-dose rivaroxaban (10 mg daily) is more effective than placebo in reducing incidence of venous thromboembolism. Rivaroxaban did not result in statistically significant reduction in incident thromboembolism at 180 days when compared to placebo and had a small, not statistically significant increase in bleeding risk; however, when only time on the drug was considered, there was an absolute reduction in VTE with rivaroxaban compared to placebo. On the other hand, the AVERT trial studied apixaban 2.5 mg twice daily versus placebo in ambulatory cancer patients at intermediate-to-high risk for venous thromboembolism (Khorana score ≥2). Prophylactic apixaban reduced the risk of VTE in these patients but increased the risk of major bleeding episodes. Major bleeding was most common in those with GI or GU malignancy. Of note, the trial populations were different, with AVERT having a significant proportion of patients with lymphoma and CASSINI having a higher proportion of pancreatic cancer.

Antithrombotic Therapy During Pregnancy

Heparins, both UFH and LMWH, are the safest therapy for venous thrombosis treatment and prevention during pregnancy. Heparin does not cross the placenta, unlike warfarin, which causes a characteristic fetal embryopathy. Warfarin also causes fetal hemorrhage and placental abruption and should be avoided during pregnancy. VTE or PE during pregnancy should be treated with intravenous UFH for 5 to 10 days, followed by an adjusted-dose regimen of subcutaneous UFH, starting with 20,000 U every 12 hours and adjusted to achieve a PTT higher than 1.5 times baseline at 6 hours after injection. An attractive alternative to UFH during pregnancy is LMWH, which can be given subcutaneously once or twice daily and does not require monitoring. Suprarenal IVC filters have also been used successfully during pregnancy without significant morbidity. In women with APS who become pregnant, therapy is critical to prevent fetal loss; aspirin is combined with prophylactic doses of either subcutaneous UFH (10,000 to 15,000 U/day in divided doses) or LMWH (to achieve an anti-Xa level of 0.1 to 0.3 U/mL). When such women have a history of thromboembolic disease, therapeutic doses of LMWH or UFH plus aspirin are employed.

Heparin should be discontinued at the time of labor and delivery, although the risk for hemorrhage is not high during delivery, especially if anti-Xa levels are less than 0.7 U/mL. One concern with residual anticoagulation at delivery is the risk for spinal hematoma with epidural anesthesia; this concern has been reported with both UFH and LMWH. The anti-Xa level that is safe for an epidural procedure is not known. Protamine sulfate can be used to neutralize UFH if the PTT is prolonged during labor and delivery; however, LMWH is only partially (10%) reversed by protamine.

Anticoagulation during the postpartum period can be carried out with heparin (either UFH or LMWH) or warfarin; neither drug is contraindicated during breast-feeding. Women receiving long-term warfarin therapy (e.g., for valvular heart disease) who wish to become pregnant need to be switched to a fully anticoagulating dose of UFH or LMWH; warfarin treatment may be restarted after delivery.

There is limited evidence to support use of DOACs in pregnancy. There are concerns about a higher incidence of miscarriages and fetal anomalies with DOACs. There is currently not enough data to show safety and suggest use of the DOACs during pregnancy, so they are not recommended.

Perioperative Anticoagulation

A common clinical problem is the management of anticoagulation in patients who require surgery. The principles of care in this situation reflect the need for adequate hemostasis during and immediately after surgical procedures as well as the critical importance of restarting anticoagulation as soon as possible postoperatively, especially because surgery itself represents a relative hypercoagulable state. The perceived risk for thromboembolism in patients with atrial fibrillation clearly affects the management of perioperative anticoagulation; in this clinical situation, the CHADS-2 score (*c*ardiac failure, *h*ypertension, *a*ge, *d*iabetes, and *s*troke) may estimate postoperative stroke risk and thus dictate the need for bridging anticoagulation with UFH/LMWH when stopping vitamin K antagonist. For patients with VTE who are anticoagulated on a short-term basis (<1 month), elective surgical procedures should be postponed; if such patients must undergo urgent surgery, discontinuation of anticoagulation and placement of a temporary IVC filter may be the best option. In most patients receiving long-term anticoagulation for VTE, preoperative heparin is not typically used; vitamin K antagonist should be discontinued for at least 4 days preoperatively to allow the INR to decrease gradually to less than 1.5, a level that is safe for surgery. Postoperatively, intravenous heparin (or subcutaneous LMWH) can be safely used for anticoagulation until therapeutic INR levels are reached after warfarin has been restarted. Increasingly, restarting a DOAC postoperatively at pre-surgery therapeutic dosing is safe and effective to avoid the need for bridging with parenteral therapy. As with all guidelines, individual patient circumstances may dictate changes. For example, institution of heparin immediately after a major surgical procedure may be contraindicated because of the high

表8.8 直接口服抗凝剂（DOAC）及其适应证	
DOAC	适应证
达比加群	直接凝血酶抑制剂，可用于治疗非瓣膜性心房颤动（预防卒中及非CNS栓塞）；VTE的维持治疗（在初始治疗后）；髋关节置换术后VTE的预防性治疗
利伐沙班	抗因子Xa活性，可用于治疗非瓣膜性心房颤动（预防卒中及非CNS栓塞）；治疗VTE及随后的预防性治疗；髋关节及膝关节术后VTE的预防性治疗
阿哌沙班	抗因子Xa活性，可用于治疗非瓣膜性心房颤动（预防卒中及非CNS栓塞）；VTE的初始或维持治疗；髋关节及膝关节术后VTE的预防性治疗
艾多沙班	抗因子Xa活性，作为维持治疗预防VTE（在初始治疗后）；用于心房颤动患者预防栓塞；已被研究用于治疗恶性肿瘤患者的VTE，其疗效不逊于达肝素（一种LMWH），但出血风险增加

CNS，中枢神经系统；VTE，静脉血栓栓塞；Xa，活化的因子X。

在预防VTE方面不逊于短疗程依诺肝素（40 mg/d，持续10天）。延长利伐沙班的使用时间［10 mg/d，持续（35±4）天］在预防VTE及其并发症方面也优于依诺肝素短疗程应用，但同样增加了出血风险。

APEX试验结果表明，与标准剂量依诺肝素治疗6～14天相比，延长贝曲沙班疗程治疗至35～42天并未显著减少急性内科疾病患者无症状近端血栓或症状性VTE的发生。

门诊高危恶性肿瘤患者的预防性抗凝治疗

CASSINI试验评估了处于血栓栓塞高风险（Khorana评分≥2分）的门诊癌症患者及小剂量利伐沙班（10 mg/d）是否能比安慰剂更有效地降低VTE的发生率。结果显示，与安慰剂相比，利伐沙班在180天时并未显著降低血栓栓塞发生率，且出血风险略增加（无统计学差异）。然而，若只考虑用药期间，与安慰剂组相比，利伐沙班组患者的VTE事件绝对减少。AVERT试验研究了阿哌沙班（2.5 mg，2次/日）在静脉血栓栓塞中高风险（Khorana评分≥2分）的门诊癌症患者中的效果。在这些患者中，预防性使用阿哌沙班虽然降低了VTE的风险，但增加了严重出血的风险。严重出血最常见于胃肠道或泌尿系统恶性肿瘤患者。值得注意的是，上述两项试验的患者人群不同，AVERT试验中有较大比例的淋巴瘤患者，而CASSINI试验中胰腺癌患者的比例更高。

妊娠期间的抗凝治疗

肝素类药物（包括UFH和LMWH）是妊娠期间治疗和预防静脉血栓形成最安全的选择。肝素不会透过胎盘，而华法林会引起特有的胎儿胚胎病，还可导致胎儿出血和胎盘早剥，故妊娠期间应避免使用华法林。妊娠期VTE或PE应采用静脉注射UFH治疗5～10天，随后用UFH皮下注射剂量调整方案，起始剂量为20 000 U，每12 h 1次，随后调整剂量至注射后6 h的APTT达到基线的1.5倍以上。LMWH是妊娠期UFH的最佳替代治疗，可每天皮下注射1次或2次，且不需要监测。下腔静脉滤器已在妊娠期患者中成功使用，且未引起明显的并发症。对于合并APS的孕妇，关键治疗是预防流产，通常给予阿司匹林联合预防剂量的皮下注射UFH（10 000～15 000 U/d，分次使用）或LMWH（使抗因子Xa水平达到0.1～0.3 U/ml）。若这些孕妇有血栓栓塞性疾病病史，应使用阿司匹林联合治疗剂量的LMWH或UFH。

肝素应在进入产程和分娩时停用，虽然分娩期间出血的风险不高，特别是当抗因子Xa水平＜0.7 U/ml时。分娩时体内残留抗凝药物有发生硬膜外麻醉后脊柱血肿的风险，这在UFH和LMWH的使用中均有报道。硬膜外麻醉下抗因子Xa的安全水平未知。如果分娩期间APTT延长，可使用硫酸鱼精蛋白中和UFH，但鱼精蛋白仅能中和部分LMWH（10%）。

产后抗凝治疗可使用肝素（UFH或LMWH）或华法林，这两类药物在哺乳期均无禁忌证。长期使用华法林（如心脏瓣膜病）的女性在备孕时需转换为足量UFH或LMWH抗凝，分娩后可重新开始华法林治疗。

目前有关妊娠期间使用DOAC的证据有限。人们担忧DOAC可能导致流产和胎儿畸形的发生率升高。目前尚无足够的数据证明妊娠期间使用DOAC的安全性及提出用药建议，因此不推荐使用。

围术期的抗凝治疗

拟行手术患者的抗凝管理是常见的临床问题。管理原则反映了手术期间和术后立即充分止血的必要性，以及术后尽快重新开始抗凝治疗的重要性，因为手术本身就是一种相对高凝状态。心房颤动患者血栓栓塞的风险可显著影响围术期的抗凝管理。在这种情况下，CHADS-2评分（心力衰竭、高血压、年龄、糖尿病和卒中）可估计术后卒中的风险，从而决定在停用维生素K拮抗剂时是否需要使用UFH/LMWH进行桥接抗凝治疗。对于接受短疗程（＜1个月）抗凝治疗的VTE患者，应推迟择期手术；若该类患者必须进行手术，停止抗凝并放置临时下腔静脉滤器可能是最佳选择。对于大多数接受长期抗凝治疗的VTE患者，术前通常不需要使用肝素；术前需停用维生素K拮抗剂至少4天，以使INR逐渐降至安全进行手术的水平（＜1.5）。术后静脉注射肝素（或皮下注射LMWH）可以安全地用于抗凝治疗，直至重新开始使用华法林后INR达标。术后按照术前的治疗剂量重新开始使用DOAC在越来越多的情况下是安全有效的，这可以避免与肠外治疗桥接。所有指南均指出，个别患者的情况可能有所不同。例如，大型外科手术后立即给予肝素可能是禁忌的，因为出血风险很高，恢复抗凝治疗

risk for hemorrhage, and reinstitution of anticoagulation may need to be delayed for 12 to 24 hours postoperatively.

Risk of postoperative VTE in patients undergoing hip or knee arthroplasty without postoperative anticoagulation is estimated at 6% by Caprini score. Thus, VTE prophylaxis is standard of care. EPCAT II 2018 showed extended thromboprophylaxis with aspirin 81 mg was noninferior to rivaroxaban 10 mg daily for 5 days in preventing symptomatic VTE in low-risk patients after total hip or knee arthroplasty.

❖ For a deeper discussion on this topic, please see Chapter 162, "Approach to the Patient with Bleeding and Thrombosis," in *Goldman-Cecil Medicine*, 26th Edition.

SUGGESTED READINGS

Adam SS, McDuffie JR, Lachiewicz PF, et al: Comparative effectiveness of new oral anticoagulants and standard thromboprophylaxis in patients having total hip or knee replacement, Ann Intern Med 159:275–284, 2013.

Barbui T, Finazzi G, Carobbio A, et al: Development and validation of an international prognostic score of thrombosis in World Health Organization-essential thrombocythemia (IPSET-thrombosis), Blood 120:5128–5133, 2012.

Basurto L, Sánchez L, Díaz A, et al: Differences between metabolically healthy and unhealthy obesity in PAI-1 level: Fibrinolysis, body size phenotypes and metabolism, Thrombosis Research vol 180:110–114, 2019.

Beer PA, Erber WN, Campbell PJ, et al: How I treat essential thrombocythemia, Blood 117:1472–1482, 2011.

Brilakis ES, Patel VG, Banerjee S: Medical management after coronary stent implantation, JAMA 310:189–198, 2013.

Carrier M, Abou-Nassar K, Mallick R, et al: AVERT Investigators. Apixaban to prevent venous thromboembolism in patients with cancer, N Engl J Med 380(8):711–719, 2019.

Cattaneo M: The platelet P2Y12 receptor for adenosine diphosphate: congenital and drug-induced defects, Blood 117:2102–2112, 2011.

Connors JM: Thrombophilia testing and venous thrombosis, N Engl J Med 377(12):1177–1187, 2017.

Cuker A, Gimotty PA, Crowtheer MA, et al: Predictive value of the 4Ts scoring system for heparin-induced thrombocytopenia, Blood 120:4160–4167, 2012.

Dobromirski M, Cohen AT: How I manage venous thromboembolism risk in hospitalized patients, Blood 120:1562–1569, 2012.

Douketis JD: Perioperative management of patients who are receiving warfarin therapy: an evidence-based and practical approach, Blood 117:5044–5049, 2011.

Khorana AA, Soff GA, Kakkar AK, et al: CASSINI Investigators. Rivaroxaban for thromboprophylaxis in high-risk ambulatory patients with cancer, N Engl J Med 380(8):720–728, 2019.

Lameijer H, Aalberts J, van Veldhuisen D, et al: Efficacy and safety of direct oral anticoagulants during pregnancy; a systematic literature review, Thrombosis Research 169:123–127, 2018.

Raskob GE, van Es N, Verhamme P, et al: Hokusai VTE Cancer Investigators. Edoxaban for the treatment of cancer-associated venous thromboembolism, N Engl J Med 378(7):615–624, 2018.

Scully M, Cataland SR, Peyvandi F, et al: HERCULES Investigators. Caplacizumab treatment for acquired thrombotic thrombocytopenic purpura, N Engl J Med 380(4):335–346, 2019.

Sobieraj DM, Lee S, Coleman CI, et al: Prolonged versus standard-duration venous thromboprophylaxis in major orthopedic surgery, Ann Intern Med 156:720–727, 2012.

Sultan AA, Tata LJ, West J, et al: Risk factors for first venous thromboembolism around pregnancy: a population-based cohort study from the United Kingdom, Blood 121:3953–3961, 2013.

Tosetto A, Iorio A, Marcucci M, et al: Predicting disease recurrence in patients with previous unprovoked venous thromboembolism: a proposed prediction score (DASH), J Thromb Haemost 366:1019–1025, 2012.

可能需要延迟至术后 12～24 h。

根据 Caprini 评分，未行术后抗凝治疗的髋关节或膝关节置换术患者发生 VTE 的风险约为 6%。因此，VTE 预防性治疗是标准治疗流程。2018 年的 EPCAT Ⅱ 试验显示，低血栓风险患者行全髋关节或膝关节置换术后长期应用阿司匹林（81 mg）在预防症状性 VTE 方面并不劣于利伐沙班（10 mg/d，持续 5 天）。

◆ 有关此专题的深入讨论，请参阅 *Goldman-Cecil Medicine* 第 26 版第 162 章"出血和血栓患者的接诊"。

推荐阅读

Adam SS, McDuffie JR, Lachiewicz PF, et al: Comparative effectiveness of new oral anticoagulants and standard thromboprophylaxis in patients having total hip or knee replacement, Ann Intern Med 159:275–284, 2013.

Barbui T, Finazzi G, Carobbio A, et al: Development and validation of an international prognostic score of thrombosis in World Health Organization-essential thrombocythemia (IPSET-thrombosis), Blood 120:5128–5133, 2012.

Basurto L, Sánchez L, Díaz A, et al: Differences between metabolically healthy and unhealthy obesity in PAI-1 level: Fibrinolysis, body size phenotypes and metabolism, Thrombosis Research vol 180:110–114, 2019.

Beer PA, Erber WN, Campbell PJ, et al: How I treat essential thrombocythemia, Blood 117:1472–1482, 2011.

Brilakis ES, Patel VG, Banerjee S: Medical management after coronary stent implantation, JAMA 310:189–198, 2013.

Carrier M, Abou-Nassar K, Mallick R, et al: AVERT Investigators. Apixaban to prevent venous thromboembolism in patients with cancer, N Engl J Med 380(8):711–719, 2019.

Cattaneo M: The platelet P2Y12 receptor for adenosine diphosphate: congenital and drug-induced defects, Blood 117:2102–2112, 2011.

Connors JM: Thrombophilia testing and venous thrombosis, N Engl J Med 377(12):1177–1187, 2017.

Cuker A, Gimotty PA, Crowtheer MA, et al: Predictive value of the 4Ts scoring system for heparin-induced thrombocytopenia, Blood 120:4160–4167, 2012.

Dobromirski M, Cohen AT: How I manage venous thromboembolism risk in hospitalized patients, Blood 120:1562–1569, 2012.

Douketis JD: Perioperative management of patients who are receiving warfarin therapy: an evidence-based and practical approach, Blood 117:5044–5049, 2011.

Khorana AA, Soff GA, Kakkar AK, et al: CASSINI Investigators. Rivaroxaban for thromboprophylaxis in high-risk ambulatory patients with cancer, N Engl J Med 380(8):720–728, 2019.

Lameijer H, Aalberts J, van Veldhuisen D, et al: Efficacy and safety of direct oral anticoagulants during pregnancy; a systematic literature review, Thrombosis Research 169:123–127, 2018.

Raskob GE, van Es N, Verhamme P, et al: Hokusai VTE Cancer Investigators. Edoxaban for the treatment of cancer-associated venous thromboembolism, N Engl J Med 378(7):615–624, 2018.

Scully M, Cataland SR, Peyvandi F, et al: HERCULES Investigators. Caplacizumab treatment for acquired thrombotic thrombocytopenic purpura, N Engl J Med 380(4):335–346, 2019.

Sobieraj DM, Lee S, Coleman CI, et al: Prolonged versus standard-duration venous thromboprophylaxis in major orthopedic surgery, Ann Intern Med 156:720–727, 2012.

Sultan AA, Tata LJ, West J, et al: Risk factors for first venous thromboembolism around pregnancy: a population-based cohort study from the United Kingdom, Blood 121:3953–3961, 2013.

Tosetto A, Iorio A, Marcucci M, et al: Predicting disease recurrence in patients with previous unprovoked venous thromboembolism: a proposed prediction score (DASH), J Thromb Haemost 366:1019–1025, 2012.

索引 Index

A

Abciximab, 192
Acanthocytes, 84
Activated partial thrombin time (aPTT), 140
Activated protein C (APC), 146
Activated protein C resistance, 194t, 202-204
Acute chest syndrome, in sickle cell disease, 86
Acute coronary syndrome
    glycoprotein IIb/IIa inhibitors in, 192
Acute leukemia, 46-66
    classifications of, 48t
Acute lymphoblastic leukemia, 48t, 52t, 60-64, 62t
Acute myeloid leukemia, 48t, 50-58, 52t, 54f-58f
    chemotherapy for, 52-54
ADAMTS13, 138
    replacement of, 202
    in thrombotic thrombocytopenic purpura, 202
Adenosine diphosphate (ADP), 192
    sideroblastic anemias in, 72
Alemtuzumab
    chronic lymphocytic leukemia, 122
Alloimmune thrombocytopenia, fetal and neonatal, 166, 166t-168t
All-*trans*-retinoic acid (ATRA), for acute promyelocytic leukemia, 58
Amyloidosis
    factor X deficiency in, 184
    primary, 130
Anagrelide, essential thrombocythemia and, 36
Anemia, 68
    aplastic, 162
    in chronic kidney disease, 78-80
    clinical presentation of, 68
    differential diagnosis of, 70f
    of inflammation, 78
    laboratory evaluation of, 68
    pernicious, 76
    with reticulocytosis, 80-90
Antibodies
    anti-β$_2$-glycoprotein I, 198, 202-204
    platelet, 164
Anticardiolipin antibodies, 198
    serologies for, 202-204
Anticoagulants
    endogenous, 144, 144f
    natural, inherited deficiency of, 194-196
Anticoagulation
    during breast-feeding, 210
    in heparin-induced thrombocytopenia, 200
    perioperative, 210-212
    during postpartum period, 210
    for venous thromboembolism, 204, 206t
Antigen-presenting cells
    for T-lymphocytes, 96
Antiphospholipid antibody syndrome (APS), 198
    diagnosis of, 198
    thrombosis in, 198
Antiplatelet therapy, 192, 192t
    platelet dysfunction caused by, 170-174, 170t, 172f, 174t
Antithrombin (AT), 144-146
    deficiency of, 194-196, 194t
    functional, 202-204
Anti-thymocyte globulin (ATG), for aplastic anemia, 14

Page numbers followed by "f" indicate figures, "t" indicate tables, and "b" indicate boxes.

A

阿昔单抗, 193
棘形红细胞, 85
活化部分凝血活酶时间（APTT），141
活化蛋白C（APC），147
活化蛋白C抵抗, 195t, 203-205
急性胸部综合征，见于镰状细胞贫血, 87
急性冠脉综合征
    糖蛋白Ⅱb/Ⅱa抑制剂，193
急性白血病, 47-67
    分型, 49t
急性淋巴细胞白血病, 49t, 53t, 61-65, 63t
急性髓系白血病, 49t, 51-59, 53t, 55f-59f
    化疗, 53-55
ADAMTS13, 139
    替代, 203
    血栓性血小板减少性紫癜, 203
腺苷二磷酸（ADP），193
    铁粒幼细胞贫血, 73
阿仑单抗
    慢性淋巴细胞白血病, 123
胎儿和新生儿同种免疫性血小板减少症, 167, 167t-169t
全反式维甲酸（ATRA），治疗急性早幼粒细胞白血病, 59
淀粉样变性
    因子X缺乏症, 185
    原发性, 131
阿那格雷，治疗原发性血小板增多症, 37
贫血, 69
    再生障碍性贫血, 163
    慢性肾脏病, 79-81
    临床表现, 69
    鉴别诊断, 71f
    炎症, 79
    实验室检查, 69
    恶性贫血, 77
    网织红细胞增多, 81-91
抗体
    抗β$_2$糖蛋白Ⅰ抗体, 199, 203-205
    血小板, 165
抗心磷脂抗体, 199
    血清学检查, 203-205
抗凝剂
    内源性抗凝剂, 145, 145f
    天然抗凝剂，遗传性缺陷, 195-197
抗凝治疗
    哺乳期, 211
    肝素诱导的血小板减少症, 201
    围术期, 211-213
    产后, 211
    静脉血栓栓塞, 205, 207t
抗原提呈细胞
    T淋巴细胞, 97
抗磷脂综合征（APS），199
    诊断, 199
    血栓形成, 199
抗血小板治疗, 193, 193t
    血小板功能障碍, 171-175, 171t, 173f, 175t
抗凝血酶（AT），145-147
    缺乏, 195-197, 195t
    功能, 203-205
抗胸腺细胞球蛋白（ATG），治疗再生障碍性贫血, 15

页码数字中，"f"代表"图"，"t"代表"表格"，"b"代表"框"。

Aplastic anemia, 12-14, 162
    clinical presentation of, 14
    definition and epidemiology of, 12
    diagnosis and differential diagnosis of, 14
    etiology of, 12
    pathology of, 12t
    treatment and prognosis of, 14
Aplastic crisis, in sickle cell disease, 86
Apoptosis, 4
Argatroban, in heparin-induced thrombocytopenia, 200
Arsenic trioxide, for acute promyelocytic leukemia, 60
Arterial thrombosis
    inessential thrombocytopenia, 200
    risk for, 190, 194t
Aspirin
    in antiplatelet therapy, 192
    clopidogrel with, 192
    platelet dysfunction caused by, 170, 170t
    prophylactic doses of UFH or LMWH with, 210
    for thrombosis, in myeloproliferative disorders, 200
Asymptomatic myeloma, 126-128
Atherothrombosis, 190-194, 204
Auer rods, 46

B

B lymphocytes, 102
    development of, 102
    lymphoid follicles, 102
    maturation of, 104f
    peripheral blood, 104
Basophils, 8, 92-94, 94f
Bence Jones protein, in multiple myeloma, 126
Bernard-Soulier syndrome, 170t, 174
Blast crisis, in CML, 40
Bleeding, 150-188
    caused by thrombocytopenia, 158-170
    clinical evaluation of, 150
    coagulation factor disorders and, 180-184
    fibrinogen disorders and, 182
    future prospectus for, 186
    laboratory evaluation of, 150-152, 152t, 154f-158f
    in liver disease, 184
    with normal laboratory values, 184-186
    platelet destruction, 162-170
    with platelet function defects, 170-178, 170t, 172f
    vascular causes of, 154-158
Bleeding time, 138, 152, 154f
Blinatumomab (BiTE), 62
Bone marrow
    hematopoiesis in, 4
    in myelodysplastic syndrome, 22-24
    in neutropenia, 100
Bone marrow biopsy, for aplastic anemia, 14
Bone marrow fibrosis, causes of, 36t
Bone marrow invasion, 160-162
Bortezomib
    in multiple myeloma, 128
    for Waldenström's macroglobulinemia, 130
Bosutinib, 42-44
Breast-feeding, anticoagulation during, 210
Burkitt lymphoma, 116

C

Cancer
    complications of, thrombosis, 198
Chédiak-Higashi syndrome, 174-176
Chemotaxis, of neutrophils, 92
Chronic granulomatous disease, 92

再生障碍性贫血，13-15，163
    临床表现，15
    定义和流行病学，13
    诊断和鉴别诊断，15
    病因，13
    病理学，13t
    治疗和预后，15
再生障碍危象，见于镰状细胞贫血，87
细胞凋亡，5
阿加曲班，肝素诱导的血小板减少症，201
三氧化二砷，治疗急性早幼粒细胞白血病，61
动脉血栓形成
    原发性血小板减少症，201
    风险，191，195t
阿司匹林
    抗血小板治疗，193
    氯吡格雷，193
    血小板功能障碍，171，171t
    预防剂量的 UFH 或 LMWH，211
    血栓形成，见于骨髓增生性疾病，201
无症状骨髓瘤，127-129
动脉粥样硬化血栓形成，191-195，205
Auer 小体，47

B

B 淋巴细胞，103
    发育，103
    淋巴滤泡，103
    成熟，105f
    外周血 B 淋巴细胞，105
嗜碱性粒细胞，9，93-95，95f
本周蛋白，见于多发性骨髓瘤，127
巨血小板综合征，171t，175
急变期危象，CML，41
出血，151-189
    血小板减少症，159-171
    临床评估，151
    凝血因子障碍，181-185
    纤维蛋白原异常，183
    未来展望，187
    实验室评估，151-153，153t，155f-159f
    肝病，185
    实验室指标正常的出血，185-187
    血小板破坏，163-171
    血小板功能缺陷，171-179，171t，173f
    血管疾病，155-159
出血时间，139，153，155f
贝林妥欧单抗（BiTE），63
骨髓
    造血，5
    骨髓增生异常综合征，23-25
    中性粒细胞减少症，101
骨髓活检，再生障碍性贫血，15
骨髓纤维化，病因，37t
骨髓侵犯，161-163
硼替佐米
    多发性骨髓瘤，129
    瓦尔登斯特伦巨球蛋白血症，131
博舒替尼，43-45
哺乳期，抗凝治疗，211
伯基特淋巴瘤，117

C

癌症
    并发症，血栓形成，199
白细胞异常色素减退综合征，175-177
趋化，中性粒细胞，93
慢性肉芽肿病，93

Chronic kidney disease (CKD)
    anemia of, 78-80
Clopidogrel
    in combination with aspirin, 192
Closure time, 138
Clot initiation, 140
Clot propagation, 140
Clotting termination, 144-146
Coagulation, 140-148
    cascade model of, 140
    laboratory testing of, 148
    models, 140-144
Coagulation factor
    disorders of, 180-184
    transfusion of, 184-186
Coagulopathy
    dilutional, 176, 184
Cobalamin (vitamin B₁₂)
    deficiency, 74-76
        causes of, 76, 76t
    intrinsic factor and, 74
    metabolic pathways of, 76f
Cold agglutinin disease, 82
    Waldenström's macroglobulinemia with, 130
Collagen
    bleeding disorders and, 154
    platelet binding to, 138
Coombs tests, 80
Cryoprecipitate, 186
Cyclooxygenase-2 (COX-2) inhibitors, platelet function and, 172
Cyclophosphamide
    for aplastic anemia, 14
Cyclosporine
    for aplastic anemia, 14
Cytokines
    hematopoiesis and, 4, 6t

D

Dasatinib, 42-44
D-dimer, 148
    in disseminated intravascular coagulation, 168
D-dimer test
    recurrence risk for thromboembolism and, 208
1-deamino-(8-D-arginine)-vasopressin (DDAVP)
    for bleeding
        caused by aspirin, 174
        in uremic platelet dysfunction, 174
    for von Willebrand disease, 178
Decitabine, for myelodysplastic syndrome, 24
Dexamethasone
    for immune thrombocytopenic purpura, 164
    for multiple myeloma, 128
Diamond-Blackfan anemia, 22-24
Diffuse large B-cell lymphoma (DLBCL), 106-108
Direct oral anticoagulants, 210t
Direct thrombin inhibitor (DTI), in heparin-induced thrombocytopenia, 200
Disseminated intravascular coagulation (DIC), 168, 168t
    cryoprecipitate for, 186
    in malignancies, 198
    microangiopathic hemolysis caused by, 82
DNA methyltransferase inhibitor therapy, for myelodysplastic syndrome, 24
Drugs
    affecting platelet function, 174, 174t
    hemolytic anemia, 80-82, 82t
    immune thrombocytopenia caused by, 164-166, 166t
    immune thrombocytopenia caused by, with heparin, 200
    neutropenia induced by, 100
    thrombocytopenia associated with, 160
Dysfibrinogenemia

慢性肾脏病（CKD）
    贫血，79-81
氯吡格雷
    联用阿司匹林，193
闭合时间，139
凝血启动，141
凝血扩增，141
凝血终止，145-147
凝血，141-149
    级联模型，141
    实验室检查，149
    模型，141-145
凝血因子
    凝血因子障碍，181-185
    输注，185-187
凝血功能障碍
    稀释性凝血功能障碍，177，185
维生素 B₁₂
    缺乏，75-77
        病因，77，77t
    内因子，75
    代谢途径，77f
冷凝集素病，83
    瓦尔登斯特伦巨球蛋白血症，131
胶原蛋白
    出血性疾病，155
    血小板结合，139
Coombs 试验，81
冷沉淀，187
环氧合酶-2（COX-2）抑制剂，血小板功能，173
环磷酰胺
    再生障碍性贫血，15
环孢素
    再生障碍性贫血，15
细胞因子
    造血，5，7t

D

达沙替尼，43-45
D-二聚体，149
    弥散性血管内凝血，169
D-二聚体检测
    复发风险，209
1-去氨基-（8-D-精氨酸）-血管升压素（DDAVP）
    出血
        阿司匹林，175
        尿毒症性血小板功能障碍，175
    血管性血友病，179
地西他滨，治疗骨髓增生异常综合征，25
地塞米松
    免疫性血小板减少性紫癜，165
    多发性骨髓瘤，129
Diamond-Blackfan 贫血，23-25
弥漫大 B 细胞淋巴瘤（DLBCL），107-109
直接口服抗凝剂，211t
直接凝血酶抑制剂（DTI），治疗肝素诱导的血小板减少症，201
弥散性血管内凝血（DIC），169，169t
    冷沉淀，187
    恶性肿瘤，199
    导致微血管病性溶血，83
DNA 甲基转移酶抑制剂治疗，治疗骨髓增生异常综合征，25
药物
    影响血小板功能，175，175t
    溶血性贫血，81-83，83t
    免疫性血小板减少症，165-167，167t
    免疫性血小板减少症，肝素，201
    中性粒细胞减少症，101
    药物相关的血小板减少症，161
异常纤维蛋白原血症

arterial disease and, 204
congenital, 182
Dyskeratosis congenita, 12

E

Eculizumab
　for paroxysmal nocturnal hemoglobinuria, 16, 84, 198
Ehlers-Danlos syndrome, 154
Elliptocytosis, hereditary, 84
Eltrombopag, 10, 14
Endocarditis
　marantic, 168
Endothelial cells
　thrombosis and, 190
　vascular
　　hemostasis and, 134
　　properties of coagulants, 138t
Eosinophilia, differential diagnosis of, 92-94, 96t
Eosinophils, 8, 92-94, 94f
Epstein-Barr virus (EBV)
　hemolytic anemia, 82
Eptifibatide, 192
Erythrocyte, hemolysis from causes extrinsic to, 82
Erythrocytosis, causes of, 32t
Erythroid cells, in myelodysplastic syndrome, 18
Erythropoietin (EPO)
　exogenous, for anemia, 10
　polycythemia vera and, 30-32
Escherichia coli
　hemolytic-uremic syndrome and, 202
Essential thrombocythemia, 34-36
　diagnostic criteria for, 34t
Evans syndrome, 164
Extramedullary hematopoiesis, 4
　in primary myelofibrosis, 36

F

Factor inhibitors, in congenital factor deficiencies, 182-184
Factor V Cambridge mutation, 194
Factor V deficiency, 182
Factor V Leiden (FVL) mutation, 194
Factor VIII
　acquired inhibitors of, 182
　liver disease and, 184
　virally inactivated concentrate, 186
Factor X deficiency, 184
Factor XI deficiency, 182
Factor XIII deficiency, 182
Fanconi anemia, 12, 162
　diagnosis of, 14
Felty syndrome, 100
Fetal loss, maternal thrombophilia and, 196-198
Fibrin clot, 146
　architecture, 146
Fibrin cross-linking, by factor XIIIa, 146
Fibrin split products, 190
　in disseminated intravascular coagulation, 168
Fibrinogen, 182
　level of, thrombin time and, 152, 152t
　loss/defects, 184
Fibrinogen disorders, 182
　dysfibrinogenemia, congenital, 182
Fibrinolysis, 146-148, 146f
　atherothrombosis and, 190
Fibrinolytic system, 146, 190
Folic acid (folate)
　deficiency of, 76
　　causes of, 76t

动脉疾病，205
先天性，183
先天性角化不良，13

E

依库珠单抗
　阵发性睡眠性血红蛋白尿症，17，85，199
埃勒斯-当洛综合征，155
遗传性椭圆形红细胞增多症，85
艾曲泊帕，11，15
心内膜炎
　非细菌性血栓性心内膜炎，169
内皮细胞
　血栓形成，191
　血管内皮细胞
　　止血，135
　　促凝剂，139t
嗜酸性粒细胞增多症，鉴别诊断，93-95，97t
嗜酸性粒细胞，9，93-95，95f
EB病毒（EBV）
　溶血性贫血，83
依替巴肽，193
红细胞，外部因素引起的溶血，83
红细胞增多症，病因，33t
红系细胞，见于骨髓增生异常综合征，19
促红细胞生成素（EPO）
　外源性EPO，治疗贫血，11
　真性红细胞增多症，31-33
大肠埃希菌
　溶血性尿毒综合征，203
原发性血小板增多症，35-37
　诊断标准，35t
伊文思综合征，165
髓外造血，5
　原发性骨髓纤维化，37

F

因子抑制物，见于先天性因子缺乏症，183-185
因子V Cambridge突变，195
因子V缺乏，183
因子V Leiden（FVL）突变，195
因子VIII
　获得性因子VIII抑制物，183
　肝病，185
　病毒灭活的浓缩物，187
因子X缺乏，185
因子XI缺乏，183
因子XIII缺乏，183
范科尼贫血，13，163
　诊断，15
Felty综合征，101
流产，母体血栓形成倾向，197-199
纤维蛋白凝块，147
　结构，147
纤维蛋白交联，因子XIIIa，147
纤维蛋白降解产物，191
　弥散性血管内凝血，169
纤维蛋白原，183
　凝血酶时间，153，153t
　缺失或缺陷，185
纤维蛋白原异常，183
　先天性异常纤维蛋白原血症，183
纤维蛋白溶解，147-149，147f
　动脉粥样硬化血栓形成，191
纤维蛋白溶解系统，147，191
叶酸
　叶酸缺乏，77
　　病因，77t

metabolic pathways of, 76f
Follicular lymphomas, 110
Fresh frozen plasma, 182

G

Genomic sequencing technologies, for myelodysplastic syndrome, 26
Glanzmann thrombasthenia, 170t, 174
Glucose-6-phosphate dehydrogenase (G6PD), 84
Glucose-6-phosphate dehydrogenase deficiency, 84-86
β 2-glycoprotein I, antibodies against, 198, 202-204
Glycoprotein IIb/IIIa, 134
    antibodies directed against, 164
    fibrinogen and, 182
    Glanzmann thrombasthenia and, 174
Glycoprotein IIb/IIIa complex (GPIIb/IIIa), 192, 192t
Graft-*versus*-host disease (GVHD)
    in stem cell transplantation, 10
Graft-*versus*-leukemia effect, 10, 46
Granulocyte-macrophage colony-stimulating factor (GM-CSF), 6-8, 96
    for fungal infections, 10
Gray platelet syndrome, 170t, 176
Growth factors, for myelodysplastic syndrome, 22

H

Haplotype, 10
Heavy-chain disease, 130
    iron deficiency anemia, 74
    MALT lymphoma and, 108
HELLP syndrome
    microangiopathichemolysis and, 82
    thrombocytopenia in, 170
Hematopoiesis, 4-28, 6t
    differentiation pathway, 4-8, 8f
        erythroid lineage, 8
        granulocyte and monocyte lineage, 8
        pluripotent stem cells in, 6-8
        stem cell plasticity in, 8
    extramedullary, in primary myelofibrosis, 36
    hematopoietic tissues, 4
    prospectus for the future, 26
    stem cell theory of, 4, 6t
Hematopoietic failure syndromes, primary, 8-26, 8t
    aplastic anemia, 12-14
    growth factors for, 10
    hematopoietic stem cell transplantation for, 10-12
    myelodysplastic syndrome, 16-26
    paroxysmal nocturnal hemoglobinuria, 14-16
Hematopoietic stem cell
    clonal disorders of, 30-66
Hematopoietic stem cell (HSC), 4
    characteristics of, 4
    plasticity of, 8
    pluripotent, 6-8
    transplantation of, 10
        sources for, 12
Hemoglobin Barts, 90
Hemoglobin C (HbC), 88
Hemoglobinopathies, 86-90
Hemoglobinuria, paroxysmal nocturnal, 84, 198
Hemolysis, as prothrombotic state, 198
Hemolytic anemia, 68
    autoimmune, 82t
    caused by
        disorders of erythrocyte enzymes, 84-86
        disorders of erythrocyte membrane, 82-84
    differential diagnosis of, 80t
    in enzyme deficiencies, 86
    hemoglobinopathies, 86-90

代谢途径，77f
滤泡性淋巴瘤，111
新鲜冰冻血浆，183

G

基因组测序技术，用于骨髓增生异常综合征，27
格兰茨曼血小板功能不全，171t，175
葡萄糖-6-磷酸脱氢酶（G6PD），85
葡萄糖-6-磷酸脱氢酶缺乏症，85-87
β₂糖蛋白I（抗β₂糖蛋白I抗体），199，203-205
糖蛋白Ⅱb/Ⅲa，135
    抗体，165
    纤维蛋白原，183
    格兰茨曼血小板功能不全，175
糖蛋白Ⅱb/Ⅲa复合物（GPⅡb/Ⅲa），193，193t
移植物抗宿主病（GVHD）
    干细胞移植，11
移植物抗白血病效应，11，47
粒细胞-巨噬细胞集落刺激因子（GM-CSF），7-9，97

    真菌感染，11
灰色血小板综合征，171t，177
生长因子，治疗骨髓增生异常综合征，23

H

单倍体基因型，11
重链病，131
    缺铁性贫血，75
    MALT淋巴瘤，109
HELLP综合征
    微血管病性溶血，83
    血小板减少症，171
造血，5-29，7t
    分化途径，5-9，9f
        红系，9
        粒细胞和单核细胞系，9
        多能干细胞，7-9
        干细胞的可塑性，9
    髓外造血，原发性骨髓纤维化，37
    造血组织，5
    未来展望，27
    干细胞理论，5，7t
造血衰竭综合征，原发性，9-27，9t
    再生障碍性贫血，13-15
    生长因子，11
    造血干细胞移植，11-13
    骨髓增生异常综合征，17-27
    阵发性睡眠性血红蛋白尿症，15-17
造血干细胞
    克隆性疾病，31-67
造血干细胞（HSC），5
    特征，5
    可塑性，9
    多能，7-9
    移植，11
        来源，13
血红蛋白巴特，91
血红蛋白C（HbC），89
血红蛋白病，87-91
阵发性睡眠性血红蛋白尿症，85，199
溶血，血栓前状态，199
溶血性贫血，69
    自身免疫性溶血性贫血，83t
    病因
        红细胞酶缺陷，85-87
        红细胞膜缺陷，83-85
    鉴别诊断，81t
    酶缺陷，87
    血红蛋白病，87-91

IgG-mediated (warm), 80-82	IgG 介导的溶血性贫血（温抗体型），81-83
IgM-mediated (cold), 82	IgM 介导的溶血性贫血（冷抗体型），83
immune, 80-82	免疫性溶血性贫血，81-83
microangiopathic, 82, 202	微血管病性溶血性贫血，83, 203
peripheral blood smear, 82	外周血涂片，83
Hemolytic-uremic syndrome (HUS), 202	溶血性尿毒综合征（HUS），203
hemorrhagic colitis in, 202	出血性结肠炎，203
microangiopathichemolysis caused by, 82	微血管病性溶血，83
Hemophilia, 140	血友病，141
A and B, 180-182	血友病 A 和血友病 B，181-183
acquired factor inhibitors in, 182	获得性凝血因子抑制物，183
factor replacement for, 182	凝血因子替代治疗，183
C, 182	血友病 C，183
Hemostasis, 150	止血，151
coagulation in, 140-148	凝血，141-149
normal, 134-148	正常止血，135-149
platelet, 138-140	血小板，139-141
vasculature physiology in, 134	血管生理学，135
Henoch-Schönlein purpura (HSP), 158	过敏性紫癜（HSP），159
Heparin	肝素
in perioperative anticoagulation, 210-212	围术期的抗凝治疗，211-213
in pregnancy, 210	妊娠期，211
resistance, 204	肝素抵抗，205
thrombocytopenia induced by, 166, 200	肝素诱导的血小板减少症，167, 201
unfractionated and low-molecular-weight, 210	普通肝素和低分子量肝素，211
for venous thromboembolism, 196, 204	静脉血栓栓塞，197, 205
malignancy-associated, 198	恶性肿瘤相关，199
for venous thromboembolism prophylaxis, 206	预防性治疗，207
Hereditary hemorrhagic telangiectasia, 158	遗传性出血性毛细血管扩张症，159
Hermansky-Pudlak syndrome, 170t, 174	赫尔曼斯基-普德拉克综合征，171t, 175
Hodgkin lymphoma, 118-120	霍奇金淋巴瘤，119-121
Homocysteine, atherothrombosis and, 190, 194t	同型半胱氨酸，动脉粥样硬化血栓形成，191, 195t
Hormone replacement, venous thromboembolism secondary to, 198	激素替代，继发静脉血栓栓塞，199
Human hemoglobins, structure and distribution of, 70t	人血红蛋白，结构和分布，71t
Human immunodeficiency virus (HIV) infection	人类免疫缺陷病毒（HIV）感染
thrombocytopenia in, 182	血小板减少症，183
Human leukocyte antigen (HLA)	人类白细胞抗原（HLA）
stem cell transplantation and, 10	干细胞移植，11
Human platelet antigen-1b (HPA-1b), 194t	人类血小板抗原-1b（HPA-1b），195t
Human T-cell lymphotropic virus type 1 (HTLV-1), 108	人类嗜 T 淋巴细胞病毒-1（HTLV-1），109
Hydroxyurea	羟基脲
for essential thrombocythemia, 36, 200	原发性血小板增多症，37, 201
for polycythemia vera, 34	真性红细胞增多症，35
for primary myelofibrosis, 36-38	原发性骨髓纤维化，37-39
for sickle cell disease, 88	镰状细胞贫血，89
Hyperhomocysteinemia, in arterial disease, 190	高同型半胱氨酸血症，见于动脉疾病，191
Hyperleukocytosis syndrome, 50	高白细胞综合征，51
Hypertension	高血压
in pregnancy	妊娠高血压
with thrombocytopenia, 170	血小板减少症，171
Hyperviscosity syndrome, Waldenström's macroglobulinemia with, 130	高黏滞综合征，瓦尔登斯特伦巨球蛋白血症，131

I

Ibritumomab tiuxetan, 114	替伊莫单抗，115
IgG-mediated (warm) hemolytic anemia, 80-82	IgG 介导的（温抗体型）溶血性贫血，81-83
IgM-mediated (cold) hemolytic anemia, 82	IgM 介导的（冷抗体型）溶血性贫血，83
Imatinib mesylate (Gleevec), 40-42	甲磺酸伊马替尼（Gleevec），41-43
Immune thrombocytopenic purpura (ITP), 164	免疫性血小板减少性紫癜（ITP），165
Immunoglobulin(s)	免疫球蛋白
IgA-associated disorders	IgA 相关疾病
Henoch-Schönlein purpura, 158	过敏性紫癜，159
IgA nephropathy, 158	IgA 肾病，159
in immune hemolytic anemia, 80	免疫性溶血性贫血，81
monoclonal (M protein), 126t	单克隆免疫球蛋白（M 蛋白），127t
Immunosuppressive therapy	免疫抑制治疗
for myelodysplastic syndrome, 22	骨髓增生异常综合征，23
Infections	感染
causing hemolysis, 82	引起溶血，83
Interferon-α	干扰素 α

for essential thrombocythemia, 36
for polycythemia vera, 34
for primary myelofibrosis, 36-38
Interleukin-11 (IL-11), 8
Intermittent phlebotomy, 34
International normalized ratio (INR), 148
International Prognostic Index (IPI), 116
International Prognostic Scoring System, for myelodysplastic disorders, 18, 20t
Intracellular killing, 92
Intravenous immunoglobulin (IVIG)
for drug-induced immune thrombocytopenia, 164
for fetal and neonatal alloimmune thrombocytopenia, 166
for immune thrombocytopenic purpura, 164
Intrinsic factor (IF), 74
Iron deficiency anemia, 72-74
Iron supplementation, oral, 74

J

Januskinase 2 (JAK2) mutation
essential thrombocythemia, 34
in myeloproliferative neoplasms, 30
polycythemia vera, 32

K

Kostmann syndrome, 98

L

Large granular lymphocytes, 104
Lead poisoning blocks, microcytic anemias, 72
Lenalidomide
for multiple myeloma, 128
for myelodysplastic syndrome, 22-24
Leukemia(s)
acute, 46-66, 48t
acutelymphoblastic, 52t, 60-64, 62t
acutelymphocytic, 120
acute myeloid, 50-58, 52t
myelodysplastic syndrome and, 16-18
acute promyelocytic, 58-60
chronic lymphocytic, 120-124
heavy-chain disease, 130
chronic myelogenous, 38-46
accelerated and blast phase, 46
chronic phase, 40-46, 42t-44t
clinical presentation of, 40, 40t
definition, epidemiology and pathology of, 38-40
diagnosis and differential diagnosis of, 40
lymphocyte infusions for, 10
prognosis of, 46
treatment of, 40-46
large granular lymphocyte, 100
lymphoid, 120-124
prospectus for future, 64-66
stem cell transplant, 10
Leukemoid reaction, 40, 96
Leukocyte adhesion deficiency, 92
Leukocytosis, 96
Leukopenia, 96
Leukoreduction, 178
Leukostasis, 50
Ligands, 134
Liver disease. *See also* Cirrhosis; Hepatitis
bleeding in, 184
Low reticulocyte count, differential diagnosis of anemia with, 72t
Lupus anticoagulant, 198
as work-up for venous thromboembolism, 202-204
Lymph node biopsy, 108

原发性血小板增多症，37
真性红细胞增多症，35
原发性骨髓纤维化，37-39
白介素-11（IL-11），9
间歇性静脉切开术，35
国际标准化比值（INR），149
国际预后指数（IPI），117
国际预后评分系统，骨髓增生异常疾病，19，21t

细胞内杀伤，93
静脉注射免疫球蛋白（IVIG）
药物诱导的免疫性血小板减少症，165
胎儿和新生儿同种免疫性血小板减少症，167
免疫性血小板减少性紫癜，165
内因子（IF），75
缺铁性贫血，73-75
补充铁剂，口服，75

J

JAK2 突变
原发性血小板增多症，35
骨髓增殖性肿瘤，31
真性红细胞增多症，33

K

Kostmann 综合征，99

L

大颗粒淋巴细胞，105
铅中毒，小细胞性贫血，73
来那度胺
多发性骨髓瘤，129
骨髓增生异常综合征，23-25
白血病
急性白血病，47-67，49t
急性淋巴母细胞白血病，53t，61-65，63t
急性淋巴细胞白血病，121
急性髓系白血病，51-59，53t
骨髓增生异常综合征，17-19
急性早幼粒细胞白血病，59-61
慢性淋巴细胞白血病，121-125
重链病，131
慢性髓细胞性白血病，39-47
加速期和急变期，47
慢性期，41-47，43t-45t
临床表现，41，41t
定义、流行病学和病理学，39-41
诊断和鉴别诊断，41
淋巴细胞输注，11
预后，47
治疗，41-47
大颗粒淋巴细胞白血病，101
淋巴细胞白血病，121-125
未来展望，65-67
干细胞移植，11
类白血病反应，41，97
白细胞黏附缺陷症，93
白细胞增多症，97
白细胞减少症，97
白细胞去除，179
白细胞淤滞症，51
配体，135
肝病 参见肝硬化；肝炎
出血，185
网织红细胞计数减低，贫血鉴别，73t
狼疮抗凝物，199
静脉血栓栓塞，203-205
淋巴结活检，109

Lymph nodes, 102, 104f
Lymphadenopathy
    causes of, 108, 108t
    cervical, 108
Lymphoblastic leukemia, acute, 48t, 52t, 60-64, 62t
Lymphoblastic lymphoma, 116
Lymphocytes, 4-6
    autoreactive, aplastic anemia and, 12
    congenital and acquired disorders of, 130
    development, function, and localization of, 102-104
    disorders of, 102-132
Lymphocytosis, 96
    reactive, 122
Lymphohistiocytosis, hemophagocytic, 170
Lymphoid follicles, 102
Lymphoid origin, neoplasia of, 104-130
Lymphoid system, 102-104
Lymphoma. *See also* Mucosa-associated lymphoid tissue
    Mediterranean, 130
    post-transplant lymphoproliferative disorder, 130
    staging evaluation for, 110t
    staging system, 110t
    subtypes, 110-116
    therapeutic agents in, 112t

M

M protein, 124, 126t
Macrocytic anemia, 74-78
Macrophage colony-stimulating factor (M-CSF), 96
Macrophages, 96
Major histocompatibility complex (MHC). *See also* Human leukocyte antigen
    stem cell transplantation and, 10
Malignancy
    thrombocytopenia associated with, 162
Mantle cell lymphoma, 116
Marantic endocarditis, 168
Marginal zone lymphomas, 114
Margination, of neutrophils, 92
Mean corpuscular volume (MCV), 70-72
Mediterranean lymphoma, 130
Megakaryocytes, 4-6
    decreased or absent, 160
Megaloblastic anemias, 74-78
    clinical manifestations of, 76-78
    treatment of, 78
Microangiopathic hemolytic anemia (MAHA), 82
Microangiopathy, thrombocytopenia accompanied by, 202
Microcytic anemias, 72-80
β_2-microglobulin
    in multiple myeloma, 126
Mixing study, of plasma, 152, 152t, 154f
Monoclonal gammopathy of uncertain significance (MGUS), 124
Monocytes, 94f, 96
Mucosa-associated lymphoid tissue (MALT), 104
    Helicobacter pylori and, 108
Multiple myeloma, 124-128
    international staging system for, 128t
Mycoplasma pneumoniae, hemolytic anemia, 82
Myelodysplastic syndrome, 16-26, 162
    clinical presentation of, 18
    definition and epidemiology of, 16
    diagnosis and differential diagnosis of, 18
    etiology of, 16-18
    prognosis of, 18-22, 20t-22t
    treatment of, 22-26
        5q minus syndrome, 22-24
        epigenetic therapy as, 24
        immunosuppressive therapy as, 22

淋巴结，103，105f
淋巴结肿大
    病因，109，109t
    颈部淋巴结肿大，109
急性淋巴细胞白血病，49t，53t，61-65，63t
淋巴母细胞性淋巴瘤，117
淋巴细胞，5-7
    自身反应性，再生障碍性贫血，13
    先天性和获得性淋巴细胞功能障碍，131
    淋巴细胞的发育、功能和定位，103-105
    淋巴细胞疾病，103-133
淋巴细胞增多，97
    反应性淋巴细胞增多，123
噬血细胞性淋巴组织细胞增生症，171
淋巴滤泡，103
淋巴细胞起源的肿瘤，105-131
淋巴系统，103-105
淋巴瘤 参见黏膜相关性淋巴样组织
    地中海淋巴瘤，131
    移植后淋巴增殖性疾病，131
    分期评估，111t
    分级系统，111t
    亚型，111-117
    治疗药物，113t

M

M蛋白，125，127t
大细胞性贫血，75-79
巨噬细胞集落刺激因子（M-CSF），97
巨噬细胞，97
主要组织相容性复合体（MHC）参见人类白细胞抗原
    干细胞移植，11
恶性肿瘤
    血小板减少症，163
套细胞淋巴瘤，117
非细菌性栓塞性心内膜炎，169
边缘区淋巴瘤，115
边集，中性粒细胞，93
平均红细胞体积（MCV），71-73
地中海淋巴瘤，131
巨核细胞，5-7
    减少或缺失，161
巨幼细胞贫血，75-79
    临床表现，77-79
    治疗，79
微血管病性溶血性贫血（MAHA），83
微血管病变，伴有血小板减少症，203
小细胞性贫血，73-81
β_2-微球蛋白
    多发性骨髓瘤，127
混合试验，血浆，153，153t，155f
意义未明单克隆丙种球蛋白血症（MGUS），125
单核细胞，95f，97
黏膜相关淋巴组织，105
    幽门螺杆菌，109
多发性骨髓瘤，125-129
    国际分期系统，129t
肺炎支原体，溶血性贫血，83
骨髓增生异常综合征，17-27，163
    临床表现，19
    定义和流行病学，17
    诊断和鉴别诊断，19
    病因，17-19
    预后，19-23，21t-23t
    治疗，23-27
        5q缺失综合征，23-25
        表观遗传学治疗，25
        免疫抑制治疗，23

lenalidomide as, 22-24
  stem cell transplantation as, 24-26, 24t
  transfusions, iron chelation, and growth factors as, 22
  World Health Organization classification of, 20t
Myelofibrosis
  primary, 36-38, 36t
  thrombocytopenia and, 160-162
Myeloid leukemia, acute, 48t, 50-58, 52t, 54f-58f
Myeloperoxidase
  of neutrophils, 92
Myelophthisis, 96
Myeloproliferative diseases (MPDs), 64
  chronic, 30
Myeloproliferative neoplasms (MPNs), 30
  classification of, 32t

N

Natural killer (NK) cells, 104
Nephrotic syndrome
  thrombosis in, 198
Neutropenia, 98-100
  differential diagnosis of, 98-100, 98t
  laboratory evaluation of, 100
  treatment of, 100
Neutrophil extracellular traps (NETS), 92
Neutrophil numbers, determinants of peripheral, 96
Neutrophilia, 96-98
  differential diagnosis of, 98t
Neutrophils, 92, 94f
  clinical disorders of, 92-100
  normal granulocyte development, structure and function of, 92-96
Nilotinib, 42-44
Non-Hodgkin's lymphomas, 104-118
  classification of, 106t
  clinical presentation of, 108
  definition and epidemiology of, 104-106
  diagnosis and differential diagnosis of, 108-110
  etiology of, 108
  pathology of, 106-108
  treatment of, 110
    for aggressive type, 114-116
    for high-grade, 116
    for indolent types, 110-114
    for mantle cell lymphoma, 116
Nonsteroidal anti-inflammatory drugs (NSAIDs)
  antiplatelet effects of, 138
  platelet dysfunction caused by, 170, 170t, 174t
Normocytic anemias, 78-80
  treatment of, 78
Nutrition
  thrombocytopenia associated with, 160

O

Omacetaxine mepesuccinate, 46
Oral contraceptives
  venous thromboembolism secondary to, 198
Osler-Weber-Rendu syndrome, 158

P

Pancytopenia, 8-10, 8t
Paroxysmal nocturnal hemoglobinuria, 14-16, 84, 198
Peripheral blood smear, 80
Peripheral blood stem cells (PBSCs), in stem cell transplantation, 10
Pernicious anemia, 76
Phagocytic cells, 96
Phagocytosis, 92
  by neutrophils, 92
Philadelphia chromosome, 30

来那度胺，23-25
  干细胞移植，25-27，25t
  输血、铁螯合剂和生长因子，23
  世界卫生组织分类，21t
骨髓纤维化
  原发性骨髓纤维化，37-39，37t
  血小板减少症，161-163
急性髓系白血病，49t，51-59，53t，55f-59f
髓过氧化物酶
  中性粒细胞，93
脊髓痨，97
骨髓增生性疾病（MPD），65
  慢性骨髓增生性疾病，31
骨髓增殖性肿瘤（MPN），31
  分类，33t

N

自然杀伤（NK）细胞，105
肾病综合征
  血栓形成，199
中性粒细胞减少症，99-101
  鉴别诊断，99-101，99t
  实验室评估，101
  治疗，101
中性粒细胞胞外诱捕网（NETS），93
中性粒细胞计数，外周中性粒细胞计数的决定因素，97
中性粒细胞增多症，97-99
  鉴别诊断，99t
中性粒细胞，93，95f
  疾病，93-101
  正常粒细胞的发育、结构和功能，93-97
尼洛替尼，43-45
非霍奇金淋巴瘤，105-119
  分类，107t
  临床表现，109
  定义和流行病学，105-107
  诊断和鉴别诊断，109-111
  病因，109
  病理学，107-109
  治疗，111
    侵袭性非霍奇金淋巴瘤，115-117
    高级别非霍奇金淋巴瘤，117
    惰性非霍奇金淋巴瘤，111-115
    套细胞淋巴瘤，117
非甾体抗炎药（NSAID）
  抗血小板作用，139
  血小板功能障碍，171，171t，175t
正细胞性贫血，79-81
  治疗，79
营养
  血小板减少症，161

O

高三尖杉酯碱，47
口服避孕药
  继发静脉血栓栓塞，199
遗传性出血性毛细血管扩张症，159

P

全血细胞减少，9-11，9t
阵发性睡眠性血红蛋白尿症，15-17，85，199
外周血涂片，81
外周血造血干细胞（PBSC），移植，11
恶性贫血，77
吞噬细胞，97
吞噬作用，93
  中性粒细胞，93
费城染色体，31

definition of, 40
Plasma
　fresh frozen, 182
Plasma cell disorders, 124-130
　rare, 130
Plasma exchange
　for hemolyticuremic syndrome, 202
　for thrombotic thrombocytopenic purpura, 202
Plasmacytic disorders, therapeutic agents in, 112t
Plasmacytoma, 124
Plasmin, 148, 190
Plasminogen activator inhibitor-1 (PAI-1), 146, 146f, 190, 204
Platelet
　alloimmunization, 166
　glycoprotein defects of, 174
　granule or secretory defects of, 174-176
Platelet count, 138
　elevated, 36
Platelet dysfunction
　acquired causes of, 170-174
　congenital causes of, 174-176
Platelet Function Analyzer-100 (PFA-100), 138, 152, 156f
Platelet refractoriness, 176-178
Platelet transfusion, 176-178
　in acute renal failure, 174
　for bleeding caused by drugs, 174
　contraindicated in thrombotic thrombocytopenic purpura, 202
　failure of, 176-178
　for immune thrombocytopenic purpura, 164
　platelet refractoriness and, 176-178
　standard, 176
Platelets, 8
　activation of, 138
　adhesion, 138-140
　bleeding time and, 138
　circulating lifetime, 138
　hemostasis, 138
　physiology, 138-140
　procoagulant properties of, 144t
　secretion, 140
　thrombosis associated with
　　atherothrombosis, 192-194, 192t
　　venous, 198-202
POEMS syndrome, 130
Polycythemia vera, 30-34, 198-200
　diagnostic criteria for, 32t
Ponatinib, 42-44
Post-transplant lymphoproliferative disorder (PTLD), 130
Prednisone. *See also* Corticosteroids
　for hemolytic anemia, 80
　for immune thrombocytopenic purpura, 164
Preeclampsia
　microangiopathichemolysis caused by, 82
　thrombocytopenia in, 170
Pregnancy
　antithrombotic therapy during, 210
　hypertension in
　　with thrombocytopenia, 170
　venous thromboembolism in, 196-198
　von Willebrand disease and, 178
Primary myelofibrosis, 36-38, 36t-38t
Promyelocytic leukemia, acute, 58-60
Protein C
　deficiency of, 196
　　in heparin-induced thrombocytopenia, 200
　levels of, 202-204
Protein S
　deficiency of, 196
　free, 202-204

定义，41
血浆
　新鲜冰冻血浆，183
浆细胞疾病，125-131
　罕见的浆细胞疾病，131
血浆置换
　溶血性尿毒综合征，203
　血栓性血小板减少性紫癜，203
浆细胞疾病，治疗药物，113t
浆细胞瘤，125
纤溶酶，149，191
纤溶酶原激活物抑制物-1（PAI-1），147，147f，191，205
血小板
　同种免疫，167
　糖蛋白缺陷，175
　颗粒或分泌缺陷，175-177
血小板计数，139
　增多，37
血小板功能障碍
　获得性病因，171-175
　先天性病因，175-177
血小板功能分析仪-100（PFA-100），139，153，157f
血小板无效输注，177-179
血小板输注，177-179
　急性肾衰竭，175
　药物诱发的出血，175
　TTP，禁忌证，203
　血小板输注失败，177-179
　免疫性血小板减少性紫癜，165
　血小板无效输注，177-179
　标准，177
血小板，9
　活化，139
　黏附，139-141
　出血时间，139
　寿命，139
　止血，139
　生理功能，139-141
　促凝特性，145t
　分泌，141
　血栓形成相关
　　动脉粥样硬化血栓形成，193-195，193t
　　静脉血栓形成，199-203
POEMS综合征，131
真性红细胞增多症，31-35，199-201
　诊断标准，33t
普纳替尼，43-45
移植后淋巴增殖性疾病（PTLD），131
泼尼松　参见皮质类固醇
　溶血性贫血，81
　免疫性血小板减少性紫癜，165
先兆子痫
　微血管病性溶血，83
　血小板减少症，171
妊娠
　抗凝治疗，211
　高血压
　　血小板减少症，171
　静脉血栓栓塞，197-199
　血管性血友病，179
原发性骨髓纤维化，37-39，37t-39t
急性早幼粒细胞白血病，59-61
蛋白C
　缺陷，197
　　肝素诱导的血小板减少症，201
　水平，203-205
蛋白S
　缺陷，197
　游离蛋白S，203-205

Prothrombin complex concentrate, 186
Prothrombin G20210A, 194, 202-204
Prothrombin time (PT), 140, 142f, 150-152, 152t, 154f
    in liver disease, 184
Prothrombotic disease states, 198
Pseudo-Pelger-Huët abnormalities, 18, 72f
Pseudoxanthoma elasticum, 154
Pulmonary embolism
    risk factors for
        acquired, 196
        inherited, 194, 194t
Purpura
    Henoch-Schönlein, 158
    immune thrombocytopenic, 164
    palpable, 158
    post-transfusion, 166-168
    senile, 158
    steroid-induced, 158
    vascular, 154
Purpura fulminans, neonatal, 196
Pyropoikilocytosis, hereditary, 84

R

Red blood cells
    congenital, membrane abnormalities, 82t
    disorders of, 68-90
    metabolism of, 84f
    normal structure and function, 68
    prospectus for future, 90
Renal failure
    in multiple myeloma, 126
Reptilase time, 182
Respiratory burst, 92
Reticulocyte count, 68
Reticulocytosis, evaluation of anemia with, 80-90
Revascularization
    coronary, antiplatelet therapies for, 192
Revised International Prognostic Scoring System (R-IPSS), for myelodysplastic syndrome, 18, 22t
Rheumatoid arthritis
    with large granular lymphocyte, 100
    neutropenia in, 100
Rituximab, 112
    for acutelymphoblastic leukemia, 60
    for factor VIII inhibitors, 184
    for immune thrombocytopenic purpura, 164
    for indolent non-Hodgkin's lymphomas, 112
    for Waldenström's macroglobulinemia, 130
Romiplostim, 10

S

Schistocytes, 82
Scurvy, 154
Sepsis
    neutropenia in, 98
Shiga-like toxin, hemolyticuremic syndrome and, 202
Sickle cell β-thalassemia, 88
Sickle cell disease, 86-88
    clinical manifestations of, 86t
Sideroblastic anemias, 72
Smoking
    venous thromboembolism and, 198
Spherocytosis, hereditary, 82-84
Spleen, lymphocytes in, 104
Splenectomy
    for immune thrombocytopenic purpura, 164
    for thrombocytopenia, 162
Spur cell anemia, 84

凝血酶原复合体浓缩物，187
凝血酶原 G20210A，195，203-205
凝血酶原时间（PT），141，143f，151-153，153t，155f
    肝病，185
血栓前疾病状态，199
假性 Pelger-Huët 畸形，19，73f
弹性纤维假黄瘤，155
肺栓塞
    危险因素
        获得性危险因素，197
        遗传性危险因素，195，195t
紫癜
    过敏性紫癜，159
    免疫性血小板减少性紫癜，165
    可触性紫癜，159
    输血后紫癜，167-169
    老年性紫癜，159
    类固醇引起的紫癜，159
    血管性紫癜，155
暴发性紫癜，新生儿，197
遗传性嗜派洛宁异形红细胞症，85

R

红细胞
    遗传性红细胞膜异常，83t
    疾病，69-91
    代谢，85f
    正常红细胞的结构和功能，69
    未来展望，91
肾衰竭
    多发性骨髓瘤，127
蛇毒凝血酶时间，183
呼吸爆发，93
网织红细胞计数，69
网织红细胞增多，贫血评估，81-91
血运重建
    冠状动脉，抗血小板治疗，193
修订的国际预后评分系统（R-IPSS），骨髓增生异常综合征，19，23t
类风湿关节炎
    大颗粒淋巴细胞，101
    中性粒细胞减少症，101
利妥昔单抗，113
    急性淋巴细胞白血病，61
    因子Ⅷ抑制物，185
    免疫性血小板减少性紫癜，165
    惰性非霍奇金淋巴瘤，113
    瓦尔登斯特伦巨球蛋白血症，131
罗米司亭，11

S

破碎红细胞，83
坏血病，155
感染中毒症
    中性粒细胞减少症，99
志贺样毒素，溶血性尿毒综合征，203
镰状细胞β-地中海贫血，89
镰状细胞贫血，87-89
    临床表现，87t
铁粒幼细胞贫血，73
吸烟
    静脉血栓栓塞，199
遗传性球形红细胞增多症，83-85
脾，淋巴细胞，105
脾切除术
    免疫性血小板减少性紫癜，165
    血小板减少症，163
棘形细胞贫血，85

Stem cell niches, 4
Stem cell transplantation
　for systemic lupus erythematosus, 198
Stem cell transplantation (SCT)
　allogeneic, 52-54
　for follicular NHLs, 114
　for primary myelofibrosis, 38
Steroid therapy
　side effects of, purpura, 154
Steroids
　for drug-induced immune thrombocytopenia, 164
　for immune thrombocytopenic purpura, 164
Stomatocytosis, hereditary, 84
Storage pool disease, 170t, 174
Surgery
　anticoagulation management in, 210-212
　venous thromboembolism and, 196
　　prophylaxis of, 206-208
Systemic lupus erythematosus (SLE)
　antiphospholipid antibodies in, 198
　immune thrombocytopenic purpura in, 162-164
　neutropenia in, 100

T

T cells, lymphocytes, 102
T lymphocytes, 102
　peripheral blood, 104
Telangiectasia, hereditary hemorrhagic, 158
Telomeres, aplastic anemia and, 12
Thalassemia, 88-90
　α-Thalassemia, 90
　β-Thalassemia, 88-90
Thalassemic syndromes, 88t
Thalidomide, for multiple myeloma, 128
Thrombin, 148
Thrombin activator fibrinolysis inhibitor (TAFI), 148
Thrombin time, 152, 152t, 154f, 182
Thrombocythemia, essential, 34-36, 198-200
Thrombocytopenia, 158-170
　bleeding time and, 138
　consumption, 170
　with decreased marrow production of platelets, 160-162, 160f
　definition of, 158-160
　differential diagnosis of, 160f
　dilutional, 170
　fetal alloimmune, 166
　heparin-induced, 166, 200
　neonatal alloimmune, 166
　with platelet destruction, 160f, 162-170
　　in disseminated intravascular coagulation, 168, 168t
　　drug-induced, 164-166, 166t
　　fetal and neonatal alloimmune, 166, 166t-168t
　　immune thrombocytopenic purpura, 164
　　immune-mediated, 162-168
　　non-immune-mediated, 168-170
　pregnancy-induced hypertension with, 170
　with sequestration of platelets, 160f, 162
Thrombocytosis, in myeloproliferative disorders, 200
Thrombolytic therapy
　for venous thromboembolism, 204
Thrombophilia, inherited, 196-198, 208
Thrombophlebitis, in Trousseau syndrome, 168
Thromboplastin, 148
Thrombopoietin (TPO), 8
Thrombosis, 190-212
　cancer-associated, 198
　clinical evaluation of, 202-204
　pathology of, 190-202
　platelet disorders and, 198-202

vascular tissues and, hemostatic regulation in, 190
Thrombotic thrombocytopenic purpura (TTP), 202
    microangiopathichemolysis caused by, 82
Tirofiban, 192
Tissue factor pathway inhibitor (TFPI), 134
Tissue-type plasminogen activator (t-PA), 146
    atherothrombosis and, 190, 204
Transfusion
    of coagulation factor, 184-186
    of cryoprecipitate, 186
    dilutional coagulopathy caused by, 176, 184
    of fresh frozen plasma, 182
    for myelodysplastic syndrome, 22
    thrombocytopenia and
        alloimmune, 166-168
        dilutional, 170
    for thrombotic thrombocytopenic purpura, 202
Translocation, in myeloproliferative neoplasms, 30
Trauma
    transfusion in, 184
    venous thromboembolism and, 196
Trousseau syndrome, 168
Tumor lysis syndrome
    in acute myeloid leukemia, 50
    with high-grade non-Hodgkin's lymphomas, 116

U

Umbilical cord blood stem cells, 12
Uremic platelet dysfunction, 174
Urokinase-type plasminogen activator (u-PA), 146

V

Vasculitis
    bleeding from, 154
    septic, 158
Vena cava filter
    in pregnancy, 210
    in trauma patients, 196, 204
    in venous thromboembolism, 204
        in perioperative anticoagulation, 210-212
Venous thromboembolism
    antithrombin deficiency and, 194-196
    cancer and, 198
    laboratory diagnostics for, 202-204, 204t
    in myeloproliferative disorders, 198
    during pregnancy, 210
    prophylaxis of, 206-210
    protein C or S deficiency and, 194
    risk factors for, inherited, 194-196, 194t
    therapy for, 204-212, 208t
Venous thrombosis, risk factors for, acquired, 196-198, 196t
Virchow triad, 190
Vitamin C, deficiency of, 154
Vitamin K
    administration of, in heparin-induced thrombocytopenia, 200
    coagulation factors and, 152
    deficiency of, 184
    replacement of, in coagulopathy, 186
von Willebrand disease, 170t, 178-180
    acquired, 180
    type 1, 178-180
    type 2, 180
    type 3, 180
von Willebrand factor (VWF), 134-138, 136f
    defects in, 180
    in factor VIII concentrate, 186

血管组织，止血调节，191
血栓性血小板减少性紫癜（TTP），203
    微血管病性溶血，83
替罗非班，193
组织因子途径抑制物（TFPI），135
组织型纤溶酶原激活物（t-PA），147
    动脉粥样硬化血栓形成，191，205
输血
    凝血因子，185-187
    冷沉淀，187
    稀释性凝血功能障碍，177，185
    新鲜冰冻血浆，183
    骨髓增生异常综合征，23
    血小板减少症
        同种免疫性血小板减少症，167-169
        稀释性血小板减少症，171
    血栓性血小板减少性紫癜，203
易位，骨髓增生性肿瘤，31
创伤
    输血，185
    静脉血栓栓塞，197
Trousseau综合征，169
肿瘤溶解综合征
    急性髓系白血病，51
    高级别非霍奇金淋巴瘤，117

U

脐带血干细胞，13
尿毒症性血小板功能障碍，175
尿激酶型纤溶酶原激活物（u-PA），147

V

血管炎
    出血，155
    感染中毒性血管炎，159
腔静脉滤器
    妊娠期，211
    创伤患者，197，205
    静脉血栓栓塞，205
        围术期的抗凝治疗，211-213
静脉血栓栓塞
    抗凝血酶缺乏症，195-197
    癌症，199
    实验室诊断，203-205，205t
    骨髓增生性疾病，199
    妊娠期，211
    预防性治疗，207-211
    蛋白质C或蛋白S缺乏，195
    遗传性危险因素，195-197，195t
    治疗，205-213，209t
静脉血栓形成，获得性危险因素，197-199，197t
Virchow三要素，191
维生素C缺乏症，155
维生素K
    肝素诱导的血小板减少症，201
    凝血因子，153
    缺乏，185
    替代治疗，凝血功能障碍，187
血管性血友病，171t，179-181
    获得性血管性血友病，181
    1型血管性血友病，179-181
    2型血管性血友病，181
    3型血管性血友病，181
血管性血友病因子（vWF），135-139，137f
    缺陷，181
    因子Ⅷ浓缩物，187

W

Waldenström's macroglobulinemia, 128-130
Warfarin, 184
    drugs affecting levels of, 208t
    in heparin-induced thrombocytopenia, 200
    international normalized ratio and, 148
    in perioperative anticoagulation, 210-212
    pregnancy and, 210
    reversal of, with fresh frozen plasma, 184-186
    skin necrosis induced by, in protein C deficiency, 196
    for venous thromboembolism, 196, 204
White cell count, 96
Wiskott-Aldrich syndrome, 176
World Health Organization (WHO)
    classification of myelodysplastic syndrome, 20t
    classification-based prognostic scoring system, for myelodysplastic syndrome, 18, 20t

W

瓦尔登斯特伦巨球蛋白血症，129-131
华法林，185
    影响华法林水平的药物，209t
    肝素诱导的血小板减少症，201
    国际标准化比值，149
    围术期的抗凝治疗，211-213
    妊娠，211
    逆转，新鲜冰冻血浆，185-187
    皮肤坏死，蛋白 C 缺陷，197
    静脉血栓栓塞，197，205
白细胞计数，97
威-奥综合征，177
世界卫生组织（WHO）
    骨髓增生异常综合征分类，21t
    基于分类的预后评分系统，骨髓增生异常综合征，19，21t